AF861705

# Inflammation:
# Mechanisms and Treatment

Proceedings of an International Meeting on
Future Trends in Inflammation IV
Organized by The European Biological Research Association
under the auspices of

The Royal Society of Medicine
The Arthritis and Rheumatism Council
The European League Against Rheumatism
The Pathological Society of Great Britain & Ireland
The British Immunology Society
The British Pharmacology Society

Held at the Royal College of Surgeons of England,
35–43 Lincolns Inn Fields, London WC2 3PN,
18th–22nd February 1980.

# Inflammation: Mechanisms and Treatment

*Proceedings of the Fourth International Meeting on Future Trends in Inflammation Organized by the European Biological Research Association and held in London, 18th–22nd February 1980*


*Edited by*

*D. A. Willoughby*

*Professor, Department of Experimental Pathology and Rheumatology, St Bartholomew's Hospital, London*

*J. P. Giroud*

*Professor, Department of Pharmacology, Hôpital Cochin, Paris*



MTP PRESS LIMITED
*International Medical Publishers*

Published by
MTP Press Limited
Falcon House
Lancaster, England


Softcover reprint of the hardcover 1st edition 1980

First Published 1980


**British Library Cataloguing in Publication Data**

International Meeting on Future Trends in
Inflammation, *4th, London, 1980*
Inflammation.
1. Inflammation – Congresses
I. Title II. Willoughby, Derek Albert
III. Giroud, J P IV. European Biological
Research Association
616.07′2 RB131

ISBN 978-94-010-9425-2 ISBN 978-94-010-9423-8 (eBook)
DOI 10.1007/978-94-010-9423-8

# Contents

CONTENTS

SECTION VI: MEASUREMENT OF HUMAN AND EXPERIMENTAL INFLAMMATION

*Chairman:* E. C. Huskisson; *Co-Chairman:* M. Lequesne

SECTION VII: IMMUNE ASPECTS

*Chairman:* T. L. Vischer; *Co-Chairman:* M. Glatt

# List of Contributors


**J.-P. ABITA**
FRA No. 4 INSERM,
UER d'Hemathologie,
Hôpital Saint Louis,
2 Place du Dr Fournier,
75475 Paris Cedex 10, France

**N. ABUAF**
Hôpital Saint-Antoine,
184 rue du Faubourg Saint-Antoine,
75571 Paris Cedex 12, France

**S. ACCARDO**
Department of Rheumatology,
University of Genoa,
Genoa, Italy

**N. R. ACKERMAN**
Institute of Biological Sciences,
Syntex Research,
Palo Alto, California 94305, USA

**H. A. AL-HABOUBI**
Department of Physiology and Pharmacology,
University of Strathclyde,
George Street,
Glasgow G1 1XW, Scotland

**Monique ANDARY**
Departement d'Immunologie Cellulaire,
Laboratoire d'Immunologie,
Hôpital Saint-Eloi,
34059 Montpellier Cedex, France

**K. R. AOKI**
Department of Pharmacology,
UCLA School of Medicine,
Los Angeles, California 90024, USA

**T. APPELBOOM**
Department of Rheumatology,
University of Brussels,
Brussels, Belgium

**M. ARNOLD**
Arbeitsgruppe Biochemie,
Max-Planck-Institut für experimentelle Kardiologie,
Sprudelhof 11,
D-6350 Bad Nauheim, West Germany

**M. ASFOUR**
Centre d'Immunologie et Biologie Parasitaire (INSERM U 167),
Institut Pasteur,
BP 3415, Lille 59019 Cedex, France

**A. AUTERI**
Department of Internal Medicine,
Medical School,
University of Siena,
Siena, Italy

**H. BAART de la FAILLE**
Institute of Dermatology,
Academic Hospital of the University of Utrecht,
Utrecht, The Netherlands

**E. H. BAART de la FAILLE-KUYPER**
Institute of Dermatology,
Academic Hospital of the University of Utrecht,
Utrecht, The Netherlands

**P. A. BACON**
The Royal National Hospital for Rheumatic Diseases,
Upper Borough Walls,
Bath BA1 1RL, England

**P. BADENOCH-JONES**
Department of Pathology,
The Royal College of Surgeons of England,
Lincoln's Inn Fields,
London WC2A 3PN, England

**P. J. BAILEY**
Department of Immunology,
Merck Institute for Therapeutic Research,
PO Box 2000, Rahway, New Jersey 07065,
USA

**M. Th. van den BARSELAAR**
Department of Infectious Diseases,
University Hospital,
Rijnsburgerweg 10,
2333 AA Leiden, The Netherlands

**W. B. van den BERG**
Department of Rheumatology,
University Hospital St Radboud,
Nijmegen, The Netherlands

**D. BERGER**
Division of Rheumatology,
Department of Medicine,
University Hospital,
CH–1211 Geneva 4, Switzerland

**J. BIGNON**
CHIC de Creteil,
Service de Pneumophtisiologie,
40 avenue de Verdun,
94010 Creteil, France

**M. E. J. BILLINGHAM**
ICI Pharmaceuticals Division,
Mereside, Alderley Park,
Macclesfield, Cheshire, England

**A. G. BIRD**
Department of Pathology,
The Medical School,
University of Newcastle upon Tyne,
Newcastle upon Tyne NE1 4LP, England

**D. BITTER-SUERMANN**
Institut für Medizinische Mikrobiologie,
Johannes-Gutenberg-Universität,
D-6500 Mainz, West Germany

**D. R. BLAKE**
Department of Medicine,
Royal Victoria Infirmary,
Newcastle upon Tyne, England

**B. M. E. von BLOMBERG-van der FLIER**
Pathological Institute,
Free University Hospital,
Amsterdam, The Netherlands

**B. BOK**
Nuclear Medicine,
Hôpital Beaujon,
Clichy, France

**M. BONNEAU**
Fondation Merieux,
17 rue Bourgelat,
69002 Lyon, France

**R. J. BONNEY**
Department of Immunology,
Merck Institute for Therapeutic Research,
PO Box 2000, Rahway, New Jersey 07065,
USA

**Barbara J. BOWMAN**
The Upjohn Company,
Kalamazoo, Michigan, USA

**Elizabeth A. BOYLE**
Anti-Inflammatory Project,
Beecham Pharmaceuticals,
Harlow, Essex, England

**D. BRADSHAW**
Department of Pharmacology,
Hôpital Cochin,
27 rue du Faubourg Saint-Jacques,
75014 Paris, France

**M. A. BRAY**
Department of Chemical Pathology,
King's College Hospital Medical School,
Denmark Hill, London SE5 8RX, England

**W. BREDIT**
Institut für Allg. Hygiene und Bakteriologie,
D-7800 Freiburg, West Germany

**Constance E. BRINCKERHOFF**
Connective Tissue Disease Section,
Department of Medicine,
Dartmouth-Hitchcock Medical Center,
Hanover, USA

**S. BRITTON**
Department of Immunobiology,
Wallenberg Laboratory,
Lilla Freskati,
S-104 05 Stockholm, Sweden

## LIST OF CONTRIBUTORS

**D. H. BROWN**
Pure and Applied Chemistry,
Strathclyde University,
Glasgow, Scotland

**J. C. BUCKLAND-WRIGHT**
Anatomy Department,
Guy's Hospital Medical School,
London, England

**R. C. BUCKNALL**
The Royal National Hospital for Rheumatic Diseases,
Upper Borough Walls,
Bath BA1 1RL, England

**Rosa CARNUCCIO**
Institute of Experimental Pharmacology,
University of Naples,
Naples, Italy

**L. CARRATELLI**
Cattedra di Seneiotica Medica,
Università di Chieti, Italy

**A. C. CARTER**
Institute of Biological Sciences,
Syntex Research,
Palo Alto, California, USA

**S. D. CARTER**
The Royal National Hospital for Rheumatic Diseases,
Upper Borough Walls,
Bath BA1 1RL, England

**I. CARUSO**
Rheumatology Service,
L. Sacco Hospital,
Milan, Italy

**E. M. CARVALHO**
Hospital Edgard Santos,
Universidade Federal da Bahia,
40000 Salvador, Bahia, Brazil

**C. H. CASHIN**
Pharmacology Department,
Roche Products Ltd.,
PO Box 6, Welwyn Garden City,
Hertfordshire, England

**A. CATS**
Department of Rheumatology,
University Medical Center,
Rijnsburgerweg 10,
2333 AA Leiden, The Netherlands

**Y.-H. CHANG**
Division of Rheumatology,
Department of Medicine,
University of California at Los Angeles,
Los Angeles, California 90024, USA

**L. CHEDID**
Department of Experimental Immunopharmacology,
Centre National de la Recherche Scientifique and Institut Pasteur,
28 rue du Docteur Roux,
75015 Paris, France

**D. CHIA**
Department of Medicine,
UCLA School of Medicine,
Los Angeles, California 90024, USA

**R. CIRILLO**
Institute of General Pathology,
University of Turin,
Corso Raffaello 30,
10125 Turin, Italy

**G. W. CIVIL**
Lilly Research Centre Ltd.,
Erl Wood Manor, Windlesham GU20 6PH,
Surrey, England

**C. B. CLAYTON**
Medical Physics Department,
Royal Victoria Infirmary,
Newcastle upon Tyne, England

**J. CLOT**
Departement d'Immunologie Cellulaire,
Laboratoire d'Immunologie,
Hôpital Saint-Eloi,
34059 Montpellier Cedex, France

**J. CNOSSEN**
Department of Pathology,
Section of Immunopathology,
University Medical Center,
PO Box 9603,
2300 RC Leiden, The Netherlands

**H. O. J. COLLIER**
Research
Miles Laboratories Ltd.,
Slough SL2 4LY, England

**N. S. CONNOR**
MRC Group in Periodontal Physiology,
Faculty of Dentistry,
University of Toronto,
Toronto, Canada

**Grace COUNTS**
Section of Rheumatology,
Department of Medicine,
Bowman Gray School of Medicine,
Winston-Salem, North Carolina 27103,
USA

**P. CUATRECASAS**
Molecular Biology Department,
Wellcome Research Laboratories,
Research Triangle Park,
North Carolina 27709, USA

**S. C. CUNNANE**
Rowett Research Institute,
Aberdeen, Scotland

**F. M. CUNNINGHAM**
Department of Chemical Pathology,
King's College Hospital Medical School,
Denmark Hill, London SE5 8RX, England

**M. CUTOLO**
Department of Rheumatology,
University of Genoa,
Genoa, Italy

**R. DALLEST**
Histocompatibility Laboratory,
Blood Bank,
Marseille 13005, France

**B. DAMERAU**
Abteilung Biochemische Pharmakologie,
Max-Planck-Institut für experimentelle Medizin,
Hermann-Rein-Strasse,
D-3400 Göttingen, West Germany

**M. DAMSTEEG**
Department of Pathology,
Section of Immunopathology,
University Medical Center,
PO Box 9603,
2300 RC Leiden, The Netherlands

**P. H.-C. DANG**
Research and Development,
Diagnostic Data Inc.,
Mountain View, California, USA

**A. DANIEL**
Faculté de Chirurgie Dentaire,
44 000 Nantes, France

**E. M. DAVIDSON**
Department of Chemical Pathology,
King's College Hospital Medical School,
Denmark Hill, London SE5 8RX, England

**P. DAVIES**
Department of Immunology,
Merck Institute for Therapeutic Research,
PO Box 2000, Rahway, New Jersey 07065,
USA

**W. DAWSON**
Lilly Research Centre Ltd.,
Erl Wood Manor, Windlesham GU20 6PH,
Surrey, England

**K. M. DEBATIN**
Institute for Immunology and Serology,
University of Heidelberg,
Im Neuenheimer Feld 305,
D-6900 Heidelberg, West Germany

**B. DELCAMBRE**
Rhumatologie,
Hôpital la Charité,
boulevard Montebello,
Lille 59037 Cedex, France

**D. DELL'ACQUA**
Rheumatology Service,
L. Sacco Hospital,
Milan, Italy

**Patricia A. DENNING-KENDALL**
Research,
Miles Laboratories,
Slough SL2 4LY, England

**D. A. DEPORTER**
Faculty of Dentistry,
The University of Toronto,
124 Edward Street,
Toronto, M5G 1G6 Ontario, Canada

**Gloria E. P. De SOUZA**
Department of Pharmacology,
Faculty of Medicine of Ribeirão Preto,
14100 Ribeirão Preto, Sao Paulo, Brazil

**T. DIAMANTSTEIN**
Immunology Research Unit,
Free University Berlin,
D-1000 Berlin 45, West Germany

**M. U. DIANZANI**
Instituto di Patologia Generale,
Corso Raffaello 30,
10125 Turin, Italy

**W. CARSON DICK**
Rheumatology Department,
Royal Victoria Infirmary,
Newcastle upon Tyne, England

## LIST OF CONTRIBUTORS

**J. T. DINGLE**
Strangeways Research Laboratory,
Wort's Causeway,
Cambridge, England

**A. C. H. M. van DINTHER-JANSSEN**
Pathological Institute,
Free University Hospital,
Amsterdam, The Netherlands

**M. DI ROSA**
Institute of Experimental Pharmacology,
University of Naples,
Naples, Italy

**N. S. DOHERTY**
Merrell National Laboratories,
Cincinnati, Ohio 45215, USA

**M. V. DOIG**
Department of Chemical Pathology,
King's College Hospital Medical School,
Denmark Hill, London SE5 8RX, England

**J.-C. DRAPIER**
Institut de Biochimie,
Université Paris-Sud,
91405 Orsay, France

**J. DUHEILLE**
Laboratoire d'Immunologie,
CHU Brabois-Nancy,
54500 Vandoeuvre, France

**J. DUNLOP**
Pure and Applied Chemistry,
Strathclyde University,
Glasgow, Scotland

**C. J. DUNN**
Synthelabo,
31 avenue P-V Couturier,
92220 Baneaux, France

**M. DUPONT**
Faculté de Chirurgie Dentaire,
44000 Nantes, France

**B. DUQUESNOY**
Rhumatologie,
Hôpital la Charité,
boulevard Montebello,
Lille 59037 Cedex, France

**K. E. EAKINS**
Pharmacology,
Wellcome Research Laboratories,
Langley Court,
Beckenham, Kent, England

**E. J. EASTHAM**
Department of Child Health,
Royal Victoria Infirmary,
Newcastle upon Tyne, England

**B. ELZINGA-CLAASEN**
Department of Infectious Diseases,
University Hospital,
Rijnsburgerweg 10,
2300 AA Leiden, The Netherlands

**D. ESNOUS**
Service d'Histologie,
CHU Cochin,
27 rue du Faubourg Saint-Jacques,
75014 Paris, France

**E. EZER**
Pharmacological Laboratory,
Chemical Works of Gedeon Richter,
H-1475 Budapest, Hungary

**J. P. FAMAEY**
Department of Rheumatology,
University of Brussels,
Brussels, Belgium

**G. FAURE**
Clinique Rhumatologique et Laboratoire d'Immunologie,
CHU Brabois-Nancy,
54500 Vandoeuvre, France

**Honor B. FELL**
Strangeways Research Laboratories,
Wort's Causeway,
Cambridge, England

**S. H. FERREIRA**
Department of Pharmacology,
Faculty of Medicine of Ribeirão Preto,
University of Sao Paulo,
14100 Ribeirão Preto, Sao Paulo, Brazil

**P. C. FINK**
Medizinische Hochschule Hannover,
Institut für klinische Chemie,
Karl-Wiechert-Allee 9,
D-3000 Hannover 61, West Germany

**L. FISNEROVA**
Department of Chemistry,
Research Institute for Pharmacy and Biochemistry,
Prague, Czechoslovakia

**Irene FLORENTIN**
Institut de Cancerologie et d'Immunogenetique,
94800 Villejuif, France

**Elsbeth Dora FLORY**
Department of Medicine,
Royal Melbourne Hospital,
3050 Victoria, Australia

**A. W. FORD-HUTCHINSON**
Department of Chemical Pathology,
King's College Hospital Medical School,
Denmark Hill, London SE5 8RX, England

**S. J. FOSTER**
ICI Pharmaceuticals Division,
Mereside, Alderley Park,
Macclesfield, Cheshire, England

**P. K. FOX**
Biochemistry Department,
Scientific Development Group,
Organon Laboratories Ltd.,
Newhouse by Motherwell,
Lanarkshire, Scotland

**J. S. FRANZONE**
Institute of General Pathology,
University of Turin,
Corso Raffaello 30,
10125 Turin, Italy

**P. FRITSCH**
CEA-IPSN,
Laboratoire de Toxicologie Expérimentale,
BP No 6,
92260 Fontenay aux Roses, France

**M. FUMAGALLI**
Rheumatology Service,
L. Sacco Hospital,
Milan, Italy

**R. van FURTH**
Department of Infectious Diseases,
University Hospital,
Rijnsburgerweg 10,
2333 AA Leiden, The Netherlands

**S. J. GADHER**
University Hospital South Manchester,
Manchester M20 8LR, England

**A. GAUCHER**
Clinique Rhumatologique,
CHU Brabois-Nancy,
54500 Vandoeuvre, France

**D. GEMSA**
Institute of Immunology and Serology,
University of Heidelberg,
Im Neuenheimer Feld 305,
6900 Heidelberg, West Germany

**R. GILLETT**
Department of Oral Pathology,
London Hospital Medical College,
London E1 2AD, England

**J. P. GIROUD**
Department of Pharmacology,
Hôpital Cochin,
27 rue du Faubourg Saint-Jacques,
75014 Paris Cedex, France

**M. GLATT**
Ciba-Geigy Ltd.,
Pharmaceuticals Division,
CH-4000 Basle, Switzerland

**E. M. GLENN**
The Upjohn Company,
Kalamazoo, Michigan, USA

**L. GLYNN**
Kennedy Institute of Rheumatology,
Hammersmith, London W6 7DW, England

**P. GORDON**
Department of Microbiology,
Loyola University Strich School of Medicine,
2160 S. First Avenue,
Maywood, Illinois 60153, USA

**M. GOUGEROT**
Laboratoire d'Immuno-Hematologie,
Hôpital Bichat,
Paris, France

**A. GOVAERTS**
Department of Immunology,
University of Brussels,
Brussels, Belgium

**A. P. GREEN**
Anti-Inflammatory Project,
Beecham Pharmaceuticals,
Harlow, Essex, England

**I. GRIFFITHS**
Rheumatology Department,
Royal Victoria Infirmary,
Newcastle upon Tyne, England

**J. GRIMOVA**
Department of Pharmacology,
Research Institute for Pharmacy and Biochemistry,
Prague, Czechoslovakia

**E. GRÜNEFELD**
Abteilung Biochemische Pharmakologie,
Max-Planck-Institut für experimentelle Medizin,
D-3400 Göttingen, West Germany

**U. HADDING**
Institut für Medizinische Mikrobiologie,
Johannes-Gutenberg-Universität,
D-6500 Mainz, West Germany

**H. HAHN**
Institute of Medical Microbiology,
Free University Berlin,
D-1000 Berlin 45, West Germany

**G. T. HAJOS**
Pharmacological Laboratory,
Chemical Works of Gedeon Richter,
H-1475 Budapest, Hungary

**N. D. HALL**
ARC Research Group,
The Royal National Hospital for Rheumatic Diseases,
Upper Borough Walls,
Bath BA1 1RL, England

**H. HANAUSKE-ABEL**
Institut für Medizinische Mikrobiologie,
Johannes-Gutenberg-Universität,
D-6500 Mainz, West Germany

**E. D. HARRIS, Jr.**
Connective Tissue Disease Section,
Department of Medicine,
Dartmouth-Hitchcock Medical Center,
Hanover, USA

**P. HASSELBACHER**
Connective Tissue Disease Section,
Department of Medicine,
Dartmouth-Hitchcock Medical Center,
Hanover, USA

**R. A. HAZELTON**
Centre for Rheumatic Diseases/University Department of Medicine,
Glasgow University,
Glasgow, Scotland

**G. A. HIGGS**
Prostaglandin Research,
Wellcome Research Laboratories,
Langley Court,
Beckenham, Kent, England

**D. HILLMAN**
Lilly Research Centre Ltd.,
Erl Wood Manor, Windlesham GU20 6PH,
Surrey, England

**I. HOLLOWAY**
Medical Physics Department,
Royal Victoria Infirmary,
Newcastle upon Tyne, England

**C. W. M. van HOLSTEIJN**
University of Utrecht,
Institute of Veterinary Pharmacology and Toxicology,
Utrecht, The Netherlands

**J.-C. HOMBERG**
Hôpital Saint-Antoine,
184 rue du Faubourg Saint-Antoine,
75571 Paris Cedex 12, France

**D. F. HORROBIN**
Institute of Innovative Medicine,
PO Box 10,
Nun's Island,
Montreal H3E 1J8, Canada

**D. A. HORWITZ**
Clinical Immunology and Rheumatology Section,
University of Southern California School of Medicine,
Los Angeles, California 90033, USA

**W. HUBER**
Research and Development,
Diagnostic Data Inc.,
Mountain View, California, USA

**E. HULSING-HESSELINK**
Department of Infectious Diseases,
University Hospital,
Rijnsburgerweg 10,
2333 AA Leiden, The Netherlands

**E. C. HUSKISSON**
Department of Rheumatology,
St Bartholomew's Hospital,
West Smithfield, London EC1A 7BE,
England

**J. M. JADIN**
Département de Biologie animale,
Faculté Universitaire Notre Dame de la Paix,
Namur, Belgium

**B. L. JEFFRIES**
Pharmacology Department,
Roche Products Ltd.,
PO Box 6, Welwyn Garden City,
Hertfordshire, England

**E. JELLUM**
Institute of Clinical Biochemistry,
Rikshospitalet,
Oslo, Norway

**June JOHNSON**
Section of Rheumatology,
Department of Medicine,
Bowman Gray School of Medicine,
Winston-Salem, North Carolina 27103, USA

**J. L. JOUVIN**
Faculté de Chirurgie Dentaire,
44000 Nantes, France

**R. W. JUBB**
Westminster Hospital,
Dean Ryle Street, Horseferry Road,
London SW1P 2AP, England

**P. JUNKER**
Section of Rheumatology,
Department of Internal Medicine,
Hvidovre Hospital,
University of Copenhagen,
Kettegaard alle 30,
2650 Hvidovre, Denmark

**Alice KAHAN**
Institut de Rhumatologie,
U-5 INSERM, ERA 337,
CNRS, Paris 75014, France

**K. KARAMANIS**
Department of Experimental Pharmacology,
Athens University Medical School,
Athens, Greece

**E. KÅSS**
Oslo Sanitetsforening,
Rheumatism Hospital,
Oslo, Norway

**V. KASSIS**
Godthåbsvaenge 23.2.th,
DK-2000 Copenhagen, Denmark

**S. H. E. KAUFMANN**
Institute of Medical Microbiology,
Free University Berlin,
D-1000 Berlin 45, West Germany

**H. U. KELLER**
Institute of Pathology,
University of Berne,
Freiburgstrasse 30,
CH-3010 Berne, Switzerland

**Julia B. KHEIFITS**
Institute of Biological Sciences,
Syntex Research,
Palo Alto, California, USA

**M. KIST**
Institut für Allg. Hygiene und Bakteriologie,
D-7800 Freiburg, West Germany

**E. A. KITCHEN**
Lilly Research Centre Ltd.,
Erl Wood Manor, Windlesham GU20 6PH,
Surrey, England

**V. KLIMETZEK**
Institute of Medical Microbiology,
Free University Berlin,
D-1000 Berlin 45, West Germany

**M. KOH**
Department of Experimental Pathology,
St Bartholomew's Hospital,
London EC1A 7BE, England

**J. KOZAK**
Medizinische Hochschule Hannover,
Institut für klinische Chemie,
Karl-Wiechert-Allee 9,
D-3000 Hannover 61, West Germany

**M. W. M. KRUIJSEN**
Department of Rheumatology,
University Hospital St Radboud,
Nijmegen, The Netherlands

**G. J. M. LAFEBER**
Department of Rheumatology,
University Medical Center,
Rijnsburgerweg 10,
2333 AA Leiden, The Netherlands

**F. LAGHI PASINI**
Department of Internal Medicine,
Medical School,
University of Siena,
Siena, Italy

## LIST OF CONTRIBUTORS

**Ch. LAIOU**
Department of Experimental Pharmacology,
Athens University Medical School,
Athens, Greece

**P. C. J. LEIJH**
Department of Infectious Diseases,
University Hospital,
Rijnsburgerweg 10,
2333 AA Leiden, The Netherlands

**Geneviève LEMAIRE**
Institut de Biochimie,
Université Paris-Sud,
91405 Orsay, France

**M. LEQUESNE**
Service de Rhumatologie,
Hôpital Leopold Bellan,
7 rue de Texel,
75014 Paris, France

**A. J. LEWIS**
Scientific Development Group,
Organon Laboratories Ltd.,
Newhouse by Motherwell,
Lanarkshire, Scotland

**G. P. LEWIS**
Department of Pharmacology,
The Royal College of Surgeons of England,
Lincoln's Inn Fields,
London WC2A 3PN, England

**J. E. LINDER**
Department of Oral Pathology,
London Hospital Medical College,
London E1 2AD, England

**N. LINHART**
Nuclear Medicine,
Hôpital Beaujon,
Clichy, France

**Petula LIVINGSTON**
Biochemistry Department,
Scientific Development Group,
Organon Laboratories Ltd.,
Newhouse by Motherwell,
Lanarkshire, Scotland

**E. LOGEMANN**
Institut für Rechtsmedizin der Universität,
Albertstrasse 9,
D-7800 Freiburg, West Germany

**B. LOPEZ-RAMOS**
Department of Immunology,
Merck Institute for Therapeutic Research,
PO Box 2000, Rahway, New Jersey 07065,
USA

**E. LORA**
Rheumatology Service,
L. Sacco Hospital,
Milan, Italy

**Ib LORENZEN**
Section of Rheumatology,
Department of Internal Medicine,
Hvidovre Hospital,
University of Copenhagen,
Kettegaard alle 30,
DK-2650 Hvidovre, Denmark

**W. LU**
Department of Oral Pathology,
London Hospital Medical College,
London E1 2AD, England

**P. M. LUNDIN**
Department of Pathology,
Sahlgren's Hospital,
S-413 45 Gothenburg, Sweden

**F. P. LUYTEN**
Department of Rheumatology,
University Hospital,
Ghent, Belgium

**A. C. M. Th. van MAARSSEVEEN**
Pathological Institute,
Free University Hospital,
Amsterdam, The Netherlands

**R. T. McCONNELL**
Molecular Biology Department,
Wellcome Research Laboratories,
Research Triangle Park,
North Carolina 27709, USA

**W. J. McDONALD-GIBSON**
Research,
Miles Laboratories Ltd,
Slough SL2 4LY, England

**B. MACE**
Service d'Histologie,
CHU Cochin,
27 rue du Faubourg Saint-Jacques,
75014 Paris, France

**R. M. McMILLAN**
Connective Tissue Disease Section,
Department of Medicine,
Dartmouth-Hitchcock Medical Center,
Hanover, USA

**F. R. MANGAN**
Anti-Inflammatory Project,
Beecham Pharmaceuticals,
Harlow, Essex, England

**M. S. MANKU**
Institute of Innovative Medicine,
PO Box 10,
Nun's Island,
Montreal H3E 1J8, Canada

**Sonia MARTINEZ**
Institute of Biological Sciences,
Syntex Research,
Palo Alto, California, USA

**R. MASSE**
Departement de Protection-Laboratoire de Toxicologie Expérimentale,
CEA-IPSN,
92542 Montrouge Cedex – BP 561, France

**G. MATHE**
Institut de Cancerologie et d'Immunogenetique,
94800 Villejuif, France

**S. C. R. MEACOCK**
Lilly Research Centre Ltd.,
Erl Wood Manor, Windlesham GU20 6PH,
Surrey, England

**M. MEIGNAN**
Hôpital H. Mondor,
Creteil, France

**C. J. L. M. MEIJER**
Department of Pathology,
Section of Immunopathology,
University Medical Center,
PO Box 9603,
2300 RC Leiden, The Netherlands

**P. MERCIER**
Histocompatibility Laboratory,
Blood Bank,
Marseille 13005, France

**P. MICHEL**
Service d'Histologie,
CHU Cochin,
27 rue du Faubourg Saint-Jacques,
75014 Paris, France

**H. MIELANTS**
Department of Rheumatology,
Academic Hospital,
B-9000 Ghent, Belgium

**Daniela MIKULIKOVA**
Experimental Therapy,
Research Institute of Rheumatic Diseases,
Piešt'any, Czechoslovakia

**J. F. A. P. MILLER**
The Walter and Eliza Hall Institute of Medical Research,
Post Office,
Royal Melbourne Hospital,
Victoria 3050, Australia

**L. MIRAM**
Institute of Biological Sciences,
Syntex Research,
Palo Alto, California, USA

**A. MISEFARI**
General Pathology,
University of Messina,
98100 Messina, Italy

**F. MONTRONE**
Rheumatology Service,
L. Sacco Hospital,
Milan, Italy

**J.-F. MORIN**
Hôpital Saint-Antoine,
184 rue du Faubourg Saint-Antoine,
75571 Paris Cedex 12, France

**H. MULLINK**
Pathological Institute,
Free University Hospital,
Amsterdam, The Netherlands

**E. MUNTHE**
Oslo City Department of Rheumatology,
Oslo, Norway

**S. NARUMIYA**
Prostaglandin Research,
Wellcome Research Laboratories,
Langley Court,
Beckenham, Kent, England

**T. NATALE**
Institute of General Pathology,
University of Turin,
Corso Raffaello 30,
10125 Turin, Italy

## LIST OF CONTRIBUTORS

**J. NEMEC**
Research Institute for Pharmacy and Biochemistry,
Prague, Czechoslovakia

**O. NEMECEK**
Department of Chemistry,
Research Institute for Pharmacy and Biochemistry,
Prague, Czechoslovakia

**P. NETTER**
Clinique Rhumatologique et Laboratoire Pharmacologie,
CHU Brabois–Nancy
L54500 Vandoeuvre, France

**D. NOLIBE**
Département de Protection,
Laboratoire de Toxicologie Experimentale,
CEA–IPSN,
92542 Montrouge Cedex – BP 361, France

**S. NORMAN**
Department of Pathology,
University of Florida,
Gainesville, Florida 32601, USA

**A. A. NORRIS**
Department of Physiology and Pharmacology,
University of Strathclyde,
George Street,
Glasgow G1 1XW, Scotland

**Gabriele OBLETTER**
Cattedra di Seneiotica Medica,
Università di Chieti, Italy

**K. OHUCHI**
Department of Biochemistry,
Faculty of Pharmaceutical Sciences,
Tohoku University,
Aoba, Aramaki,
Sendai 980, Japan

**M. OKA**
Department of Medicine,
Keio University,
Japan

**J. OORT**
Pathological Institute,
Free University Hospital,
Amsterdam, The Netherlands

**C. A. OTTAWAY**
Department of Bacteriology and Immunology,
Western Infirmary,
University of Glasgow,
Glasgow G11 6NT, Scotland

**R. M. J. PALMER**
Department of Pharmacology,
Wellcome Research Laboratories,
Langley Court,
Beckenham, Kent, England

**G. PAPADIMITRIOU**
The Royal National Hospital for Rheumatic Diseases,
Upper Borough Walls,
Bath BA1 1RL, England

**F. PARANT**
Department of Experimental Immunotherapy,
Institut Pasteur,
28 rue du Docteur Roux,
75015 Paris, France

**M. PARANT**
Department of Experimental Immunotherapy,
Institut Pasteur,
28 rue du Docteur Roux,
75015 Paris, France

**D. M. V. PARROTT**
Department of Bacteriology and Immunology,
Western Infirmary,
University of Glasgow,
Glasgow G11 6NT, Scotland

**C. M. PEARSON**
Division of Rheumatology,
Department of Medicine,
University of California at Los Angeles,
Los Angeles, California 90024, USA

**Monique PELLETIER**
Department of Pharmacology,
Hôpital Cochin,
27 rue du Faubourg Saint-Jacques,
75014 Paris, France

**T. di PERRI**
Department of Internal Medicine,
Medical School,
University of Siena,
Siena, Italy

**Paola PERSICO**
Institute of Experimental Pharmacology,
University of Naples,
Naples, Italy

**J.-F. PETIT**
Institut de Biochimie,
Université Paris–Sud,
91405 Orsay, France

**A. PINTO**
Institute of Experimental Pharmacology,
University of Naples,
Naples, Italy

**A. POMPIDOU**
Service d'Histologie,
CHU Cochin,
24 rue du Faubourg Saint-Jacques,
75014 Paris, France

**J. P. PONCY**
CEA–IPSN,
Laboratoire de Toxicologie Expérimentale,
BP No 6,
92260 Fontenay aux Roses, France

**O. PONTANO**
Cattedra di Seneiotica Medica,
Università di Chieti, Italy

**B. F. PONTZ**
Institut für Medizinische Mikrobiologie,
Johannes-Gutenberg-Universität,
D–6500 Mainz, West Germany

**N. A. PORTER**
Department of Chemistry,
Duke University,
Durham, North Carolina, USA

**J. POUREL**
Clinique Rhumatologique,
CHU Brabois–Nancy,
54500 Vandoeuvre, France

**L. B. A. van de PUTTE**
Department of Rheumatology,
University Hospital St Radboud,
Nijmegen, The Netherlands

**D. RAMAN**
Rheumatology Department,
Royal Victoria Infirmary,
Newcastle upon Tyne, England

**V. D. RAMANATHAN**
Department of Pathology,
The Royal College of Surgeons of England,
Lincoln's Inn Fields,
London WC2A 3PN, England

**M. RAULO**
Hôpital Saint-Antoine,
184 rue du Faubourg Saint-Antoine,
75571 Paris Cedex 12, France

**H. G. REMOLD**
Harvard Medical School,
Boston, Massachusetts, USA

**R. RIBEIRO DOS SANTOS**
Department of Parasitology,
Faculty of Medicine of Ribeirão Preto,
14100 Ribeirão Preto, Sao Paulo, Brazil

**E. F. J. RING**
The Royal National Hospital for Rheumatic Diseases,
Upper Borough Walls,
Bath BA1 1RL, England

**G. RIVEAU**
Laboratory of Experimental Immunopharmacology,
Centre National de la Recherche Scientifique and Institut Pasteur,
Paris, France

**M. ROCH-ARVEILLER**
Department of Pharmacology,
Hôpital Cochin,
27 rue du Faubourg Saint-Jacques,
75014 Paris, France

**Lise-Lotte RÖCKERT**
Department of Pathology,
Sahlgren's Hospital
413 45 Gothenburg, Sweden

**N. A. ROHLOFF**
The Upjohn Company,
Kalamazoo, Michigan, USA

**Z. ROUBAL**
Department of Biochemistry,
Research Institute for Pharmacy and Biochemistry,
Prague, Czechoslovakia

**B. ROUVEIX**
Institut de Pharmacologie,
Paris, France

LIST OF CONTRIBUTORS

**H. ROUX**
Department of Rheumatology,
Hôpital de la Conception,
Marseille 13385 Cedex 4, France

**S. ROVIDA**
Istituto di Statistica Medica e Biometria,
University of Genoa,
Genoa, Italy

**M. RUSSO**
Unidade de Ensino e Pesquisa,
Hospital Universitario,
Universidade de Sao Paulo,
and
Microbiologia e Imunologia,
Instituto de Ciencias Biomedicas,
Sao Paulo, Brazil

**S. A. SAEED**
Research,
Miles Laboratories Ltd.,
Slough SL2 4LY, England

**M. G. SAIFER**
Research and Development,
Diagnostic Data Inc.,
Mountain View, California, USA

**J. A. SALMON**
Prostaglandin Research Department,
Wellcome Research Laboratories,
Langley Court,
Beckenham, Kent, England

**E. SAMANTA**
Department of Rheumatology,
University of Genoa,
Genoa, Italy

**M. SANDEN**
Department of Pathology,
University of Gothenburg,
Sahlgren's Hospital,
S-413 45 Gothenburg, Sweden

**F. SANTORO**
Centre d'Immunologie et Biologie Parasitaire
(INSERM U 167),
Institut Pasteur,
BP 3415, Lille 59019 Cedex, France

**J. SANY**
Service de Consultation de Rhumatologie
Sociale,
Centre Gui-De-Chauliac,
Hôpital Saint–Eloi,
34059 Montpellier Cedex, France

**H. SATO**
Department of Biochemistry,
Faculty of Pharmaceutical Sciences,
Tohoku University,
Aoba, Aramaki,
Sendai 980, Japan

**W. SCHAPER**
Arbeitsgruppe Biochemie,
Max-Planck-Institut für experimentelle
Kardiologie,
Sprudelhof 11,
D-6350 Bad Nauheim, West Germany

**M. SCHARDT**
Department of Medicine,
Swiss Research Institute,
Davos CH 7270, Switzerland

**R. J. SCHEPER**
Pathological Institute,
Free University Hospital,
Amsterdam, The Netherlands

**H. U. SCHORLEMMER**
Institut für Medizinische Mikrobiologie,
Johannes-Gutenberg-Universität,
D-6500 Mainz, West Germany

**A. D. SEDGWICK**
Department of Experimental Pathology,
St Bartholomew's Hospital,
West Smithfield, London EC1 7BE, England

**J. L. SELPH**
Pharmacology Department,
Wellcome Research Laboratories,
Research Triangle Park,
North Carolina 27709, USA

**L. SENA**
Institute of General Pathology,
University of Turin,
Corso Raffaello 30,
10125 Turin, Italy

**Anastasia SFIKAKIS**
Department of Experimental Pharmacology,
Athens University Medical School,
Athens, Greece

**P. SFIKAKIS**
First Department of Propedeutic Medicine,
King Paul Hospital,
Athens University Medical School,
Athens, Greece

**M. E. SHIPLEY**
Department of Rheumatology and Rehabilitation,
King's College Hospital,
London, England

**M. I. SIEGEL**
Molecular Biology Department,
Wellcome Research Laboratories,
Research Triangle Park,
North Carolina 27709, USA

**M. M. SIMON**
Institute of Immunology and Genetics,
German Cancer Research Center,
Heidelberg, West Germany

**W. SLUITER**
Department of Infectious Diseases,
University Hospital,
Rijnsburgerweg 10,
2333 AA Leiden, The Netherlands

**M. J. H. SMITH**
Department of Chemical Pathology,
King's College Hospital Medical School,
Denmark Hill, London SE5 8RX, England

**W. E. SMITH**
Pure and Applied Chemistry,
Strathclyde University,
Glasgow, Scotland

**E. SORKIN**
Department of Medicine,
Swiss Research Institute,
Davos CH 7270, Switzerland

**Anita STURM**
Department of Immunology,
Merck Institute for Therapeutic Research,
PO Box 2000, Rahway, New Jersey 07065,
USA

**R. D. STURROCK**
Centre for Rheumatic Diseases/
University Department of Medicine,
Glasgow University,
Glasgow, Scotland

**K. SUGIO**
Department of Biochemistry,
Faculty of Pharmaceutical Sciences,
Tohoku University,
Aoba, Aramaki,
Sendai 980, Japan

**S. S. SUYKENS**
Department of Rheumatology,
University Hospital,
Ghent, Belgium

**L. SZPORNY**
Pharmacological Laboratory,
Chemical Works of Gedeon Richter,
H-1475 Budapest, Hungary

**M. THOMPSON**
Rheumatology Department,
Royal Victoria Infirmary,
Newcastle upon Tyne, England

**M. J. THOMSON**
Anti-Inflammatory Project,
Beecham Pharmaceuticals,
Harlow, Essex, England

**Patricia A. THROWER**
Department of Rheumatology,
St Bartholomew's Hospital,
West Smithfield, London EC1 7BE, England

**G. TILL**
Institute of Immunology and Serology,
University of Heidelberg,
Im Neuenheimer Feld 305,
D-6900 Heidelberg, West Germany

**A. J. TOMOLONIS**
Institute of Biological Sciences,
Syntex Research,
Palo Alto, California, USA

**M. V. TORRIELLI**
Institute of General Pathology,
University of Turin,
Corso Rafaello 30,
10125 Turin, Italy

**W. TREADWAY**
Section of Rheumatology,
Department of Medicine,
Bowman Gray School of Medicine,
Winston-Salem, North Carolina 27103, USA

**Z. TRNAVSKA**
Department of Biochemistry,
Research Institute of Rheumatic Diseases,
Piešt'any, Czechoslovakia

**K. TRNAVSKY**
Department of Experimental Therapy,
Research Institute of Rheumatic Diseases,
Piešt'any, Czechoslovakia

LIST OF CONTRIBUTORS

**J. E. TRUAX**
Pharmacology Department,
Wellcome Research Laboratories,
Research Triangle Park,
North Carolina 27709, USA

**S. TSURUFUJI**
Department of Biochemistry,
Faculty of Pharmaceutical Sciences,
Tohoku University,
Aoba, Aramaki,
Sendai 980, Japan

**J. L. TURK**
Department of Pathology,
The Royal College of Surgeons of England,
Lincoln's Inn Fields,
London WC2A 3PN, England

**R. TURNER**
Section of Rheumatology,
Department of Medicine,
Bowman Gray School of Medicine,
Winston-Salem, North Carolina 27103, USA

**D. VARONOS**
Department of Experimental Pharmacology,
Athens University Medical School,
Athens, Greece

**L. VECCHIET**
Cattedra di Seneiotica Medica,
Università di Chieti, Italy

**Diana VENZA-TETI**
General Pathology,
University of Messina,
98100 Messina, Italy

**G. VERBRUGGEN**
Department of Rheumatology,
University Hospital,
Ghent, Belgium

**E. M. VEYS**
Department of Rheumatology,
Academic Hospital,
De Pintelaan 135,
B-9000 Ghent, Belgium

**R. VINEGAR**
Pharmacology Department,
Wellcome Research Laboratories,
Research Triangle Park,
North Carolina 27709, USA

**T. L. VISCHER**
Division of Rheumatology,
Department of Medicine,
University Hospital,
CH-1211 Geneva 4, Switzerland

**W. VOGT**
Max-Planck-Institut für experimentelle Medizin,
Hermann-Rein-Strasse 3,
D-3400 Göttingen, West Germany

**J. R. WALKER**
Department of Allergy,
Lilly Research Centre Ltd.,
Erl Wood Manor, Windlesham GU20 6PH,
Surrey, England

**H. van WEELDEN**
Department of Dermatology,
State University Hospital,
Utrecht, The Netherlands

**E. A. WEST, III**
Section of Rheumatology,
Department of Medicine,
Bowman Gray School of Medicine,
Winston-Salem, North Carolina 27103, USA

**D. D. WHITE**
Biochemistry Department,
Scientific Development Group,
Organon Laboratories Ltd.,
Newhouse by Motherwell,
Lanarkshire, Scotland

**P. C. WILKINSON**
Bacteriology and Immunology Department,
University of Glasgow,
Glasgow G11 7LG, Scotland

**D. M. WILLIAMS**
Department of Oral Pathology,
The London Hospital Medical College,
London E1 2AD, England

**L. D. WILLIAMS**
Research and Development,
Diagnostic Data Inc.,
Mountain View, California, USA

**D. A. WILLOUGHBY**
Department of Experimental Pathology,
St Bartholomew's Hospital,
London EC1A 7BE, England

**Vivienne R. WINROW**
ARC Research Group,
The Royal National Hospital for Rheumatic Diseases,
Upper Borough Walls,
Bath BA1 1RL, England

**J. H. WISSLER**
Arbeitsgruppe Biochemie,
Max-Planck-Institut für experimentelle Kardiologie,
Sprudelhof 11,
D-6350 Bad Nauheim, West Germany

**D. E. WOOLLEY**
Department of Biochemistry,
University of South Manchester,
Withington Hospital,
Manchester, England

**R. A. WOUTERSEN**
Central Institute for Toxicology and Nutrition, TNO,
PO Box 360,
3700 AJ Zeist, The Netherlands

**J. WYBRAN**
Department of Immunology,
University of Brussels,
Brussels, Belgium

**P. YOUINOU**
Hôpital Saint-Antoine,
184 rue du Faubourg Saint-Antoine,
75571 Paris Cedex 12, France

**J. ZAAGSMA**
Department of Medicinal Chemistry,
Section of Molecular Pharmacology,
Faculty of Science,
Free University,
Amsterdam, The Netherlands

**I. J. ZEITLIN**
Department of Physiology and Pharmacology,
University of Strathclyde,
George Street,
Glasgow G1 1XW, Scotland

**M. ZIFF**
Department of Internal Medicine,
University of Texas Health Sciences Center,
5323 Harry Hines Boulevard,
Dallas, Texas 75235, USA

**Th. L. van ZWET**
Department of Infectious Diseases,
University Hospital
Rijnsburgerweg 10,
2333 AA Leiden, The Netherlands

# Preface

This report on Future Trends in Inflammation IV records another of the multidisciplinary meetings organized by the European Biological Research Association. The organizers wish to record their thanks to all the participants and delegates who made this such an enjoyable meeting.

Our thanks are due to a number of members of the pharmaceutical industry who so kindly donated funds. These funds were used to provide grants for young research workers to attend this meeting. Many people have kindly given their time and help to make this congress possible. It is impossible to list them by name, but we are profoundly grateful. We were dubious at the outset as to whether to hold this meeting in a period when many other meetings are being organized on inflammation. The enthusiastic attendance proves that we were right in going ahead.

The next international meeting will be held in France in 1983. For further details please contact:

Professor J. P. Giroud
Department of Pharmacology,
Hôpital Cochin
75014 Paris, France

D. A. Willoughby
J. P. Giroud

# Section I
# Future Trends

CHAIRMAN: L. Chedid
CO-CHAIRMAN: Dame Honor Fell

# 1

# The participation of mononucleur phagocytes in immune based inflammatory processes with special reference to their secretory responses

P. DAVIES AND R. J. BONNEY (USA)

## INTRODUCTION

Since the last meeting in this series, considerable new information regarding the functions of mononuclear phagocytes in host defence systems and the expression of chronic inflammation has been gathered[25]. Consequently, certain concepts regarding the roles played by macrophages in the inflammatory process have been elaborated further. These concern roles for macrophages in (a) the afferent limb of the immune response in relation to antigen processing and presentation to cells of the lymphoid system[21]; and (b) the effector arm of the immune response where they respond to products of lymphoid cells by secreting a variety of mediators directed towards the resolution of host defence responses. In this brief review we will be concerned predominantly with the role of the macrophage in the effector arm of immune responses.

## THE RECOGNITION OF LYMPHOCYTE PRODUCTS BY MACROPHAGES

The products of lymphocytes which have responded to immunogenic stimuli react with macrophages in a number of ways directed towards the efficient removal of the stimulus. Most important among these are lymphokines and antibodies, the latter forming immune complexes in the presence of specific antigen.

## LYMPHOKINES

Lymphokines constitute a number of high molecular weight products produced by both T and B lymphocytes as a result of stimulation with antigens or mitogens[3]. These substances have a broad spectrum of biological effects, several of which are mediated through the agency of macrophages[4]. Macrophages possess binding sites for certain lymphokines such as migration inhibitory factor (MIF) and macrophage activation factor (MAF)[4]. Glycolipids are considered important constituents of such receptors with the removal of L-fucose abolishing responses to MIF and MAF. Also, treatment of macrophages with α-L-fucosidase or trypsin abolish their responsiveness to MIF and MAF. This effect is reversible, responsiveness being restored after some time in culture[16]. Much remains to be learned concerning the precise nature of lymphokines modulating macrophage function as well as the properties of the surface determinants of macrophages to which they bind.

## STIMULATION OF SECRETORY PRODUCT FORMATION BY MACROPHAGES RESPONDING TO LYMPHOKINES

Macrophages exposed to lymphokines in tissue culture show a wide variety of morphological, functional and biochemical changes[4]. Included among these responses is the secretion of a number of products relevant to inflammatory processes (Table 1.1).

**Table 1.1** Stimulation of macrophage secretion by lymphokines

| *Responding macrophage population* | *Product* | *Reference* |
|---|---|---|
| Resident mouse peritoneal | plasminogen activator | 10, 13, 26 |
| Oil-induced guinea pig peritoneal | collagenase | 15, 27 |
| Resident mouse peritoneal | lysosomal enzymes | 14 |
| BCG-induced guinea pig peritoneal | prostaglandins | 7 |
| Human peripheral blood monocytes | procoagulant factor | 18 |
| Human peripheral blood monocytes | C2 | 11 |
| Human peripheral blood monocytes | Stimulant of prostaglandin and collagenase production by synoviocytes | 6 |

The release of hydrolytic enzymes such as collagenase, plasminogen activator and lysosomal enzymes together with prostaglandins may make significant contributions to the role played by macrophages at sites of delayed hypersensitivity responses. Lymphokines may also modulate the way in which macrophages affect other cell types in their pericellular environment. Dayer *et al.*, have found that lymphokines stimulate the release of a substance from human peripheral blood monocytes which increases the synthesis of prostaglandins and collagenase by human rheumatoid synovial cells.[6]

## ANTIGEN–ANTIBODY COMPLEXES

The role of immune complexes in the pathogenesis of acute and chronic inflammation has been widely investigated and described. Receptors for both immunoglobulins and immune complexes on macrophages have been characterized[29]. Studies with macrophages from various species indicate that there is class and sub-class specificity for immunoglobulin binding to macrophages. For example, human monocytes bind $IgG_1$ and $IgG_3$ while murine macrophages bind $IgG_{2a}$ and $IgG_{2b}$.It is now clear that at least two Fc receptors exist in murine macrophages, the one binding monomeric and immune aggregates of $IgG_{2a}$ (FcR1) while the other binds immune aggregates of $IgG_1$ and $IgG_{2b}$ (FcR11). The former receptor is inactivated by trypsin but the latter is not 8, 22, 28. Variants of the macrophage cell line, J774, have been isolated which lack the receptor (FcR11) for $IgG_1$ and $IgG_{2b}$ [24]. Unkeless[23] has also produced a monoclonal antibody toFcR1 and shown that it inhibits rosetting of antibody coated erythrocytes to macrophages, macrophage cell lines as well as lymphocytes. The availability of such a monoclonal antibody provides the opportunity for the purification of Fc receptors by affinity chromatography. The purification of such a receptor should facilitate investigations of the mechanism of interaction of immune complexes with macrophages and the consequent effects of this interaction on macrophage functions.

**Table 1.2** Stimulation of macrophage secretion by immune complexes

| *Responding macrophage population* | *Product* | *Reference* |
|---|---|---|
| Resident mouse peritoneal | lysosomal enzymes | 2 |
| Resident mouse peritoneal | prostaglandins | 1 |
| Human monocytes | procoagulant factor | 17 |
| Human monocytes | oxygen metabolites | 9 |

Several inflammatory mediators are secreted by macrophages in response to immune complexes. (Table 1.2). Macrophages from several sources release lysosomal enzymes in a selective manner in response to immune complexes (for review see Davies and Bonney[5]). Immune complexes cause the release of oxygen metabolites such as superoxide and hydroxyl radicals[9]. Macrophages also secrete considerable amounts of arachidonic acid oxygenation products upon exposure to immune complexes. Studies in this laboratory[1] have shown that resident mouse peritoneal macrophages exposed to immune complexes synthesize and release both prostaglandin $E_1$ and 6-ketoprostaglandin $F_{1\alpha}$ in a concentration and time-dependent manner. There are increasing indications that macrophages are involved in the activation of the blood coagulation system and the deposition of fibrin that is frequently seen during chronic inflammatory response. Studies from several laboratories indicate that macrophages contain procoagulant activity, the level of which can be significantly increased and released into the pericellular environment by exposure to a variety of stimuli, including immune complexes and lymphokines[17, 18].

## COMPLEMENT RECEPTORS

Macrophages possess trypsin labile C3b receptors which can be detected by the binding of 19S antibody-coated erythrocytes in the presence of complement. The function of the C3b receptor has been associated with attachment of C3b coated ligands to the cell acting synergistically with antibody to mediate phagocytosis[20]. C3b has also been shown to initiate the selective release of lysosomal hydrolases from macrophages, a response thought to be initiated by binding to C3b receptors[19].

C5a initiates a number of responses in phagocytic cells, the most widely studied being chemotaxis. This response is initiated, by extremely low concentrations of this product, of complement activation through binding to high affinity receptors. In addition, C5a has been shown to stimulate the selective release of lysosomal hydrolases and a neutral protease from alveolar macrophages[12]. This response is relatively slow, occurring over a period of many hours. C5a is a peptide containing 74 amino acids. In biological fluids its carboxy terminal arginine residue is rapidly removed to form $C5a_{desarg}$, a molecule which retains the biological activity of C5a. This biological stability suggests that $C5a_{desarg}$ is an important inflammatory mediator by virtue of its chemotactic activity and ability to stimulate secretion of hydrolytic enzymes in phagocytic cells.

## CONCLUDING REMARKS

The participation of macrophages in immune-based chronic inflammatory responses appears to be facilitated by the presence of specific recognition sites for products of immune responses on their plasma membranes. This allows rapid binding of immune complexes which are then efficiently interiorized, particularly when C3b is bound to the complex with subsequent digestion and degradation within secondary lysosomes. The interaction with lymphokines leads to widespread cellular activation directed towards the more effective limitation and resolution of the inflammatory process. Secretion of a variety of products is a concomitant of the response of macrophages to immune complexes and lymphokines. These products contribute to regulation and resolution of chronic inflammatory responses and in chronic inflammatory diseases may be responsible for certain aspects of the abnormal cellular proliferation and irreversible tissue damage that occurs. It is therefore clear that a precise understanding of the mechanism by which macrophages recognize and react to products of lymphocytes participating in immune-based inflammatory responses will be critical to establishing approaches to controlling the adverse consequences associated with chronic inflammatory diseases.

## References


1 Bonney, R. J., Naruns, P., Davies, P. and Humes, J. L. (1979). Antigen-antibody complexes stimulate the synthesis and release of prostaglandins by mouse peritoneal macropahges. *Prostaglandins*, **18,** 605

2 Cardella, C. J., Davies, P. and Allison, A. C. (1974). Immune complexes induce selective release of lysosomal hydrolases from macrophages *in vitro*. *Nature (London)*, **247,** 46

3 Cohen, S., Pick, E. and Oppenheim, J. J. (1979). *Biology of Lymphokines*. (New York: Academic Press)

4 David, J. R. and Remold, H. G. (1979). The activation of macrophages by lymphokines. In Cohen, S. Pick, E. and Oppenheim, J. J. (eds.) Biology of Lymphokines p. 121. (New York: Academic Press)

5 Davies, P. and Bonney, R. J. (1980). The secretion of hydrolytic enzymes by mononuclear phagocytes. In Weissmann, G. (ed.) *Handbook of Inflammation Vol. 2*, p. 497 New York, North Holland Elsevier

6 Dayer, J. M., Breard, J., Chess, L. and Krane, S. M. (1979). Participation of monocytes, macrophages and lymphocytes in the production of a factor that stimulates collagenase and prostaglandin release by rheumatoid synovial cells. *J. Clin. Invest.*, **64,** 1386

7 Gordon, D., Bray, M. A. and Morley, J. (1976). Control of lymphokine production by prostaglandins. *Nature (London)*, **262,** 401

8 Heusser, C. H., Anderson, C. L. and Grey, H. M. (1977). Receptors for IgG: Subclass specificity of receptors on different mouse cell types and the definition of two distinct receptors on a macrophage cell line. *J. Exp. Med.*, **145,** 1316

9 Johnston, R. B. Jr. Lehmeyer, J. E. and Guthrie, L. A. (1976). Generation of superoxide anion and chemiluminescence by human monocytes during phagocytosis and on contact with surface bound-immunoglobulin G. *J. Exp. Med.*, **143,** 1551

10 Klimetzek, V. and Sorg, C. (1977). Lymphokine-induced secretion of plasminogen activator by murine macrophages. *Eur. J. Immunol.*, **7,** 185

11 Littman, B. H. and Ruddy, S. (1977). Production of the second component of complement by human monocytes: Stimulation by antigen-activated lymphocytes or lymphokines. *J. Exp. Med.*, **145,** 1344

12 McCarthy, K. and Henson, P. M. (1979). Induction of lysosomal enzyme secretion by alveolar macrophages in response to the purified complement fragments C5a and $C5a_{des\text{-}arg}$.

13 Newman, W., Gordon, S., Hammerling, U., Senik, A. and Bloom, B. R. (1978). Production of migration inhibition factor (MIF) and an inducer of plasminogen activator (IPA) by subsets of T cells in MLC. *J. Immunol.*, **120,** 927

14 Pantalone, R. M. and Page, R. C. (1975). Lymphokine-induced production and release of lysosomal enzymes by macrophages. *Proc. Natl. Acad. Sci.*, (*USA*), **72,** 2091

15 Pantalone, R. M. and Page, R. C. (1977). Enzyme production and secretion by lymphokine-activated macrophages. *J. Reticuloendothel. Soc.*, **21,** 343

16 Remold, H. G. (1973). Requirement for α-L-fucose on the macrophage membrane receptor for MIF. *J. Exp. Med.*, **138,** 1065
17 Rothberger, M., Zimmerman, T. S., Spiegelberg, H. L. and Vaughan, J. H. (1977). Leukocyte procoagulant activity. Enhancement of production *in vitro* by IgG and antigen-anitbody complexes. *J. Clin. Invest.*, **59,** 549
18 Rothberger, H., Zimmerman, T. S. and Vaughan, J. H. (1978). Increased production and expression of tissue-thromboplastin-like procoagulant activity *in vitro* by allogeneically stimulated lymphocytes. *J. Clin. Invest.*, **62,** 649
19 Schorlemmer, H. U. and Allison, A. C. (1976). Effects of activated complement components on enzyme secretion by macrophages. *Immunology*, **31,** 781
20 Silverstein, S. C., Steinman, R. S. and Cohn, Z. A. (1977). Endocytosis. *Ann. Rev. Biochem.*, **46,** 669
21 Unanue, E. R. and Rosenthal, A. S. (1980). *Macrophage Regulation of Immunity*. New York: Academic Press,
22 Unkeless, J. C. (1977). The presence of two Fc receptors on mouse macrophages: evidence from a variant cell line and differential trypsin sensitivity. *J. Exp. Med.*, **145,** 931
23 Unkeless, J. C. (1979). Characterization of a monoclonal antibody directed against mouse macrophage and lymphocyte Fc receptors. *J. Exp. Med.* **150,** 580
24 Unkeless, J. C., Kaplan, G., Plutner, H. and Cohn, Z. A. (1979). Fc receptor variants of a macrophage cell line. *Proc. Natl. Acad. Sci. (USA)* **76,** 1400
25 Van Furth, R. (ed.) (1980). *Proceedings of the Third Leiden Conference on Mononuclear Phagocytes*. (The Hague: Martinus Nijhoff BV)
26 Vassalli, J. D. and Reich, E. (1977). Macrophage plasminogen activator: Induction by products of activated lymphoid cells. *J. Exp. Med.*, **145,** 429
27 Wahl, L. M., Wahl, S. M., Mergenhagen, S. E. and Martin, G. R. (1975). Collagenase production by lymphokine-activated macrophages. *Science*, **187,** 261
28 Walker, W. S. (1976). Separate Fc receptors for immunoglobulins $IgG_{2a}$ and $IgG_{2b}$ on an established cell line of mouse macrophages. *J. Immunol.*, **116,** 911
29 Zuckerman, S. H. and Douglas, S. D. (1979). Dynamics of the macrophage plasma membrane. *Ann. Rev. Microbiol*, **33,** 267

# Discussion

**Dr I. F. Skidmore (UK)** asked whether Dr Davies had attempted to block prostaglandin production with steroids, and if so, what effect actinomycin D would have.

**Dr Davies** said that he would predict that a steroid inhibitory effect would be blocked by actinomycin D but they had not yet discovered conditions appropriate to product blockage of the steroid effect without also blocking prostaglandin production.

In response to a comment by Dr Chedid that indomethacin did not apparently block the release of endogenous pyrogen or lymphocyte activating factor in the presence of low levels of prostaglandin, he said that the problem was complicated. In some situations prostaglandins appeared to be essential for inducing the release of certain molecules, for example, collagenase. However, this appeared to be true only for the induction phase. The secretion phase appeared to proceed independently of prostaglandin. On the other hand, there were instances where supra-pharmacological doses of prostaglandin would inhibit the release of certain mediators.

**Professor C. Pearson (USA)** asked what evidence existed that macrophages released more than one type of interferon and how this related to the immunomodulatory effect.

**Dr Davies** said that the release of interferon from macrophages had been studied by groups other than his own but so far its relation to the immunomodulatory effect did not seem to have been fully established.

**Professor T. L. Vischer (Switzerland)** asked whether macrophage activated states were reversible.

**Dr Davies** said that in talking about macrophage activation one had to define the source of the cells and whether they had been elicited in any particular way that needed specifying. One also needed to define the culture conditions and whether they received further stimulation within the culture environment. He did not know of any circumstances in which a macrophage population could be induced first to produce and then to stop producing prostaglandin and finally to produce it once more. Their own attempts to produce such switching on and off had been unsuccessful. Although pharmacological agents would inhibit the release of mediators, such inhibition seemed irreversible.

**Professor D. A. Willoughby (UK)** asked Dr Davies to speculate on appropriate directions for future therapy. Among various possibilities one might attempt to inhibit chemotactic factors; to inhibit factors controlling cell secretion or to impede the ability of cells to move into an inflamed area. One might also choose to inhibit the transformation of monocytes into macrophages and he wondered which, among this catalogue of possibilities, gave the best possibilities for intervention.

**Dr Davies** said that in looking at secretory products there was no single substance the inhibition of which would necessarily represent a therapeutic advance. One had to look individually at such secretory products, define the conditions under which they were produced, and attempt to modulate such conditions pharmacologically. Only then could one start to speculate on which interventions were most appropriate. As to chemotaxis, it was also essential for the host defence mechanism that cells be allowed to accumulate at sites of inflammation because this was one of their major functions. Possibly it might be a good idea to search for ways of increasing their specificity and efficiency at such sites and to prevent the spill-over phenomena (as they presently seemed) leading to tissue damage and proliferation so characteristic of chronic inflammatory lesions.

# 2

# Future trends in mechanisms of cartilage destruction (Abstract)

J. T. DINGLE (UK)

Very recent research at the Strangeways Laboratory, Cambridge, has demonstrated that chondrocyte function may be controlled, at least in part, by the release from adjacent synovial tissue of factors, provisionally named *catabolins*, that can act directly on living cartilage cells. Our work during the last year has led to the identification of human and animal catabolins and substantial purification of a catabolin from porcine synovium. We have shown that it is highly effective in producing almost total (~ 90%) resorption of cartilage matrix in organ culture by the indigenous chondrocytes. It seems possible that catabolin may have a substantial role in arthritis in causing the characteristic articular cartilage erosion. Pharmacological control of this novel mechanism could be of importance in modulating the course of arthritic disease.

# Discussion

**Dr P. Davies (USA)** asked if there was any indication as to the target cell specificity of catabolin. Was it specific only for chondrocytes or could it affect other cells? He wondered whether the hypothesis advanced for destruction of proteoglycan by membrane associated enzymes in chondrocytes might be equally true for the cells in the advancing front of the pannus.

**Dr Dingle** thought it very likely that catabolin might be active in systems other than synovial cartilage. However, such an action would not be easy to demonstrate. It was readily shown in cartilage preparations where loss of metachromasia and proteoglycan could be observed, but it was difficult to know how to measure such an action in tissue such as skin or cornea where fibroblasts were reacting with other fibroblasts. As to specificity, catabolin was certainly species specific. Human catabolin acted on bovine cartilage but the reverse was not true. Rabbit catabolin was active on rabbit but not on bovine cartilage, and they had not been able to demonstrate any effect in chick. Thus, there was certainly species specificity, but he had no evidence for tissue specificity.

**N. R. Ackerman (USA)** asked about the role of catabolin in cartilage. He wondered if it might be inducing enzyme secretion and if so, whether it might be possible to antagonize such secretion, for example, with chelating agents. There was some evidence of chelating agents being able to inhibit autolysis of rabbit ear cartilage maintained in culture.

**Dr Dingle** had no direct information on any enzymes that might be released by catabolin. They had refrained from measuring proteases and similar enzymes since it was their belief that measurement of enzymes released in a culture system gave very little information about conditions occurring at or near the cell surface. They had performed only a few experiments on pharmacological control. Indomethacin had no effect on catabolin production. There was some evidence from Dame Honor Fell's work that steroids might interfere with catabolin production but they did not appear to inhibit the effect of catabolin in cartilage. They had no information on other therapeutic agents.

**Dr Tonneson (Denmark)** asked what was the oxygen and glucose content of the system, and whether catabolin was normally present in synovial tissue.

**Dr Dingle** said that the medium used was a conventional BTJ5 medium with 20% oxygen and 1 mg/ml of glucose. The question of whether catabolin was normally present in synovial membrane could not at present be answered. They were attempting to purify it to the point where it would be possible to raise an anti-serum to locate its presence by immunoassay. Their present methods involved abnormal tissue and so far their results showed only that the tissue had the capacity to produce the molecule. They did not know whether it would produce it normally *in vivo*.

**Dame Honor Fell (Co-Chairman)** said that they had originally wanted to quantify the amount of synovial tissue present in cultures but it was impossible to cut equivalent explants of synovium. Their procedure was, therefore, to remove and mince the synovial villi and the cultures contained quantities of the pooled mince which behaved in certain respects like an inflammatory tissue without the invading cells. There was a very active repair process, coupled with considerable breakdown of collagen material. She believed that it was because the synovium was in this particular state that it caused the breakdown effects observed when it was associated with cartilage.

**Dr S. S. Kirwar (USA)** asked whether catabolin arose in any particular cell type in the synovial tissue.

**Dr Dingle** said that they had used chopped synovium which contained histiocytes, fibroblasts and other cells, and so it was impossible to answer the question.

**Dame Honor Fell** said that the tissue also contained the so-called A cells, which in some earlier work they had found to be identical in certain respects with tissue macrophages. They might be responsible for some of the activity observed. There were a great many of them in the explants and they could mitose in culture.

**Dr C. J. Dunn (France)** asked what effect might be expected to result from the injection of catabolin into an animal knee joint, and whether such a procedure would result in inflammation.

**Dr Dingle** had no reason to suppose that catabolin *per se* would be involved in the inflammatory process. He was simply suggesting that it was the product of damaged, repairing or stimulated synovial cells, macrophages or fibroblasts. As to conditions within a joint, he thought it unlikely that such a low molecular weight material as catabolin would remain in the joint for any length of time. Indeed, they would greatly welcome some slow release system that could keep it there.

**Dr G. Gordon (USA)** asked Dr Dingle to speculate on what would happen when the irresistible force of a pannus continuing to grow met the immovable object of a cartilage no longer lysed because catabolin had been inhibited.

**Dr Dingle** said that he was not able to answer the question, if only because they did not know exactly what pannus is. However, because of experiments which he and the co-chairman had performed many years previously, in which vitamin A stimulated chick limb bone rudiments, and bearing in mind the co-chairman's findings on late stage catabolin experiments in which chondrocytes apparently turned into cells resembling fibroblasts that would proliferate, it was worth speculating that part of the pannus at least might be derived from cartilage. This suggestion raised interesting possibilities, but he was not prepared to speculate further.

# 3

# New developments in leukocyte chemotaxis research: a survey

P. C. WILKINSON (SCOTLAND)

A book such as this presents a suitable opportunity for appraisal of recent progress in the study of the locomotion and chemotaxis of leukocytes, a study that has gained momentum during the past decade, but that has for many years fascinated biologists and medical scientists and will see its centenary during the 1980s[1]. Over the past few years there have been a number of major developments. Firstly, the locomotor reactions of leukocytes to chemoattractants are now defined with better precision than formerly. Both conceptually and in the laboratory, we can now distinguish *chemotaxis*, as a reaction by which chemical substances determine the direction of leukocyte locomotion, from *chemokinesis*, as a reaction by which they determine its rate[2]. Since positive chemotactic reactions cause cells to accumulate, and positive chemokinetic reactions may cause them to disperse, the practical distinction between these two reactions is important. Secondly, these years have seen the definition of classes of binding sites on the leukocyte surface for various categories of chemotactic factors which are discussed below. Thirdly, a beginning has been made in explaining the process of transduction, by which binding of a chemotactic factor to the cell surface signals a locomotor event in the cell. The locomotor events themselves, which are mediated by microfilament systems consisting of actin and myosin, actin-binding protein and other related proteins, are not yet understood in detail at the molecular level[3].

## CELL SURFACE BINDING SITES FOR CHEMOTACTIC FACTORS

Table 3.1 lists various categories of chemotactic factor. This is not a complete list, which would have to be very long, but it suggests some of the types of material that can excite directional locomotion and includes factors which have been especially useful for binding studies and studies of transduction processes. For use in such studies, a chemotactic factor needs to be well purified chemically, readily available in quantity, and have good biological activity. Many groups are at present working with the synthetic formylated peptide chemotactic factors first described by Schiffmann *et al*[4] and which fulfil these criteria. These are a series of dipeptides[4] or tripeptides[5] which are formylated at the N-terminal amino group, and which frequently have methionine as the N-terminal residue. The C-terminal residues require to be hydrophobic for full activity, and the commercially available type-example of such peptides has become N-formyl-methionyl-leucyl-phenylalanine (f-Met-Leu-Phe).

**Table 3.1** Categories of chemotactic factor

| |
|---|
| Low molecular weight |
| formylated peptides |
| lipids: arachidonic acid derivatives |
| eosinophilotactic peptides |
| Intermediate molecular weight |
| C5a and C5-derived peptides |
| High molecular weight |
| $\alpha_s$- and $\beta$-caseins |
| denatured proteins (e.g. serum albumin, haemoglobin) |
| lectins |
| lymphokines |
| Cell-surface immune reactions |
| cells carrying specific antibody migrate in presence of specific antigen |

The possible, but not proven, biological significance of these formylated peptides lies in the fact that prokaryotes commence ribosomal synthesis of a new protein with formyl-methionine, which may later be cleaved. Since eukaryotic protein synthesis does not proceed in this way (except in mitochondria), this may provide a recognition system for distinguishing prokaryotic invaders from eukaryotic cells.

Formylated peptides bind saturably and with high affinity (Table 3.2) to the surfaces of rabbit or human neutrophils[6–10] and induce vigorous locomotor responses which are chemotactic in the true sense[11]. The most active show maximal efficacy at concentrations around $10^{-9}$ mol/l. There are definable populations of receptors for these peptides on the neutrophil surface. Binding of peptide may be followed by rapid internalization of receptors[12]. Of potential therapeutic interest is the fact that peptides with competitive antagonist activity have been described. These include CBZ-Phe-Leu[13], an antagonist with activity at fairly high concentrations ($ID_{50} = 10^{-4}$ mol/l), and Boc-Phe-Leu-Phe-Leu-Phe[14] which acts at lower concentrations ($ID_{50} = 6.8 \times 10^{-8}$ mol/l). There is also a wide range of peptides with partial agonist activity[15]. It is perhaps difficult to visualize therapeutic situations in which competitive antagonists of chemotactic factors derived from pathogenic bacteria would be useful, but, if similar antagonists can be found for chemotactic factors which attract leukocytes into auto-destructive lesions, they might be of considerable use to the clinician. This is a possibility for the future.

**Table 3.2** Affinities of chemotactic factors for neutrophils and number of cell-surface binding sites

| *Factor* | *Species* | *$K_a$ (L/M; approx.)* | *Number of binding sites* | *Reference* |
|---|---|---|---|---|
| f-Nle-Leu-Phe | rabbit | $10^9$ | $10^5$ | 6. Aswanikumar *et al.*, 1977 |
| f-Met-Leu-Phe | human | $10^8$ | $2\times10^3$ | 10. Williams *et al.*, 1977 |
| f-Nle-Leu-Phe-Nle-Tyr-Lys | human | $10^9$ | $1.2\times10^5$ | 12. Niedel *et al.* 1979 |
| C5a | human | $2\times10^8$ | $1–3\times10^5$ | 16. Chenoweth and Hugli, 1978 |
| $\alpha_s$-casein | rabbit | $2\times10^5$ | $5\times10^6$ | 24. Wilkinson and Allan, 1978 |
| Alkali-denatured HSA | rabbit | $10^6$ | $10^6$ | 24. Wilkinson and Allan, 1978 |
| Native HSA | rabbit | non-saturable low-affinity binding | | 24. Wilkinson and Allan, 1978 |

Mainly because of difficulties in preparing large enough quantities in high yield, studies of the interaction of complement-derived chemotactic factors with the cell surface have proceeded more slowly than those with the formyl peptides. Chenoweth and Hugli[16] have defined receptors on human neutrophils for C5a (Table 3.2), which are not identical with the receptors for formyl peptides and are not blocked by formyl peptides. Neither does C5a block the formyl-peptide receptors[6,10]. In the hands of Hugli and colleagues, C3a has no chemotactic activity[17]. Removal of the C-terminal arginine residue from C5a produces a peptide (C5a-desarg) which has chemotactic activity in agarose assays[18] but is poorly active in filter assays unless serum protein is added. It will be most interesting if competitive antagonists can be developed which block the receptors for complement peptides. These could have therapeutic potential in, for example, immune complex mediated inflammatory lesions with complement-dependent neutrophil infiltrations.

The singular efficacy of complement as a chemotactic system probably lies, not only in the efficacy of C5a as compared to other chemotactic factors, but even more in the fact that, in plasma-containing media, gradients of C5a are renewable at the gradient source. For example, in an assay using *Candida albicans* spores as gradient source, very accurate orientation and rapid chemotaxis and phagocytosis by surrounding neutrophils was seen[19]. Complement is continuously being activated on the surface of the spore, either by anti-*Candida* antibody or by alternative pathway activation. Without this continuous activation, the gradient would be likely to decay rapidly, leading

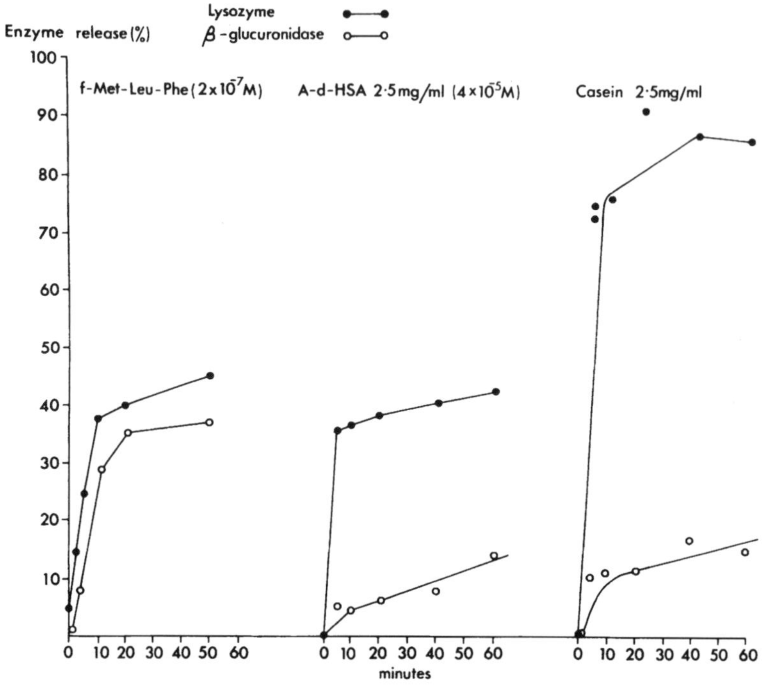


**Figure 3.1** Release of lysozyme and ß-glucuronidase from rabbit peritoneal neutrophils induced by chemotactic factors. Note that f-Met-Leu-Phe causes equal release of both, but that the proteins induce preferential release of lysozyme

to non-recognition of the micro-organisms by neutrophils after a short time, and to a smaller neutrophil accumulation at the lesion.

We have been interested for some years in the chemotactic properties of a number of proteins with exposed hydrophobic sidegroups. These include proteins such as $\alpha_s$ or β-casein[20,21], proteins with synthetic hydrophobic sidegroups conjugated to them[22], small hydrophobic peptides such as succinyl-melittin[23] and denatured proteins such as serum albumin or globin[24,25]. The biological significance of recognition of this group of molecules may lie in the requirement for clearance of denatured proteins or products of tissue damage from the body, usually under circumstances where there is no florid inflammation. Such proteins are rapidly cleared by liver macrophages when injected into the circulation[26]. Binding sites for alkali-denatured serum albumin can be demonstrated on human neutrophils[24], although the binding is of lower affinity than that of C5a or formyl peptides (Table 3.2). Good orientation of human neutrophils towards alkali-denatured serum albumin or to α- and β-casein can be demonstrated in orientation chambers (unpublished observations). Serum albumin in its native state shows low affinity binding to neutrophil surfaces and is not chemotactic. It does, however, have good chemokinetic activity, probably because it coats surfaces on which neutrophils move and provides a surface that is optimal for cell adhesion[27,28]. The role of the substratum in leukocyte movement is discussed in more detail below.

Another group of chemoattractant molecules of current interest comprises lipids such as the hydroxyeicosatetraenoic acids (HETE) which are produced by the action of lipoxygenases on arachidonic acid. The chemoattractant activity of these was first described by Turner *et al.*[29] and they provide a series of molecules known to be produced in inflammation which could have potential pathological importance, although this remains to be shown. The position of the hydroxyl group on the fatty acid molecule is of importance, since Goetzl *et al.*[30] have shown that the order of chemoattractant activity for neutrophils is 5-hydroxy > 8,9-> 11,12-hydroxy. Recent work suggesting an important role for lypoxygenase-generated products of arachidonic acid in chemotactic transduction is discussed below. See also new work on leukotriene B (Ford-Hutchinson *et al.*, this volume).

## CHEMOTACTIC FACTORS AS ACTIVATORS OF OTHER CELL FUNCTIONS

It is now well established that contact of chemotactic factors with the neutrophil surface activates not only directional locomotion but a variety of other events (Table 3.3). Formyl peptides and C5a have been shown to act as metabolic activators judged by superoxide production, increase in chemoluminescence and hexose monophosphate shunt activity[31-35] although HETE

**Table 3.3** Activation of neutrophil functions by chemotactic factors

| *Function activated* | *Formyl peptides* | *C5a* | *Casein and denatured proteins* | *HETE* | *Arachidonic acid* |
|---|---|---|---|---|---|
| Chemotaxis | + | + | + | + | NT |
| Enzyme release | | | | | |
| β-glucuronidase | + | + | weak | no | + |
| lysozyme | + | + | + | NT | + |
| proteases | + | | + | NT | NT |
| HMP shunt activation | + | + | no | no | NT |
| Superoxide production | + | NT | NT | no | NT |
| $H_2O_2$ production | + | NT | NT | no | NT |
| Transient aggregation | + | + | NT | NT | + |

NT = not tested

apparently does not stimulate metabolic activity[30] and casein apparently has little effect in increasing hexose monophosphate shunt activity[36]. Another important effect of chemotactic factors is to induce release of hydrolytic enzymes into the medium by exocytosis of specific or azurophil granules.

Both formyl peptides and C5a induce rapid release (within 5 min) of lysozyme and of β-glucuronidase[5,37] but the cells need to be treated with cytochalasin B for these peptides to induce enzyme release. Neutrophils on surfaces coated with immunoglobulin release enzymes without a requirement for cytochalasin B, as was shown by Henson[38].

Miss G. Bradley and I have recently studied enzyme release induced by protein chemotactic factors. These induce rapid release of lysozyme and slow release of β-glucuronidase (Figure 3.1) and a cytochalasin-independent release of proteases is induced by $\alpha_s$ and β-caseins and by alkali-denatured serum albumin (unpublished observations), Venge[39] reported casein-induced release of chymotrypsin-like cationic proteases by human neutrophils. In our recent, unpublished, observations we have shown that these released proteases can digest chemotactic proteins such as casein and denatured albumin. Thus movement of neutrophils on surfaces coated with these proteins may be facilitated by proteolytic cleavage of adhesion sites, although we do not have evidence for such a mechanism as yet.

**Signal transduction**

There are interesting new findings on events that follow immediately upon binding of formylated peptides to the surfaces of neutrophils and that may be important for signal transduction. One of the first of these events is release of arachidonic acid from the cells, possibly by the action of a cellular phospholipase A[40]. The increase in phospholipid degradation is associated with a decreased incorporation of [$^3$H]methyl groups into membrane lipids. Addition of exogenous arachidonic acid to neutrophils causes a specific increase in membrane permeability to calcium[41]. It is possible that lipoxygenase-activated products play a role in transduction. An inhibitor of lipoxygenase-generated metabolic pathways, nordihydroguaiaretic acid (NDGA) inhibited the increase in calcium permeability induced by arachidonate[41], also that induced by f-Met-Leu-Phe in rabbit neutrophils. Thus arachidonate released from neutrophils on contact with chemotactic factors may be activated by lipoxygenases, thus inducing changes in membrane ion permeability necessary for transduction.

Ion fluxes are now believed to play an important role in chemotactic signal transduction. F-Met-Leu-Phe induces an immediate influx of $Na^+$ into neutrophils, followed by a delayed $Na^+$ efflux and $K^+$ influx[43], the latter probably being dependent on $Na^+K^+$ATPase pumping activity[44]. F-Met-Leu-Phe also induces fluxes of $Ca^{2+}$ whose direction depends on the extracellular $Ca^{2+}$ concentration[43–47], and functions such as locomotion and exocytosis are probably dependent on these fluxes. Calcium bound to the inner surface of the neutrophil plasma membrane is released on addition of f-Met-Leu-Phe[48] and may thus be made available in the cytoplasm for use in calcium-dependent contractile events. In macrophages, electrophysiological changes can be detected on addition of f-Met-Leu-Phe[49] in the form of a small brief depolarization followed by a more prolonged and deeper hyperpolarization. The role of cyclic nucleotides in chemotactic signal transduction is still unclear. It has now been reported by several groups that addition of chemotactic factor induces a brief (1 min) rise, followed by a fall, in intracellular cyclic AMP levels[50–52] and there are reports of a more sustained rise in cyclic GMP levels[50,53], however, there is no clear evidence about how this relates to the chemotactic response. Several groups have suggested that drugs which raise intracellular cyclic GMP levels also enhance locomotion of neutrophils or monocytes to attractants[54–56]. Among these drugs is levamisole, which can reverse chemotactic deactivation *in vitro*[15], and, more interestingly, has been shown to reverse the depression in locomotion of human neutrophils and monocytes induced by a variety of viruses including herpes simplex[57] both if the neutrophils were treated with levamisole *in vitro*, and in a proportion of patients treated with the drug *in vivo*. Levamisole was also found to reverse the chemotactic defect in children with hyperimmunoglobulin E syndrome[58].

## CHEMOTAXIS AND ADHESION TO SUBSTRATA

We turn now from these biochemical events to consideration of locomotion and chemotaxis as phenomena that take place on a surface: the cell crawling towards its goal along a substratum. This is important because, however active the chemotactic factor and however sophisticated the cellular sensory apparatus, the capacity of the cell to move at all and the speed at which it will move will depend on the substratum onto which it is placed. Cell movement requires a balance between attachment and detachment. If either predominates, poor movement will result. Most proteins bind well to glass, tissue culture plastic or the cellulose esters of which micropore filters used in chemotaxis assays are made. However, peptides bind poorly or in a way that does not promote cell locomotion[24]. Cells on protein-free surfaces show almost no locomotor response to formylated peptides or to C5a[59]. If serum albumin is added to the medium, a chemotactic response to these peptides is seen[60] and, indeed, serum albumin on its own induces chemokinetic, but not chemotactic, locomotion[27,28].

This is due to substratum-bound albumin as can readily be shown by coating a substratum with albumin, then washing it free of all fluid-phase protein. Under these conditions, leukocytes will not only locomote chemokinetically on the surface, but will respond chemotactically to peptide chemotactic factors added to the fluid phase[60]. Dierich *et al.*[61] showed that neutrophils moving into filters towards casein would move as far on a casein-coated filter as when the casein was diffusing from a fluid-phase source from below the filter. Wilkinson and Allan[60] set up gradients of protein chemotactic factors across filters, then carefully washed the filters so that the only gradient remaining was of protein attached to the filter. Under these conditions, human neutrophils showed chemotactic responses as judged by checkerboard assays.

We have recently tried to repeat this using a visual assay. A gradient of casein was set up across an orientation chamber as described by Zigmond[11] and the coverslip was then carefully washed free of fluid-phase protein. Human neutrophils were then allowed to adhere to the coverslip and their locomotion was filmed. Table 3.4 shows that, on the side of the coverslip nearest to the casein source, neutrophils showed a net flux towards the source. On the side of the coverslip furthest from the source, no net flux was observed. Presumably the diffusion of this high molecular-weight attractant had not advanced sufficiently far for the gradient to influence the cells on this part of the coverslip. Thus there is now evidence from both filter and visual assays that neutrophils can respond to substratum-bound gradients of proteins.

This is reminiscent of the observations of Carter[62,63] on haptotaxis; the locomotion of fibroblasts from points of low adhesiveness on the substratum to points of high adhesiveness. However, it seems unlikely that leukocyte chemotaxis is a special case of haptotaxis as defined by Carter[63]. Keller *et al.*[52] showed that cells moving up a gradient towards a complement-derived peptide did not change their adhesiveness and Smith *et al.*[64] showed a reduc-

**Table 3.4** Analysis of displacement of human neutrophils in a substratum-bound gradient of casein on a glass coverslip

| | *Number of cells analysed* | *Mean time during which cells were observed* (s) | *Mean displacement towards gradient source* (μm/min) | *Mean square displacement towards* (μm² m⁻¹) |
|---|---|---|---|---|
| Cells in sector within μm of gradient source | 25 | 328 | +5.3 | +55.8 |
| Cells in sector further than μm of gradient source | 29 | 394 | +0.3 | −8.1 |

Casein (1 mg/ml, Merck) was allowed to diffuse from one trough across the bridge of a Zigmond orientation chamber for 15 min. The fluid-phase casein was then carefully washed away and the coverslip was removed. Human blood neutrophils ($2 \times 10^6$/ml) were then allowed to adhere to the casein-coated coverslip and their subsequent locomotion was filmed in a chamber containing Hanks-HEPES buffer + HSA (1 mg/ml) using time-lapse cinematography. The tracks taken by the cells were traced and the mean displacement in an axis perpendicular to the gradient source was calculated for the whole population studied. The mean square displacement was also calculated. Note positive displacement of cells near the gradient source, and the lack of net displacement of cells further away.

tion in adhesiveness of rabbit neutrophils in optimal concentrations of $\alpha_s$- and β-caseins, denatured serum albumin and formylated peptides, which is the opposite of what the haptotactic mechanism would suggest.

## CONCLUSIONS

In summary, developments during the past few years have included the first reports defining the binding sites for chemotactic factors. These sites have only been studied by measuring the binding of chemotactic factors to the surfaces of neutrophils and have not yet been isolated as molecular species. There is considerable interest in calcium as a messenger and possibly as a controlling ion for microfilament function, but we do not yet have any knowledge of how transduction processes are linked to the microfilament system. Leukocyte locomotion is crucially dependent on adhesion to substrata and the nature of this adhesion determines the capacity of the cell to show chemokinetic and chemotactic responses to signals from its environment.

## References


1 Leber, T. (1888). Uber die Entstehung der Entzündung und die Wirkung der entzundungerregenden Schädlichkeiten. *Fortschr. Med.* **4,** 460

2 Keller, H. U., Wilkinson, P. C., Abercrombie, M., Becker, E. L., Hirsch, J. G., Miller, M. E., Ramsey, W. S., and Zigmond, S. H. (1977). A proposal for the definition of terms related to locomotion of leucocytes and other cells. *Clin. Exp. Immunol.,* **27,** 377

3 Stossel, T. P. (1978). The mechanism of leukocyte locomotion. In Gallin, J. I. and Quie, P. G. (eds.) *Leukocyte Chemotaxis*, p. 143. (New York: Raven Press)

4 Schiffmann, E., Corcoran, B. A. and Wahl, S. A. (1975). N-formyl methionyl peptides as chemoattractants for leukocytes. *Proc. Nat. Acad. Sci. (USA),* **72,** 1059

5 Showell, H. J., Freer, R. J., Zigmond, S. H., Schiffmann, E., Aswanikumar, S., Corcoran, B. and Becker, E. L. (1976). The structure-activity relations of synthetic peptides as chemotactic factors and inducers of lysosomal enzyme secretion for neutrophils. *J. Exp. Med.,* **143,** 1154

6 Aswanikumar, S., Corcoran, B., Schiffmann, E., Day, A. R., Freer, R. J., Showell, H. J., Becker, E. L. and Pert, C. B. (1977). Demonstration of a receptor on rabbit neutrophils for chemotactic peptides. *Biochem. Biophys. Res. Commun.*, **74,** 810

7 Niedel, J., Wilkinson, S. and Cuatrecasas, P. (1979). Receptor-induced uptake and degradation of$^{125}$I-chemotactic peptides by human neutrophils. *J. Biol. Chem.*, **254,** 10700

8 Unpublished observations (1980)

9 Sha'afi, R. I., Williams, K., Wacholtz, M. C. and Becker, E. L. (1978). Binding of the chemotactic synthetic peptide [$^{3}$H]formyl-nor-leu-leu-phe to plasma membrane of rabbit neutrophils. *FEBS Lett.* **91,** 305

10 Williams, L. T., Synderman, R., Pike, M. C., and Lefkowitz, R. J. (1977). Specific receptor sites for chemotactic peptides on human polymorphonuclear leukocytes. *Proc. Natl. Acad. Sci (USA).*, **74,** 1204

11 Zigmond, S. H. (1977). Ability of polymorphonuclear leukocytes to orient in gradients of chemotactic factors. *J. Cell Biol.*, **75,** 606

12 Niedel, J. E., Kahane, I, and Cuatrecasas. P. (1979). Receptor-mediated internalization of fluorescent chemotactic peptide by human neutrophils. *Science,* **205,** 1412

13 O'Flaherty, J. T., Showell, H. J., Kreutzer, D. L., Ward, P. A. and Becker, E. L. (1978). Inhibition of *in vivo* and *in vitro* neutrophil responses to chemotactic factors by a competitive antagonist. *J. Immunol.*, **120,** 1326

14 Aswanikumar, S., Schiffmann, E., Corcoran, B. A., Pert, C. B., Morell, J. L. and Gross, E. (1978). Antibiotics with agonist and antagonist chemotactic activity. *Biochem. Biophys. Res. Commun.*, **80,** 464

15 Wilkinson, P. C. (1979). Synthetic peptide chemotactic factors for neutrophils: the range of active peptides, their efficacy and inhibitory activity, and susceptibility of the cellular response to enzymes and bacterial toxins. *Immunology*, **36,** 579

16 Chenoweth, D. E. and Hugli, T. E. (1978). Demonstration of specific C5a receptor on intact human polymorphonuclear leukocytes. *Proc. Nat. Acad. Sci. (USA).*, **75,** 3943

17 Fernandez, H. N., Henson, P. M., Otani, A. and Hugli, T. E. (1978). Chemotactic response to human C3a and C5a anaphylatoxins. I. Evaluation of C3a and C5a leukotaxis *in vitro* and under simulated *in vivo* conditions. *J. Immunol.*, **120,** 102

18 Chenoweth, D. E., Rowe, J. G. and Hugli, T. E. (1979). A modified method for chemotaxis under agarose. *J. Immunol. Meth.*, **25**, 337

19 Allan, R. B. and Wilkinson, P. C. (1978). A visual analysis of chemotactic and chemokinetic locomotion of human neutrophil leucocytes. *Exp. Cell Res.*, **111**, 191

20 Wilkinson, P. C. (1972). Characterization of the chemotactic activity of casein for neutrophil leucocytes and macrophages. *Experientia*, **28**, 105

21 Wilkinson, P. C. (1974). Surface and cell membrane activities of leukocyte chemotactic factors. *Nature (London)*, **251**, 58

22 Wilkinson, P. C. and McKay, I. C. (1972). The molecular requirements for chemotactic attraction of leucocytes by proteins. Studies of proteins with synthetic side groups. *Eur. J. Immunol.*, **2**, 570

23 Wilkinson, P. C. (1977). Succinyl bee venom melittin is a leukocyte chemotactic factor. *Nature (London)*, **267**, 713

24 Wilkinson, P. C. and Allan, R. B. (1978). Binding of protein chemotactic factors to the surfaces of neutrophil leukocytes and its modification with lipid-specific bacterial toxins. *Mol. Cell Biochem.*, **20**, 25

25 Wilkinson, P. C. (1973). Recognition of protein structure in leukocyte chemotaxis. *Nature (London)*, **244**, 512

26 Thorbecke, G. J., Maurer, P. H., and Benecerraf, B. (1960). The affinity of the reticulo-endothelial system for various modified serum proteins. *Br. J. Exp. Pathol.*, **41**, 190

27 Wilkinson, P. C. and Allan, R. B. (1978). Assay systems for measuring leukocyte locomotion: an overview. In Gallin, J. I. and Quie, P. G. (eds.) *Leukocyte Chemotaxis*, p. 1. (New York: Raven Press)

28 Keller, H. U., Wissler, J. H., Hess, M. W. and Cottier, H. (1978). Distinct chemokinetic and chemotactic responses in neutrophil granulocytes. *Eur. J. Immunol.*, **8**, 1

29 Turner, S. R., Tainer, J. A. and Lynn, W. S. (1975). Biogenesis of chemotactic molecules by the arachidonate lipoxygenase system of platelets. *Nature (London)*, **257**, 680

30 Goetzl, E. J., Brash, A. R., Tauber, A. I., Oates, J. A. and Hubbard, W. C. (1980). Modulation of human neutrophil function by mono-hydroxy-eicosatetraenoic acids. *Immunology* (In press)

31 Goetzl, E. J. and Austen, K. F. (1974). Stimulation of human neutrophil leukocyte aerobic glucose metabolism by purified chemotactic factors. *J. clin. Invest.*, **53**, 591

32 Hatch, G. E., Gardner, D. E. and Menzel, D. B. (1978). Chemiluminescence of phagocytic cells caused by *N*-formylmethionyl peptides. *J. Exp. Med.*, **147**, 182

33 Lehmeyer, J. E., Snyderman, R. and Johnston, R. B. (1979). Stimulation of neutrophil oxidative metabolism by chemotactic peptides: influence of calcium ion concentration and cytochalasin B and comparison with stimulation by phorbol myristate acetate. *Blood*, **54**, 35

34 Simchowitz, L. and Spilberg, I. (1979). Generation of superoxide radicals by human peripheral neutrophils activated by chemotactic factor. Evidence for the role of calcium. *J. Lab. Clin. Med.*, **93**, 583

35 Becker, E. L., Sigman, M. and Oliver, J. M. (1979). Superoxide production induced in rabbit polymorphonuclear leukocytes by synthetic chemotactic peptides and A23187. *Am J. Pathol.*, **95**, 81

36 Anderson, R., Glover, A., and Rabson, A. R. (1978). The effect of chemotactic factors and agents which influence neutrophil movement in anaerobic glycolysis and hexose monophosphate shunt activity. *Immunology*, **35**, 141

37 Goldstein, I., Hoffstein, S., Gallin, J. and Weissmann, G. (1973). Mechanisms of lysosomal enzyme release from human leukocytes. Microtubule assembly and membrane fusion induced by a component of complement. *Proc. Natl. Acad. Sci (USA).*, **70**, 2916

38 Henson, P. M. (1971). The immunologic release of constituents from neutrophil leukocytes. I. The role of antibody and complement on non phagocytosable surfaces or phagocytosable particles. *J. Immunol.*, **107**, 1535

39 Venge, P. (1979). Kinetic studies of cell migration in a modified Boyden chamber: dependence on cell concentration and effects of the chymotrypsin-like cationic protein of human granulocytes. *J. Immunol.*, **122**, 1180

40 Hirata, F., Corcoran, B. A., Venkatasubramanian, K., Schiffmann, E. and Axelrod, J. (1979). Chemoattractants stimulate degradation of methylated phospholipids and release of arachidonic acid in rabbit leukocytes. *Proc. Nat. Acad. Sci. (USA).*, **76**, 2640

41 Volpi, M., Naccache, P. H. and Sha'afi, R. I. (1980). Arachidonate metabolites increase the permeability of the plasma membrane of neutrophils to calcium. *Biochem. Biphys. Res. Commun.* (In press)

42 Naccache, P. H., Showell, H. J., Becker, E. L. and Sha'afi, R. I. (1979). Pharmacological differentiation between the chemotactic factor induced intracellular calcium redistribution and transmembrane calcium influx in rabbit neutrophils. *Biochem. Biphys. Res. Commun.*, **89**, 1224

43 Naccache, P., Freer, R. J., Showell, J. H., Becker, E. L. and Sha'afi, R. I. (1977). Transport of sodium, potassium and calcium across rabbit polymorphonuclear leukocyte membranes: effect of chemotactic factor. *J. Cell Biol.*, **73**, 428

44 Becker, E. L., Talley, J. V., Showell, H. J., Naccache, P. H. and Sha'afi, R. I. (1978). Activation of the rabbit polymorphonuclear leukocyte membrane $Na^+K^+$-ATPase by chemotactic factor. *J. Cell Biol.*, **77**, 329

45 Gallin, J. I. and Rosenthal, A. S. (1974). The regulatory role of divalent cations in human granulocyte chemotaxis: evidence for an association between calcium exchanges and microtubule assembly. *J. Cell Biol.*, **62**, 594

46 Boucek, M. M. and Snyderman, R. (1976). Calcium influx requirement for human neutrophil chemotaxis: inhibition by lanthanum chloride. *Science*, **193**, 905

47 Petroski, R. J., Naccache, P. H., Becker, E. L. and Sha'afi, R. I. (1979). Effect of chemotactic factors on calcium levels of rabbit neutrophils. *Am. J. Physiol.*, **237**, C43

48 Naccache, P. H., Volpi, M., Showell, H. J., Becker, E. L. and Sha-afi, R. I. (1979). Chemotactic factor-induced release of membrane calcium in rabbit neutrophils. *Science*, **203**, 461

49 Gallin, E. K. and Gallin, J. I. (1977). Interaction of chemotactic factors with human macrophages. Induction of transmembrane potential changes. *J. Cell Biol.*, **75**, 277

50 Anderson, R., Glover, A., Koornhof, H. J. and Rabsen, A. R. (1976). *In vitro* stimulation of neutrophil motility by levamisole: Maintenance of cGMP levels in chemotactically stimulated levamisole-treated neutrophils. *J. Immunol.*, **117**, 428

51 Jackowski, S. and Sha'afi, R. I. (1979). Response of adenosine cyclic 3',5'-monophosphate level in rabbit neutrophils to the chemotactic peptide formyl-methionyl-leucyl-phenylalanine. *Mol. Pharmacol.* **16**, 473

52 Keller, H. U., Wissler, J. H. and Ploem, J. (1979). Chemotaxis is not a special case of haptotaxis. *Experientia*, **35**, 1669

53 Hatch, G. E., Nichols, W. K. and Hill, H. R. (1977). Cyclic nucleotide changes in human neutrophils induced by chemoattractants and chemotactic modulators. *J. Immunol.*, **119**, 450

54 Estensen, R. D., Hill, H. R., Quie, P. G. and Hogan, H. D. (1977). Cyclic GMP and cell movement. *Nature (London)*, **245**, 458

55 Sandeler, J. A., Gallin, J. I. and Vaughan, M. (1975). Effects of serotonin, carbamylcholine and ascorbic acid on leukocyte cGMP and chemotaxis. *J. Cell Biol.*, **67**, 480

56 Gallin, J. I., Sandeler, J. A., Clyman, R. I., Mangamiello, V. C. and Vaughan, M. (1978). Agents that increase cyclic AMP inhibit accumulation of cGMP and depress human monocyte locomotion. *J. Immunol.*, **120**, 492

57 Rabson, A. R., Whiting, D. A., Anderson, R., Glover, A. and Koornhof, H. J. (1977). Depressed neutrophil motility in patients with recurrent herpes simplex virus infections. *In vitro* restoration with levamisole. *J. Infect. Dis.*, **135**, 113

58 Wright, D. G., Kirkpatrick, C. H. and Gallin, J. I. (1977). Effects of levamisole on normal and abnormal leukocyte locomotion. *J. Clin. Invest.*, **59**, 941

59 Wilkinson, P. C. (1976). A requirement for albumin as carrier for low molecular weight leucocyte chemotactic factors. *Exp. Cell Res.*, **103**, 415

60 Wilkinson, P. C. and Allan, R. B. (1978). Chemotaxis of neutrophil leukocytes towards substratum-bound protein attractants. *Exp. Cell Res.*, **117**, 403

61 Derich, M. P., Wilhelm, D. and Till, G. (1977). Essential role of surface bound chemoattractant in leukocyte migration. *Nature (London)*, **270**, 351

62 Carter, S. B. (1965). Principles of cell motility: the direction of cell movement and cancer invasion. *Nature (London)*, **208**, 1183

63 Carter, S. B. (1967). Haptotaxis and the mechanism of cell motility. *Nature (London)*, **213**, 256

64 Smith, R. P. C., Lackie, J. M. and Wilkinson, P. C. (1979). The effects of chemotactic factors on the adhesiveness of rabbit neutrophil granulocytes. *Exp. Cell Red.*, **122**, 169

# Discussion

**Dr A. W. Ford-Hutchinson: (UK)** said that their recent results might help to explain the apparent discrepancies between the effects of HETE and arachadonic acid. They had examined polymorphonuclear leukocytes (PMN) treated with calcium ionophore and found that the major biologically active lipoxygenase product was, in fact, leukotriene B or 5,12-dihydroxyeicosatetranoic acid, which was a very potent chemokinetic and aggregatory substance for PMNs, active down to doses as low as 10 pg/ml. It also caused neutrophil degranulation. As yet they had not examined whether it was a chemotactic agent.

**Dr P. Davies (USA)** asked what was the relative concentration of stimuli such as C5a or f-Met-Leu-Phe required to stimulate movement compared to that required to release enzymes or stimulate superoxide production. He also wondered in the experiments with PMN releasing enzymes whether Dr Wilkinson had used cytochalasin B.

**Dr Wilkinson** said that the concentrations of formyl peptides required for stimulation depended upon the assay. In a locomotion assay the concentration was $10^{-9}$mol/l; in an orientation assay it was $10^{-8}$ but the amount required for enzyme release was considerably greater. This was also true with the protein chemotactic factors, although there the difference did not seem to be so great and one needed only ten-fold higher concentrations of protein to obtain optimal protease release rather than to obtain chemotaxis. One interesting feature of cytochalasin B is that this molecule was required to obtain protease release with the low molecular-weight chemotactic factor but it was not required for release of those proteins that bound to surfaces. It was not clear what actions cytochalasin B had. If a cell were on a suitable surface it would secrete quite readily without cytochalasin B having to be added.

# 4

# Future trends in free radical studies

W. HUBER (USA)

Free radical mediated events *in vivo*, particularly as related to inflammation, have been and are likely to remain for the foreseeable future intimately wedded to the active species derived from molecular oxygen, or, as it is more properly called, dioxygen. Since the discovery of the superoxide dismutating activity of metalloprotein enzymes (SOD) having copper, manganese or iron at their active site, and that of the selenium containing glutathione peroxidase, these ubiquitously occurring endogenous enzymes and the active species they regulate have been the subject of a veritable landslide of investigations[1–5]. To properly assess *future trends* at this juncture, I think it is important to have a brief look first at 'what is what' in our present knowledge of this Janus-faced role of oxygen centred free radicals in tissue.

The appearance of blue-green algae on earth was a dramatic event, in that these organisms were the first capable of true photosynthesis. They could use water as a source of reducing power and liberate free oxygen into the environment, making the rise of the enormous variety of aerobic creatures in the biosphere possible. It is ironic that in evolution a molecule that became the staff of life for so many would also be toxic for them.

Ground state oxygen contains two unpaired electrons and therefore is spin restricted. As a consequence, it will follow univalent pathways of reduction whenever energetically possible, leading to the superoxide anion ($O_2^-$), as inversion of electronic spin states is a relatively slow process in comparison to the lifetime of collision complexes.

The benefits of energy yield and participation in biosynthetic reactions and the detriment of toxicity both stem from oxygen's propensity for stepwise reductions. Suitable biological control mechanisms have evolved to keep the steady-state concentrations of $O_2^-$ and $H_2O_2$ vanishingly small under normal conditions by the use *in vivo* of scavengers of $O_2^-$, $H_2O_2$, OH• and $^1O_2$ (Table

4.1). The play thus involves two main sets of characters, the oxygen free radicals and related active species, and the scavengers which keep things under control during the multitude of actions and interactions being performed intra- and extracellularly during the metabolic journey from molecular oxygen to water.

**Table 4.1** Representative scavengers* for $H_2O_2$, $O_2^-$, $OH\bullet$, $^1O_2$

| Hydrogen Peroxide | Superoxide ion | |
|---|---|---|
| catalase | Superoxide dismutases (SOD) | |
| glutathione peroxidase | $Cu^{2+}$ $Zn^{2+}$ SOD | |
| Other peroxidases | $Mn^{2+}$ SOD | |
| | $Fe^{3+}$ SOD | |
| | tyrosamine | |
| | tiron (dihydroxybenzene-disulfoniacid) | |
| **Hydroxyl Radical** | **Singlet oxygen** | |
| butanol, ethanol | β-Carotene | compounds that react rapidly |
| mannitol | histidine | with $^1O_2$ are not specific for |
| benzoate | cholesterol | it and those that are specific |
| dimethyloxyethane | bilirubin | for it do not react rapidly |
| | 2,5-dimethylfurane | (Foote, 1977) |
| | diazabicylo-octane | |

*Scavengers may themselves be converted into free radicals, which may exhibit their own toxicity in biological systems

It is less than 60 years since the first attempts were made to relate oxygen toxicity to the accumulation of its reduction product $H_2O_2$. In 1931 Haber and Willstätter[6] were the first to postulate $O_2^-$ and its complementary acid, hydroperoxyl radical $HP_2^{\cdot}$ as short-lived transients during radiolysis of oxygenated solutions. Similarities between the lethality of oxygen and of ionizing radiation led Gerschman *et al.*[7] to the proposal that the basic course of oxygen toxicity was due to the uncontrolled reactions of free radicals. Pulse radiolysis experiments in frozen solutions by Czapski[8] and his co-workers established the existence of $O_2^-$ and $HP_2^{\cdot}$ and the dependence of their decay pattern on pH. The possible involvement of $O_2^-$ in biological reactions was first proposed by Fridovich and Handler[9] to explain reactions of xanthine oxidase-xanthine on aerobic sulphite auto-oxidation. By now a large body of work has clearly established that the univalent reduction of molecular oxygen to $O_2^-$ is a commonplace event in biological oxidation[1]. Enzymes, enzymatic co-factors, cell organelles and phagocytozing cells all form or participate in the formation of $O_2^-$. The enzymes associated with the generation of $O_2^-$ are oxidoreductases and a representative selection is presented in Table 4.2. The amount of $O_2^-$ formed during the consumption of oxygen seems to depend upon how intact the subcellular structures are and has been shown to range from 17% (*S. faecalis* extracts) to <1% (submitochondrial particles).

$O_2^-$ represents the conjugate base of the weak acid $HO_2^{\cdot}$ or hydroperoxyl radical with a p$k_a$ of 4.8. The solvation of $O_2^-$ in water is very strong and its heat of solution is near – 100 kcal/mol. Even in the gas phase it binds up to 3 mole-

**Table 4.2** Representative biological systems involved in generation of detectable superoxide ion in presence of oxygen

| Cells | Oxidoreductases |
|---|---|
| PMNs | xanthine oxidase |
| macrophages | aldehyde oxidase |
| monocytes | galactose oxidase |
| | amine oxidase |
| Organelles | dihydro-orate oxidase |
| mitochondria, SMPs | tryptophan-2, 3-dioxygenase |
| microsomes | flavoprotein-dehydrogenases |
| nuclei | ferredoxin-NADPH reductase |
| | rubredoxin-NADPH reductase |
| Other proteins | cytochrome-NADPH reductase |
| cytochrome P-450 | |
| iron-sulphur proteins | |
| haemoglobin | |
| Classes of organic compounds | |
| quinones, polyphenols, flavins, thiols, methional | |

**Table 4.3** Some reactions of superoxide ion of potential biological importance

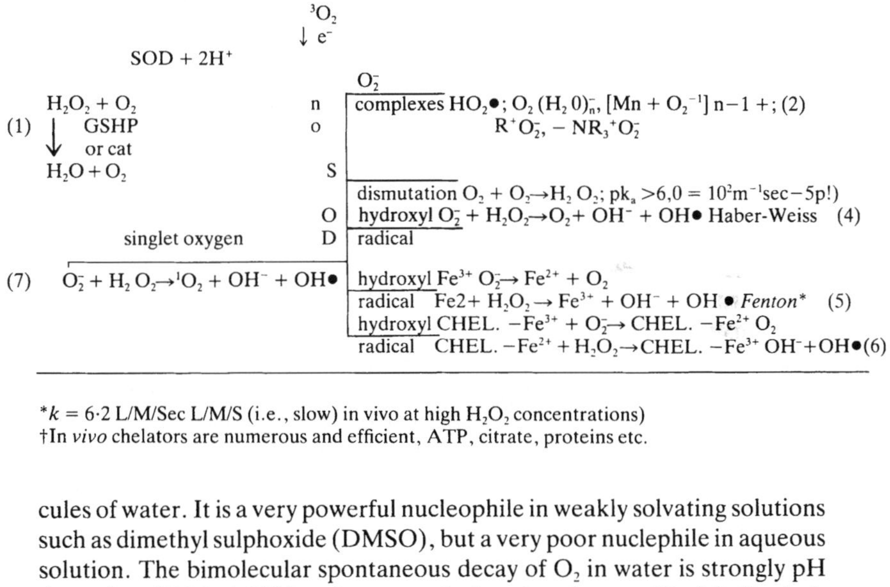


*$k$ = 6·2 L/M/Sec L/M/S (i.e., slow) in vivo at high $H_2O_2$ concentrations)
†In *vivo* chelators are numerous and efficient, ATP, citrate, proteins etc.

cules of water. It is a very powerful nucleophile in weakly solvating solutions such as dimethyl sulphoxide (DMSO), but a very poor nuclephile in aqueous solution. The bimolecular spontaneous decay of $O_2$ in water is strongly pH dependent (Table 4.3(3)) and comparatively rather slow at pH>6.0. Catalasis of this dismutation by Cu–Zn SOD, in contrast, is not pH dependent above the p*k* value of $O_2^-$ i.e. pH 4.8. The interaction of $O^{1}{}_2^-$ with the $H_2O_2$ formed by its spontaneous dismutation has potentially very damaging biological consequences, as one of the reaction products is the hydroxyl radical ($OH^{\cdot}$), which is one of the most potent oxidants known. This so-called Haber–Weiss reaction

(Table 4.3(4)) has recently been shown to be thermodynamically possible, although slow, compared with competing reactions such as the disappearance of OH by reactions with $H_2O_2$ Catalysis by redoxactive metal ions in form of organic chelates appears more likely *in vivo* (Table 4.3(6)), although a Fenton-type reaction, i.e. the generation of powerful oxidizing species from the reduction of peroxide by metal ions, remains a possibility when relatively high concentrations of $H_2O_2$ are available (Table 4.3(5)). Finally, another potent oxidizing species, singlet oxygen, may be formed as a sequel of $O_2^-$ reactions (Table 4.3(7))

As the available evidence clearly demonstrates that oxygen-derived active species, if unchecked, can present a grave danger for the integrity of the molecular fabric of life, evolution, not surprisingly, had provided suitable defences for respiring cells. The keystone of these defences is provided by three specific types of enzymes: catalases, peroxidases and superoxide dismutases, which scavenge, respectively, $H_2O_2$ and $O_2^-$. In man, a selenium enzyme, glutathione peroxidase, discovered by Mills in 1957[10], and catalase, are the two principal converters of hydroxperoxides and functionally appear to exert their effects in separate compartments, with catalase occurring mostly in the peroxisomes[11]. Both enzymes occur in most human cells and are very effective, so that the steady state level of $H_2O_2$ is probably very low. In contrast, their serum concentration, as well as that of the SOD's, is negligible, a factor of importance in superoxide pathology.

It is an oddity of protein biochemistry that the cuprein, Cu–Zn metalloproteins, first described by Mann and Keilin in 1939[12], remained molecules in search of functions for nearly 30 years. Then they were assigned, in short order, not one but two important properties. We discovered in 1965 their potent anti-inflammatory efficacy upon parenteral administration[13] and McCord and Fridovich in 1969 discovered their superoxide dismutase activity[14].

Superoxide dismutases (SOD) are based on copper and zinc or on manganese or iron. They seem to occur in all respiring organisms, with the copper–zinc enzyme characteristically found only in the cytosol of eukaryotic cells. The manganese and iron enzymes occur mostly in bacteria and are closely homologous in amino acid sequence, but are quite different as proteins from the copper–zinc enzyme, with which they share only the superoxide dismutating function[15]. The manganese enzyme is also found in mammals where it occurs within the mitochondrial matrix and in certain species (man, baboon) also in the cytosol of liver cells[16]. The combination of SOD's and peroxidases thus represents a first line of defence against endogenous oxygen toxicity by controlling $O_2^-$ and $H_2O_2$ levels in an attempt to eliminate the toxic hazards inherent in the formation of hydrogen radicals and singlet oxygen.

One significant result of the work with SODs is the recognition that $O_2^-$ and inflammation appear to be intimately related. This is based on two major bodies of information: (1) that SOD is an anti-inflammatory agent, a fact well established by now through double-blind controlled trials in man and animals[17], and (2) that phagocytozing cells liberate superoxide radical[18]. The polymorphonuclear leukocytes (neutrophilic granulocytes) and the monocytes in the blood are able to leave the circulation and sense their way to a site of inflammation where they can accumulate in large numbers. Each of these cell types can ingest foreign material, generate microbicidal products and release presynthesized hydrolytic enzymes (and other antimicrobial proteins) into the vicinity of the ingested pathogens.

In neutrophils, the hexose-monophosphate shunt is the NADPH delivery system for the oxidase and for the glutathione redox system, and the shunt activity is stimulated manyfold during phagocytosis[19]. Conversion of $O_2^-$ to $H_2O_2$ in these systems is probably brought about after the enzyme system located in the plasma membrane reduces $O_2$ to $O_2^-$, which then may react with the protons to form form $H_2O_2$ without any enzyme.

The $V_{max}$ of 9.72 nmol of $O_2$/min/$10^7$ cells is sufficient to account for the net oxygen uptake observed during PMN phagocytosis of a wide variety of particles[20]. The stoichiometry of NADPH oxidation and $O_2^-$ production indicated two pathways of electron release from the enzyme: a univalent pathway resulting in $O_2^-$ generation, and a divalent pathway leading directly to $H_2O_2$ formation. The combination of the two, perhaps with derived $OH^\cdot$ and $^1O_2$, together with the cellular myeloperoxidase seems to represent the microbicidal system of these cells[21].

This essential body defence, unfortunately, has ill consequences too. Phagocytozing cells generate $O_2^-$ randomly over their surface, driven by subsurface enzyme system(s) based on NADPH[22], even though the immediate need for $O_2^-$ is in the phagocytozing vacuoles only. Thus, $O_2^-$ and $H_2O_2$ can destroy their generating cells[23] and also damage membranes of adjacent cells and fibres, an event that has a singularly damaging potential because SODs and peroxidases are virtually absent from extracellular fluids[24,25]. Consider the following scenario: local trauma or infection results in inflammation and in the release of substances which attract phagocytes. These leukocytes migrate to the site, become activated and proceed to generate $O_2^-$ and $H_2O_2$, damaging their membranes and those of adjacent cells in the process with the release of lysosomal inflammants, causing further inflammation, followed by further influx of phagocytes and release of still more $O_2^-$ and $H_2O_2$. This self-exacerbating process maintains the inflammation, which continues until stopped.

SOD's *in vitro* have been found to protect fully or in part against the effects of oxygen free radicals on the events of biogical importance listed in Table 4.4. These include membrane damage, inflammation, nucleic acid degradation and a host of single reactions, such as oxidation of thiols, lipids, flavins, porphyrins and catecholamines. Others involve arylepoxides, hydroxydopamine and radiomimetic chemotherapeutic agents. It is evident then that the SOD's have provided valuable tools to get a clearer insight into a large variety

**Table 4.4** Effects on systems of biological importance postulated for $O_2^-$ and/or OH•

| Multi-component | Single component |
|---|---|
| membrane damage | lipid peroxidation |
| inflammation | polysaccharide degradation |
| nucleic acid degradation | oxydation of: thiols, flavins, porphyrins, catecholamines |
| ageing acceleration | toxicity of: adriamycin, bleomycin, *cis*-platinum, Paraquat, streptonigrin |
| radiation damage | arylperoxides→cancer |
| ozone toxicity | hydroxydopamine→neurotoxicity |

of biologically important events caused by or related to $O_2^-$ formation. The effect of SOD, however, does not tell one whether the $O_2^-$ is the initiator of a chain of events or the proximal agent.

The anti-inflammatory effect of Cu–Zn SOD's in a wide variety of different diseases in animal and man, their pharmacological specificity (Table 4.5) and their bio-availability (Table 4.6)[26] appear to be a strong and valid argument supporting the *in vivo* role of oxygen free radicals as a cause of inflammation.

**Table 4.5** Some pharmacological effects of orgotein

| | |
|---|---|
| Orgotein IS | anti-inflammatory<br>anti-superoxide ($O_2^-$)<br>anti-viral* |
| Orgotein is NOT | analgesic<br>antipyretic<br>immunosuppressant<br>infection promoting |
| Orgotein does NOT | potentiate effects of barbiturates or alcohol<br>interfere with wound healing |

*Herpes simplex; parainfluenza-3

**Table 4.6** Bioavailability of orgotein SOD-activity in animals* (mouse, rat, guinea pig, dog, man)

| *Serum level* | *Hours after injection* *i.v.* | *s.c.* *i.m.* |
|---|---|---|
| maximum | 0.01 | 2–3 |
| <10% of maximum | 0.3–1.0 | 6–10 |
| *t* ½[3]‡ | 0.10–0.25 | 3–4 |
| | (0.5)† | (5–6)† |

* Thin-gel agarose electrophoreses (250 V, 10 mamp, 15–20 min) followed by NBT-riboflavin zymograms
†Values for man
‡Initial half-life for I.V. 'half-life' after peak concentration for s.c. and i.m.

Therapy with extracellular SOD's appear to resolve it by virtue of their removal.

Inflammatory diseases in man shown to date to respond to therapy with parenterally administered bovine Cu–Zn SOD are listed in Table 4.7. The potential spectrum is already broad, with musculoskeletal and urological applications proven in considerable detail, and ophthalmological and dermatological indications investigated sufficiently to establish considerable promise[27].

**Table 4.7** Human diseases responding to therapy* with bovine Cu–Zn superoxide dismutase (orgotein)

| | |
|---|---|
| Double-blind, randomized | |
| | rheumatoid arthritis; osteoarthritis; Duchenne muscular dystrophy; side effects of high-dose radiation therapy |
| Open drug | |
| *controlled* | chronic cystitis; post-operative radiation; induratio penis plastica (Peyronie's disease) |
| *uncontrolled* | inflammatory musculoskeletal diseases; uveitis; choroiditis; keratitis dendritica; atopic eczema, herpes simplex lesions; Paraquat poisoning (?) |

*Systemic and/or local injections

The risk factor for the use of Cu–Zn SOD as a parenteral drug is very low for the patient, lower by orders of magnitude than the risk factors of any of the presently available steroidal, non-steroidal, or slow-acting anti-rheumatic drugs. From its clinical profile, Cu-Zn SOD emerges as a drug with the specific action spectrum of a true anti-inflammatory agent, free of analgesic activity and devoid of general pharmacological effects[28].

It is apparent from the scenario presented here that the role of oxygen free radicals in physiological and pathological events is vast. As in any rapidly developing field, the future is full of fascinating and challenging potential. The sheer mass of it gives one no choice but to pick and choose, and any selections will no doubt, betray personal bias.

Future work in the area of oxygen-derived active species will have to address itself to a series of problems which are presently subject to rather intensive debate. Table 4.8 is an attempt to identify the ones considered of major importance. Among others, the question of why $O_2^-$ displays unusual reactivity in *in vitro* biochemical systems, but not in well-defined chemical experiments, is one for which a satisfactory answer must be obtained before we can assign the definitive role for $O_2^-$ in *in vivo* manifestations of oxygen toxicity. Despite this disparity, the best proof so far of involvement of $O_2^-$ in biological processes is the inhibition by SOD.

The solution will probably come from the recognition that the reactivity of $O_2^-$ is always that of its complexes with metal ions or protons either with the

**Table 4.8** Suggested future trends in oxygen-free radical studies. Small amounts of and short exposures to oxygen-free radicals can cause large biological effects

| Action mechanisms | |
|---|---|
| *Detrimental* | |
| membranes | lethal, partial, delayed damage due to increased lifetime of $O_2^-$ in 'structured' (aprotic) multilayers; disturbance to respiratory system; ageing |
| lipids | mechanism(s) of peroxidation and contribution to membrane injury; cleavage of fatty esters without peroxidation: validity *in vivo*; effect on prostaglandin synthesis |
| xenobiotic | decompartmentalization of metal ion(s) by drugs, toxic chemicals or viruses, with subsequent OH• formation |
| Beneficial | exploration of physiological roles of oxygen-free radicals:- enzymatic redox mechanisms; oxidative photophosphorylation; respiratory electron transfer chain |

naked $O_2^-$, the solvated form $O_2(H_2O)_n^-$ or the conjugate acid[29] $HO_2^{\cdot}$. Another biologically important reaction of $O_2^-$ is that with positively charged species. These can vary from protons and metal ions to organic cations. Furthermore, each of these ion pairs can be solvated or even solvent separated. In addition, formation of ion pairs such as $-NR_3^{\cdot}O_2^-$ are distinct possibilities in lipid membranes. Altogether one is faced with nearly a dozen possible species which can be present in an *in vivo* locale.

In this contest it is important to remember that aqueous phases in and around cell structures should be considered as 'structured' water[30]. As $O_2^-$ becomes more stable the more non-protic the solvent is, generation in biological systems with 'structured' water may well increase its lifetime appreciably, and have its toxicity.

The influence of the environment upon the reactivity of oxygen free radicals achieves an added dimension if one considers their sites of generation in the mammalian body. In this context, the copious generation of $O_2^-$ by phagocytes is of particular interest, as they appear without fail at sites of trauma and infection. The generating site appears to be in a particulate fraction, located in the plasma membrane of the leukocyte. It is most probably an NADPH oxidase which remains nearly inactive in the resting cell, but upon arrival of NADPH from the cytosol and oxygen from the exterior becomes an efficient $O_2^-$ producer, consuming about 38% of the oxygen of the respiratory burst and releasing up to 90% of this outside of the cell in form of $O_2^-$ and $H_2O_2$[19]. The observed damage may result from direct action or via intermediaries which are toxic. If damage is extensive, the cell may die. If damage is slight, effects may be delayed. Experiments with reconstituted cells and liposomes in different environments are needed to assess the relevance to *in vivo* events.

The large proportion of polyunsaturated lipids in cell membranes and the propensity of such lipids to undergo oxidation by a free radical chain mechanism has resulted in a large number of *in vitro* investigations, employing micelles, vesicles and reconstituted cells, and using protection by SOD and/or catalase as indicators for the degree of attack by oxygen free radicals. The results which recently have been reviewed by Fridovich[31] show that *in vitro* enzymatically produced $O_2^-$ and $H_2O_2$ damage the cell membrane and that the proximal attacking agent is $OH^{\cdot}$ and $^1O_2$ or subsequent reactants, such as hydroperoxides, epoxides or ozonides. Of relevance for such a mechanism are observations showing that the initial insult can be brief and still lead to cell leakage and/or lysis many hours later. If the concept of organized water in tissue being more aprotic is valid. Nielan's[32] demonstration that $O_2^-$ cleaved glycerylesters of long-chain fatty acids in aprotic solvents could result *in vivo* in de-esterification without peroxidative side reactions. Such a mechanism, for instance, could increase the rate of biosynthesis of prostaglandin by making arachidonic acid, which is stored as phosphatidyl esters, available to prostaglandin synthetase.

More aprotic behaviour of membrane-bound 'structured' water should also lead to a rethinking of the ability of SOD to quench $^1O_2$ *in vivo* in special situations. This has previously been dismissed out of hand for kinetic reasons, based on the reaction rate of $^1O_2$ in unhindered aqueous systems[31].

The essential physiological roles of oxygen free radicals also need to be explored. The occurrence and possible participation of $O_2^-$ during oxidative photophosphorylation suggests an essential role of this species with the obligatory requirement of biological sources of $O_2^-$.

The wide distribution of superoxide dismutase and the dispute over its role, either dismutating $O_2^-$ or quenching $^1O_2$, still leaves the possibility open that $^1O_2$ may be generated from $O_2^-$ as a potential toxic agent, but nevertheless playing an obligatory role in some metabolic oxidation reactions. This is evident from the number of enzymatic redox mechanisms which have been shown to involve $O_2^-$. It was also suggested that $O_2^-$ has an essential function in the electron transfer chain in the respiratory system, providing an alternate energy source[1]. Superoxide dismutase would here merely serve as a regulating enzyme. Solving these questions will have far reaching consequences towards the comprehension of the function of oxygen and superoxide in particular, in biological systems.

The functional specificity of SODs, glutathione peroxidase and catalase *in vivo* as the principle scavengers of $O_2^-$ and $H_2O_2$ has also become a subject of spirited debate. Some principal areas for future research are listed in Table 4.9. They revolve around two major topics: (1) is control of oxygen free radicals in mammals the true and only biological function of SOD's, glutathione peroxidase and catalase? (2) What are the capabilities of these three enzymes when given exogenously to be effective and safe as drugs in the treatment of pathology caused by oxygen free radicals, and diseases perhaps not directly related to but derived from free radical events?

Catalysed $O_2^-$ dismutation is an inherent property of the metal ions $Cu^{2+}$,

**Table 4.9** Suggested future trends in studies with superoxide dismutases and peroxidases SODS and peroxidases have other *in vivo* functions and properties

| |
|---|
| Endogenous SODs |
| intracellular abundance indicating other functions? |
| Exogenous Cu–Zn SODs |
| treatment of disease; control of drug toxicity; role in ageing; PMN mobilization; action mechanisms |
| Exogenous GSH-peroxidase |
| protection of membrane lipids; scavenging of chemical mutagens |
| **Needed** |
| Potent, specific, membrane-permeable, non-toxic inhibitor(s) of SODs and peroxidases |
| sensitive, specific and quantitatively reproducible mammalian models of induced or spontaneous disease |
| Data on *in vivo* synthesis of SODs and peroxidases |

$Fe^{3+}$ and $Mn^{2+}$, and *in vitro* has been observed at high efficiency for a variety of organic chelates with these metals. The structural features required for this activity are only three: (1) a free co-ordination position for binding $O_2^-$, (2) a redox potential of approximately −0.1 to 0.8 V, and (3) metal ion valence alteration occurring faster than spontaneous dismutation.

Based on these and related considerations, Fee[33] has suggested that the dismutase activity of the SOD's possibly resulted from coincidences rather than evolutionary design. The *in vivo* instability of metal complexes other than the SOD's is a major argument against this contention. *Indeed* the truly remarkable stability of Cu–Zn SOD's under *in vivo* conditions very much suggests a 'last stand' defence of evolutionary design. On the other hand, certain aerobic bacterial (*M. lepramurium*) and plant cells (corn, peas, oat seedlings) contain SODs at 1.5–10% of their soluble proteins[34,35] Also, the drug effects of exogenous Cu–Zn remain long after demonstrable SOD activity has disappeared from the body[26]. New experimental approaches are clearly needed to resolve these discrepancies. Thought should be given to whether the relative intracellular abundance and extracellular therapeutic efficacy of Cu–Zn SOD's indicates a role in the general protection of tissue against injury. Use as a storage and buffer source of Cu and Zn for use in newly synthesized metalloproteins has been suggested[33] but seems less likely since the Cu–Zn SOD's hold their metals under physiological conditions so tightly chelated that even dialysis against 1 mM EDTA does not remove them.

It seems that exogenously administered SOD's will become increasingly more important as drugs for the treatment of diseases with inflammatory components. Clinical use to date is limited to bovine Cu–Zn SOD, as the necessary toxicological and pharmacological background data are still lacking for other SOD's. Much work remains to be done before it will be possible to decide whether and how appropriate peroxidases can be made into useful drugs. Apart from their obvious role as regulators of aberrations of intracellular $H_2O_2$ and other hydroxperoxides, accumulation of GSH-peroxidase *in vitro* has shown a potential to (1) protect unsaturated lipids in biomembranes, (2) interact with the arachidonic acid cascade in prostaglandin synthesis, and (3) scavenge chemical mutagens[5] The latter postulate is based on observations relating selenium availability to the incidence of cancer, which indicates that the anti-cancer activity of selenium is not cytostatic, but rather prevents some early step during carcinogenesis which could be a peroxide-mediated mutation[36]

Bovine Cu–Zn SOD, as already mentioned, had been found to be effective as a drug in a wide spectrum of diseases with inflammatory components. Among these, ophthalmological, dermatological and respiratory diseases, as well as muscular diseases in addition to Duchenne muscular dystrophy, invite closer attention. Such exploration, to be fruitful, must be done with carefully controlled, double-blind trials, as responses to injections of placebo, in our experience, can be not only beneficial, but also long lasting.

The response of the inflammatory syndrome to exogenous Cu–Zn SOD is taking on another dimension by our discovery that injections of SOD mobilize PMNs into the circulation, as well as into the injection site[37]. PMN appearance at the injection site and in the circulation reaches a peak several hours after the injection, when the SOD content has already dropped to a small fraction of the initial level. Bovine Cu–Zn SOD is not chemotactic *per se in vitro* (Boyden chamber)[38], hence the PMN mobilizing effect appears to require mediators present in tissue and circulation. In view of these data and the demonstration of membrane stabilization by bovine Cu–Zn SOD[25] it is intriguing to speculate whether the disease controlling effect is the product of moving ample amounts of PMNs to the injured site while protecting these cells against premature leakage or lysis at the site.

Protection by parenteral Cu-Zn SOD against the toxic effects of xenobiotic substances, including radiomimetic drugs, is being increasingly demonstrated. Paraquat (methylviologen), a non-selective herbicide, forms radicals which react avidly with dioxygen to form $O_2^-$ and the paraquat cation. When ingested it is highly toxic to animals, with the lung eventually the most damaged organ, leading to death by anoxia[39]. Exogenous SOD ameliorates or inhibits the toxic effect[40]. In man, in our experience high-dose treatment with exogenous SOD (about 60 mg/day), given both systemically and by inhalation, has to commence no later than 24 h after paraquat ingestion and to assure survival should be accompanied by the best supportive therapy available to remove excess paraquat from the system[41].

The radiomimetic drugs, bleomycin, *cis*-platinum and adriamycin, seem to exert their tissue toxicity by similar radical mechanisms[42–44]. In parallel to the inhibition by exogenous SOD of toxic side effects occurring during radiation therapy of malignancies[45], we find that in laboratory animals the toxic effects on lung, kidney and heart, respectively, can be ameliorated by therapy with exogenous Cu–Zn SOD[46]. This occurs, at least in animal models, without interfering with the tumourolytic efficacy of these drugs, which is not necessarily surprising as the anti-cancer effect is thought to come about by interaction with cellular nucleic acids.

$O_2^-$ has been linked frequently to the process of ageing[47,48] by virtue of its crosslinking effects on fibres; its disturbance of the cellular respiratory system; by lipid and other peroxidative processes leading to an increase in cellular inclusion bodies, and its possible promotion of mutagenesis. We are trying to assess the ageing potential of $O_2^-$ in lifetime studies in normal laboratory animals by comparing animals treated with exogenous Cu–Zn SOD against placebo treated controls. In a pilot study, 40 mice and 20 rats, equally divided as to sex, were injected once per week with SOD at 1.0 mg/kg s.c., the control animals receiving placebo. All animals were weighed weekly and observed 6 days/week. The animals were treated either until they became moribund or until the size of a group entered into the study had been reduced to 30% or less. Under these conditions, the lifespans and weight gains of treated mice or rats were not significantly different from those of appropriate control groups throughout the 2.5 year observation period. Appearance, as well as histopathological findings, did not show any differences between the groups. In addition, lesions were observed in various organs of both treated and control animals and these showed no consistent pattern of association of abnormalities. On the other hand, the pattern of tumour occurrence does not suggest any tendency for tumour induction or promotion by SOD.

A more elaborate lifetime study involving 550 albino mice is now under way and, hopefully, will provide statistically valid information on whether daily SOD injections (s.c) at three dose levels (2, 6, 18 mg/kg) will improve ageing parameters such as longevity, appearance, weight, tissue and body fluid composition, as well as tumour incidence, when compared against placebo. The animals will be observed daily, weighed weekly, and observed ophthalmologically at 0, 6, 12 and 18 months. At base line, interim sacrifice (12 months) and at termination complete haematology, clinical chemistry and microscopic examination on 42 different organs and tissues will be performed.

Studies along the lines presented in Table 4.9 would greatly benefit by the availability of specific enzyme inhibitors and bioassays. Non-toxic, membrane-permeable inhibitors would permit us to measure the rate of intracellular production of oxygen free radicals and provide much needed information on how these processes proceed in whole cells and/or subcellular organelles, and how they respond to exogenous SOD's and/or peroxidases, which could be interiorized in the form of liposomes.

Animal models of induced inflammation, numerous as they are, all suffer from lack of specificity and poor day to day reproducibility of response to inflammatory and anti-inflammatory agents. This experimental 'noise' is sizable and occurs even though all conditions are rigidly controlled, making valid assessment of all but large differences a practical impossibility. Solutions will probably come from a clearer understanding of how laboratory animals of the same species and strain vary from day to day in their responses to insults such as induced inflammation and to therapy and/or prophylaxis to counteract such insults. As a contribution to the solution of these problems, we have explored together with E. C. Huskisson the use of inflammatory osteoarthritis of the knee as an *in vivo* model disease for the evaluation of anti-inflammatory drugs[49] This worked well for exogenous SOD, but this approach is, of course, limited to soluble drugs that can be injected locally because they are free of tissue toxicity at the doses used.

As so frequently occurs in a rapidly developing field, the available evidence had created more questions than answers. Progress will require conceptual and methodological approaches spanning the spectrum of investigations from physical chemistry to the human clinic.

In closing, two facts should be considered.

Firstly, if one equates the effects in living matter of ionizing radiation with that of oxygen free radicals, the remarks voiced more than two decades ago by men like J. A. V. Butler and L. G. Gray seem peculiarly appropriate: namely, that comparatively small doses can produce such marked biological changes, although, in general, much larger doses are required to produce easily observable chemical changes. Thus, the 'big problem' is still very much with us. Yet we all feel sure that the study of the influence of oxygen free radicals will yield profound consequences for the theories of ageing of carcinogenesis and of heredity.

Secondly, an unexpected and stimulating result coming from worldwide studies during the last decade is the demonstration that oxygen free radicals are intimately involved in inflammation and possibly other disease. From this flows my concept that the road is now open for the development of a series of truly new drugs, based on rigidly purified intracellular components and their derivatives, which are usable across species. These will be much more akin to the molecules directly participating in biological mechanisms than to synthetic drugs. They will be more truly specific, and, last but not least, most of them will be toxicologically and immunologically very safe.

## References

*1 Bors, W., Saran, M., Lengfelder, E., Spöttc, R. and Michel, C. (1974). The relevance of the superoxide anion radical in biological systems. *Curr. Top. Radia. Res. Q.*, **9**, 247

2 Fee, J. A. and Valentine, J. S. (1977). Chemical and physical properties of superoxide. In Michelson, A. M., McCord, J. M. and Fridovich, I. (eds.), *Superoxide and Superoxide Dismutases*, pp. 19–60. (London: Academic Press)

3 Willson, R. L. (1979). Hydroxyl radicals and biological damage in vitro: What relevance in vivo? In *Oxygen Free Radicals and Tissue Damage*. Ciba Symp. 65, new series, pp. 19–42. (Amsterdam: Excerpta Medica)

4 Fridovich, I. (1976). Superoxide dismutase and the chemistry of hydrogen peroxide. In

* The literature on oxygen free radicals and their biological scavengers has recently been reviewed extensively. The reader should consult the reviews listed as references 1–5 for further details.

Pryor, W. A. (ed.) *Free Radicals in Biology*, Vol. I pp. 239–277. (New York: Academic Press)

5 Flohé, L. (1979). Glutathione peroxidase: fact and fiction. In *Oxygen Free Radicals and Tissue Damage*. Ciba Symp. 65, new series, pp. 95–122. (Amsterdam: Excerpta Medica)

6 Haber, F. and Willstätter, R. (1931). Unpaarigkeit und Radikalketten in Reaktionsmechanismus organischer und enzymatischer Vorgänge. *Chem. Berichte*, **64**, 2844

7 Gerschman, R., Gilbert, D. L., Nye, S. W., Dwyer, P. and Fenn, W. O. (1954). Oxygen poisoning and x-irradiation. A mechanism in common. *Science*, **119**, 623

8 Czapski, G. (1971). Superoxide anion: pulse radiolysis in frozen solutions. *Ann. Rev. Phys. Chem.*, **22**, 171

9 Fridovich, I. and Handler, P. (1958). Xanthine oxidase III. Sulfite oxidation as an ultrasensitive assay. *J. Biol. Chem.*, **233**, 1578

10 Mills, G. C. (1957). Hemoglobin catabolism. I. Glutathione peroxidase, an erythrocyte enzyme which protects hemoglobin from oxidative breakdown. *J. Biol. Chem.*, **229**, 189

11 Sies, H. (1974). Biochemistry of the peroxisome in the liver cell. *Angew. Chem. Int. Ed. Engl.*, **13**, 706

12 Mann, T. and Keilin, D. (1939). Hemocuprein and hepatocuprein. *Proc. R. Soc. London, Ser. B*, **126**, 303

13 Huber, W., Schulte, T. L., Carson, S., Goldhamer, R. E. and Vogin, E. E. (1968). Some chemical and pharmacological properties of a novel antiinflammatory protein. *Toxicol. Appl. Pharmacol.*, **12**, 308

14 McCord, J. M. and Fridovich, I. (1969). Superoxide dismutase. An enzymic function for erythrocuprein (Hemocuprein). *J. Biol. Chem.*, **244**, 6049

15 Steinman, H.M. and Hill, R. L. (1973). Sequence homologies among bacterial and mitochondrial superoxide dismutases. *Proc. Natl. Acad. Sci.* (USA), **70**, 3725

16 Weisiger, R. A. and Fridovich, I. (1973). Superoxide dismutase: Organelle specificity. *J. Biol. Chem.*, **248**, 3582

17 Menander-Huber, K. B. (1979). Double-blind controlled clinical trials in man with bovine Cu-Zn superoxide dismutase (orgotein). In Bannister, W. H. and Bannister, J. V. (eds.) *The Significance of Superoxide and Superoxide Dismutase. Vol. II: Biological and Clinical Aspects.* (New York: Elsevier in press)

18 Johnston, R. B. Jr., Keele, B. B. Jr., Misra, H. P., Webb, L. S., Lehmeyer, J. E. and Rajagopalan, K. V. (1975). Superoxide anion generation and phagocytic bactericidal activity. In Bellanti, J. A. and Dayton, D. H. (eds.) *The Phagocytic Cell in Host Resistance*, pp. 61–75. (New York: Raven Press)

19 Roos, D. and Weening, R. S. (1979). Defects in the oxidative killing of microorganisms by phagocytic leukocytes. In *Oxygen Free Radicals and Tissue Damage*. Ciba Symp. 65, new series, pp. 225–262. (Amsterdam: Excerpta Medica)

20 Badwey, J. A. and Karnovsky, M. L. (1979). Production of superoxide and hydrogen peroxide by an NADH-oxidase in guinea pig polymorphonuclear leukocytes. *J. Biol. Chem.*, **254**, 11530

21 Klebanoff, S. J. and Rosen, H. (1979). The role of myeloperoxidase in the microbicidal activity of polymorphonuclear leukocytes. In *Oxygen Free Radicals and Tissue Damage*. Ciba Symp. 65, new series, 262–283. (Amsterdam: Excerpta Medica)

22 Babior, B.M. and Kipnes, R. S. (1977). Superoxide-forming enzyme from human neutrophils: evidence for a flavin requirement. *Blood*, **50**, 517

23 McCord, J. M. and Salin, M. L. (1977) Self-directed cytotoxicity of phagocyte-generated superoxide free radical. In Rossi, F., Patriarca, P. L. and Romeo, D. (eds.) *Movement, Metabolism, and Bactericidal Mechanisms of Phagocytes*. pp. 257–264. (Padua: Piccin)

24 McCord, J. M. (1974). Free radicals and inflammation: protection of synovial fluid by superoxide dismutase. *Science*, **185**, 529

25 Huber, W. and Saifer, M. G. P. (1977). Orgotein, the drug version of bovine Cu-Zn superoxide dismutase. I. A summary account of safety and pharmacology in laboratory animals. In Michelson, A. M., McCord, J. M. and Fridovich, I. (eds.) *Superoxide and Superoxide Dismutases* pp. 517–536. (New York: Academic Press)

26 Huber, W., Menander-Huber, K. B., Saifer, M. G. P. and Williams, L. D. (1979). Bioavailability of superoxide dismutase: Implications for the anti-inflammatory action mechanism of orgotein. *Agents Actions Suppl.* (In press)

27 Menander-Huber, K. B. and Huber, W. (1977). Orgotein, the drug version of bovine Cu-Zn superoxide dismutase. II. A summary account of clinical trials in man and animals. In Michelson, A. M., McCord, J. M. and Fridovich, I. (eds.) *Superoxide and Superoxide Dismutases*, pp. 537–549. (New York: Academic Press)
28 Huber, W. (1979). Orgotein (bovine Cu-Zn superoxide dismutase) an anti-inflammatory protein drug: Discovery, toxicology and pharmacology. *Eur. J. Rheumatol. Suppl.* (In press)
29 Hill, H. A. O. (1979). The identity of superoxide radical anion species. In *Oxygen Free Radicals and Tissue Damage* Ciba Symp. 65, new series, pp. 363–366. (Amsterdam: Excerpta Medica)
30 Tanford, C. (1961). *Physical Chemistry of Macromolecules*. p. 317. (New York: Wiley).
31 Fridovich, I. (1979). Superoxide dismutases: Defense against endogenous superoxide radical. In *Oxygen Free Radicals and Tissue Damage*. Ciba Symp. 65, new series pp. 77–93. (Amsterdam: Excerpta Medica)
32 Niehaus, W. G. (1978). A proposed role of superoxide anion as a biological nucleophile in the deesterification of phospholipids. *Bioorg. Chem.*, **7**, 77
33 Fee, J. A. (1979). On the question of superoxide toxicity and the biological function of superoxide dismutases. In *Third International Symposium on Oxidases and Related Oxidation-Reduction Systems*. (Albany: New York)
34 Ichihara, K., Kuzonose, E., Kuzonose, M. and Mori, T. (1977). Manganese superoxide dismutase content of mycobacterium lepramurium. *J. Biochem.*, **81**, 1427
35 Giannopolitis, C. N. and Ries, J. K. (1977). Cu-Zn superoxide dismutases content of seedlings of corn, peas and oats. *Plant Physiol.*, **59**, 309
36 Schrauzer, G. N., White, D. A. and Schneider, C. J. (1977). Cancer mortality correlation studies. III. Statistical associations with dietary selenium intakes. *Bioinorg. Chem.*, **7**, 23
37 Huber, W., Saifer, M. G. P. and Williams, L. D. (1979). Superoxide dismutase pharmacology and orgotein efficacy: New perspectives. In Bannister, W. H. and Bannister, J. V. (eds.) *The Significance of Superoxide and Superoxide Dismutase. Vol. II: Biological and Clinical Aspects*. (New York: Elsevier, in press)
38 Ward, P. A. (1974). Personal communication
39 Smith, L. L., Rose, M. S. and Wyatt, I. (1979). The pathology and biochemistry of paraquat. In *Oxygen Free Radicals and Tissue Damage*. Ciba Symp. 65, new series, pp. 321–341. (Amsterdam: Excerpta Medica)
40 Autor, A- P. (1974). Reduction of paraquat toxicity by superoxide dismutase. *Life Sci.*, **14**, 1309
41 Huber, W. and Menander-Huber, K. B. (1979). Unpublished observations
42 Lown, J. W. and Sim, S. (1977). The mechanism of the bleomycin-induced cleavage of DNA. *Biochem. Biophys. Res. Commun.*, **77**, 1150
43 Goodman, J. and Hochstein, P. (1977). Generation of free radicals and lipid peroxidation by redox cycling of adriamycin and daunomycin. *Biochem. Biophys. Res. Commun.*, **77**, 797
44 McGinness, J. E., Proctor, P. H., Demopoulos, H. B., Hokanson, J. A. and Kirkpatrick, D. S. (1978). Amelioration of cis-platinum nephrotoxicity by orgotein (superoxide dismutase). *Physiol. Chem. Phys.*, **10**, 267
45 Edsmyr, F., Huber, W. and Menander, K. B. (1976). Orgotein efficacy in ameliorating side effects due to radiation therapy. I. Double-blind, placebo-controlled trial in patients with bladder tumors. *Curr. Ther. Res.*, Clin. Exp., **19**, 198
46 Williams, L. D., Dang. P. H. C., Gerstl, B. and Huber, W. (1979). Unpublished results
47 Harman, D. (1956). Ageing: A theory based on free radical and radiation chemistry. *J. Gerontol.*, **11**, 298
48 Fridovich, I. (1977). Oxygen is toxic! *Bioscience*, **27**, 462
49 Menander-Huber, K. B., Huskisson, E. C. and Huber, W. (1978). Inflammatory osteoarthritis as an *in vivo* model disease in man for the evaluation of anti-inflammatory drugs. In *International Congress of Inflammation*. (Bologna: Italy, Oct 31–Nov 3) Abstract P2/44

# Discussion

**Dr P. Gordon: (USA)** questioned Dr Huber's suggestion that SOD enhanced circulating neutrophils because it mobilized neutrophils from their sites. If the superoxide (not the dismutase) generated leukotactic principles for neutrophils, specifically lipid peroxide, the event which he was describing might result from a fall in their distribution in the bloodstream. If the superoxide signals were 'turned off' in the peripheral regions of the body, there might be reduced penetration of PMNs into the foci of inflammation.

**Dr Huber** said that this was possible but what one observed on i.p. injection of a few milligrams of SOD per rat was a massive migration into the peritoneal cavity with a concomitant increase in circulating PMNs of over 100%. The differences were highly significant.

**Dr Gordon (USA)** was amazed to learn that the toxic effect of some anti-cancer agents which acted by generating superoxide were suppressed by SOD whereas the anti-tumour effects were not.

**Dr Huber** said that extracellular SOD did not penetrate the cell membrane. It was too large a molecule. The toxic effects of the anti-cancer agents occurred in organs different from sites where the tumours were usually situated. For *cis*-platinum, toxicity was seen in the kidney; for bleomycin in the lung and for adriamycin in the heart. These toxic effects seemed to be mediated through superoxides but penetration of the chemotherapeutic agent into the cell was required for it to have an effect on nucleic acids.

**Dr W. C. Dick (UK)** asked at what evolutionary stage was the superoxide dismutase mechanism believed to have appeared.

**Dr Huber:** said that it seemed to have developed when the first oxygen-using animals appeared on earth. Oxygen was not only the staff of life but it was also toxic with its two unpaired electrons. Since all living processes depended on oxygen, the system which avoided oxygen's intracellular toxic effects had to be maintained at all costs, and this accounted for the system's stability.

# 5

# Future trends in the immunopathology of rheumatoid arthritis

M. ZIFF (USA)

In the immunopathology of rheumatoid arthritis (RA), two reactions occur simultaneously. One is an exudative, immune complex-induced reaction which is most obviously manifest in the synovial effusion. This phase of RA has been well described[1]. In this reaction there is activation of complement with the generation of chemotactic factors, lowering of complement levels and exudation of polymorphonuclear (PMN) cells. Lysosomal enzymes are released from both the phagocytic lining cells of the synovial membrane and from the polymorphonuclear cells of the effusion. These enzymes participate in the amplification of the immune complex phase of rheumatoid synovitis, mainly by activation of components of the complement sequence. This immune complex phase of rheumatoid synovitis contributes in a major fashion to the symptomatology of the disease. It is also responsible, through the release of proteolytic enzymes and collagenase into the joint fluid, for much of the erosion of cartilage which occurs in this disease.

A second phase of RA is the cellular phase which occurs in the sub-lining layer of the synovial membrane. In this phase, mononuclear cells gather in the sub-lining layer in a perivascular distribution[2,3]. Here they undergo blastic transformation, and secrete lymphokines[4] and immunoglobulins (Igs)[5]. Among these Igs are IgG–rheumatoid factor (IgG–RF)[6] and IgM–rheumatoid factor (IgM–RF)[5]. The lymphokines act to further propagate the cellular immune response in the sub-lining layer, and the rheumatoid factors form immune complexes which participate in the immune complex phase of the disease. Thus, in a sense, the sub-lining layer infiltrates serve as a factory for the production of agents which on the one hand stimulate further proliferation of the cellular phase of the disease, and, on the other, for the production of agents required for the immune complex phase of the disease.

## THE IMMUNE COMPLEX PHASE

### Role of IgG–RF complexes

A large literature has emphasized the importance of IgG–RF in the pathogenesis of rheumatoid synovitis and in the development of systemic complications in this disease. Beginning with the work of Kunkel *et al*[7]. evidence has accumulated that the serum of certain patients with RA contains IgG complexes of intermediate size. Although present at levels demonstrable in the analytical ultracentrifuge in the serum of some patients with uncomplicated classical RA, these complexes are more commonly found in the sera of patients with systemic complications[8–12].

The recent availability of newly developed assays for immune complexes has stimulated interest in the quantitation by these techniques of IgG–RF complexes in the sera of patients with RA and the systemic complications of RA. Zubler and co-workers[13] have noted increased C1q binding in density gradient fractions of RA serum containing immune complexes of intermediate size (14–24S) and Gabriel and Agnello[14] using a monoclonal RF competitive binding method demonstrated binding activity in fractions sedimenting as low as 8S. Hurd and co-workers[12] found increased C1q binding, although not monoclonal RF binding, in the sera of patients with Felty's syndrome which was not observed in sera of patients with uncomplicated RA, suggesting that Felty's syndrome is characterized by IgG–RF complexes of larger size.

### IgG–RF complexes of rheumatoid synovial fluid

Of major importance has been the observation that IgG–RF complexes are largely responsible for the lowering of complement levels, which is characteristic of RA synovial effusions[16]. These complexes activate the classical complement pathway[17]; they may also activate the alternate pathway[18]. In addition, they react with IgM–RF[19] to form larger immune complexes which may be phagocytozed by synovial lining phagocytic cells[20] and by polymorphonuclear cells[21]. The phagocytosis of these complexes is associated with the formation of inclusions and the release of lysosomal enzymes. By virtue of these reactions and the secondary reactions which follow, IgG–RF complexes initiate the immune complex phase of rheumatoid synovitis.

Pope and co-workers[22] have studied the composition of the IgG–RF containing intermediate complexes of RA plasma. These were separated by gel filtration, pepsin digested and the $F(ab')_2$ fragments examined for their capacity to react with normal IgG using the ultracentrifuge. All of the $F(ab')_2$ reacted with normal IgG indicating that all of the IgG in the intermediate complexes had anti-IgG activity. On this basis, it was concluded that the intermediate complexes are self-associated IgG–RF complexes. Self-association of IgG–RF rather than association of IgG–RF with non-rheumatoid factor IgG occurs preferentially because two bonds rather than one can form between individual IgG–RF molecules when these react with each other.

**Rheumatoid factor synthesis in the synovial membrane**

With regard to the local synthesis of RF in the synovial membrane, the work of Natvig and co-workers is of particular interest[6,23]. These workers found a predominance of IgG staining plasma cells in the RA synovial membrane; and 30–60% of these plasma cells were IgG–RF synthesizing cells. This work suggests that the RA synovial membrane plays an important role in the synthesis of IgG–RF. It would also explain the fact that the immune complexes are present in synovial effusions in somewhat larger concentrations than in serum (see below).

**In vitro synthesis of rheumatoid factor**

Efforts have been made to quantify the synthesis of IgM–rheumatoid factor (IgM–RF) *in vitro*. Vaughan *et al.*[24] have attempted this using a Jerne plaque technique employing reduced and alkylated rabbit IgG haemolysin to coat the red blood cells of sheep. Only small numbers of IgM–RF producing cells were demonstrated in the peripheral blood mononuclear cells (PBM) of patients with RA, although moderate numbers were seen in patients with rheumatoid vasculitis and in patients with severe joint exacerbations. Larger numbers were found in the bone marrow.

**Comparison of immune complex levels in the serum and synovial fluid**

Using the monoclonal RF (MRF) binding assay, which measures the level of 'aggregated IgG', there was an increase in immune complex levels in the synovial fluid as compared to serum[25]. This was marked in some cases but of borderline significance in the entire group of patients examined. Also, Zubler and co-workers[13] found moderately greater immune complex levels in the synovial fluid than in the serum by the Clq binding assay in seropositive RA patients. Halla *et al.*[26] also detected immune complexes in higher concentration in the synovial fluid than in the serum. Finally, Hay *et al.*[27] have recently found higher levels of IgG–RF and IgM–RF complexes in the synovial fluid than in the serum. These findings suggest a significant contribution of local synthesis to the IgG–RF concentration in the RA synovial fluid.

**Radio-immunoassay methods for IgG–RF and IgM–RF**

Radio-immunoassay methods for IgG–RF and IgM–RF have recently become available. In the method described by Hay *et al.*[28], antiglobulins are bound to rabbit IgG bound to the surface of plastic tubes. The amount of antiglobulin bound is determined by adding [$^{125}$I]antihuman IgG or IgM. More recently, Carson *et al.*[29] have modified this method to make it more specific for IgG–RF and IgM–RF. To assay IgG–RF, the Fc region of IgG has been substituted as antigen and to quantitate IgG–RF binding, [$^{125}$I]rabbit F(ab')$_2$ antihuman antibody, specific for the Fd portion of IgG, has been used. IgM–RF was similarly measured using IgG as a first coat and [$^{125}$I] rabbit F(ab')$_2$ antihuman IgM to quantitate the IgM–RF binding.

### Future trends

Although it is apparent from the immunofluorescent studies cited that the rheumatoid synovial membrane synthesizes significant quantities of IgG–RF and IgM–RF, direct measurements of the amounts of those auto-antibodies synthesized as a fraction of the total IgG and IgM synthesized have not received more than preliminary study. Smiley *et al.*[5], cultivating rheumatoid synovial tissue pieces, found that an average of 9% of the IgM synthesized *in vitro* had properties of IgM–RF. In preliminary experiments, Lochead *et al.*[30] subsequently found that up to 5% of the IgG synthesized had IgG–RF activity. However, when Gilliland *et al.*[31] analysed culture supernants of a cell line derived from rheumatoid synovium, they found, by measuring the binding of the newly synthesized IgG to human and rabbit IgG, that most of the newly synthesized IgG had the properties of IgG–RF. With the availability of recently developed radio-immunoassay techniques for IgG–RF and IgM–RF[28,29], it will be possible to repeat the preceding studies with modern quantitative methods and determine accurately the contribution of the synovial tissue to IgG–RF and IgM–RF production.

## THE IMMUNOLOGIC TRIGGER IN RHEUMATOID SYNOVITIS

### IgG as a possible antigen

Most studies of the action of IgG, usually heat-aggregated IgG, on the immune response in RA have dealt with the cellular immune response, i.e. with lymphocyte transformation and the production of migration inhibitory factors against leukocytes and macrophages. Results have been variable, but positive evidence of stimulation in such systems has been observed by Clot *et al.*[32] and Fröland and Garder[33], studying leukocyte migration inhibition, and Kinsella[34] and Dorner *et al.*[35] studying lymphocyte transformation.

Little attention has been given to antibody production by RA lymphocytes in response to aggregated IgG (IgG–agg). Johnson *et al.*[36] have presented evidence for the presence of conformationally altered IgG in RA patients and suggested that such IgG has the capacity to stimulate B cells directly via an Fc receptor. Yamasaki and Ziff[37] have shown that *in vitro* synthesis of Ig by lymphocytes of RA patients is stimulated by IgG–agg in the presence of fresh seropositive autologous serum. The possibility that IgG–agg might react with suppressor T cells to inhibit their ability to suppress B-cell function must also be kept in mind[38].

**Polyclonal B cell activation in relation to rheumatoid factor synthesis**

The occurrence of RFs in patients with a variety of infectious and other hypergammaglobulinaemic states may, at least in part, be the result of polyclonal B-cell activation (PBA). IgM–RF activity has been noted in association with hypergammaglobulinaemia in the course of sarcoidosis, tuberculosis, viral hepatitis and parasitic infestations. Experimentally, RF has been induced after repeated injections of heat-killed *Escherichia coli*[39] or streptococci[40].

The polyclonal activation of B cells to stimulate auto-antibody formation has recently been actively investigated in the mouse. The induction of anti-DNA antibody was first observed following the injection of bacterial lipopolysaccharide (LPS) into various strains of mice[41]. Polyclonal B-cell activators like dextran sulphate and PPD have also stimulated this change[42]. IgM–RF has also been induced by repeated injections of LPS into responder mouse strains[43].

An interesting form of PBA has recently been studied in a number of laboratories. This is the phenomenon of Epstein–Barr virus (EBV) induced B cell lymphoblastoid cell line formation. Interest in this form of PBA is based on two observations. First is the observation of Alspaugh and co-workers[44] that EBV infection of normal peripheral blood lymphocytes induces the development in these cells of lymphoblastoid cells lines which contain a 'rheumatoid arthritis associated' nuclear antigen (RANA) against which most patients with RA have precipitating (RAP) antibodies. Second is the observation of Slaughter and co-workers[45] that RA lymphocytes form RF producing cell lines more rapidly than normal lymphocytes.

Rheumatoid factor production in EBV infected cultures of peripheral blood mononuclear cells (PBM) has been studied by Slaughter *et al.*[45] Both normal and RA mononuclear cells produced increased amounts of IgM–RF in response to the polyclonal stimulatory action of EBV on the B cell population, but greater amounts were produced by the RA mononuclear cells. Dr Hugo Jasin in our laboratory[46] has examined the effect of pokeweed mitogen (PWM), a T cell dependent polyclonal activator of B cell function, on rheumatoid factor synthesis *in vitro*. Although there was active synthesis of IgM–RF in such cultures, the synthesis of IgM–RF in PWM stimulated normal control cultures exceeded that of the similarly stimulated rheumatoid cultures significantly. Presumably, with PWM there is either a block in T cell mediated activation of precursor B cells for rheumatoid factor synthesis, or continuous activation of B lymphocyte precursors *in vivo* may result in depletion of such cells.

**Future trends**

The identity of the stimulating agent in the RA synovial membrane which is responsible for the blastic transformation and Ig synthesis which takes place in this tissue is unknown. Of interest in connection with the possible role of IgG as an antigen is the observation of Roitt[47] that 95–98% of the weight of immune complexes isolated from RA synovial effusions could be accounted for by IgG, IgM and complement components. He could find no significant amounts of other material which might represent exogenous antigen. However, because of the insufficient and often conflicting data available, it is necessary to leave open the possibility that IgG plays an antigenic role in rheumatoid synovitis.

There continues to be an active interest in a possible role for Epstein–Barr virus in the aetiology of RA. Depper *et al.*[48] have recently confirmed the observation of Slaughter *et al.*[45] that rheumatoid PBM generate lymphoblastoid B cell lines more rapidly than normal PBM. By examining the outgrowth times of the B cell containing fraction in the presence and absence of the T cell fraction, they determined that the short outgrowth time of rheumatoid cell lines was due to a deficiency of suppressor T cells which regulate the formation of lymphoblastoid cell lines. Thus we have evidence of a new type of suppressor cell deficiency in connective tissue disease, a deficiency of suppressor cells which regulate lymphoblastoid cell line formation. Presumably this is basically a deficiency of cells which regulate EBV polyclonal B cell activation. It has recently been shown that this deficiency is not limited to RA, since short outgrowth times have also been demonstrated in patients with multiple sclerosis[49].

Two groups[50,51] have recently reported that there is marked generation of suppressor T cells for B cell activation during EBV infection in infectious mononucleosis. It was observed that PBM from patients with infectious mononucleosis contained substantial numbers of suppressor T cells, which, when co-cultured with normal B cells, inhibited the synthesis of polyclonal Ig induced by EBV or PWM. This is in contrast to the deficiency of suppressor T cells for EBV stimulation of B cells in RA. The basis for the deficiency of suppressor T cells for EBV induced B cell transformation in RA is deserving of further study.

**Genetic factors**

That there is a familial aggregation of rheumatoid factors has been known since 1958[52,53]. Recently, Stastny[54] demonstrated a markedly increased frequency of HLA–Dw4 in RA using the mixed lymphocyte reaction typing procedure and Gibofsky and co-workers[55], the increased frequency of HLA–DRw4 by serum histocompatibility typing. It will be important to relate the RA histocompatibility marker with a corresponding phenotypic abnormality which predisposes to the rheumatoid state. There is at present no information regarding this relationship. It could represent a genetic predisposition to react to an as yet unidentified exogenous antigen or to autologous IgG. On the other hand, it might relate to the capacity of a virus such as EBV to induce the formation of neo-antigens in genetically susceptible individuals. It is of interest in this connection that Catalano *et al.*[56] have noted a relationship between the prevalence of RA and the prevalence of the RA precipitin (RAP) in two populations with differing prevalence of RA. In the American Chippewa Indian tribe, the prevalence of RA is about 5% and in caucasians about 1%. The frequency of the RAP was 40% in the Chippewas and 10% in the caucasians ($p = 0.002$). This suggests that there may be a genetic aspect to the deficiency of T lymphocyte suppression of EBV transformation in RA.

A number of reports have demonstrated a deficiency of suppressor T cells for nonspecific Ig synthesis in patients with active systemic lupus erythematosus. Such deficiency has not been demonstrated as yet in RA, although, as noted above, a deficiency of suppressor T cells has been observed for the formation of B cell lines. It is possible that future investigation may demonstrate a T suppressor cell deficiency with regard to an as yet unidentified antigen which is related to the Dw4 marker in RA. It is unlikely to be a specific deficiency for EBV in view of the fact that a shortened outgrowth time for cell line formation has also been noted in multiple sclerosis.

## SUMMARY

Two types of immunopathological reaction occur simultaneously in the rheumatoid joint. The two reactions occur side by side and may be mutually interdependent. One is an immune complex induced reaction which is most obviously manifested in the synovial effusion. The other is a cellular reaction which occurs in the sub-lining layer of the synovial membrane. In the cellular reaction, mononuclear cells gather in the sub-lining layer of the synovial membrane in a perivascular distribution and undergo blastic transformation with eventual formation of plasma cells which secrete immunoglobulins and lymphokines. Among the immunoglobulins secreted is the IgG form of rheumatoid factor.

IgG–rheumatoid factor forms self-associated complexes which can be demonstrated in the synovial effusion, These complexes activate the classical complement sequence and produce lowering of complement levels in the synovial effusion. There is evidence from immunofluorescent staining data that a significant fraction of the IgG which is synthesized by the rheumatoid synovial membrane is IgG–rheumatoid factor. This is consistent with the observation that the immune complex levels present in synovial effusions are somewhat larger than in the serum. Newly developed radio-immunoassay techniques will in the future permit accurate measurements of the production of IgG–rheumatoid factor and IgM–rheumatoid factor in the synovial tissue both on an absolute basis and as a percentage of the respective amounts of IgG and IgM synthesized. This is desirable information in order to quantitate the contribution of local synthesis of these auto-antibodies to the synovial fluid levels.

Future investigation, it may be presumed, will also provide information which will help to identify the antigen or mitogen which is responsible for the extensive cellular immune response and immunoglobulin synthesis which takes place in the rheumatoid synovium.

There has been an active recent interest in the role of polyclonal activators such as Epstein-Barr virus in rheumatoid synovitis. Patients with RA have a high incidence of an antibody to an Epstein–Barr virus (EBV) induced nuclear antigen known as the rheumatoid associated nuclear antigen (RANA). EBV has also been shown to produce B cell lymphoblastoid cell lines from rheumatoid peripheral blood mononuclear cells more rapidly than from normal PBM. This has been demonstrated to be due to a deficiency of suppressor T cells for EBV stimulation of B cell transformation. There also appears to be a relationship between the prevalence of RA in different populations and the prevalence of EBV antibodies in these populations, presumably reflecting the ease with which antibodies to the resident EBV antigens are formed. The basis for the deficiency of suppressor T cells for EBV-induced B cell transformation in RA is deserving of future study.

With the association of RA with the HLA–Dw4 genetic marker, the relationship between this marker and possible aetiological factors in RA becomes an important subject for investigation. As techniques for relating genetic markers on immunoreactive cells to the immune response develop, the elucidation of the immunopathologic significance of the Dw4 marker in RA will be of great interest.

## References


1 Zvaifler, N. J. (1971). Immunoreactions in rheumatoid synovial effusions. *J. Exp. Med.*, **134** (Suppl), 2765

2 Kobayashi, I. and Ziff, M. (1973). Electron microscopic studies of lymphoid cells in the rheumatoid synovial membrane. *Arthritis Rheum.*, **16**, 471

3 Ishikawa, H. and Ziff, M. (1976). Electron microscopic observation of immunoreactive cells in the rheumatoid synovial membrane. *Arthritis Rheum.*, **19**

4 Stastny, P., Rosenthal, M., Andreis, M. *et al.* (1976). Lymphokines in the rheumatoid joint. *Arthritis Rheum.*, **18**, 237

5 Smiley, J. D., Sachs, C. and Ziff, M. (1968). *In vitro* synthesis of immunoglobulin by rheumatoid synovial membrane. *J. Clin. Invest.*, **47**, 624

6 Munthe, E. and Nativig, J. B. (1972). Immunoglobulin classes, subclasses and complexes of IgG rheumatoid factor in rheumatoid plasma cells. *Clin. Exp. Immunol.*, **12**, 55

7 Kunckel, H. G., Muller-Eberhard, H. J., Fudenberg, H. H. *et al.* (1961). Gamma globulin complexes in rheumatoid arthritis and certain other conditions. *J. Clin. Invest.*, **40**, 117

8 Jasin, H. E., LaSpallito, J. J. and Ziff, M. (1970). Rheumatoid hyperviscosity syndrome. *Am. J. Med.*, **49**, 484

9 Pope, R. M., Fletcher, M. A., Mamby, A. *et al.* (1975). Rheumatoid arthritis associated with hyperviscosity syndrome and intermediate complex formation. *Arch. Intern. Med.*, **135**, 281

10 Andreis, M., Hurd, E. R., LaSpallito, J. J. *et al.* (1978). Comparison of the presence of immune complexes in Felty's Syndrome and rheumatoid arthritis. *Arthritis Rheum.*, **21**, 310

11 Tomasi, J. B. Jr., Fudenberg, H. H. and Fenby, N. (1962). Possible relationship of rheumatoid factors and pulmonary disease. *Am.J.Med.*, **33,** 243
12 Theofliopoulos, A. N., Burtonboy, G., LaSpallito, J. J. *et al.* (1974). IgM rheumatoid factor and low molecular weight IgM. An association with vasculitis. *Arthritis Rheum.*, **17,** 272
13 Zubler, R. H., Nydegger, U., Perrin, L. H. *et al.* (1976). Circulating and intra-articular immune complexes in patients with rheumatoid arthritis. Correlation of $^{125}$I-C1q binding activity with clinical and biological feature of the disease. *J.Clin.Invest.*, **57,** 1308
14 Gabriel, A. J. and Agnello, V. (1977). Detection of immune complexes. The use of radioimmunoassays with C1q and monoclonal rheumatoid factor. *J.Clin.Invest.*, **59,** 990
15 Hurd, E. R., Chubick, A., Jasin, H. E *et al.* (1979). Increased C1q binding immune complexes in Felty's syndrome: comparison with uncomplicated rheumatoid arthritis. *Arthritis Rheum.*, **22,** 697
16 Winchester, R. J., Agnello, V. and Kunkel, H. G. (1970). Gamma globulin complexes in synovial fluids of patients with rheumatoid arthritis. Partial characterization and relationship to lowered complement levels. *Clin.Exp.Immunol.*, **6,** 689
17 Winchester, R. J., Agnello, V. and Kunkel, H. G. (1969). The joint-fluid gamma G-globulin complexes and their relationship to intraarticular complement diminution. *Ann.N.Y.Acad.Sci.*, **168,** 195
18 Ruddy, N., Fearon, D. J. and Austin, K. F. (1978). Depressed synovial fluid levels of properdin and properdin factor B in patients with rheumatoid arthritis. *Arthritis Rheum.*, **18,** 289
19 Hannestad, K. (1967). Presence of aggregated gamma-G-globulin in certain rheumatoid synovial effusions. *Clin. Exp. Immun.*, **2,** 511
20 Kinsella, J. D., Baum, J. and Ziff, M. (1970). Studies of isolated synovial lining cells of rheumatoid and non rheumatoid synovial membranes. *Arthritis Rheum.*, **13,** 734
21 Hurd, E. R., LoSpalluto, J. J. and Ziff, M. (1970). Formation of leukocytes in clusters in normal polymorphonuclear cells incubated with synovial fluid. *Arthritis Rheum.*, **13,** 724
22 Pope, R. M., Teller, D. C. and Mannik, M. (1974). The molecular basis of self-association of antibodies to IgG (rheumatoid factors) in rheumatoid arthritis. *Proc.Nat.Acad.Sci.(USA),* **71,** 517
23 Nativg, J. B., Munthe, E. and Pable, J. (1975). Evidence for intracellular component-fixing complexes of IgG rheumatoid factor in rheumatoid plasma cells. *Rheumatology,* **6,** 167
24 Vaughn, J. T., Chibara, T., Moore, T. L. *et al.* (1976). Rheumatoid factor-producing cells detected by direct hemolytic plaque assay. *J.Clin.Invest.*, **58,** 933
25 Lutha, H. S., McDuffie, F. C., Hunder, G. G. *et al.* (1975). Immune complexes in sera and synovial fluids of patients with rheumatoid arthritis. Radioimmunoassay with monoclonal rheumatoid factor. *J.Clin.Invest.*, **56,** 438
26 Halla, J. T., Volanakis, J. E. and Schrohenloher, E. E. (1979). Immune complexes in rheumatoid arthritis sera and synovial fluids. A comparison of three methods. *Arthritis Rheum.*, **22,** 440
27 Hay, F. C., Nineham, L. J., Perumal, R. *et al.* (1979). Intra-artucular and circulating immune complexes and antiglobulins (IgG and IgM) in rheumatoid arthritis; correlation with clinical features. *Ann.Rheum.Dis.*, **38,** 1
28 Hay, F. C., Nineham, L. J. and Roitt, I. M. (1975). Routine assay for detection of IgG and IgM antiglobulins in seronegative and seropositive rheumatoid arthritis. *Br.Med.J.*, **3,** 203
29 Carson, D. A., Lawrence, S., Catalono, M. A. *et al.* (1977). Radioimmunoassay of IgG and IgM rheumatoid factors reacting with human IgG. *J.Immunol.*, **119,** 295
30 Lochead, J. A., Smiley, J. E. and Ziff, M. (1971). Prolonged immunoglobulin synthesis by rheumatoid synovium in culture: quantitation of rheumatoid factor (RF) production. *Arthritis Rheum.*, **14,** 171
31 Gilliland, B. C., Ford, D. K. and Mannik, M. (1978). Synthesis by an established lymphocyte cell line from a rheumatoid synovium. *Arthritis Rheum.*, **21,** 330
32 Clot, J., Sany, J. and Verre, H. (1973). Aspects de l'immunité a médiation cellulaire dans la polyarthrite rheumatoide. I. Etude de caracterisation de la reponse vis-à-vis des immunoglobulines G non dênaturées. *Pathol.Biol.*, **21,** 465
33 Froland, S. S. and Granarder, P. I. (1973). The effect of IgG *in vitro* on leukocytes from patients with rheumatoid arthritis. *Scand.J.Immunol.*, **2,** 385
34 Kinsella, T. D. (1974). Enhancement of human lymphocyte transformation by aggregated

human gamma globulin. *J. Clin. Invest.*, **53**, 1108

35 Dorner, R. W., Gantner, G. E. Jr., Goldschmidt, J. *et al.* (1974). Stimulation of lymphocyte transformation by autologous serum fractions from patients with rheumatoid arthritis. *Immunology*, **27**, 781

36 Johnson, P. M., Watkins, J. and Wolborow, E. J. (1975). Antiglobulin production to altered IgG in reheumatoid arthritis. *Lancet*, **1**, 611

37 Yamasaki, K. and Ziff, M. (1977). Enhancement of *in vitro* immunoglobulin synthesis of rheumatoid lymphocytes by aggregated human gamma globulin. *Arthritis Rheum.*, **20**, 679

38 Moretta, L., Webb, S. R., Gross, C. E. *et al.* (1977). Functional analysis of two human T cell subpopulations: help and suppression of B cell responses by T cells bearing receptors for IgM or IgG. *J. Exp. Med.*, **146**, 184

39 Abruzzo, J. L. and Christian, C. L. (1961). The induction of a rheumatoid factor-like substance in rabbits. *J. Exp. Med.*, **114**, 791

40 Bokisch, V. A., Bernstein, D. and Krause, R. M. (1972). Occurrence of 19s and 7s anti-IgGs during hyperimmunization of rabbits with streptococci. *J. Exp. Med.*, **136**, 799

41 Fournie, G. J., Lambert, P. H. and Meischer, P. A. (1974). Release of DNA in circulating blood and induction of anti-DNA lipopolysaccharides. *J. Exp. Med.*, **140**, 1189

42 Izui, S., Eisenberg, R. A. and Dixon, F. J. (1979). IgG anti-DNA-rheumatoid factor complexes in sera from autoimmune MRL/I mice. *Arthritis Rheum.*, **22**, 625 (Abstract)

43 Izui, S., Eisenberg, R. A. and Dixon, F. J. (1980). (In press)

44 Alspaugh, M. A., Jensen, F. C., Rabin, M. *et al.* (1976). Lymphocytes transformed by Epstein–Barr virus. Induction of nuclear antigen reactive with antibody in rheumatoid arthritis. *J. Exp. Med.*, **147**, 1018

45 Slaughter L., Carson, D. A., Jensen, F. C. *et al.* (1978). *In vitro* effects of Epstein–Barr virus on peripheral blood mononuclear cells from patients with rheumatoid arthritis and normal subjects. *J. Exp. Med.*, **148**, 1429

46 Jasin, H. E. and Ziff, M. (1980) (In preparation)

47 Riott, I. M. (1977) International Congress on Rheumatology, San Francisco, California

48 Depper, J. M., Bardwick, R. P., Bluestein, H. G. *et al.* (1979). Abnormal regulation of Epstein–Barr virus transformation of rheumatoid lymphoid cells. *Arthritis Rheum.*, **22**, 605

49 Fraser, K. B., Millar, J. H. D., Haire, M., *et al.* (1979). Increased tendency to spontaneous *in vitro* lymphocyte transformation in clinically active multiple sclerosis. *Lancet*, **2**, 715

50 Toscato, G., Magrath, I., Broder, S. *et al.* (1979). Immunoregulatory cell function in Epstein-Barr virus induced infectious mononucleosis. *Clin. Res.*, **27**, 476A

51 Haynes, B. F., Schooley, R. T., Payling-Wright, C. *et al.* (1979). Emergence of suppressor T cells of immunoglobulin (Ig) production during acute Epstein-Barr virus (EBV)-induced infectious mononucleosis (IM). *Clin. Res.*, **27**, 327A

52 Ziff, M., Schmid, F. R., Lewis, A. J. *et al.* (1958). Familial occurrence of the rheumatoid factor. *Arthritis Rheum.*, **1**, 392

53 Lawrence, J. S., Valkenburg, H. A., Brenner, J. M. (1970). Heberden Dration, 1969: Rheumatoid arthritis – nature or nurture? *Ann. Rheum. Dis.*, **29**, 357

54 Stastyny, P. (1977). HLA-D typing in rheumatoid arthritis. *Arthritis Rheum.*, **20**, 545

55 Gibofsky, A., Winchester, R. J., Patarroy, M. *et al.* (1978). Disease associations of the Ia-like human alloantigens: contrasting patterns in rheumatoid arthritis and systemic lupus erythematosus. *J. Exp. Med.*, **148**, 1728

56 Catalano, M. A., Carson, D. A., Lotze, M. *et al.* (1979). Antibodies to Epstein–Barr virus related nuclear antigens in 2 groups at different risks for rheumatoid arthritis. *Clin. Res.*, **27**, 322A

# Discussion

**Dr E. Munthe: (Norway)** asked whether it was possible that immune complexes stimulated T cells. In particular, he wondered whether anything was known about the possible relationship of high molecular weight substances such as IgM–rheumatoid factor and smaller IgG intermediate complexes in their ability to stimulate T cells.

**Dr Ziff** said that activation of T cells from lymphoblasts in the synovial membrane was probably not related to immune complexes. The fundamental question is whether some other mitogen or antigen such as EB virus stimulated this blastic transformation in the synovial membrane. However, he doubted whether the transformation was due to IgG complexes.

**Dr A. Cats: (Netherlands)** noted that complement was depressed in the synovial fluid of patients with rheumatoid arthritis but not in the circulation and he asked Dr Ziff to comment on this discrepancy.

**Dr Ziff** said that there were indeed differences between synovial fluid and serum. IgG–rheumatoid factor complexes were present in sera but their concentrations were low in comparison with those in synovial fluid. There was continual ingress of complement into the synovial effusion and he suspected that the levels of these complexes were higher in the fluid because they were made locally. A major question for the future was to try to understand this process.

# 6

# Future trends in anti-rheumatic drugs

E. C. HUSKISSON (UK)

The past few years have seen definite improvements in anti-inflammatory drugs. There are more compounds available. There are drugs which are much safer and better tolerated than the older anti-inflammatory drugs like aspirin. There are drugs which are much more convenient than aspirin, some of which can be taken as a single daily dose. There are drugs which act on some aspect of the disease process in rheumatoid arthritis and may alter the outcome of the disease. There are drugs for gout which make the management of this disease relatively easy and very successful. The future will certainly bring more drugs, although many will be similar to existing compounds. It would be good to see some different drugs. It would also be good to have treatments for osteoarthritis and rheumatoid arthritis which were as effective as the current treatment of gout.

**Non-steroidal anti-inflammatory drugs**

It does not take a crystal ball to show that many more new anti-inflammatory drugs will be made available over the course of the next few years. This is amply justified by individual variation in response. It is now clear that individual variation is the major determinant both of the effectiveness of non-steroidal anti-inflammatory drugs and also of their toxicity. The mechanism of this individual variation remains unexplained. It is more difficult to predict whether the newer, non-steroidal anti-inflammatory drugs will be any better than those which are currently available. There have been two major changes in the group over the past few years. The first was the arrival of drugs like the propionic acid derivatives which were substantially better tolerated. The second was the arrival of drugs which were substantially more convenient. These include a number of compounds which can be taken either once or twice daily.

Recommendations about the number of doses required per day have been based on the pharmacokinetics of individual compounds. Flurbiprofen and indomethacin with short half-lives are given 3–4 times daily. Piroxicam and benoxaprofen with long half-lives are given once daily. It must, however, be said that pharmacokinetic studies have been disappointing in relation to drugs in this class. There is clearly no relationship between the duration of action of indomethacin and its plasma half-life. A large dose at night has a large effect in the following morning and lasts until the following afternoon, but plasma concentrations have fallen to a very low level within 12 h. Thus, there is no correlation between plasma levels of these compounds and their effects and plasma levels do not explain individual variation in response. It may therefore be that even drugs with short plasma half-lives can be given once or twice daily and it is unwise to predict the effects of drugs on the basis of their plasma levels.

Better understanding of the complexities of the pathways of prostaglandin synthetase is likely to lead to compounds with actions on different prostaglandin intermediates. It is more difficult to predict whether such compounds will be any different in man. It could be that compounds with a predominantly cellular action have advantages over inhibitors of the cyclo-oxygenase or lipoxygenase pathways. It remains disappointing that no anti-inflammatory drug has been shown to influence the outcome of a chronic inflammatory process like rheumatoid arthritis. This statement is based upon clinical impression and no formal trials have yet been carried out.

The proliferation of compounds with essentially similar actions must eventually end, although further small improvements can no doubt be made. With more new compounds, some old drugs must be discarded and some must be used more selectively for those indications in which they have particular advantages.

**Corticosteroids**

The limitations of corticosteroids are well known. They cause Cushing's disease. There is nevertheless one difference between their action and that of the non-steroidal anti-inflammatory drugs. Corticosteroids are universally effective in diseases like polymyalgia rheumatica and display no individual variation in response. For this reason alone, it might be worth persuing a class of non-steroidal anti-inflammatory drugs with steroid-like activity. Individual variation is a problem.

**Analgesics**

The limitations of analgesics are also well known. The absence of anti-inflammatory activity is an obvious disadvantage in a group of diseases in which inflammation is prominent. These compounds are also taken in excess for suicidal purposes and many, including aspirin, paracetamol and drugs which depress the central nervous system, are dangerous. It seems that the non-steroidal anti-inflammatory drugs may be safer in this respect. For example, propionic acid derivatives make good analgesics and may be safer for the suicidal. It is likely that new compounds will emerge with better analgesic potency but less anti-inflammatory activity and these may be still more useful as simple analgesics.

**Specific treatment for rheumatoid arthritis**

Further progress is likely in the field of drugs with specific actions in rheumatoid arthritis. These compounds act slowly, improve extra-articular features of the disease as well as joint symptoms and signs, reduce erythrocyte sedimentation rate (ESR) and rheumatoid factor and may alter the outcome of the disease. Penicillamine and immunosuppressive drugs certainly slow down the rate of radiological progression. There is unfortunately no agreement as to what these drugs should be called. They are variously called *long-acting, slow-acting, remission-inducing, basic, specific, second-, third-* or *fourth-line drugs*. None of these titles is perfect and the nature and the mode of action of these compounds remain completely unknown. It is not inappropriate to follow an old pharmacological principle and call them *penicillamine-like drugs*. Penicillamine remains the leader of the field. It has advantages over gold, immunosuppressive agents and chloroquine and none of the newer arrivals in the field (like levamisole) have been shown to be superior to penicillamine. Clinicians have become much more skilful with penicillamine and an optimal dosage schedule has probably at last been reached. Nevertheless, there is room for more studies of different dosage regimes and particularly of the toxic manifestations. Many of these, like the proteinuria and drug-induced systemic lupus erythematosus, seem to be mediated by immune complexes. A study of the mechanisms of these adverse reactions could lead to ways of avoiding them. It could also lead to a greater understanding of the fundamental actions of this compound in rheumatoid arthritis. This is particularly so since these side effects are in many cases disease related. Patients with rheumatoid arthritis seem to be much more liable to various complications than patients with other diseases.

Patients with rheumatoid arthritis also respond quite differently to levamisole and two serious complications, neutropenia and vasculitis, make it unwise to give this drug on a 3- or 7-day regime. Treatment with a single weekly dose appears to be much safer, although intermittent treatment brings a new problem. There is a significant incidence of febrile reactions which occur after each individual dose. Nevertheless, levamisole is comparable in potency to penicillamine and represents another possible alternative.

New thiol compounds are likely to receive further attention. 5-thiopyridoxine has been shown to be effective in rheumatoid arthritis and potentially a useful alternative to penicillamine. The disulphide compound, pyritinol, has also been shown to be effective and these compounds may be substantially less toxic than penicillamine.

It is still not clear whether anti-inflammatory drugs can also show penicillamine-like activity. Two clinical trials showed such an action with alclofenac while one failed to show such an effect. One trial has shown this type of effect with fenclofenac and this awaits confirmation. Clozic certainly appears to have a rather different action from most anti-inflammatory drugs. If these properties can be confirmed, this represents a useful class of compound for further development.

**Specific therapy for osteoarthritis**

Two features have changed in osteoarthritis. First is a recognition of the importance of inflammation and the role of anti-inflammatory drugs in controlling the symptoms of the disease. They do more than simply relieving pain. Second is the realization that there are fundamental biochemical abnormalities in cartilage which might be amenable to drug therapy. It is impossible at the present time to identify the primary biochemical abnormality of the disease. It could be related to mineral deposition or proteoglycan formation or could be something quite different. These mechanisms are nevertheless clues for the development of penicillamine-like drugs for this common and important disease. The actions of diphosphonates have been well established in animal models of inflammation and it remains to see their effects in osteoarthritis. They should have action in diseases associated with hydroxyapatite formation. It does not seem unreasonable to expect new drugs for pyrophosphate deposition, just as we have allopurinol for urate deposition.

As mechanisms for other diseases become clearer, we should expect the development of new drugs with quite different actions which will be appropriate for particular diseases. It does not seem that the rheumatic diseases will be solved by attacking the final common pathway: inflammation. It seems that each will need its own magic bullet, acting on a more fundamental aspect of the disease process.

# Discussion

**A. W. Ford-Hutchinson (UK)** May I suggest a possible mechanism of action for alclofenac. Our metabolic studies on the drug have shown that it produced an epoxide intermediate which was a powerful alkylating agent. It might also give rise to one of the active metabolites of cyclophosphamide. In addition to its anti-inflammatory action it therefore appeared to be exerting a mild immunosuppressive effect.

**Dr P. Gordon: (USA)** Thymopoietin should probably be distinguished from levamisole in that the latter is an immunomodulator and not an immunopotentiator. There is considerable evidence for striking immunosuppression induced by levamisole as a result of enhanced T suppressor function. The suggestion has been put forward that levamisole's action is due to non-specific stimulation of an inadequately functioning region of the lymphocyte system. My group have shown that mice treated with ether anaesthesia during immunization with human erythrocytes showed a considerable cellular immune response which levamisole suppressed. I am not sure what effect thymopoietin has, but I understand it to be a stimulator of T cell function, in contrast to levamisole, which had clearly immunosuppressive properties but without the total effects exerted by cytotoxic agents.

**Dr Tonnesson: (Denmark)** Could synovectomy alter the course of rheumatoid arthritis.

A large trial in UK showed that synovectomy of the knee did not appear to exert any long term effects. One study has shown that synovectomy of the metacarpal joints in the hand had some effect on the disease, but I think that its influence was probably small.

# Section II
# Review of Current Developments

CHAIRMAN: J. L. Turk
CO-CHAIRMAN: E. Munthe

# 7

# A review of mechanism of action of steroid and non-steroid anti-inflammatory drugs

S. TSURUFUJI, K. SUGIO, H. SATO AND K. OHUCHI (JAPAN)

The present article will review our work on the anti-exudative action of steroidal and non-steroidal anti-inflammatory drugs. In the light of present knowledge, both steroidal and non-steroidal anti-inflammatory drugs appear to inhibit production of pro-inflammatory prostaglandins (PGs) in a variety of biological systems involving cultured cells and isolated tissues maintained under appropriate incubation conditions[1–6]. Glucocorticoids appear to inhibit PG production or its release from the cells by suppression of the action of phospholipase $A_2$ or by some unknown mechanisms[7–9]. Non-steroidal anti-inflammatory drugs such as indomethacin block cyclo-oxygenase[10,11]. However, it remains to be established whether decrease in the production or release of prostaglandins takes place at the inflammatory locus in parallel with the inhibition of the vascular permeability response.

Apart from the prostaglandin hypothesis, a glucocorticoid dependent gene expression hypothesis has also been investigated as a possible mechanism of the anti-exudative effect of the steroid anti-inflammatory drugs.

## Carrageenin air pouch inflammation

*Materials and methods*

In order to investigate the above question, an experimental model of inflammation, the carrageenin air pouch method was established in our laboratory[12,13] (Figure 7.1). Male Sprague-Dawley strain rats 6 weeks old were injected with 8.0 ml of air s.c. on the back. 24 h later, 4.0 ml of 2% carrageenin (Seakem No. 202) solution in 0.9% NaCl was injected into the air sac so formed, in order to induce an inflammatory response. At any time after the injection of carrageenin, exudate fluid in the carrageenin air pouch can be withdrawn, in order to measure vascular permeability in the inflammation locus or to determine PG levels in the exudate. For the measurement of vascular permeability, rats were injected i.v. with 1.0 $\mu$Ci of [$^{131}$ I]-human serum albumin and 30 min later exudate fluids were withdrawn to measure radioactivity[13]. Determination of the concentration of PGE in the exudate samples was performed by radio-immunoassay [14,15]. Drugs to be tested were administered through a stomach tube as suspensions in distilled water. Control animals were given the vehicle only. In the case of dexamethasone treatment, the drug was administered 2 h prior to the application of the inflammatory agent carrageenin and radio-iodinated serum albumin was injected i.v. 2.5 h after commencement of the inflammation. In the experiments using indomethacin, the drug was administered 4 h after the injection of carrageenin and radioactive serum albumin was injected i.v. 3.5 h after administration of the drug. In each case animals were sacrificed 30 min after the injection of the labeled albumin by cutting the carotid artery under light ether anaesthesia. The entire exudate fluid was collected to measure leakage of the radioactive serum albumin into the whole exudate fluid. The PGE level in the exudate was also assayed.

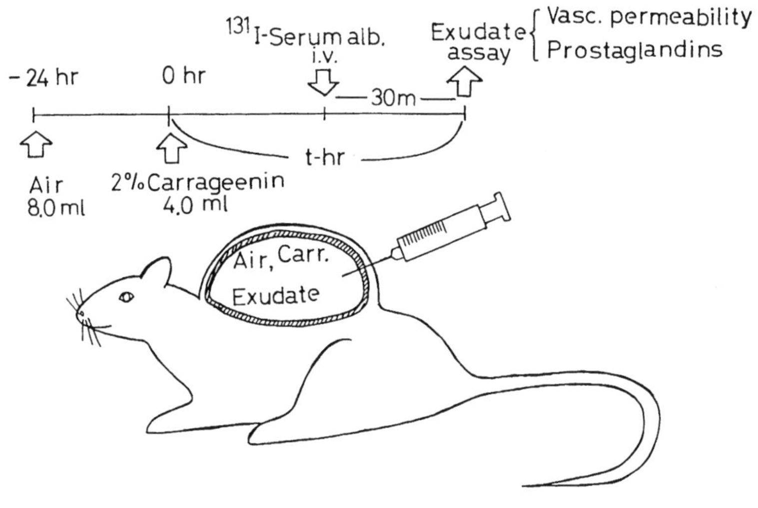


**Figure 7.1** Carrageenin air pouch inflammation. Air is injected s.c. into the backs of rats. Carrageenin solution is injected into the air sac 24 h later. At any time after the injection of the carrageenin, inflammatory exudate fluid in the carrageenin air pouch can be sampled to measure vascular permeability and prostaglandin levels in the exudate. The vascular permeability is determined in terms of the leakage of [$^{131}$I]human serum albumin injected i.v.

## RESULTS

The results are summarized in Figure 7.2. Both indomethacin and dexame-

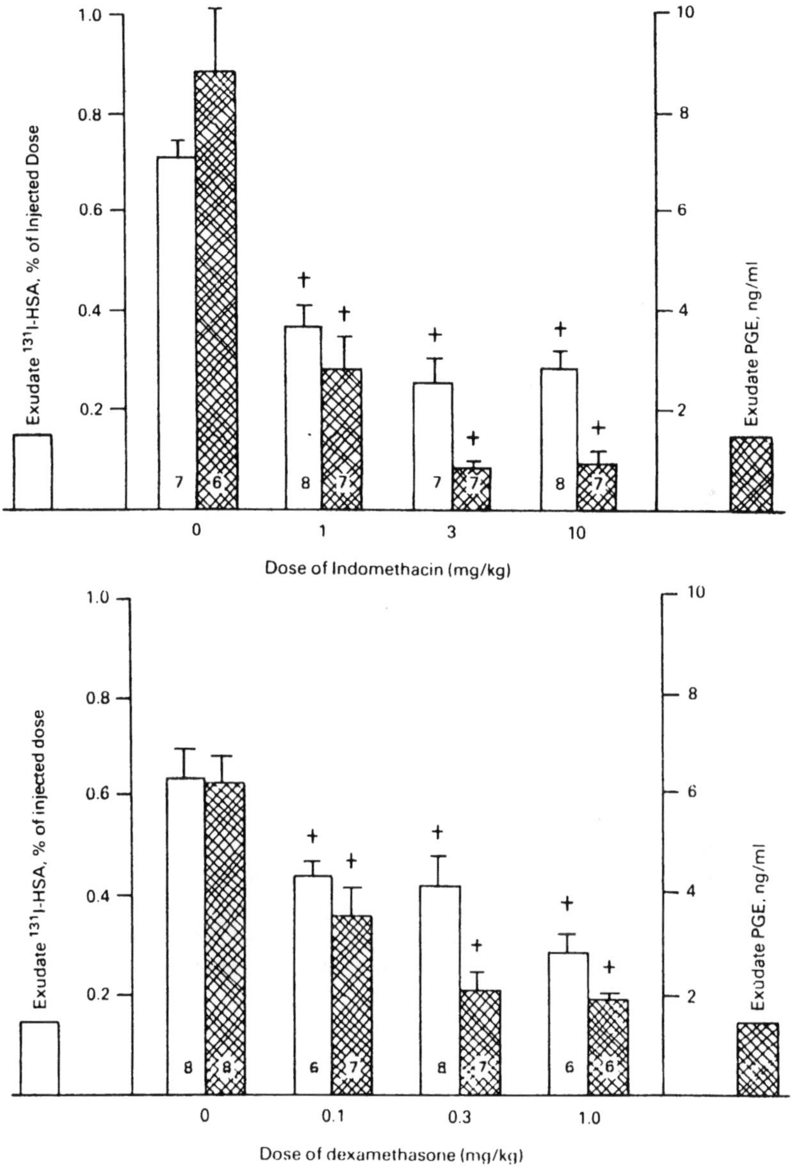


**Figure 7.2** Effect of the drugs on PGE level in the exudate and on vascular permeability in the acute stage of the carrageenin air pouch inflammation (a) indomethacin; (b) dexamethasone). The exudate fluid was taken 8 h after the injection of carrageenin in the case of indomethacin and 3 h for dexamethasone. The vertical bars show SEM. Statistically significant differences from the controls are indicated + ($p < 0.005$). Numbers in the columns indicate the numbers of the rats used

thasone exerted a dose-dependent inhibitory effect on the PGE levels in the exudate. Vascular permeability in the inflammatary locus was also inhibited in parallel with the reduction of PGE levels in both the dexamethasone and indomethacin groups. These results appear to indicate that steroidal and non-steroidal anti-inflammatory drugs share a common mechanism responsible for their anti-exudative effect in the acute phase of the carrageenin induced air pouch inflammation. In other words, the concept that inhibitory effects on the production of pro-inflammatory substances such as E prostaglandins are responsible for the anti-exudative action of both the steroidal and non-steroidal anti-inflammatory drugs appears to be acceptable.

**Effects of anti-inflammatory drugs on the vascular permeability response induced by chemical mediators**

In this series of experiments male DDY mice 6–7 weeks old were used. In order to provoke vascular permeability responses, mice were injected in their right footpad with a chemical mediator such as serotonin, bradykinin or PGE, or a mixture of PGE and bradykinin and 5 $\mu$l of Tyrode's solution. Tyrode's solution was injected into the left footpad as a control. These chemical mediators produced rapidly growing footpad oedema which reached maximum swelling within 12 min. Thereafter the tissue oedema declined quickly and disappeared by 2 h. Tyrode's solution did not produce any tissue swelling at the end of the 12 min period. Footpad thickness was measured by a dial gauge calliper calibrated in 1/100 mm graduations. Difference in the footpad thickness between the right and left foot was taken as an index of the footpad reaction.

In order to evaluate inhibitory effects of indomethacin and dexamethasone against vascular permeability responses induced by various chemical mediators, indomethacin was administered orally and dexamethasone was injected s.c. before the injection of the mediators in the footpads. On the basis of appropriate preliminary experiments, time course studies were performed in an attempt to determine a suitable time interval between dexamethasone treatment (at the dose of 0.5 mg/kg s.c. in 2.5% ethanol solution) and injection of serotonin or bradykinin in the footpad. In accordance with the results summarized in Figure 7.3, dexamethasone was administered 3 or 4 h before the injection of various chemical mediators in the footpad (unless otherwise stated) in all the following experiments. In the case of indomethacin, the drug was administered orally 1 h before the injection of the chemical mediators, in accordance with pharmacokinetic data in the literature[16], in an attempt to produce a maximum blood concentration of the drug coincidentally with the production of the vascular permeability response.

As indicated in Figure 7.4, indomethacin failed to inhibit the vascular permeability responses induced by serotonin, bradykinin, PGE and a mixture of PGE, and bradykinin, even if a dose as high as 30 mg/kg was applied. On the other hand, dexamethasone brought about a dose-dependent suppression of

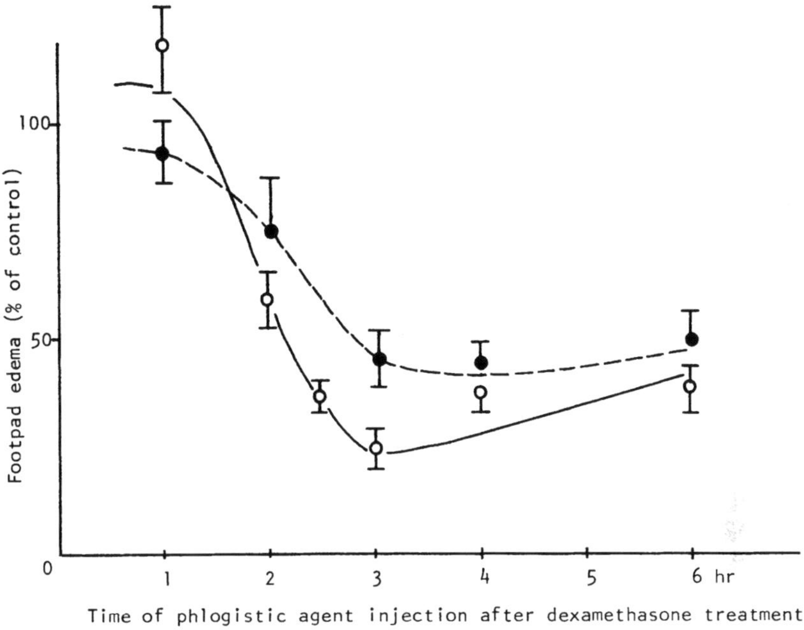


**Figure 7.3** Time course studies on the appearance of the anti-exudative effects of dexamethasone in bradykinin- and serotonin-induced footpad oedema in mice. Dexamethasone was injected s.c. at time 0. Footpad oedema was measured 12 min after the injection of bradykinin (3.0 μg) or serotonin (0.3 μg) into the footpad
●--------● Bradykinin ○———○ Serotonin

the footpad oedema with all of the inflammatory agents investigated, as shown in Figure 7.5.

It is evident, therefore, that anti-inflammatory steroids have the capability of suppressing the pro-inflammatory actions of various chemical mediators, in addition to their inhibitory potency against the production of prostaglandins, whereas indomethacin is unable to counteract chemical mediators.

Majno *et al*[17] indicated that histamine, serotonin and bradykinin provoke vascular permeability responses by inducing contraction of vascular endothelial cells in the venules. Contraction of the endothelial cells makes their intercullular gaps expand so as to cause plasma exudation and resultant tissue oedema. Therefore, the target for the anti-exudative action of the steroids against serotonin- and bradykinin-induced oedema appears to be vascular endothelial cells in the venules.

## Requirement for gene expression in the anti-exudative action of glucocorticoids

In respect to the mechanisms underlying a variety of physiological effects of

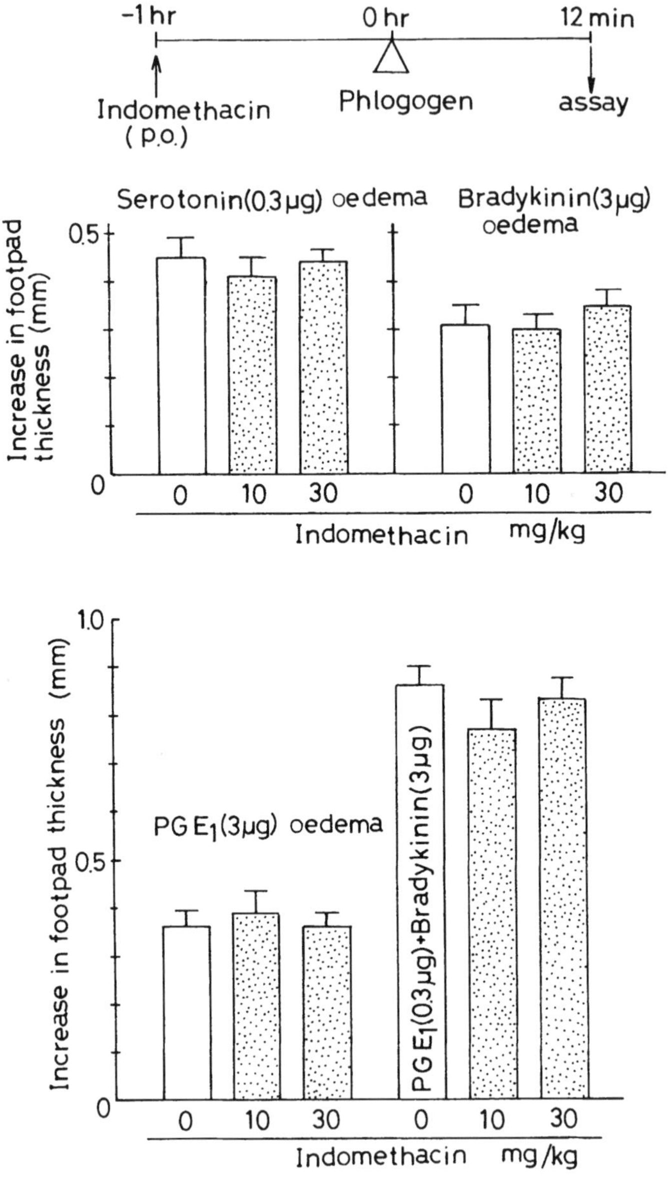


**Figure 7.4** Effects of indomethacin on the footpad oedema provoked by serotonin, bradykinin, $PGE_1$ or a mixture of $PGE_1$ and bradykinin

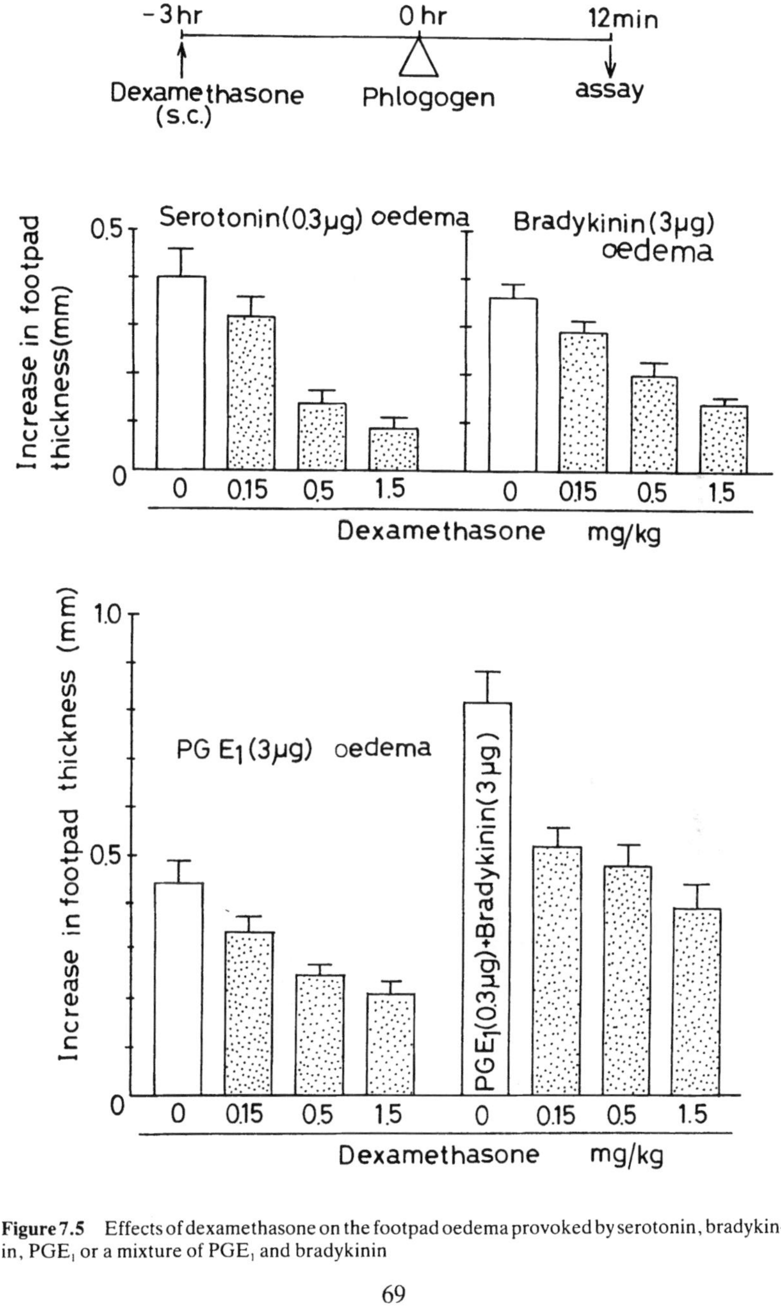


**Figure 7.5** Effects of dexamethasone on the footpad oedema provoked by serotonin, bradykinin, $PGE_1$ or a mixture of $PGE_1$ and bradykinin

various steroid hormones, sex steroids, mineralocorticoids and glucocorticoids, the roles of gene expression and steroid hormone receptors are generally recognized, on the basis of a large body of experimental evidence to be of considerable importance[18–20]. However, a review article on peripheral effects of glucocorticoids[21] suggests that it is still unclear whether the pharmacological actions of the glucocorticoids, such as the anti-inflammatory action, require binding of the steroid to the cytoplasmic receptor with a series of subsequent processes for the activation of specific genetic codes.

Recent studies on the mechanisms underlying the inhibitory action of glucocorticoids on prostaglandin production have revealed that RNA and protein synthesis inhibitors such as actinomycin D, puromycin and cycloheximide interfere with the inhibitory effect of such steroids on prostaglandin production[22–24]. The induction by steroids of inhibitory proteins or peptides capable of inhibiting the production of prostaglandin in antigen challenged lungs and activated macrophages had also been suggested[23,24]. However, as already noted, dexamethasone has the capability of inhibiting bradykinin-, serotonin- and prostaglandin-induced exudative responses, although indomethacin a potent inhibitor of prostaglandin synthesis, fails to inhibit the exudative processes induced by these chemical mediators. It has also been reported frequently in the literature that indomethacin is unable to suppress vascular permeability responses induced by bradykinin and serotonin[25–28]. It is therefore reasonable to assume that mechanisms other than inhibition of the production of prostaglandin should be responsible for the anti-exudative actions of anti-inflammatory steroids in bradykinin- and serotonin-induced vascular permeability responses. On the basis of these considerations and assuming that the target cells for the anti-exudative actions of the steroids are indeed vascular endothelial cells in the venules, we have attempted to test the gene expression hypothesis for the mechanism of the anti-exudative action of dexamethasone in bradykinin- and serotonin- induced footpad oedema in mice.

Figure 7.6 shows that steroid hormone receptors are found in the cytoplasm in a variety of target cells when they are not occupied by the hormone. After binding of the receptors with the hormone, the hormone-receptor complex is activated to enter the nucleus. In the case of the tissue culture hepatoma cells investigated intensely by Tomkins *et al.*[29,30] anti-glucocorticoid compounds such as progesterone, 17α-methyltestosterone and fluoxymesterone were found to interfere with the appearance of the glucocorticoid effect by a competitive inhibition against the binding of the hormone with its cytoplasmic receptor.

After the hormone–receptor complex is translocated from the cytoplasm into the nucleus, the complex binds to the nuclear chromatin, so as to induce transcription and production of hormone specific messenger RNAs[19]. As a consequence, hormone specific proteins synthesized on polyribosomes through translation of specific mRNAs exert hormone specific physiological

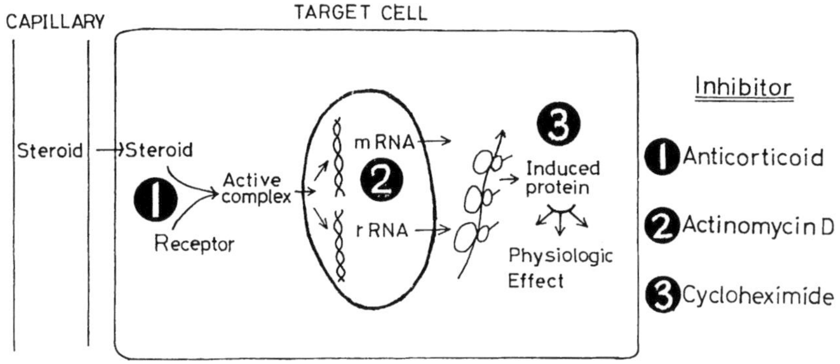


**Figure 7.6** General model for the mechanism of steroid hormones and interference by anti-glucocorticoids, actinomycin D and cycloheximide with the physiological effects of glucocorticoid hormones

effects. Actinomycin D, as an inhibitor of DNA dependent RNA synthesis, and cycloheximide or puromycin, as inhibitors of protein synthesis, have therefore been widely used in order to block manifestation of the physiological effects of various steroid hormones[19]. Such blockade to the appearance of hormone actions is generally accepted as evidence to indicate a requirement for gene expression in these hormone actions. Experiments involving these concepts were performed in our laboratory using:

(1) Progesterone, 17α-methyltestosterone and fluoxymesterone as anti-glucocorticoids in an attempt to interfere with binding of the anti-inflammatory steroid to its hypothetical cytoplasmic receptor.

(2) Actinomycin D in an attempt to block DNA-dependent RNA synthesis.

(3) Cycloheximide to block the synthesis of hypothetical anti-inflammatory proteins[31,32].

*Blockade by anti-glucocorticoids, actinomycin D and cycloheximide of the anti-exudative effects of dexamethasone in serotonin- and bradykinin-induced footpad oedema in mice.*

Following the findings of Tomkins *et al.* in hepatoma tissue culture cells[29,30], the three steroidal compounds progesterone, 17α-methyltestosterone and fluoxymesterone were also selected as anti-glucocorticoids in the present experiments. In addition, androstenedione was also tested as an inactive steroid control[29,30]. All test compounds were administered s.c. in suspensions in sesame oil 1 h before s.c. injection of dexamethasone. Bradykinin or serotonin was injected in the footpad of mice 3 h after the application of dexamethasone and footpad oedema was assayed 12 min after the injection of each inflammatory agent. The results are summarized in Table 7.1. In such experimental conditions all three anti-glucocorticoid compounds effectively neutralized the anti-exudative action of dexamethasone, while androstenedione, which was reported by Tomkins to be an inactive compound was also inert in the present biological systems.

**Table 7.1** Effects of various non-corticoid steroids on the anti-exudative action of dexamethasone in bradykinin- and serotonin-induced footpad œdema in mice

| *Treatment** (*s.c.*) | *Footpad œdema* | | *Time of each treatment before inflammatory injection (h)* |
|---|---|---|---|
| | *Bradykinin* (% of control) | *Serotin* (% of control) | |
| None (control) | 100 | 100 | — |
| Dexamethasone (0.5 mg/kg) alone | 45.0 | 34.2 | 3 |
| Progesterone (100 mg/kg) | | | 4 |
| Dexamethasone (0.5 mg/kg) | 87.1 | 65.8 | 3 |
| Methyltestosterone (100 mg/kg) | | | 4 |
| Dexamethasone (0.5 mg/kg) | 87.8 | 73.8 | 3 |
| Fluoxymesterone (100 mg/kg) | | | 4 |
| Dexamethasone (0.5 mg/kg) | | 71.4 | 3 |
| Androstenedione (200 mg/kg) | | | 4 |
| Dexamethasone (0.5mg/kg) | 47.1 | 36.5 | 3 |

*Each non-corticoid steroid alone did not cause any significant change in footpad œdema.
Non-corticoid steroids were injected 1 h before dexamethasone injection. Footpad œdema was provoked 3 h after dexamethasone treatment by subplanter injection of bradykinin (3 $\mu$g) or serotonin (0.3 $\mu$g) and assayed 12 min later.

In addition to the studies with anti-glucocorticoids, the effects of the RNA synthesis inhibitor actinomycin D and the protein synthesis inhibitor cycloheximide on the anti-exudative actions of dexamethasone were also investigated. Actinomycin D or cycloheximide was injected twice, at the same time as the dexamethasone injection and then 1.5 h later, in an attempt to maintain their inhibitory effects for at least 3 h after the injection of dexamethasone. Bradykinin or serotonin was also injected into the footpad of mice 3 h after the application of dexamethasone and footpad oedema was again assayed 12 min after the injection of each of these inflammatory agents. The results are summarized in Table 7.2. Both actinomycin D and cycloheximide completely blocked the anti-exudative actions of dexamethasone.

*Time relationships in the effects of anti-glucocorticoids, actinomycin D and cycloheximide on the anti-exudative actions of dexamethasone*

The finding that anti-glucocorticoids, actinomycin D and cycloheximide have the capability, in appropriate situations, of blocking the anti-exudative

**Table 7.2** Blockade by actinomycin D and cycloheximide of anti-exudative action of dexamethasone in bradykinin- and serotonin-induced footpad œdema in mice

| *Treatment** (*s.c.*) | *Footpad œdema* *Bradykinin* (% of control) | *Serotonin* (% of control) |
|---|---|---|
| None (control) | 100 | 100 |
| Dexamethasone (0.5 mg/kg) alone | 34.1 | 36.2 |
| Actinomycin D (1 mg/kgX2) Dexamethasone (0.5 mg/kg) | 90.2 | 100.0 |
| Cycloheximide (6 mg/kgX2) Dexamethasone (0.5 mg/kg) | 109.4 | 95.6 |

*Actinomycin D alone or cycloheximide alone did not cause any significant change in the footpad œdema.
Actinomycin D or cycloheximide were administered s.c. at the time of and 1.5 h after the injection of dexamethasone, and footpad œdema was provoked 3 h after dexamethasone treatment as described in Table 7.1.

actions of dexamethasone is consistent with the concept that the anti-exudative effect of the glucocorticoid depends not only upon the binding of the corticoid to its receptor but also upon DNA-dependent RNA synthesis and new protein synthesis. This suggests a role for glucocorticoid-specific gene expression in the manifestation of the anti-exudative action of the corticosteroid. If we assume the validity of the gene expression hypothesis in the anti-exudative effect of the steroid, then the time course of the manifestation of the steroid effect appears of great significance (Figure 7.3). It seemed unlikely that a hypothetical anti-inflammatory protein would already have been synthesized at 1 h after the application of dexamethasone, since the anti-exudative action has not appeared by that time. On the other hand, such a hypothetical anti-inflammatory protein does appear to have been synthesized by 3 h after the application of the steroid. In good agreement with this concept is the fact that treatment with cycloheximide 1 h after dexamethasone blocked the steroid action, while cycloheximide at 3 h failed to block the anti-exudative action of dexamethasone (Table 7.3). All of these experimental results appear to indicate that glucocorticoid receptors and glucocorticoid stimulation of gene expression play essential roles in the manifestation of the anti-exudative actions of dexamethasone.

In marked contrast to the case of cycloheximide, application of anti-glucocorticoids 1 h after the injection of dexamethasone was too late to block the anti-exudative effect of the steroid as shown in Table 7.3. Such observations appear to indicate that nuclear binding of dexamethasone would have already occurred within 1 h after the injection, although an anti-inflammatory protein would have not been produced in any significant quantity. This appears consistent with the finding that specific nuclear binding of steroids can occur even within 5 min and events subsequent to the binding are mainly responsible for the time lag in the manifestation of glucocorticoid responses[18].

**Table 7.3** Time relationships in the effects of anti-glucocorticoids, actinomycin D and cycloheximide on the anti-exudative action of dexamethasone against bradykinin and serotonin œdema in the footpads of mice

| *Treatment** (*s.c*) | *Time of each treatment after dexamethasone treatment* (h) | *Footpad œdema* *Bradykinin* (% of control) | *Serotonin* (% of control) |
|---|---|---|---|
| None (control) | — | 100 | 100 |
| Dexamethasone (0.5 mg/kg) alone | 0 | 33.3 | 31.4 |
| Dexamethasone (0.5 mg/kg)<br>Cycloheximide (3 mg/kg) | 0<br>1 | 87.9 | 93.6 |
| Dexamethasone (0.5 mg/kg)<br>Cycloheximide (3 mg/kg) | 0<br>3 | 36.4 | 36.1 |
| Dexamethasone (0.5 mg/kg)<br>Actinomycin D (1 mg/kg) | 0<br>3 | 41.2 | |
| Dexamethasone (0.5 mg/kg)<br>Methyltestosterone (100 mg/kg) | 0<br>1 | 47.0 | 24.4 |
| Dexamethasone (0.5 mg/kg)<br>Progesterone (100 mg/kg) | 0<br>1 | 47.0 | |

*Each non-cortisoid steroid, actinomycin D or cycloheximide alone did not cause any significant change in the footpad œdema.

### *Role of gene expression in the effect of hydrocortisone on granulomatous inflammation*

Apart from the effect of dexamethasone on the footpad oedema induced by bradykinin and serotonin, we also investigated whether induction of specific mRNA is essential for the anti-exudative action in carrageenin induced granuloma pouch inflammation in rats[33]. Actinomycin D was used as a tool for suppressing DNA dependent RNA synthesis. Puromycin was also used in order to explore whether *de novo* synthesis of a hypothetical anti-inflammatory steroid. Vascular permeability was measured as the leakage into granuloma pouch exudate of radio-iodinated human serum albumin which was injected i.v.

Significant dose-dependent inhibition of vascular permeability was observed 5 h after the local injection of hydrocortisone over the range 0.5–15 mg/kg. Time course study for the anti-exudative action of the steroid indicated that inhibition of vascular permeability was not attained until 1 h after the injection of the steroid and that the inhibition reached a statistically significant level at 2 h and was maintained for a further 10 h. When puromycin or actinomycin D was injected in the granuloma pouch prior to the application of hydrocortisone, or during the time lag of 1 h after steroid treatment, both substances almost completely blocked the anti-exudative action of the steroid. On the other hand, when puromycin or actinomycin D were administered after the appearance of the anti-exudative effect of the steroid, the vascular permeability suppressing action of the steroid was not inhibited. These results also tend to confirm the concept that gene expression under the influence of glucocorticoids is responsible for their anti-exudative action in the granulomatous stage of carrageenin air pouch inflammation.

Although indomethacin is effective in suppressing the vascular permeability response in the acute stage of this same inflammation, it is unable to suppress the exudative process in the chronic proliferative stage (granulomatous stage) of the inflammation. In addition, exudate levels of PGE, $PGE_2$, $PGF_2$, 6-$KPGF_1$ alpha and $TXB_2$ in the chronic proliferative stage have been shown to decrease with the passage of time, in spite of definite increases in the vascular permeability. These observations indicate that the mechanisms for the anti-exudative actions of the glucocorticosteroids are somewhat different from those for indomethacin.

## CONCLUSION

It is unlikely that prostaglandins play any role either in the exudative processes in the chronic proliferative stage of carrageenin air pouch inflammation or in the bradykinin- and serotonin-induced vascular permeability responses. Consequently, a hypothetical anti-inflammatory protein synthesized under the influence of the steroid is suggested as being able to exert anti-exudative effects without affecting prostaglandin production in the inflammatory tissues.

### References


1 Vane, J. R. (1971). Inhibition of prostaglandin synthesis as a mechanism of action for aspirin-like drugs. *Nature (London), New Biol.* **231,** 232

2 Flower, R., Gryglewski, R., Herbaczynska-Cedro, K. *et al.* (1972). Effects of anti-inflammatory drugs on prostaglandin biosynthesis. *Nature (London), New Biol.*, **238,** 104

3 Kantrowtiz, F., Robinson, D. R., McGaire, M. B. *et al.* (1975). Cortiscosteroids inhibit prostaglandin production by rheumatoid synovia. *Nature (London)*, **258,** 737

4 Gryglewski, R. J., Panczenko, B., Korbut, R. *et al.* (1975). Corticosteroids inhibit prostaglandin release from perfused mesenteric blood vessels of rabbit and from perfused lungs of sensitized guinea pig. *Prostaglandins*, **10,** 343

5 Tam, S., Hong, S. C. and Levine, L. (1977). Relationships, among the steroids, of anti-inflammatory properties and inhibition of prostaglandin production and arachidonic acid release by transformed mouse fibroblasts. *J. Pharmacol. Exp. Ther.* **203,** 162

6 Floman, Y. and Zor, U. (1976). Mechanism of steroid action in inflammation: inhibition of prostaglandin synthesis and release. *Prostaglandins*, **12,** 403

7 Hong, S. L. and Levine, L. (1976). Inhibition of arachidonic acid release from cells as the biochemical action of anti-inflammatory corticosteroids. *Proc. Natl. Acad. Sci. (USA)*, **73,** 1730

8 Blackwell, G. J., Flower, R. J., Nijkamp, F. P. *et al.* (1978). Phospholipase A2 activity of guinea-pig isolated perfused lungs: stimulation, and inhibition by anti-inflammatory steroids. *Br. J. Pharmacol.*, **62,** 79

9 Chang, J., Lewis, G. P. and Piper, P. J. (1977). Inhibition by glucocorticoids of prostaglandin release from adipose tissue *in vitro*. *Br. J. Pharmacol.*, **59,** 425

10 Yamamoto, S., Ogino, N., Ohki, S. *et al.* (1977). Enzymological studies on prostaglandin biosynthesis. In Karashe, N. and Fried, J. (eds.) *Biochemical Aspects of Prostaglandins and Thromboxanes*, pp. 1–13. (New York: Academic Press)

11 Hamberg, M. and Samuelsson, B. (1974). Prostaglandin endoperoxides. Novel transformations of arachidonic acid in human platelets. *Proc. Natl. Acad. Sci. (USA)*, **71,** 3400
12 Fukuhara, M. and Tsurufuji, S. (1969). The effect of locally injected anti-inflammatory drugs on the carrageenin granuloma in rats. *Biochem. Pharmacol.*, **18,** 475
13 Tsurufuji, S., Sugio, K. and Endo, Y. (1977). Inhibition of vascular permeability by cycloheximide in granulomatous inflammation. *Biochem. Pharmacol.*, **26,** 1131
14 Chang, W. C., Murota, S. and Tsurufuji, S. (1975). Contents of Prostaglandin E in the exudate of rat carrageenin granuloma. *Japan. J. Pharmacol.*, **25,** 219
15 Ohuchi, K., Sato, H. and Tsurufuji, S. (1976). The content of prostaglandin E and prostaglandin F2alpha in the exudate of carrageenin granuloma of rats. *Biochim. Biophys. Acta*, **424,** 439
16 Wiseman, E. H. (1974). Drug kinetic studies with nonsteroidal antiinflammatory agents in animals and man. In Scherrer R. A. and Whitehouse, M. W. (eds.) *Antiinflammatory Agents, Chemistry and Pharmacology*, pp. 235–243. (New York: Academic Press)
17 Majno, G., Shea, S. M. and Leventhal, M. (1969). Endothelial contraction induced by histamine-type mediators: an electron microscopic study. *J. Cell. Biol.*, **42,** 647
18 Baxter, J. D. and Forsham, P. H. (1972). Tissue effects of glucocorticoids. *Am. J. Med.*, **53,** 573
19 Chan, L. and O'Malley, B. W. (1976). Mechanism of action of the sex steroid hormones. *N. Engl. J. Med.*, **294,** 1322, 1372, 1430
20 Baxter, J. D. and Funder, J. W. (1979). Hormone receptors. *N. Engl. J. Med.*, **301,** 1149
21 Leung, K. and Munck, A. (1975). Peripheral actions of glucocorticoids. *Ann. Rev. Physiol.*, **37,** 245
22 Danon, A. and Assouline, G. (1978). Inhibition of prostaglandin biosynthesis by corticosteroids requires RNA and protein synthesis. *Nature (London)*, **273,** 552
23 Flower, R. J. and Blackwell, G. J. (1979). Anti-inflammatory steroids induce biosynthesis of a phospholipase A2 inhibitor which prevents prostaglandin generation. *Nature (London)*, **278,** 456
24 DiRosa, M. and Persico, P. (1979). Mechanism of inhibition of prostaglandin biosynthesis by hydrocortisone in rat leucocytes. *Br. J. Pharmacol.*, **66,** 161
25 Daum, A. and Römer, D. (1970). Die Wirkung von Antiphlogistica auf die durch Bradykinin induzierte Permeabilitätserhöhung in der Ratten haut und an der Rattenpfote. *Nauyn-Schmiedebergs Arch. Pharmakol.*, **266,** 313
26 Ikeda, K., Tanaka, K. and Katori, M. (1975). Potentiation of bradykinin-induced vascular permeability increase by prostaglandin E2 and arachidonic acid in rabbit skin. *Prostaglandins*, **10,** 747
27 Williams, T. J. and Peck, M. J. (1977). Role of prostaglandin-mediated vasodilation in inflammation. *Nature (London)*. **270,** 530
28 Williams, T. J. (1979). Prostaglandin $E_2$, prostaglandin $I_2$ and the vascular changes of inflammation. *Br. J. Pharmacol.*, **65,** 517
29 Samuels, H. H. and Tomkins, G. M. (1970). Relation of steroid structure to enzyme induction in hepatoma tissue culture cells. *J. Mol. Biol.*, **52,** 57
30 Rousseau, G. G., Baxter, J. D. and Tomkins, G. M. (1972). Glucocorticoid receptors: relations between steroid binding and biological effects. *J. Mol. Biol.*, **67,** 99
31 Tsurufuji, S., Sugio, K. and Takemasa, F. (1979). The role of glucocorticoid receptor and gene expression in the anti-inflammatory action of dexamethasone. *Nature (London)*, **280,** 408
32 Tsurufuji, S., Sugio, K., Takamasa, F. and Yoshizawa, S. (1980). *J. Pharmacol. Exp. Ther.* (In press)
33 Tsurufuji, S. and Kazuo, S. (1978). Molecular mechanisms in the manifestation of anti-inflammatory activity of glucocorticoids. *Eur. J. Rheumatol. Inflammation.*, **1,** 226

# Discussion

**I. F. Skidmore: (UK)** I would like to refer to results which support Dr Tsurufuji's approach. It is possible to take a range of steroids designed primarily as anti-inflammatory agents and their rank order of potency proves to be identical to a series of biological responses which include the following: vasoconstriction in man when the steroid was applied topically; anti-inflammatory action in rheumatoid arthritis; anti-inflammatory activity in rats for both acute and chronic inflammation; inhibition of neutrophil accumulation in the carboxymethyl cellulose pouch; inhibition of neutral proteinase release from mouse macrophages; inhibition of the production of thromboxane $A_2$ in infused guinea pig lung; inhibition of prostaglandin production by rheumatoid synovial cells; glycogen accumulation in mouse liver, and thymus involution in the mouse. This is very strong evidence that a common receptor is involved in all of these responses although it does not indicate that a common mechanism of action is involved. One must not automatically draw the conclusion that because the same host receptor might be involved in all of these processes then they all involved host binding in the nucleus. In other words, one must not assume that the same protein was involved in all cases. Nonetheless, although they were diverse mechanisms involved in the anti-inflammatory action of steroids, it does seem likely that they had a common action at the receptor level. Using the carboxymethyl cellulose pouch and measuring sensitivity to actinomycin D to determine the rank order correlation of a range of steroids we have also found that inhibition of neutrophil accumulation in the rat by steroids is certainly a specific receptor mediated process.

**Dr Tsurufuji** agreed that the mechanisms of anti-inflammatory action of steroids must be very diverse. So far I have only suggested that glucocorticoids differ in their anti-inflammatory action in respect to the exudative response induced by certain chemical mediators. One can only speculate, but I feel that this mechanism might have great importance and that it might at least partly explain the difference in clinical efficacy between steroid and non-steroid drugs.

**Professor C. M. Pearson: (USA)** asked whether, after the steroid sticks to the receptor in the cytoplasm, there was a breakdown of the corticosteroid so that only a portion of it entered the nucleus to exert its effect. In particular, he wondered what that portion might be.

**Dr Tsurufuji** said that he did not know.

**Dr Tonneson (Denmark)** said that Dr Tsurufuji's technique of injecting air and labelled albumin means that one must inevitably measure the product of blood flow permeability. The amount of labelled albumin would depend upon blood flow, and he wondered what was the concentration of non-labelled serum albumin in the exudate.

**Dr Tsururfuji** had not determined this quantity. In order to investigate the effects of dexamethasone or indomethacin it had not proved necessary to determine the absolute concentration of plasma protein in the exudate. In addition, determination of the non-labelled albumin concentration was of little value. He measured the influence of anti-inflammatory drugs on vascular permeability 30 min after albumin injection and during this time no change in plasma albumin concentration in the exudate would occur.

**Professor A. Bennett (UK)** noted that Dr Tsurufuji appeared to obtain an increase in footpad thickness 1 h after dexamethasone injection in his serotonin experiments. He wondered if this was evidence of a biphasic response.

**Dr Tsurufuji** said that this was due to experimental variation in the serotonin results. Experiments with bradykinin showed no such variation.

# 8

# Review of immunotherapy in rheumatoid arthritis

E. M. VEYS AND H. MIELANTS (BELGIUM)

In the present state of knowledge about the immunopathology of rheumatoid arthritis (RA), the failure to eliminate an unknown antigen has been postulated in several models. A defective macrophage function might be the cause of the persistence of non-degradable bacterial fragments (peptidoglycan) in the macrophage after successful phagocytosis and so produce a paradoxical hyperinflammatory response due to the continued existence of a positive tendency to inflammation[1]. In the infective theories, there is either short-term infection altering cells or tissue antigens and the infective agent then disappears leaving a self-perpetuating auto-immune response to altered self-antigens, or the infection can be persistent and is then responsible for perpetuation of pathology.

In the 'target' model, the virus infects joint cells. The resulting cell damage, or alteration of cell function, together with an intense but finally ineffective immunological reaction against the infected or altered cell, constitutes the disease. Another possibility is that the virus infects and alters the function of the effector cells of the immune system, T or B lymphocytes or macrophages. Alteration of B cells leads to excessive production of antibodies, and infection of T cells results in a loss of regulation of B-cell functions[2]. If the disordered inflammatory events are considered to be a failure of antigen elimination, new directions for therapeutic intervention in RA become justified and immunomodulating agents such as levamisole have to be investigated for effectiveness in this disease.

## LEVAMISOLE PHARMACOLOGY

In therapeutic doses of 2.5 mg/kg, levamisole restores to normal functions of T lymphocytes, polymorphonuclear and mononuclear phagocytes, especially when these functions are initially impaired. These effects have been shown by *in vivo* as well as *in vitro* studies[3]. Levamisole also restores delayed skin hypersensitivity in anergic patients and cell-mediated responses in elderly subjects and in patients with some immune deficiency diseases as well as in animals receiving immunosuppressive therapy. The activity of the drug in adjuvant arthritis in rats has been studied in detail by Trabert *et al*[4]. The data are contradictory to those mentioned above, since levamisole accentuates the severity of the disease. In this model levamisole consequently not only restores impaired cellular immune responses but also enhances an already activated system. The schedule used is important, since the authors found that continuous therapy may result in a loss of efficacy in adjuvant arthritis. These data may certainly be of paramount importance in the future to explain some kind of responses in patients with RA.

Levamisole seems to have no direct effect on B lymphocytes, but in case of increased B-cell activity it may be reduced to normal as is shown by decreased numbers of Ig-bearing or EAC-rosette forming cells and the normalization of antibody levels. This action seems to result from an improvement in the regulatory function of T cells on B cells, and a stimulatory effect upon T suppressor cells. *In vivo* the drug is capable of restoring thymic function in nude and thymectomized mice and in children with primary immune deficiencies[5]. Finally, levamisole has a favourable influence on the course of autoimmune diseases in animals. It can, for example, prevent or delay the development of disease in young NZB/NZW mice. In advanced diseases it is less efficient but maintains the remission induced by cyclophosphamide[6].

## CLINICAL ACTIVITY IN RA

Although the multitude of trials performed with levamisole in RA were useful and necessary to establish the activity of the drug in this disease, it must be realized that the majority of information available about activity and toxicity in the short term comes from the EULAR trial[7] and from the *Multicenter Study*[8].

In the EULAR Study, two dose schedules for levamisole (150 mg either 3 days per week or 7 days per week) were compared with each other and with placebo over a period of 6 months. The total number of subjects amounted to 110 controls, 124 patients on 7 days per week and 129 patients on 3 days per week. Statistical analysis showed no difference between the two dosage regimens of levamisole for all variables investigated. After 3 months, patients treated with levamisole had improved significantly more than the placebo group. At 6 months the effect was even more pronounced and a highly significant difference was observed for all variables measured (Figure 8.1).

In this trial hardly any factors influencing responsiveness or adverse reac-

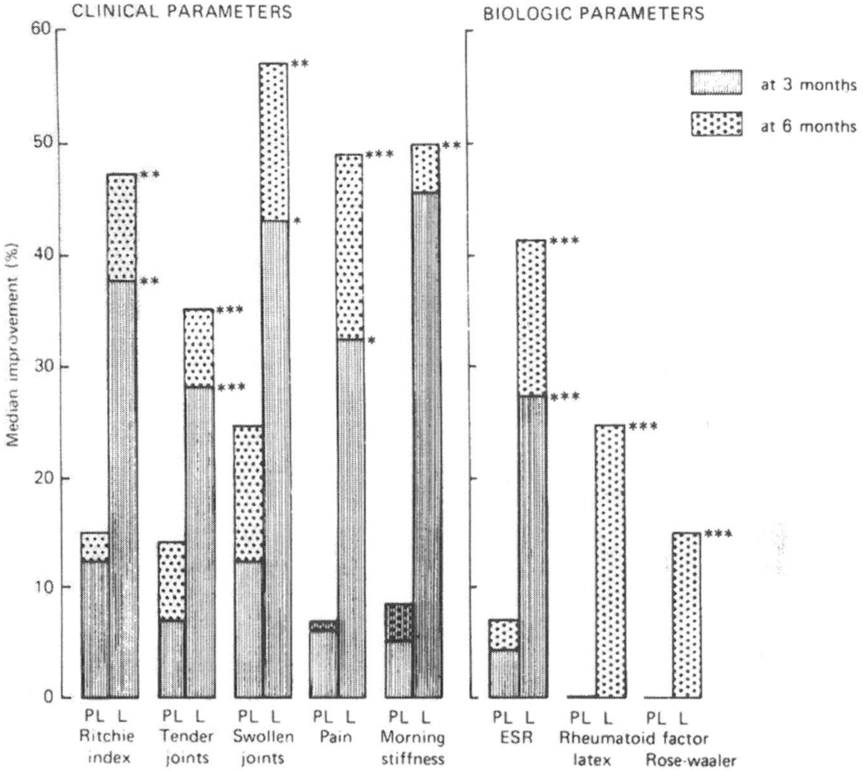


**Figure 8.1** Median improvement of clinical and biological parameters observed in the EULAR Trial (PL = placebo; L = levamisole). The asterisks indicate the degree of statistical significance

tions were found except that improvement occurred significantly more frequently in patients with few radiological changes and patients who had never received basic anti-rheumatic therapy than in patients with advanced disease and who had previously been treated with other basic anti-rheumatic drugs. As will be stressed later, major side effects occurred at the same frequency with both regimens used in the EULAR Study. Serious idiosyncratic reactions, particularly agranulocytosis, limit uncontrolled use of levamisole in practice in the conditions used in this trial.

After Di Perri *et al.* [8] showed that a once weekly dose of levamisole restores reduced E rosette lymphocytes in RA for 5–6 days and after Veys and Mielants[9] showed that this treatment schedule allowed early detection of agranulocytosis, a new Multicenter Trial[10] was started to evaluate the effectiveness of a single weekly treatment with 50 mg (43 patients) or 150 mg (44 patients) levamisole in RA patients. The design of the study, patient selection and data analysis were essentially the same as in the EULAR Study. After 3 months both groups had significantly improved to a comparable degree (Figure 8.2).

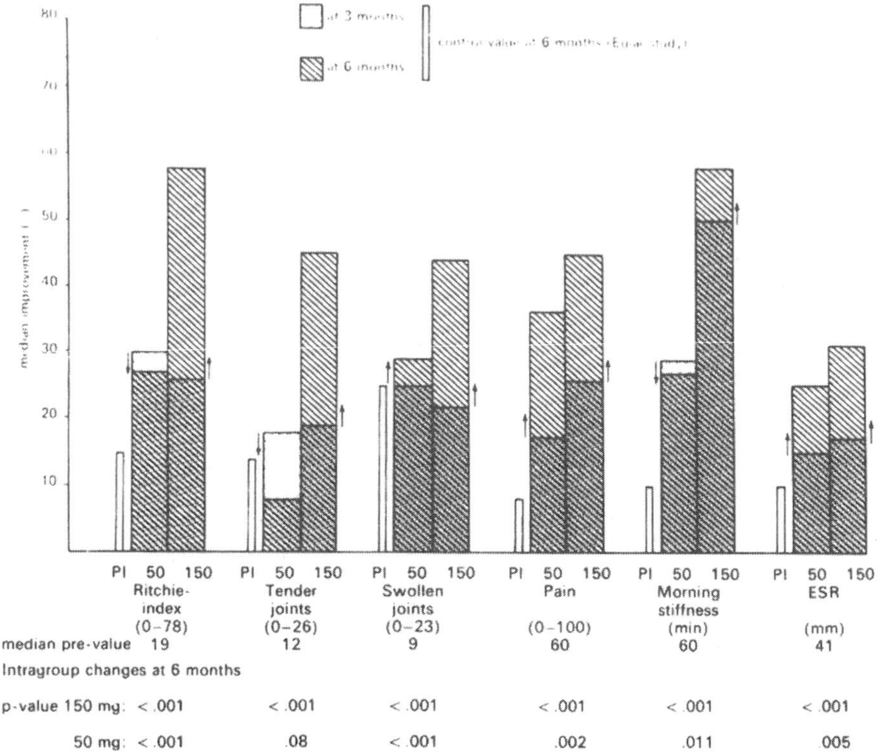


**Figure 8.2** Median improvement of clinical parameters and of sedimentation rate observed in the Multicentre Trial comparing administration of levamisole once weekly at dosages of 150 mg and 50 mg. The control values at 6 months of the placebo group of the EULAR Study are also presented

After 6 months, only patients on 150 mg had further improved in all measures. It must be stressed that for this study, the same control data were used as in the EULAR Study, so that, strictly speaking, no comparison is available between placebo and a once weekly dose of 150 mg levamisole in this investigation. Recent trials included placebo patients and confirmed these data. It also appeared that once weekly administration was as effective as 3 or 7 day/week regimens, but with significantly fewer side effects.

## TREATMENT SCHEDULES

More than 6 years have passed since the first use of levamisole in the treatment of rheumatoid arthritis and many different schedules have been suggested. Such variations have been justified by the search for a compromise between drug activity and toxicity. However, we must admit that the optimal regimen is probably still to be found. The major reason for altering the continuous treatment regimen was the attempt to reduce the incidence of the major side effect of levamisole in RA, i.e. agranulocytosis. Consequently, 150 mg/day levamisole was given in our group, only on the first 4 days of the week and the beneficial effects seemed to be comparable with those obtained on continuous treatment, but long term it seemed that the major side effect occurred just as frequently with both regimens. These data were confirmed by the EULAR Trial. It clearly appears from this study that these schedules are therefore unacceptable because of the high incidence of agranulocytosis in patients under treatment.

The Multicenter Study using a once weekly dose proves the effectiveness of this schedule. Leukocyte counts performed 10–14 h after intake of the drug allow early detection of high risk patients for agranulocytosis[11]. We therefore suggested that the drug should be given in one single dose of 150 mg, 10 h prior to performing a white blood cell count. With this low dosage, the proportion of patients likely to develop agranulocytosis remained at about 5%, but they could be detected before this occurred. It is extremely important that the physician has the result of the white blood cell count after each dose and before giving the next dose to the patient. It seems that a single weekly dose of 150 mg represents an optimal balance of efficacy and toxicity and can be proposed as the best scheme for future therapy. If that schedule is, however, still ineffective after 3–6 months, it then seems reasonable to increase it to 150 mg given on 2 non-consecutive days per week, with appropriate white blood cell counts once per week.

## ADVERSE REACTIONS

The adverse reactions mentioned in the EULAR Study[7] and in the Multicenter Trial[8] are presented in Table 8.1 and correspond very closely to those reported in a review on adverse reactions observed in 988 RA patients treated with levamisole[12]. Levamisole does not cause liver or renal toxicity and all adverse reactions are reversible on withdrawal of the drug. Sensori-neural reactions are rare but necessitate the interruption of treatment in some cases since they give rise to excitation with persistent insomnia. Gastrointestinal intolerance cannot be related directly to the use of the drug and is seen at the same incidence in patients treated with placebo in double blind studies. No severe stomach lesions were reported on levamisole treatment.

The so-called *idiosyncratic reactions* definitely seem to be drug related. Skin rashes are infrequent, especially in the 1 day/week schedule, but require withdrawal of the drug in some cases. In other cases challenge with the drug after a period of interruption does not cause the reappearance of the skin lesions. Mouth ulcers are infrequent and are rarely the cause of discontinuation of treatment. Flu-like illness with fever is more common and is

**Table 8.1** Adverse reactions observed in the two Multicenter Trials, in which four different schedules of levamisole administration were used

| | *No. patients* | | *No. patients* | |
|---|---|---|---|---|
| | 50 mg ($N$ = 45) | 150 mg ($N$ = 48) | 7days/week ($N$ = 124) | 3 days/week ($N$ = 129) |
| Gastrointestinal intolerance | 3 (7%) | 4 (9%) | 25 (20%) | 22 (17%) |
| Skin rash | 0 — | 1 (2%) | 32 (26%) | 31 (24%) |
| Agranulocytosis | 1 (2%) | 0 — | 4 (3.2%) | 3 (2.3%) |
| Flu-like illness, fever | 9 (20%) | 14 (29%) | 13 (10.5%) | 14 (11%) |
| Mouth ulcers | 1 (2%) | 0 — | 11 (9%) | 8 (6%) |
| Neurologic | 1 (2%) | 2 (4%) | 4 (3%) | 9 (7%) |
| Proteinuria | 0 — | 1 (2%) | — | — |
| Patients with adverse reactions | 10 (22%) | 19 (40%) | 65 (53%) | 61 (48%) |

found in 20% of the patients in the double blind study comparing 2 dosages on a 1 day/week schedule. This side effect is frequently associated with leukotoxicity.

Agranulocytosis is the most important adverse reaction to levamisole because it is potentially dangerous. The reaction is reported in short-term studies in 3% of the RA patients treated with levamisole. In the long term we found this frequency to be much higher. Agranulocytosis occurs suddenly, with disappearance of neutrophils from the peripheral blood. The blood cell count presents a dramatic fall of granulocytes. Although the percentage of lymphocytes is increased, their total number is also markedly depressed. The bone marrow is emptied to the level of the granulocytes, but complete recovery occurs within 1–2 weeks after interruption of treatment. Levamisole probably acts as a hapten on the leukocyte membrane of sensitized patients (Type II immune reaction). Agranulocytosis occurs after very variable periods of treatment, ranging from a few weeks to 2 years. Sero-positive RA patients carrying the HLA–B27 antigen carry a high risk[13].

**Early detection of high risk patients to agranulocytosis**

Mielants and Veys[11] have analysed the change in white blood cells in the course of a controlled re-challenge of RA patients who had previously presented agranulocytosis to levamisole (Figure 8.3). Leukocytes and granulocytes decrease 6 h after intake of the drug and non-segmented granulocytes simultaneously increase in peripheral blood. Ten hours after intake the changes were most pronounced and after 24–48 h the blood counts were back to normal initial values. These data have prompted the actual treatment schedule used in most centres, i.e. the intake of one single dose of 150 mg levamisole one day/week followed by the monitoring of white blood cells 10 h after drug intake. It is extremely important that the physician knows the result of the blood count before the patient takes the following dose of levamisole.

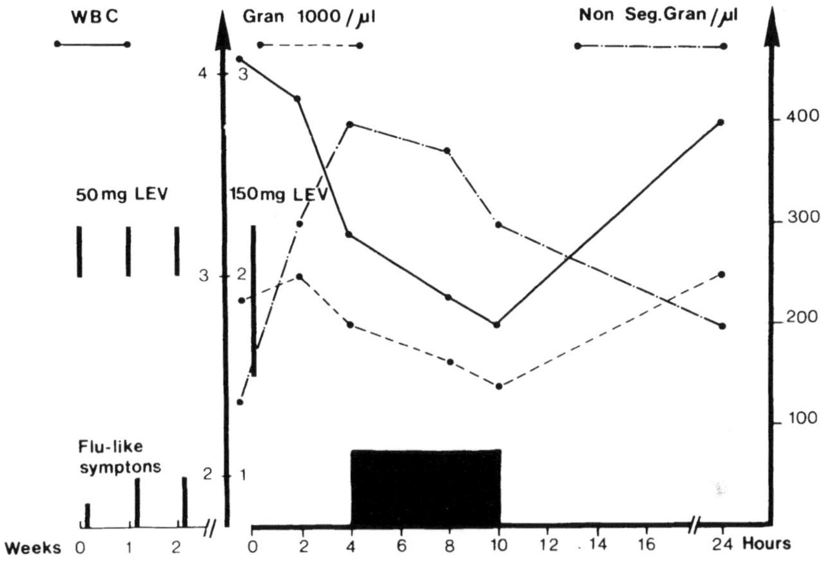


**Figure 8.3** Change in the white blood cells in the course of a rechallenge of an RA patient who had previously presented agranulocytosis to levamisole (WBC = white blood cell counts; GRAN = granulocytes; Non Seg. Gran. = non segmented granulocytes; Lev = levamisole

## LONG-TERM STUDY

Two hundred and one patients with a classic or definite RA according to the ARA criteria were treated with levamisole in our Department (Figure 8.4). All of them had active disease at the outset of the treatment. No other basic anti-rheumatic drugs were used. The patients continued to take the analgesic or anti-inflammatory drugs they have been using prior to admission; change of these drugs during the treatment period was avoided as much as possible. Paients were evaluated at the start, and every 3 or 6 months. Assessments included the Ritchie index, the number of swollen joints, duration of morning stiffness and erythrocyte sedimentation rate by the Westergren method. A patient was considered to be in remission if the number of swollen joints and the morning stiffness had fallen to zero. A patient was considered as significantly improved if he presented

(1) A decrease of swelling and tenderness by 2 gradations or to zero in 30% of the active joints with no activity in inactive joints, or

(2) An improvement of swelling and tenderness in 50% of active joints with involvement of previously inactive joints in less than 10% of those initially active joints.

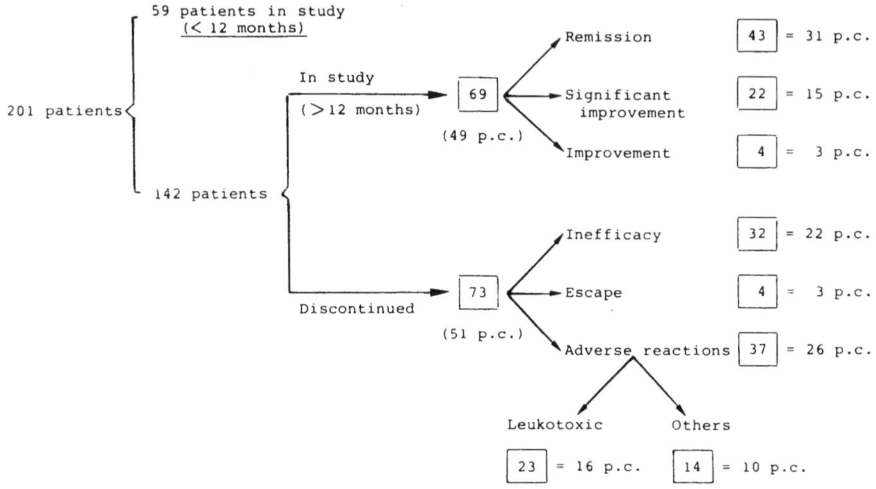


**Figure 8.4** Summary of results in the long-term study

A patient was considered as improved if the investigator maintained the patient on the same basic anti-rheumatic drug. Fifty nine patients still under levamisole treatment were excluded from the study since the duration of treatment is at present less than 1 year.

### Treatment schedules

RA patients treated with levamisole before June 1977 received the drug at the dose of 150 mg daily, or on 3, 4 or 7 consecutive days/week. From June 1977 the schedule of a single intake of 150 mg 1 day/week (including control of white blood cell count 10 h after intake) was introduced. In patients not responding to the drug after 3–6 months, the dosage was increased to 150 mg for 2 non-consecutive days/week. Definite inefficacy was assumed for patients not responding to this regimen after 3 months. We do not have experience with an initial schedule of 2 non-consecutive days/week.

### Adverse reactions

Only adverse reactions requiring discontinuation of treatment were considered in this analysis (agranulocytosis, rash, mouth ulcers and flu-like illness).

Temporary side effects disappearing despite continuation of treatment were not listed (sensori-neural reactions, gastrointestinal symptoms and leukopenia), nor were adverse reactions that subsided after a short interruption of treatment and did not reappear (rash, mouth ulcers, flu-like illness and sensori-neural reactions).

## RESULTS

### Clinical responses

Of the 141 patients analysed in the study (Figure 8.4), 69 are still on levamisole treatment (49%). According to earlier definitions, the responses are distributed as follows : remission, 43 patients (31%); significant improvement, 22 patients (15%); improvement, 4 patients (3%). The mean duration of treatment was 20 months (range, 12–72 months). Figure 8.5 shows that the relative proportion of patients in remission increases for periods of treatment exceeding 18 months. These data indicate that patients frequently continue to improve during the first 2 years of treatment, and that the plateau of activity is not achieved after 6 months as reported in literature[14].

### Inefficacy (*Figure 8.6*)

Levamisole treatment was discontinued for inefficacy in 32 patients (22%). The mean duration of treatment was 10 months (range 3–29 months). In 12 patients the treatment was stopped after more than 1 year. Eight of these cases responded initially to the drug but relapsed despite continuation of treatment and failed to recover even after changing the schedule from 1 to 2 days/week. In 10 patients there was no response at all (14%).

### Loss to follow-up

Four patients (3%) were lost to follow-up after 6–9 months of treatment. Three of them were in clinical remission at the last registration of data.

### Adverse reactions (*Figure 8.6*)

Levamisole administration had to be interrupted for adverse reactions in 37 cases (26%). The most frequent adverse reactions were leukotoxic side effects which occurred in 23 patients (16 %). The nature and incidence are listed in Table 8.2. The mean duration of treatment before the occurrence of leukotoxicity was 7.4 months (range, 2–30 months) and for other side effects 9.3 months (range 3–31 months). Since leukotoxic adverse reactions occurred after more than 2 years in some cases, it is mandatory to control white blood cell count 10 h after intake of levamisole uniformly throughout the entire treatment. We propose every 2 weeks in patients on a 1 day/week schedule and every week in patients on a 2 non-consecutive day/week schedule. Figure 8.6 shows that after 1 year the number of withdrawals is nearly

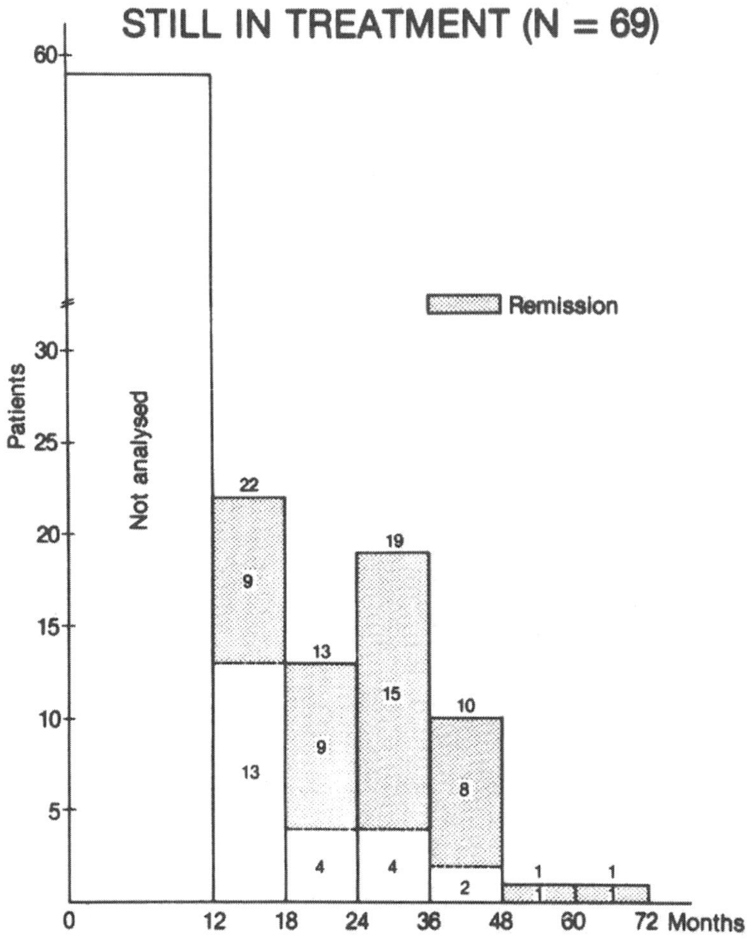


**Figure 8.5** Duration of drug administration in patients still on levamisole treatment

the same for adverse reactions as for inefficacy. Side effects frequently occur in patients presenting marked improvement; 12 patients out of the 23 with leukotoxicity and 7 patients out of the 14 with other adverse reactions were cleared at the moment of withdrawal. (Figure 8.7)

## SCHEDULES

The schedules in patients still on treatment and in patients in whom drug administration was interrupted for inefficacy are presented in Table 8.3. Fifty out of 69 patients who benefited from the treatment are actually on a 1 day/

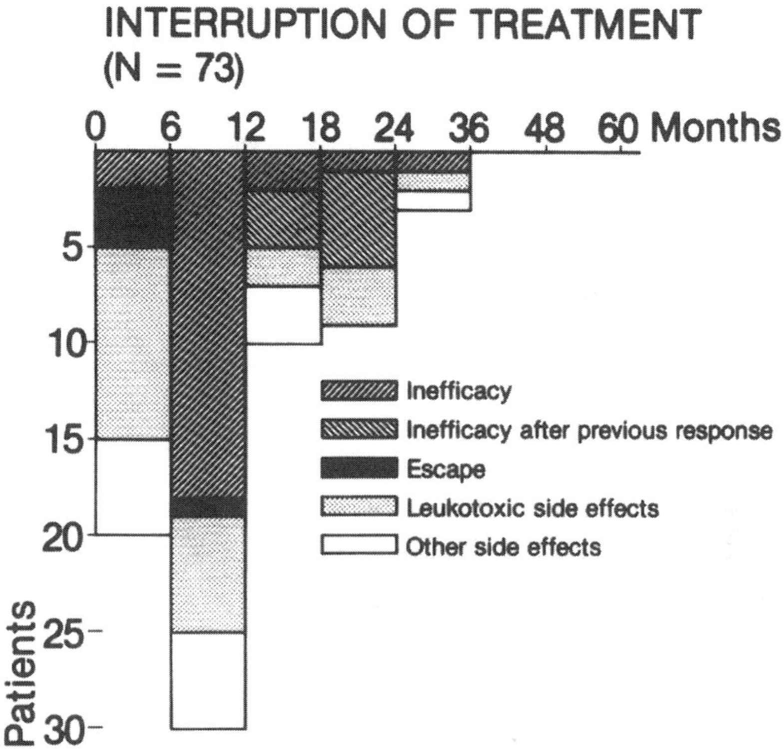


**Figure 8.6** Duration of drug administration in patients in which levamisole treatment was interrupted for adverse reactions or inefficacy

week schedule, and 16 are on a higher regimen. Fourteen patients receive levamisole on 2 non-consecutive days/week but this scheme was never used initially in the Department. In seven patients not responding to a 1 day/week schedule, an increase to 2 days/week was followed by a good response. In seven other patients the 1 day/week schedule was accompanied by a marked improvement but a relapse occurred under treatment. A new response was then obtained by increasing the regimen to 2 days/week. Twenty six patients still on treatment were started on schedules of 3, 4 or 7 days/week. Only two of them are actually still on higher schedules than 1 or 2 days/week. Twenty four patients thus responded very well to a decrease of the scheme. After a primary period of treatment on 1 day/week, an increase to 2 days was necessary in some of them to achieve or to maintain the initial response.

With regard to adverse reactions, Table 8.2 reveals that flu-like illness seems to be more frequent on a 1 day/week schedule and that allergic vasculitis (Figure 8.8) was only encountered on high regimens. Figure 8.9 shows interesting data on variation of the schedules. In 56 patients the regimen was

**Table 8.2** Nature and incidence of adverse reactions observed in a long-term study on 142 patients. The schedules at the moment of occurrence of side effects are also listed

| *Withdrawals for adverse reactions* | | *Schedules* (days) | | | |
|---|---|---|---|---|---|
| | | 7 | 4 | 2 | 1 |
| Skin vasculitis | 2 | 1 | 1 | | |
| rash | 2 | | | 1 | 1 |
| ulcus cruris | 1 | | | | 1 |
| Mouth ulcers | 3 | | 1 | 1 | 1 |
| Flu-like illness | 5 | | | 1 | 4 |
| Sensori-neural (excitation) | 1 | | | | 1 |
| Leukotoxicity | 23 | 1 | 8 | 1 | 13 |
| Total | 37 (26%) | 2 | 10 | 4 | 21 |

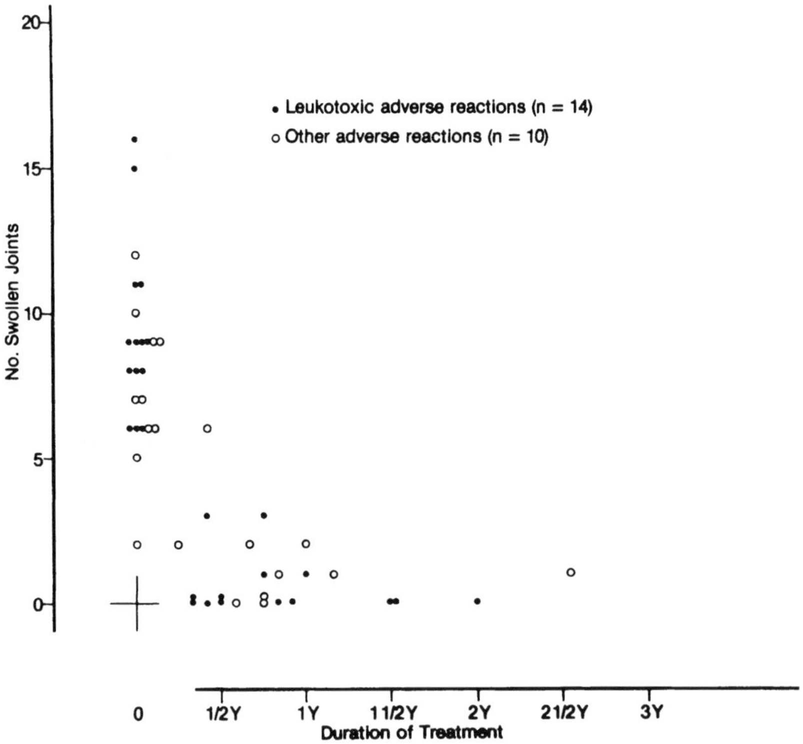


**Figure 8.7** Change of number of swollen joints during treatment in patients withdrawn for adverse reactions. A dramatic decrease of this variable is observed in a large number of the patients

**Table 8.3** Schedules in patients still on treatment and in patients in which the levamisole administration was interrupted for inefficacy. Initial and actual regimens or schemes at the moment of interruption are reported

| | *Schedules (days/week)* | | | | | | | |
|---|---|---|---|---|---|---|---|---|
| | *At start* | | | | *At last evaluation* | | | |
| | 7 | 4 or 3 | 2 | 1 | 7 | 4 or 3 | 2 | 1 |
| Remission | 5 | 12 | 0 | 26 | 0 | 1 | 5 | 37 |
| Significant improvement | 0 | 7 | 0 | 15 | 0 | 1 | 6 | 15 |
| Improvement | 1 | 1 | 0 | 2 | 0 | 0 | 3 | 1 |
| Inefficacy | 5 | 8 | 0 | 11 | 4 | 5 | 6 | 9 |
| Inefficacy after previous response | 0 | 4 | 0 | 3 | 0 | 0 | 4 | 4 |

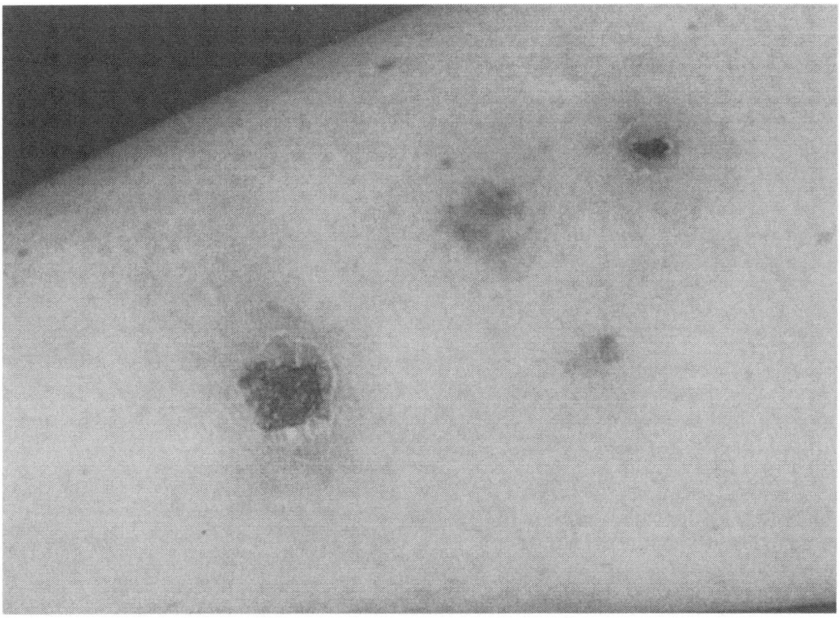

**Figure 8.8** Allergic vasculitis on the forearm of an RA patient treated with levamisole

not changed and 38 of them are still in remission or present a significant improvement. All of them are on a 1 day/week regimen. Seventeen of the 23 patients in whom the schedule was decreased are still doing very well. An increase from 1 to 2 days was applied to 13 patients but only seven of them responded to this variation. A new increase following an initial decrease had a beneficial effect in three of the five patients. It was possible to return to a 1 day/week schedule after an earlier increase to induce a beneficial response in two cases. Two patients discontinued the treatment on their own initiative, since they were in complete remission, but they relapsed and new drug intake was necessary to reinduce the remission.

| Schedule | Remission and Sign. Improv. | Improvement | Inefficacy after response | Inefficacy | Total |
|---|---|---|---|---|---|
| 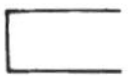 | 36 | 2 | 1 | 17 | 56 |
| 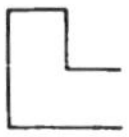 | 16 | 1 | 4 | 2 | 23 |
| 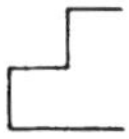 | 6 | 1 | 2 | 4 | 13 |
| 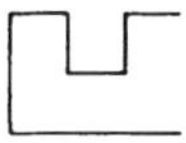 | 3 | 0 | 1 | 1 | 5 |
| 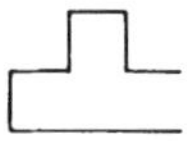 | 2 | 0 | 0 | 0 | 2 |
| 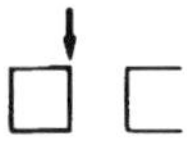 | 2 | 0 | 0 | 0 | 2 |
| 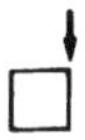 | 2 Agranulocytosis | 0 | 17 Adverse react. | 2 Adverse reactions | 21 |

**Figure 8.9** Variation of the schedules in the long-term study. No quantitative value may be attributed to the schedule diagrams; only variations of the schemes are indicated. The first line represents patients maintained on a constant scheme, the second line represents patients in which the schedule was decreased, and so on

Only 2 of the 21 patients in whom interruption of the treatment was necessary for side effects have remained in remission for more than 3 years after interruption without any drug intake. These 2 patients had agranulocytosis for more than 2 weeks. The hypothesis can be advanced that agranulocytosis had influenced some lymphocyte clones, directly implicated in the aetiopathogenesis of the disease. In 17 patients in whom the treatment was interrupted for adverse reactions the initial response was followed by a relapse. Follow-up was possible in 14 patients. The duration of remission after interruption ranged from 6 weeks to 3 years. No correlation was found between the duration of treatment and the duration of remission after interruption in these cases ($r = 0.14$, Figure 8.10).

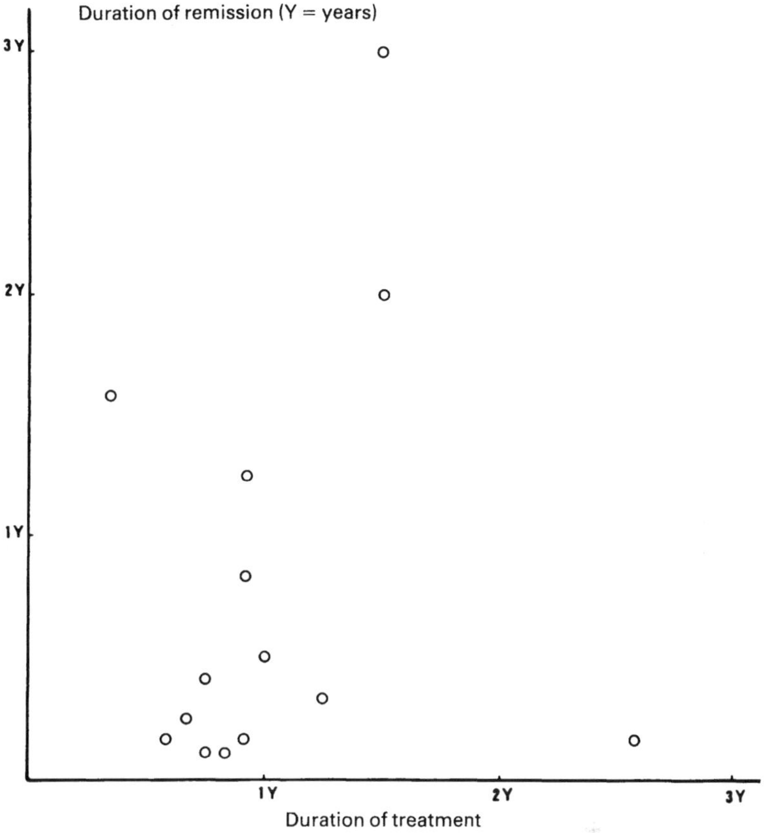


**Figure 8.10** Relation between the duration of remission (years, ordinate) in patients in which levamisole treatment was interrupted for adverse reactions and the duration of drug administration (years, abscissa)

## MECHANISM OF ACTION OF LEVAMISOLE

A number of chemical modes of action have been suggested for levamisole, which may act in various ways to produce its therapeutic effects and perhaps also the unwanted adverse reactions.

### (1.) Cyclic nucleotide stimulation

Agents increasing intracellular cyclic AMP, such as β-adrenergic agents, depress cellular functions. Drugs inducing an increase of intracellular cyclic GMP, such as cholinergic agents like acetylcholine and imidazole, augment the proliferative and secretory functions of cells involved in immune and inflammatory processes. Levamisole mimics the action of other stimulators of cyclic GMP and in this way improves cellular functions, although it also causes a decrease in the B lymphocyte activity of EAC-rosette formation[15]. However, all the actions of the drug cannot be explained by this mechanism, since the differentiation of immature T lymphocytes is a cyclic AMP-dependent activity.

**(2.) Thiols**

A metabolite of levamisole, OMPI ((±)-2-oxo-3(2-mercaptoethyl)-5-phenylimidazolidine), has a free sulphydryl group formed by the opening of the sulphur-containing ring in levamisole. It is known that auto-oxidative necrosis of cells in culture induced by a glutathione depletion is inhibited by levamisole and to a greater degree by OMPI. It has therefore been suggested that levamisole might act by providing a radical scavenger for the multiplying immunocytes and so induce immunoregulatory effects[16].

**(3.) Levamisole: a thymomimetic agent?**

There is a striking parallelism between the effects of levamisole and those of thymic hormone(s) in tests designed to investigate maturation of effector functions of T lymphocytes, polymorphonuclear and mononuclear phagocytes, and also in therapeutic studies to reconstitute immunodeficiencies in animals and in children. It is proposed that levamisole interacts with thymopoietin receptors on effector lymphocytes, polymorphonuclear and mononuclear phagocytes and influences cell metabolism by altering the cyclic AMP/GMP ratio in the cell. There is no certain evidence of common receptor sites for levamisole and thymopoietin, but the structural similarity between levamisole and the active site of thymopoietin and the fact that the two compounds have cholinergic activity both support this hypothesis[17].

## THYMOPOIETIN AS A TREATMENT IN RA?

On the basis of this theory Veys and Mielants in Ghent, in collaboration with Huskisson in London, Rosenthal in Zurich and Vischer in Geneva, are performing a clinical study to investigate the activity of pentapeptide thymopoietin 32–36 (TP5). The study is composed of three stages : in the first double blind portion, 1 mg TP5, administered i.m. once weekly ($N = 15$) was compared with placebo ($N = 15$). In the second part 50 mg TP5 was administered i.v. once weekly ($N = 23$) in an open study, and in a third part 50 mg TP5 given i.v. once weekly was compared with a levamisole group (150 mg once weekly). Publication of the results is currently in preparation.

## CONCLUSIONS

Levamisole administration was followed by a dramatic decrease of disease activity in 49% of patients in a long-term evaluation (mean duration of treatment was 20 months). Although levamisole intake was accompanied by various side effects and a group of RA patients did not respond to the treatment (22%), this drug represents a useful addition to the therapeutic arsenal for RA. It is important to note that interruption of drug administration is followed by complete reversibility of all adverse reactions within a couple of days. No nephrotoxicity or hepatotoxicity was found. The best schedule for levamisole treatment in RA is probably not yet found, but in order to combine optimal activity and safety, we recommend the 1 day/week schedule (with measurement of white blood cell count 10 h after intake of the drug) at least every 2 weeks. Increase of the schedule to 2 non-consecutive days/week is advised if no clinical response is obtained after 3–6 months. Despite the fact that levamisole shows beneficial effects in RA (in which immunological impairment is postulated) the question remains unsolved as to the mechanism to which this effect may be attributed.

## SUMMARY

The drugs with a 'specific' action in RA can be subdivided into:

(1) A group the mechanism of which remains totally unknown (Gold salts and d-penicillamine).

(2) A group inducing a reduction of immune responses (immunosuppressives and thoracic duct drainage).

(3) A group restoring some immunologically impaired functions (transfer factor, BCG and levamisole).

The authors have only discussed the last group, and since the clinical data on transfer factor and BCG are so scarce (especially in a controlled situation), this review has been restricted to recent data about the use of levamisole in RA. In several controlled studies levamisole proved to be effective in RA certain cases. It appears from long-term studies that the clinical improvement induced by this drug can be maintained for a long time. In the authors' series, 69 out of 142 cases (49%) on levamisole treatment showed an improvement lasting more than 1 year. Discontinuation of drug administration is in many cases followed by an early exacerbation of disease activity. Toxicity has been discussed in detail and the early reversibility of all adverse reactions by interruption of treatment has been stressed. Early detection of high risk patients likely to develop agranulocytosis is possible with the once weekly intake of the drug (150 mg) followed by white blood cell count and differentiation 10 h later. Recent data confirm that this scheme is effective in RA.

One of the most important problems remains finding markers among a subgroup of RA patients in order to predict who is likely to benefit from such drug treatment. Despite the fact that levamisole shows beneficial effects in RA, in which immunological impairment is postulated, the question remains unsolved as to the mechanism to which this effect may be attributed.

## References


1 Snyderham, R., Pike, M. C. and Altman, L. C. (1975). Abnormalities of leukocyte chemotaxis in human disease. *Ann. N. Y. Acad. Sci.*, **256,** 386

2 Harmion, B. P. (1978). Infection, autoimmunity and rheumatoid arthritis. In Zvaifler, N. J. (ed.) *Clinics in Rheumatic Diseases. Immunology*, pp. 565–586. (London, Philadelphia, Toronto: Saunders)

3 Symoens, J. and Rosenthal, M. (1977). Levamisole in the modulation of the immune response : the current experimental and clinical state. *J. Reticulo-endothelial Soc.*, **21,** 175

4 Trabert, U., Rosenthal, M. and Muller, W. (1976). The effect of levamisole on adjuvant arthritis in the rat. *J Rheumatol.*, **3,** 166

5 Symoens, J., De Cree, J., Van Bever, W. and Janssen, P. A. J. (1979). *Pharmacological Properties of Drug Substances. Vol. 2.* (Washington: American Pharmaceutical Association Academy of Pharmaceutical Sciences)

6 Zulman, J., Michalski, J., McCombs, C., Greenspan, J. and Talal, N. (1978). Levamisole maintains cyclophosphamide induced remission in murine lupus erythematosus. *Clin. Exp. Immunol.* **31,** 321

7 Multicenter Study Group (1978). Levamisole in rheumatoid arthritis. A randomised double-blind study comparing two dosage regimens of levamisole with placebo. *Lancet*, **2,** 1007

8 Di Perri, T., Auteri, A., Pasini, F. L. *et al.* (1978). A weekly oral dose of levamisole in the treatment of rheumatoid arthritis associated with E-rosette lymphocyte reduction. *Eur. J. Rheumatol.* **1,** 155

9 Veys, E. M. and Mielants, H. (1978). Early detection of high-risk rheumatoid arthritis patients under one day/week levamisole administration. *Eur. J. Rheumatol.*, **1,** 261

10 Multicenter Study Group (1978). A multicentre randomized double-blind study comparing two dosages of levamisole in rheumatoid arthritis. *J. Rheumatol.*, **5** (Suppl. 4), 5

11 Mielants, H. and Veys, E. M. (1978). A study of the hematological side-effects of levamisole in rheumatoid arthritis, with recommendations. *J. Rheumatol.*, **5** (Suppl. 4), 77

12 Symoens, J., Veys, E., Mielants, H. and Pinals, R. (1979). Adverse reactions to levamisole. *Cancer Treatment Rep.*, **62,** 1721

13 Veys, E. M., Mielants, H. and Rosenthal, M. (1977). Agranulocytosis, levamisole and HLA-B27. *Lancet*, **2,** 764

14 Veys, E. M. and Mielants; H. (1978). Experience and recommendations for treatment schedule of levamisole in rheumatoid arthritis. *J. Rheumatol.*, **5** (Suppl. 4), 31

15 Renoux, G. and Renoux (1977). Roles of the imidazole or thiol moiety on the immunostimulant action of levamisole. In Chirigos, M. A. (ed.) *Control of Neoplasia by Modulation of the Immune System*. pp. 67–80. (New York : Raven Press)

16 De Brabander, M., Aerts, F., Geuens, G., Van Ginckel, A., Van De Veire, R. and Van Belle, H. (1978). Dl-2–oxo–3(2–mercaptoethyl)–5–phenylimidazolidine. A sulfur metabolite of levamisole that interacts with microtubules. *Chem. Biol. Interactions,* **23,** 45

17 Goldstein, G. (1978). Mode of action of levamisole. *J. Rheumatol.,* **5** (Suppl. 4), 143

# Discussion

**Professor J. L. Turk: (Chairman)** asked if the studies reported by Professor Veys had been performed according to a controlled double-blind protocol and whether he had obtained objective assessment of the efficacy of levamisole.

**Professor Veys** said that the EULAR Trial and the Multicenter Trial were both double-blind. The long-term study was not. It was controlled but open. As to objective assessment, all trials followed the standard procedures for investigating patients with rheumatoid arthritis and he did not know what other objective measures could be applied. However, it was of interest that levamisole also influenced the patient's immunological responses.

**Professor D. A. Horwitz (USA)** wished to make a comment on macrophage function in rheumatoid arthritis. Some years previously with Dr Allison, in UK he had developed an assay of human monocyte cytotoxicity and current work in his laboratory suggested that such monocyte cytotoxicity was depressed in rheumatoid arthritis. He had been involved in the single dose levamisole trial for some 6 months and had found a correlation between depressed monocyte cytotoxicity and the patient's response to the drug. Of 27 patients treated, 22 had responded and almost all of them had had depressed monocyte cytotoxicity, which improved as their condition improved. Patients who did not respond to the drug were those who had had normal monocyte cytotoxicty from the beginning.

**Dr N. R. Ackerman: (USA)** asked for more information on the dosing schedule and results obtained with thymopoietin.

**Professor Veys** said that the results were very preliminary but with the 23 patients evaluated so far it seemed that administration of 50 mg thymopoietin i.v. once weekly did permit some patients to respond, although this was not the case for the once weekly i.m. injection of 1 mg thymopoietin. So far they had no data at all on the comparison of thymopoietin with levamisole. An important point was that some patients who stopped thymopoietin treatment presented marked exacerbation of the disease with the rapid appearance of subcutaneous nodules and skin vascular lesions.

**Dr E. Munthe: (Co-Chairman)** said that they had observed leukocytosis during the first months of levamisole treatment in their studies.

**Professor Veys** said that he had never seen a true increase in leukocyte count after the beginning of treatment, although he had seen exacerbation of the clinical signs during the first 8 weeks in several patients. What he did sometimes observe was leukopenia following levamisole, but he mentioned it as an individual side effect since on continuing treatment such patients present potential cases of agranulocytosis. It was therefore better to consider leukocyte side effects as one phenomenon and to withdraw treatment accordingly.

In answer to a question on whether levamisole affected the course of the disease, more specifically whether it affected erosion or had an influence on the cartilage, Professor Veys said that he did not know. They did not have X-ray data and those were the only data that would permit such an evaluation.

# 9

# Crystal deposition disease

G. FAURE, A. GAUCHER, P. NETTER,
J. POUREL AND J. DUHEILLE (FRANCE)

The number of crystalline compounds whose presence has been demonstrated in articular and periarticular structures has rapidly increased during the past 20 years thanks to progress in techniques of observation and identification. Their origin and the pathophysiological role which they play in the rheumatic disorders in which they are implicated are far from being well understood. Some effects ascribed to crystals might be only of incidental importance. This topic will be reviewed under four different headings:

1 The identification of crystals.
2 The different crystals implicated in rheumatic disorders.
3 The pathophysiological consequences of inflammation and articular degeneration.
4 The source of crystals.

**Identification of crystals**

Crystals of monosodium urate have been known since the invention of the optical microscope but it was McCarty[1,2] and Hollander who asserted that they were present in the articular effusions of subjects suffering from acute gouty arthritis. These workers used polarized light microscopy, techniques which are still in daily use, but their power of identification are limited. The same techniques were used to demonstrate the presence of crystals other than monosodium urate, i.e., calcium pyrophosphate dihydrate and apatite. McCarty[1,2] identified calcium pyrophosphate dihydrate as a mixture of triclinic and monoclinic forms by the use of X-ray diffraction on powder patterns and infrared spectroscopy.

More recently, crystals were searched for using transmission electron microscopy but many technical problems arise as crystals vanish during preparation and sectioning of samples and transmission electron microscopy only allows observation of crystal ghosts. The techniques of scanning electron microscopy and of scanning transmission electron microscopy made it possible to detect even isolated microcrystals and to examine their morphologies. In conjunction with X-ray microanalysis, it can be used for identification of crystals by means of elemental analysis and determination of element ratios. We have used the Weissenberg technique to obtain a monocrystalline identification for large $CaHPO_4$ crystals and to determine the crystalline parameters. These techniques allow detection of tiny and isolated microcrystals that would have gone undetected by any other technique. Scanning electron microscopy should perhaps be able to establish the real frequency of calcium and phosphorus compounds in inflammatory disorders.

**The different crystals implicated in rheumatic disorders**

Monosodium urate can usually be observed in synovial fluid inside phagocytic cells as fine needles 6 μm long covered with an extension of the cell membrane. In the chalky material issuing from ulcerated tophi, and *in situ* in a tophus obtained at surgery, monosodium urate crystals were apparent as small needles with tapered or rod-like ends (Figure 9.1).

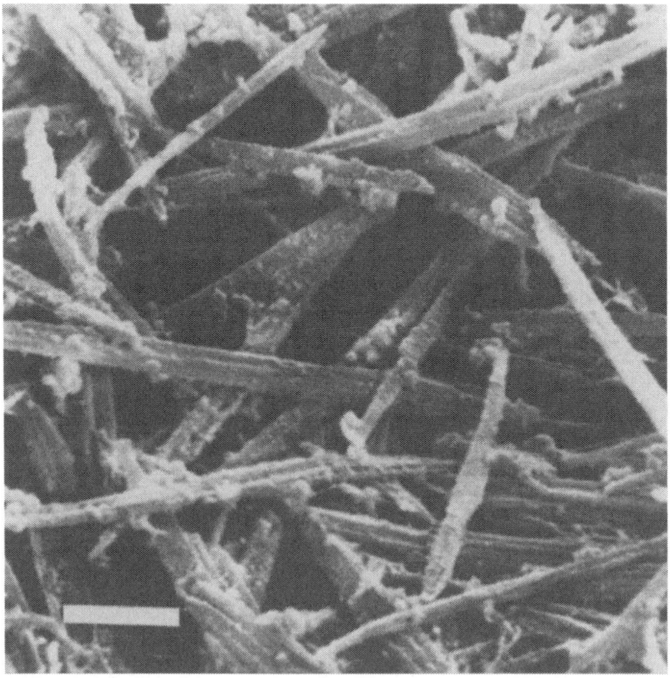

**Figure 9.1** Monosodium urate monohydrate crystals in a large paratendinous tophus (bar = 2.5 μm)

Triclinic calcium pyrophosphate dihydrate was obtained after concentration of the formed constituents from synovial fluid. They were $5 \times 2 \times 2\,\mu m$ rhomboidal structures with the characteristics of triclinic holoedrism. In cartilage and meniscal fibrocartilage, triclinic calcium pyrophosphate dihydrate also appears as rhomboidal structures connected with collagen fibres (Figure 9.2). X-ray diffraction made it possible to identify the presence of monoclinic calcium pyrophosphate dihydrate in synovial fluid. This compound appears as elongated rods clearly different from the triclinic form.

Apatite was identified by Dieppe and co-workers in synovial fluid from osteoarthritic patients and on the synovial membrane. Previously, McCarty had identified by X-ray diffraction the 'shiny coins' which he had seen by light microscopy. These products obtained from shoulder calcific tendonitis appear as rock-like structures (Figure 9.3). Dicalcium hydrogen phosphate or brushite, also first identified by McCarty, was found in cases of destructive arthropathies, on the surface of articular tissues and in the cartilage (Figure 9.4). Other crystals have been reported in the joints including octacalcium phosphate and cholesterol that look like plates but are not inflammatory. Corticosteroid esters do not have morphological characteristics so specific or so recognizable as do natural crystals (Figure 9.5).

**Pathophysiological consequences of crystals**

Crystals induce arthropathies or are associated with inflammatory arthritis and degenerative arthropathies and they have inflammatory properties. Clinical situations such as gout, pseudogout or bursitis provide evidence of this fact but crystals also exist in articular tissues and tendon sheaths without inflammation. Many inflammation experimental models have been designed to confirm these properties and to test the action of non-steroidal anti-inflammatory drugs in man, or in such animals as the dog and rat. Mediators of inflammation have been measured in synovial fluid or in specific models. Hageman factor, histamine, kinins and prostaglandins have been found but they are not a *sine qua non* for crystal synovitis. Recently, it was shown that calcium pyrophosphate dihydrate and hydroxyapatite are significant activators, as is monosodium urate. Complement derived chemotactic factors and a specific glycopeptide have been studied, as they are able to attract phagocytic cells. The cellular interaction with crystals mainly involves polymorphonuclear phagocytes. It is recognized that crystals are phagocytozed and rupture phagolysosomes from within leading to cell death and to release of LDH and lysosomal enzymes during acute inflammatory crisis. The role of surface IgG adsorbed from human serum has been emphasized by Kozin. Phagocytosis of crystals is enhanced by IgG absorbed onto the crystal surface with the Fc end of the molecule available to Fc receptors on phagocytic cells.

However, very little is known at present about the relationship between chronic inflammation and crystals or the relationship between crystal and articular degeneration. A scheme has been designed by Dieppe and Willoughby

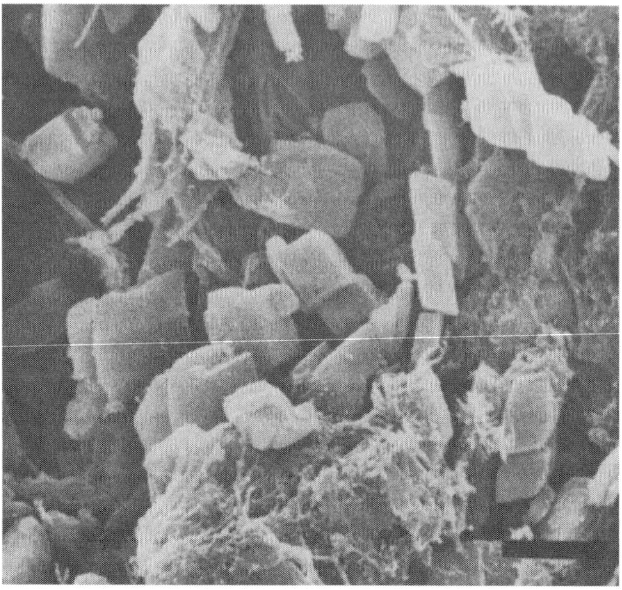

**Figure 9.2** Triclinic calcium pyrophosphate dihydrate crystals scattered among collagen fibres in a calcified meniscus (bar = 2 μm)

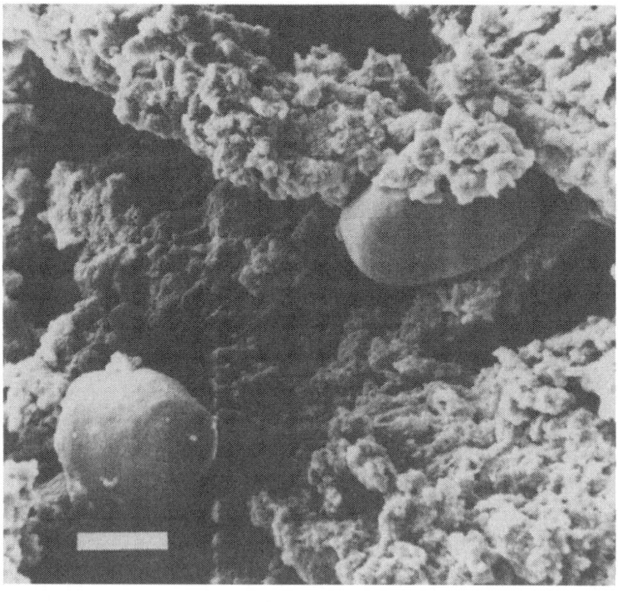

**Figure 9.3** Agglomerates of apatite microcrystals from tendon calcification in the chronic stage (bar = 10 μm)

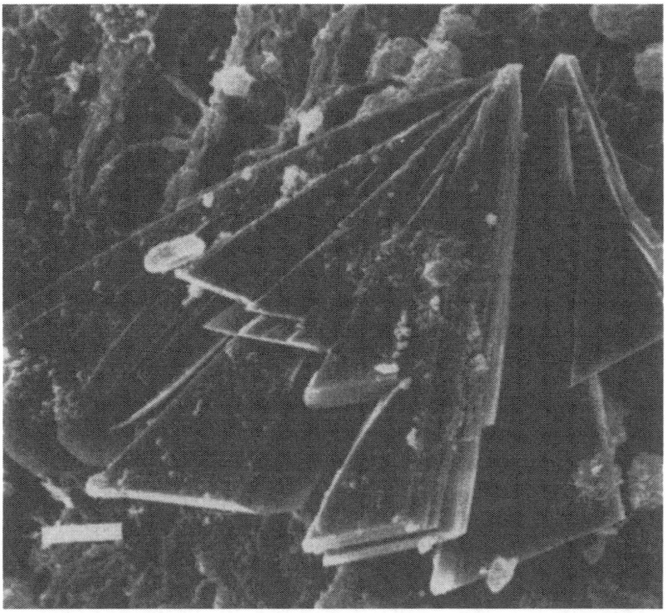

**Figure 9.4** Calcium hydrogen phosphate dihydrate crystals in the form of arrowheads (bar = 5 μm)

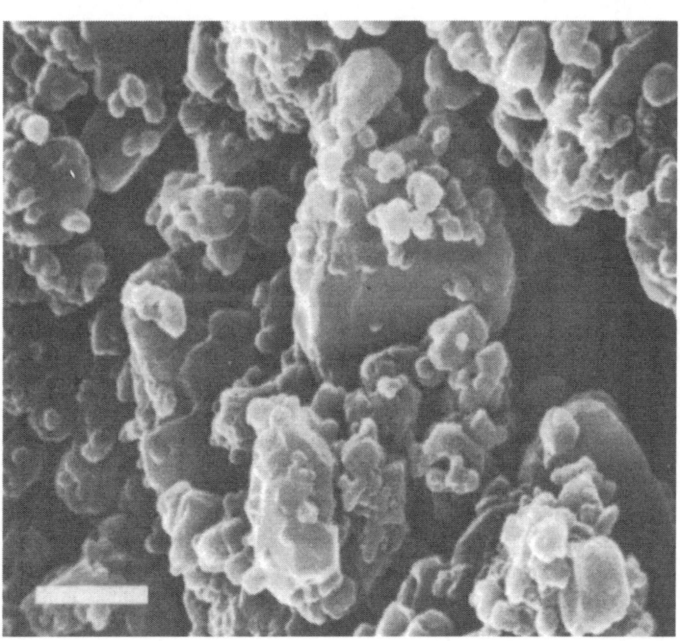

**Figure 9.5** Commercial preparation of corticosteroid microcrystals (bar = 2.5 μm)

to unify osteoarthritis and crystal deposition and as McCarty stated, three possibilities exist:

1 Crystals and cartilage degeneration both stem from a common underlying, probably metabolic, abnormality.
2 Crystal phase formation follows degenerative change.
3 As in gout, crystal deposition precedes cartilage degeneration.

In the group of hereditary diffuse articular chondrocalcinoses which we are studying[3,4], joints are not very damaged in spite of large deposits of crystals. However, these are made of very small (less than 2 $\mu$m) triclinic calcium pyrophosphate dihydrate crystals. These results are not consistent with crystal formation following degenerative changes, but the two other hypothesis remain possible.

**Source of crystals**

Urate metabolic disturbances are now well known and precipitation of monosodium urate crystals occurs in hypersaturated media. Calcium phosphate crystal formation is more puzzling, and a metabolic disturbance of pyrophosphate metabolism may be looked for. PPi level was found elevated in synovial fluid and lowered during pseudogouty crisis, but an elevated joint fluid PPi is not specific for CPPD deposition. Elevated blood PPi levels have been found but this was not confirmed by Russel or by Mc Carty. A metabolic defect is to be searched for in patients with an hereditary diffuse disease form. Pathological study of cartilage from one of these patients confirms that calcium pyrophosphate dihydrate crystals do precipitate in the cartilage matrix outside chondrocyte lacunae. They accumulate in intermediate layer of cartilage and from pseudotophi containing huge amounts of crystals. Transformation of one calcium phosphate compound is possible in specific physical conditions and association of different calcium phosphate crystals has been reported *in vivo*. Precursors of calcium pyrophosphate dihydrate were studied by Pritzker in hydrogels. We also observed synthetic calcium pyrophosphate precursors through scanning electron microscopy[4], but for the moment the definition of naturally occurring compounds is not improved. Ultrastructural confirmation by Ali of the presence of mineral apatite nodules in osteoarthritic cartilage is important because of the origin of this mineral. Establishing the source of crystals may therefore be at hand, even if the mechanism of corticosteroid flares post-injection is not understood and cannot be foreseen.

**Acknowledgments**

The authors wish to thank B. Malaman and J. Steinmetz (Laboratoire de Chimie du Solide associé au C.N.R.S., Professor B. Roques, Université de Nancy I) for X-ray diffraction of crystals. Synthetic pyrophosphate crystals were kindly provided by R. Russel and P. Hearn. Financial support has come from Université de Nancy I, and ATP I.N.S.E.R.M. 76–79–108.

## References

1 McCarty, D. J. (1979). Pathogenesis and treatment of crystal-induced inflammation. In McCarty (ed.) *Arthritis and Allied Conditions*, pp. 1245–1261. (Philadelphia: Lea and Febiger)

2 McCarty, D. J. (1979). Calcium pyrophosphate crystal deposition disease. Pseudogout: articular chondrocalcinosis. In McCarty, D. J. (ed.) *Arthritis and Allied Conditions*, pp. 1276–1299. (Philadelphia: Lea and Febiger)

3 Faure, G., Netter, P. and Gaucher, A. (1979). *Microscopie électronique à balayage et pathologie articulaire. Etude de la membrane synoviale humaine.*(Paris: Merck Sharp et Dohme Chibret)

4 Faure, G., Netter., P. Malaman, B., Steinmetz, J., Duheille, J. and Gaucher A. (1980). Scanning electron microscopy study of microcrystals implicated in human rheumatic diseases. SEM 1980/III 163.176. (AMF O'Hau (Chicago) SEM Inc.)

# Discussion

**Professor J. L. Turk** (Chairman) asked whether the crystals could be activating Hageman factor which could then cause plasminogen conversion to plasmin, activation of C3 and the presence of C3 breakdown products resulting in inflammation. In short, was complement involved? He believed that there was evidence that apatite was one of the substances that would activate Hageman factor.

**Dr Faure** said that experimental evidence does exist on Hageman factor and coagulation factors but the data were not clear. A range of different mediators could have a place in the activation of inflammation in acute crises.

**Dr. E. Munthe (Co-Chairman)** drew attention to the extra-articular precipitation of calcium pyrophosphate crystals along tendons. The salts can be found in the absence of any cartilage and even when there were no signs of degenerative changes in the tendons themselves.

**Dr Faure** said that such calcification was probably evidence of a diffused metabolic disease. They were studying such metabolic disturbances in collaboration with workers in San Diego and New York. There was a possibility that the hereditary form of the disease was different from the sporadic form that appeared in elderly patients.

**Dr Barry; (New Zealand)** said that patients with low levels of magnesium in the system sometimes developed chondrocalcinosis. He wondered whether magnesium levels had been measured in patients with crystal deposition disease.

**Dr Faure** had not studied magnesium blood levels in his patients but those he had examined showed no evidence of disease usually associated with chrondrocalcinosis.

**Dr A. Fam (Canada)** said that in experimental studies, cholesterol crystals had been found to be inflammatory. He wondered whether cholesterol crystals played a role in human joint disease such as clinical arthritis.

**Dr Faure** said that in man, cholesterol crystals were not considered to be inflammatory but he could not give a definite answer to the question.

**Dr E. Munthe (Norway)** asked whether there were any experimental data on the activation of macrophages by crystals. Could one distinguish between activation of the cells and phagocytosis of crystals by macrophages with subsequent rupture of the cell and release of enzymes.

**Dr Faure** had no personal experience relating to this question but he believed that the interaction of monocytes or macrophages with crystals would be an important future trend in the study of crystal deposition disease.

In answer to a question about the size of the crystals in synovial fluid, synovial membrane and cartilage in patients suffering from gout, he said that there were no differences between crystals in the articular structure and the synovial fluid. The sizes were similar. However, for CPPD crystals there was a wide range of sizes from 1–20 $\mu m$ in length. In experimental models Dunn had shown that small crystals were more inflammatory than larger ones but he did not know whether this effect had clinical importance.

# 10

# T-cell dependent inflammatory responses

J. F. A. P. MILLER (AUSTRALIA)

Delayed type hypersensitivity (DTH) is a T-cell dependent inflammatory response at the site of antigen deposition, usually in the skin. It reaches its peak intensity 24–48 h after initiation and is characterized by a mononuclear cell infiltration. T cells, but not B cells nor immune serum, can transfer the reaction to naive animals. The measurement of the intensity of DTH involves quantifying the inflammatory response at the site of antigen deposition. Redness and induration can be measured in man and in certain animals such as the guinea pig. In mice, ear thickness increase or footpad swelling may be used. Alternatively, a radioactive precursor of DNA ([$^{125}$I]UdR) can be injected systemically to label the progenitors of the mononuclear cells which enter inflammatory sites. The intensity of the DTH reaction in a defined site, such as an ear where antigen is injected intradermally, will be proportional to the radioactivity obtained. The results may be expressed as the ratio of the radioactivity of the challenged (left, L) ear to the unchallenged (right, R) ear (L/R[$^{125}$I]UdR uptake)[1].

This presentation will deal with recent work in two areas of importance to an understanding of T-cell function: the influence of the major histocompatibility complex (MHC) on T-cell activation, and the analysis of specific and non-specific T-cell factors by cell fusion.

### MHC influence on DTH

The T cells involved in DTH belong to a defined sub-set distinguishable, according to several criteria, from T cells which subserve other immunological reactions[2]. For example, the various sub-sets of T cells can be distinguished according to surface markers (antigens of the Ly series in mice) and to their control by genes of the major histocompatibility complex (MHC, Table 10.1). The MHC (*H*-2 in mice or *HLA* in man) is a cluster of genes coding for structures or antigens (glycoproteins) many of which are expressed on the surface membrane of most cells. For the purpose of this discussion, the *H-2* complex can be divided into two main regions. The genes of the peripheral regions *H-2K* and *H-2D*, code for antigens present on most cells, and were originally discovered because of their capacity to provoke graft rejection. The genes of the central *I* region code for *I*-associated (*Ia*) antigens and are distributed among 5 sub-loci (so far detected): *I-A*, *I-B*, *I-J*, *I-E* and *I-C*.

**Table 10.1** T cell sub-sets

| *T cell sub-sets* | *Function* | *Cell surface markers* | *MHC restriction* |
|---|---|---|---|
| $T_D$ | DTH | Ly-1$^+$, *Ia*$^-$ | *I-A* for protein antigens |
| $T_H$ | help B cells produce IgG antibody | Ly-1$^+$, some are *Ia*$^+$ | *I-A* |
| $T_C$ | kill specific targets after contact | Ly-2,3$^+$, *Ia*$^-$ | *H-2K*, *H-2D* |
| $T_S$ | suppress responses of other lymphocytes | Ly2,3$^+$, *I-J*$^+$ | *I-J* |

The MHC exerts a profound influence on T cell functions. Thus, the frequency of alloreactive T cells (i.e. T cells with reactivities directed to antigens coded by MHC genes in non-identical members of the same species) is 100–1000 times greater than the frequency of T cells reactive to non-MHC coded antigens. Different T-cell sub-sets exhibit the phenomenon of MHC restriction as described below. The MHC-linked *Ir* genes influence the responsiveness of T cells or T-cell dependent functions. Finally, there are *I*-region coded determinants on antigen specific 'helper' or 'suppressor' factors which can be released or extracted from $T_H$ and $T_S$ cells, respectively.

Most immune phenomena associated with T cells are subject to *H-2* restriction, i.e., identity at certain *H-2* gene products is required between cells responsible for immune induction of T cells (antigen-presenting 'stimulator' (cells) and targets of immune T cells. For example, $T_D$ cells cannot be activated by soluble forms of antigen. On the contrary, the antigen must be presented on the surface of some 'stimulator' cell such as an epidermal cell (perhaps the epidermal cells of Langerhans) in the case of contact sensitivity, or a macrophage (for other forms of DTH). The $T_D$ cells, activated as a result of appropriate antigen presentation, have their reactivities directed not to antigen alone but to antigen as well as a component, on the surface of the antigen-presenting cell, coded by the MHC. This was demonstrated in two types of experiments. One involved the transfer of sensitized cells into various strains of naive mice. These were challenged with soluble antigen which was presumably taken up by antigen presenting cells. According to the strains used, these cells may or may not have differed in their MHC from the donors of the sensitized T cells. Successful transfer occurred only when there was matching, at certain MHC regions, between donors and recipients[3]. In the case of protein or polypeptide antigens, the MHC region involved in restriction was *I-A*; in the case of contact chemicals it was *H-2K, H-2D* or *I-A*.

The second type of experiment used a more direct approach. The immunizing and/or the challenging antigen were both associated with macrophages *in vitro* (by antigen-pulsing and washing techniques) and these cells were given to the mice. For the successful elicitation of DTH to protein antigens, identity at *I-A* was required between the antigen-pulsed macrophages used for sensitization and those used for challenge of the sensitized mice[4,5] (Table 10.2).

**Table 10.2** Elicitation of DTH by KLH-pulsed Mph injected intradermally is restricted by *I* region products expressed on the surface of the Mph

| *Sensitized* mice* | *KLH-pulsed† Mph* | *MHC compatibility* | *L/R]*[125]*I] UdR uptake* |
|---|---|---|---|
| C57BL | CBA | completely allogeneic | 1.3 ± 0.1† |
| B10.A | B10.BR | *K*-end | 3.2 ± 0.4 |
| B10.A | B10.D2 | *D*-end | 1.5 ± 0.1† |
| CBA | B10.A (4R) | *H-2K* and *IA* | 2.4 ± 0.2 |
| A.SW | A.TL | *H-2K* | 1.1 ± 0.1† |
| B10.A (4R) | A.TL | *IA* | 3.5 ± 0.4 |
| B10.A (4R) | B10.A (5R) | *IB* | 1.4 ± 0.2‡ |
| B10.A (5R) | CBA | *IJ* and *IE* | 1.5 ± 0.1† |
| B10.A (2R) | BALB/c | *IC* and *S* | 1.5 ± 0.1‡ |
| A.TH | A.TL | *H-2K* and *H-2D* | 1.2 ± 0.1‡ |

*Mice were sensitized with keyhole limpet haemocyanin (KLH) in CFA.
†These KLH-pulsed Mph could elicit DTH in sensitized syngeneic mice.
‡No significant difference between this value and that in non-sensitized mouse ($p > 0.05$).
Data from reference 10.

The intimate relationship between T cell activation and MHC components hints at the following generalization. First, MHC molecules should have the ability to associate closely with other proteins on cell surfaces. Evidence in favour of this is rapidly accumulating (e.g. viral antigens[6]; bacterial antigens[7]; parasite antigens[8] and minor histocompatibility antigens[9]). Secondly, the T-cell system must have evolved from cells with a self-surveillance function: screening MHC-coded self 'histocompatibility' antigens on cell surfaces for their association with foreign material must have become the primary function of the T cell. Division of labour among the various T-cell sub-sets occurred as the complexity of the system increased. It is beyond the scope of this presentation to discuss these points further. They do, however, pinpoint the MHC genes as one level at which immunoregulation by T lymphocytes must be occurring. Since some form of association between antigen and MHC gene products is essential for T-cell recognition and activation, a 'non-permissive' interaction between a particular antigenic determinant and an MHC component must lead to low or non-responsiveness. The extensive polymorphism of MHC gene products would thus allow most individuals of a given species to respond adequately to one or other determinants of a complex antigen (for further references see review by Miller[10]).

**Analysis of T cell factors by cell fusion**

Since Köhler and Milstein[11] introduced the technique of cell fusion to produce monoclonal antibodies, efforts have been made to immortalize clones of antigen-specific T cells by hybridization with T lymphoma cell lines (e.g. Taniguchi and Miller[12]). This should permit the collection of sufficiently pure material to elucidate the structure of T cell antigen recognition molecules and of factors such as 'lymphokines' which are involved in the inflammatory response of DTH.

In order to obtain functional T-cell hybridomas, three major problems have had to be resolved. First, a particular antigen-specific T cell of a given sub-set should be enriched. This can be done in several ways depending on properties exhibited by a given T-cell sub-set. For example, suppressor T cells have been enriched by their ability to bind to antigen coated dishes (Taniguchi and Miller[13]) and the T cells that transfer DTH by velocity sedimentation (*vide infra*). Secondly, the parent tumour line should be selected against, subsequent to fusion. This is usually achieved with biochemical mutant lines by chemical selection procedures in medium containing hypoxanthine, aminopterine and thymidine, but it can also be done with nonmutant lines by sorting cells (with the fluorescence activated cell sorter), (FACS) with a given surface marker as well as cells containing more than twice the normal number of chromosomes[14]. Thirdly, screening assays should be developed (see Table 10.3) to permit rapid characterization of the hybridomas obtained. Some of these points will now be illustrated from work attempting to hybridize cells involved in DTH.

**Table 10.3** Some screening tests for functional T cell hybrids

| |
|---|
| Karyotype: chromosome numbers, chromosome markers |
| Surface markers: Thy-1, Ly, *I-J*, *Ia*, *H-2*, *Ig* |
| Antigen binding: fluorescence, radioactivity |
| Anti-idiotype or anti-$V_H$ binding if B and T cells share idiotypes or $V_H$ regions |
| Cloned DNA probe for $V_H$ region expression |
| MIF production after antigen-pulsed macrophages or mitogens |
| Help or suppression of immune functions *in vivo* or *in vitro* |

Enrichment of cells able to transfer DTH was achieved with velocity sedimentation techniques. First, B cells and adherent cells, from lymph nodes of mice sensitized to the antigen keyhole limpet haemocyanin (KLH), were removed by passage through an anti-immunoglobulin column. The non-adherent cells (mostly T cells) were then separated on the basis of their sedimentation velocity (s) at unit gravity using a stabilizing buffered step gradient. $10^6$ cells from different fractions were tested for their ability to transfer DTH to naive recipients. Responses could be obtained with cells with $s = 6$ mm/h, whereas transfer of as many $16 \times 10^6$ of the smaller cells ($s =$ 3–5 mm/h) did not give a positive DTH reaction. The enriched DTH population was then fused to the T lymphoma cell line BW 5147 using polyethylene glycol. Subsequent to fusion and chemical selection, the hybrid cells were examined for chromosome numbers, surface markers and ability to bind KLH specifically. A number of hybridomas did bind KHL (as detected by the FACS) and of these, some were $I\text{-}J^+$, i.e., exhibited a marker characteristic of suppressor T cells (Table 10.4). In fact, both cells and supernantant from this particular hybrid could suppress the induction of DTH to KLH *in vivo* in mice (Table 10.5). The fact that a suppressor T-cell hybrid was obtained by fusing cells from lymph nodes of mice sensitized for DTH shows that immunization is associated with the activation of more than one particular sub-set of T cells.

**Table 10.4** Lymph node cells of KLH-sensitized CBA mice enriched by velocity sedimentation and fused with BW 5147 T lymphoma

| *Hybrid line* | *Chromosome number* | *Percentage of cells showing* | | | | |
|---|---|---|---|---|---|---|
| | | *Ig* | *Thy 1.2* | *I-J^k^* | *KLH* binding* | *HGG† binding* |
| L6-20 | 80 | <1 | >95 | — | <1 | — |
| L6-20-2 | — | <1 | >95 | — | 63 | — |
| 28 other sub-clones | — | — | 75–95 | — | <1 | — |
| K21 | 75 | <1 | 68 | — | 9 | — |
| K21–5 | — | <1 | 89 | — | 15 | <1 |
| K21-10 | — | <1 | 73 | — | 36 | <1 |
| K21-11 | — | <1 | 76 | — | 33 | <1 |
| K21-30 | — | <1 | 69 | — | 33 | <1 |
| 15 other sub-clones | — | <1 | 59–91 | — | <5 | <1 |
| 137 | 78 | <1 | >95 | 55 | 47 | <1 |
| 137–10 | — | <1 | — | — | 56 | <1 |
| 137-10-9 | — | <1 | — | 56 | 31 | <1 |
| 137-10-11 | — | <1 | — | 44 | 20 | <1 |
| 1-23 | 78 | <1 | >95 | <1 | <1 | <1 |

*KLH = keyhole limpet haemocyanin †HGG = human gammaglobulin

**Table 10.5** Suppression of induction of DTH to KLH by T cell hybridomas

| *Treatment of mice* | *L/R[^125^I]-UdR uptake* |
|---|---|
| 50 μg KLH-CFA* | 5.9 ± 0.8 |
| 50 μg KLH-CFA + 0.5 ml sn 137–10 i.v. | 1.5 ± 0.2 |
| 50 μg KLH-CFA + 3 × $10^7$ 137-10 cells i.v. | 2.0 ± 0.4 |
| 50 μg KLH-CFA + 0.5 ml sn 1-23 i.v. | 5.2 ± 0.4 |
| 50 μg KLH-CFA + 3 × $10^7$ 1-23 cells i.v. | 4.8 ± 0.5 |

*KLH = keyhole limpet haemocyanin; CFA = complete Freund's adjuvant

Other hybrids could be stimulated by mitogens to produce noncellular factors able to help B cells produce antibody[15] or able to inhibit the migration of macrophages (Arnold and Miller, unpublished).

The production of cloned specific and functional T cell lines by hybridization procedures offers great advantages for the reproducible, large-scale production of various materials for chemical analyses. Among these are antigen-specific factors, such as the T cell surface antigen recognition molecules, and non-antigen specific factors, such as the lymphokines involved in the production of DTH inflammatory lesions.

## References

1 Vadas, M. A., Miller, J. F., Gamble, J. *et al.* (1975). A radioisotopic method to measure delayed type hypersensitivity in the mouse. I. Studies in sensitized and normal mice. *Int.Arch.Allergy Appl.Immunol.*, **49**, 670

2 Miller, J. F., Vadas, M. A., Whitelaw, A. *et al.* (1975). A radioisotopic method to measure delayed type hypersensitivity in the mouse. II. Cell transfer studies. *Int.Arch.Allergy Appl.Immunol.*, **49**, 693

3 Vadas, M. A., Miller, J. F., Whitelaw, A. *et al.* (1977). Regulation by the H-2 gene complex of delayed type hyersensitivity. *Immunogenetics*, **4**, 137

4 Smith, F. I., Mottram, P. and Miller, J. F. A. P. (1979). *Scand. J. Immunol.*, *10*, 343

5 Mottrom, P. and Miller, J. F. A. P. (1980). *Eur. J. Immunol.*, *10*,165

6 Helenius, A., Morein, B., Fries, E. *et al.* (1978). Human (HCA-A and HLA-B) and murine (H-2K and H-2D) histocompatibility antigens and cell surface receptors for Semliki Forest virus. *Proc.Nat.Acad.Sci. (USA).*, **175**, 3846

7 Klareskog, L., Bank, G., Forsgren, A. *et al.* (1978). Binding of HLA antigen-containing liposomes to bacteria. *Proc.Nat.Acad.Sci. (USA).*, **75**, 6197

8 Sher, A., Hall, B. F. and Vadas, M. A. (1978). Acquisition of murine major histocompatibility complex gene products by schistosomula of *Schistosoma mansoni*, *J. Exp. Med.*, **148**, 46

9 Smith, F. I. and Miller, J. F. A. P. (1979). Delayed-type hypersensitivity to allogenic cells in mice. III. Sensitivity to cell surface antigens coded by the major histocompatibility complex and by other genes. *J.Exp.Med.*, **150**, 965

10 Miller, J. F. (1979). Influence of the major histocompatibility complex on T-cell activation. *Adv. Cancer Res.*, **29**, 1

11 Köhler, G. and Milstein, C. (1975). Continuous cultures of fused cells secreting antibody of predefined specificity. *Nature* (*London*), **256**, 495

12 Taniguchi, M. and Miller, J. F. A. P. (1978). Specific suppressive factors produced by hybridomas derived from the fusion of enriched suppressor cells and a T lymphoma cell line. *J.Exp.Med.*, **148**, 373

13 Taniguchi, M. and Miller, J. F. A. P. (1977). Enrichment of specific suppressor T cells and characterization of their surface markers. *J.Exp.Med.*, **146**, 1450

14 Arnold, B., Battye, F. L., and Miller, J. F. A. P. (1979). An improved method for selecting T cell hybridomas by the fluorescence-activated cell sorter. *J.Immunol.Meth.*, **29**, 353

15 Schrader, J. W., Arnold, B. and Clark-Lewis, J. (1980). A con A-stimulated T-cell hybridoma releases factors affecting haematopoietic colony-forming cells and B-cell antibody responses. *Nature* (*London*), **283**, 197

# Discussion

**Professor J. L. Turk: (Chairman)** said that Professor Miller's work was indicative of future trends in delayed hypersenstivity research. Of particular interest was the role of the $T_H$ region and the idiotype of the cells. He wondered how long it would be before data accumulated in these areas.

**Professor Miller:** said that many workers using a variety of experimental designs are producing data suggesting idiotype sharing between T and B lymphocytes. However, his own group had never been able to show the presence of idiotype markers on any of the T-cell hybrids which they had.

**Dr R. Scheper: (Netherlands)** asked why clonal selection had not been used to obtain higher concentrations of antigen specific T cells.

**Professor Miller:** said that they had actually adopted such an approach. *In vitro* culture of normal cells with antigen had allowed them to select antigen-specific cells over a period of weeks, and cells which had been adapted *in vitro* produced more stable hybrids than cells taken directly when they were fused with lymphocyte lines.

**Professor Turk:** said that the identity of the T suppressor cell had always been a problem. In human beings it is the $T\gamma$ cell but there is increasing evidence to suggest that this was not a true T cell, although it has some T-cell characteristics. Following purification, in the electron microscope it looks very much like a cell of the mononuclear phagocyte series. In the guinea pig there seems to be two types of suppressor cell, one behaving like a T cell and the other behaving like a B cell or perhaps a macrophage with a cytophilic antibody on its surface. He wondered whether Professor Miller had examined separated T suppressor cells by electron microscopy to establish that they were in fact lymphocytes and not macrophages.

**Professor Miller:** had not performed such studies but had referred to other work in which, on electron microscopy, suppressor hybrids certainly resembled mononuclear lymphocytes which bound antigen. The identity, at least of the suppressor cell which bound to antigen coated dishes, had certainly not been evaluated. It might be a macrophage which could blind antigen and present it in association with *I-J* to the real suppressor T cell which was also trapped by the same binding technique.

**Professor Turk:** said that it had come as a shock to some workers who had used markers without considering their cellular morphology to discover that a cell with all the characteristics of a T cell which forms an E rosette under the electron microscope occasionally turns out strongly to resemble a macrophage.

# 11

# Arachidonic acid peroxidation in inflammation and its inhibition as a mechanism for anti-inflammatory activity

G. HIGGS AND K. EAKINS (UK)

---

It is 10 years since arachidonic acid metabolism was first associated with the development of the inflammatory response. The detection of prostaglandin release in experimental inflammation[1] and anaphylaxis[2] initiated a series of experiments in which arachidonic acid peroxidation was demonstrated in numerous inflammatory conditions in animals and man. In parallel with these studies, prostaglandins were shown to have potent inflammatory properties. It is now generally accepted that prostaglandins, along with vasoactive amines and kinins are the most likely chemical mediators of vascular responses in acute and chronic inflammation[3]. An important stimulus to this area of research came with the discovery that aspirin and other non-steroid anti-inflammatory drugs selectively inhibit prostaglandin symthesis[4-6]. This led Vane to propose his now famous theory that inhibition of prostaglandin biosynthesis explains the therapeutic and toxic effects of aspirin-like drugs[4]. The other major group of anti-inflammatory drugs, the coricosteroids, do not have a direct effect on arachidonate metabolizing enzymes but they are thought to interfere with the release of fatty acids from phospholipids[7-10]. The role of prostaglandins in inflammation and the effects of prostaglandin synthetase inhibitors have been comprehensively reviewed by Ferreira and Vane[11].

Much of the early work with prostaglandins and inflammation concerned the detection and effects of stable products of arachidonate metabolism. Since 1969, however, it has been evident that there are unstable intermediates formed during the generation of prostaglandins[2]. In the mid-1970s

Samuelsson and his colleagues identified two cyclic endoperoxides[12] which are known to occupy a pivotal role as intermediates in the synthesis of stable prostaglandins, thromboxanes[13] and prostacyclin[14] each of which have different biological properties. The pharmacology and endogenous roles of these unstable cyclo-oxygenase products have been discussed by Moncada and Vane[15].

In 1974 an alternative route of arachidonate oxygenation was demonstrated with the discovery of a platelet lipoxygenase[16,17]. Similar enzyme systems have been reported in other tissues such as lung[18] and leukocytes[19]. Lipoxygenases synthesize a series of hydroperoxy and hydroxy acids, some of which have been detected in inflammation. The possibility that this route of metabolism is a source of inflammatory mediators is now being investigated. Further interest in this area has been stimulated by the proposal that arachidonate lipoxygenase initiates the formation of slow reacting substances released in immediate hypersensitivity reactions[20].

### Cyclo-oxygenase pathways

The initial reaction in the cyclo-oxygenase pathway[21,22] is abstraction of hydrogen at C-13 and peroxidation at C-11. This step is followed by addition of oxygen at C-15 and ring closure between C-8 and C-12 (Figure 11.1) to form the cyclic endoperoxides [12] $PGG_2$ and $PGH_2$. If cyclization does not occur, 11-hydroxy eicosatetraenoic acid (11-HETE) is formed via the corresponding hydroperoxy acid. Alternatively, abstraction of hydrogen at C-13 also facilitates peroxidation at C-15, in which case 15-HETE would result. Cyclic endoperoxides can then be converted to thromboxanes, prostacyclin, the stable prostaglandins or a 17C hydroxy acid (HHT) plus malondialdehyde (Figure 11.1).

### Cyclo-oxygenase products in inflammation

Stable prostaglandins, mainly from the E series and predominantly $PGE_2$, have been detected in many types of inflammatory response (for a review see reference 11). The discovery of other products of arachidonate cyclo-oxygenase has led to the investigation of their production in inflammation. Thromboxane generating enzymes have been detected in polymorphonuclear (PMN) leukocytes[23-25] macrophages[26,27] and granuloma tissue[28]. Prostacyclin is the major cyclo-oxygenase product synthesized by blood vessel walls[14,29] and is also produced by macrophages[30] and granuloma tissue.[31] These reports demonstrate that thromboxanes and prostacyclin, as well as the stable prostaglandins, can be generated by inflammatory tissues *in vitro*. Recent work has also provided evidence that prostaglandin endoperoxides are metabolized via thromboxane or prostacyclin synthetase during inflammatory responses *in vivo*. Thromboxane $B_2$ ($TXB_2$) and 6-oxo-$PGF_{1\alpha}$, the stable breakdown products of thromboxane[13] $A_2$ and prostacyclin[32], respectively (Figure 11.1) have been detected in carrageenin induced inflammatory

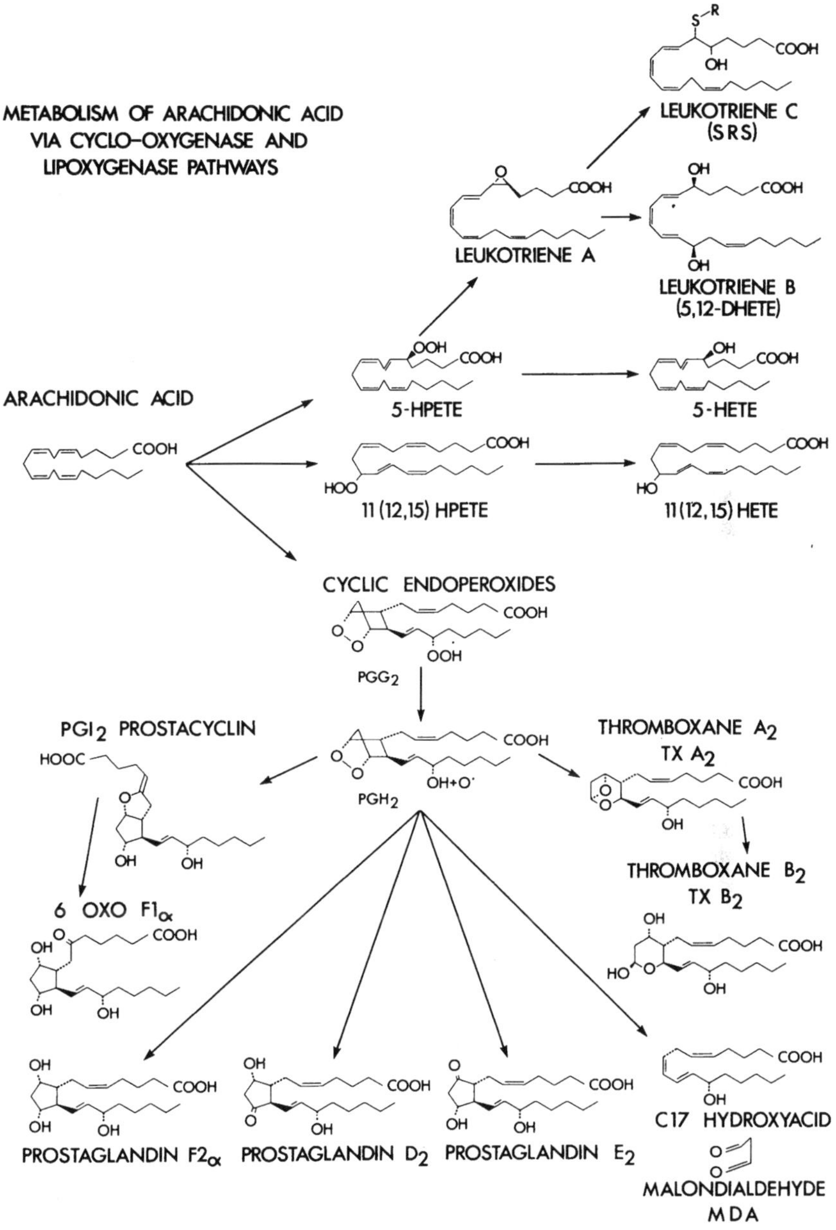


**Figure 11.1** Metabolic pathways of arachidonic acid (1979)

exudates in rats[33]. $TXB_2$ has also been found in joint fluids aspirated from patients with rheumatoid arthritis[34].

Concentrations of $PGE_2$ and 6-oxo-$PGF_{1\alpha}$ in inflammatory exudates collected from 4 h to 48 h follow a similar pattern but $PGE_2$ levels are approximately double those of 6-oxo-$PGF_{1\alpha}$ (Table 11.1). Maximum cyclo-oxygenase activity appears from 8 h to 48 h, although thromboxane concentrations reach a peak at 12 h and rapidly decline (Table 11.1). Between 48 h and 8 days, synthesis of all three products decreases to less than 35% of maximum values.

**Table 11.1** Concentration of cyclo-oxygenase products in inflammatory exudates collected from subcutaneously implanted sponges in rats 33

| | ng/ml (mean±SEM) | | |
|---|---|---|---|
| *Time* | *$PGE_2$** | *6-oxo-$PGF_{1\alpha}$** | *$TXB_2$** |
| 12 h | 43±14 | 23±2.8 | 74±11 |
| 24 h | 65±17 | 33±6.7 | 17±5.4 |
| 48 h | 63±16 | 27±6.6 | 4.8±1.8 |
| 4 days | 44±3.2 | 25±2.0 | 5.7±1.4 |
| 8 days | 22±1.2 | 4.2±0.7 | 6.4±0.7 |

*Values obtained by radioimmunoassay; data from Higgs and Salmon[33]

**Table 11.2** Relative vasodilator or vasodepressor activity of prostaglandin $E_2$, prostacyclin ($PGI_2$) and 6-oxo-$PGF_{1\alpha}$

| *Preparation* | *$PGI_2$* | *$PGE_2$* | *6-oxo-$PGF_{1\alpha}$* | *Reference* |
|---|---|---|---|---|
| Dog mesentery | 1 | 0.02–1 | <0.0001 | 35 |
| Dog hind limb | 1 | 2–15 | <0.0001 | 35 |
| Rat systemic blood pressure | 1 | 0.125–0.25 | 0.008 | 36 |
| Rabbit systemic blood pressure | 1 | 0.5 | 0.0004 | 36 |
| Rat gastric mucosa | 1 | 0.1 | | 37 |
| Rabbit skin | 1 | 1 | <0.0001 | 38 |
| Hamster cheek pouch | 1 | 0.012 | 0.043 | 39 |

## Activity of cyclo-oxygenase products in inflammation

Some of the most convincing evidence that prostaglandins are involved in inflammation is based upon their potent actions on vascular smooth muscle. Prostaglandin $E_2$ is vasodilator and its production in inflammation contributes to the characteristic erythema seen in acute inflammation. Prostacyclin also has strong vasodepressor and vasodilator properties, being more potent than $PGE_2$ in most vascular beds (Table 11.2).

Oedema formation is the result of an interaction between mediators which separately cause vasodilatation and increased vascular permeability[40]. The combined actions of the two different types of mediator result in enhanced oedema formation[41,42]. The vasodilator component of plasma exudation in rabbit skin is reduced by cyclo-oxygenase inhibitors[38] and is most likely due to the local release of $PGE_2$ and prostacyclin. Like $PGE_2$, prostacyclin induces rat paw oedema[43,44] and enhances the effects of other mediators in carrageenin induced oedema[43] or bradykinin induced plasma exudation[38].

Prostaglandins of the E series are hyperalgesic and they enhance the pain-producing activity of other inflammatory mediators such as bradykinin[45,46]. Prostacyclin is more potent than $PGE_2$ in producing hyperalgesia[43,47] but its effects are shorter lasting[47]. Carrageenin induced hyperalgesia is reversed by cyclo-oxygenase inhibitors administered before or after the inflammatory stimulus. This suggests that the response is mediated by the production of a short acting cyclo-oxygenase product such as prostacyclin rather than $PGE_2$[47].

Cyclic AMP regulates leukocyte function and the elevation of neutrophil cyclic AMP results in the inhibition of movement of these cells[48]. Prostacyclin is the most potent adenyl cyclase stimulator among the prostanoids[49,50] and concentrations of prostacyclin as low as 1–100 ng/ml prevent PMN leukocyte chemotaxis *in vitro*[51]. Furthermore, intravenous infusions of prostacyclin inhibit the characteristic margination and adherence of leukocytes in inflamed venules in the hamster cheek pouch[52]. These observations indicate that prostacyclin protects blood vessel walls against leukocyte adherence as well as platelet aggregation[53]. It is interesting that total leukocyte numbers in 8-day inflammatory exudates are at their highest when prostacyclin production is at its lowest[33].

The role of thromboxane $A_2$ in inflammation is difficult to assess in view of its very short half-life. However, thromboxane production has been detected in phagocytozing PMNs[23–25] and aggregating platelets[13] and these cells may be the source of thromboxane $B_2$ detected in inflammatory exudates[33,34]. $TXA_2$ is a potent aggregator of platelets[13] and is a powerful vasoconstrictor[54]. These properties may help to prevent haemorrhage in inflammation. There are no reports of the effects of thromboxane $A_2$ in inflammation but thromboxane $B_2$ has been reported to be chemotactic for mouse PMNs[55] and may, therefore, be involved in the accumulation of cells at an inflammatory site. $TXB_2$ is not, however, chemotactic for human leukocytes[56].

It has been suggested that the generation of free radicals during cyclo-oxygenase metabolism may lead to inflammatory effects[57]. The radical scavenger MK447 facilitates the conversion of $PGG_2$ to $PGH_2$ (Figure 11.1) by removal of a free oxygen radical. The hypothesis that this is the mechanism of the anti-inflammatory activity of MK447 is not, however, supported by evidence that $PGG_2$ is less potent than $PGE_2$ in producing rat-paw oedema[58] or plasma exudation in rabbit skin[40]. It seems most likely, therefore, that the inflammatory properties of the cyclic endoperoxides are due mainly to their conversion to prostacyclin or $PGE_2$.

The only other cyclo-oxygenase product which remains to be discussed in this section is the 17C hydroxy acid, 12-L-hydroxyheptadecatrienoic acid (HHT). HHT has less chemotactic activity than other hydroxy acids[56] but it does stimulate T-lymphocyte chemokinesis in conditions where lipoxygenase products, stable prostaglandins and thromboxanes are inactive[59]. This property may influence the function of these immune cells in inflammatory responses.

**Lipoxygenase pathways**

The major product of arachidonic acid oxygenation in platelets is 12-L-hydroxyeicosatetraenoic acid (12-HETE; Figure 11.1) which is generated by a lipoxygenase[16,17]. This discovery has led to the identification of a number of mono-, di- and tri-hydroxy acids synthesized in different tissues. It is unlikely that platelets play an important part in the development of inflammation as the inflammatory response proceeds virtually unimpaired in thrombocytopaenic animals[60]. The activity of leukocyte lipoxygenases, however, may well have a bearing on inflammation.

Polymorphonuclear leukocytes convert arachidonic acid to 5-HETE via the corresponding hydroperoxy acid[19] (Figure 11.1). Samuelsson and his colleagues have now proposed that 5-HPETE is an intermediate in the formation of a family of compounds, each containing a conjugated triene structure[20,61] (Figure 11.1). These products, named leukotrienes, include 5-12 di-HETE and leukotriene C which is formed by the addition of cysteine or a cysteine-containing peptide to the 5–6 epoxide of arachidonic acid[62].

**Lipoxygenase products in inflammation**

Whereas the evidence for cyclo-oxygenase activity in inflammation is substantial, there are few reports, as yet, of lipoxygenase products in inflammatory conditions. When the recently discovered hydroxy acids and leukotrienes become available for use as standards, the assay of these substances in biological fluids such as inflammatory exudates will be possible. Despite the relative infancy of these investigations, and the problems of assay, there are already some indications that lipoxygenase is activated in inflammatory conditions in experimental animals and man. When arachidonic acid is injected into a site of developing granuloma in the rat, a significant proportion is converted to hydroxy acids[63]. Furthermore, 12-HETE has been detected in the inflamed skin of patients with psoriasis[64] and production of 12-HETE in this disease is reduced by anti-inflammatory glucocorticoids[65].

Leukocytes produce a number of hydroxy acids as well as the leukotrienes. Incubation of PMN leukocytes with the calcium ionophore A23187 selectively enhances peroxidation in the C-5 position of arachidonic acid[66] and it is possible that a similar lipoxygenase activation occurs in inflammation.

## Inflammatory activity of lipoxygenase products

The discovery in 1975 that 12-HETE is chemotactic for PMN leukocytes[67] stimulated the investigation of lipoxygenase as a possible source of mediators of cell migration. 12-HETE is chemotactic for human eosinophils and neutrophils and has a weaker effect on monocytes[68]. The monohydroxy acids produced by leukocytes are chemokinetic and 5-HETE is more potent than 12-HETE[69,70]. The most potent chemokinetic hydroxy acid so far tested[71] appears to be leukotriene B (5-12 di-HETE). In terms of peak activity, the chemotactic properties of these lipoxygenase products are comparable with those of the complement fraction[68] C5a. It is possible that lipoxygenase activation could represent an amplification mechanism in local cell accumulation.

The biological activities of leukotrienes remain to be investigated, but preliminary evidence *in vitro*[20] indicates that leukotriene C is a slow reacting substance (SRS). Release of SRS in immediate hypersensitivity reactions has been studied for many years[72], but the chemical identity of these substances has proved elusive. It is possible that leukotrienes are important in inflammatory responses as well as in increased anaphylactic mediator release.

## Anti-inflammatory drugs

### *Cyclo-oxygenase inhibitors*

Prostacyclin and $PGE_2$ are produced in experimental inflammation in sufficient amounts to contribute to the erythema, oedema and hyperalgesia which is characteristic of acute inflammation. The selective inhibition of cyclo-oxygenase by drugs such as indomethacin and aspirin[4-6] explains their anti-inflammatory actions[4].

A number of cyclo-oxygenase inhibitors have a differential effect on leukocyte migration into subcutaneously implanted sponges in rats[73,74]. Indomethacin, aspirin and flurbiprofen enhance the accumulation of cells in inflammatory exudates at doses which significantly reduce prostaglandin production, but inhibit cell migration at higher doses[74,75] (Figure 11.2). The inhibition of cyclo-oxygenase may divert substrate towards the production of chemotactic lipoxygenase products which then account for increased leukocyte migration (Figure 11.2). The subsequent inhibition of leukocyte migration at higher doses may be explained by a non-specific inhibition of arachidonic acid peroxidation.

Sodium salicylate and phenylbutazone also potentiate leukocyte migration, but at doses which have no effect on prostaglandin production[74]. Some non-steroid anti-inflammatory drugs cause an increase in the total products of lipoxygenase[76] and this may be an alternative explanation of the enhanced leukocyte migration seen with low doses of these drugs. The theory that effects on leukocyte migration are mediated through lipoxygenase is sup-

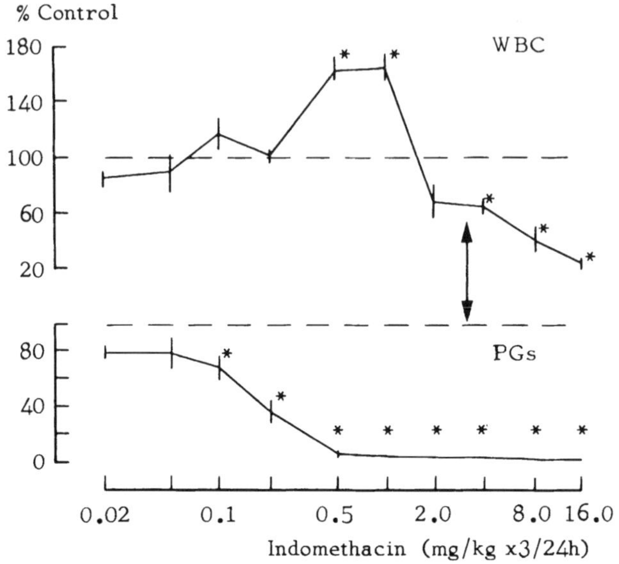


**Figure 11.2** The effect of indomethacin on total leukocyte numbers (WBC) and prostaglandin concentrations (PGs) in inflammatory exudates collected by the subcutaneous implantation of carrageenin impregnated sponges in rats. The exudates are collected at 24 h and the drug is given orally at the time of implantation, 8 h later, and 3 h before removal of the sponge. Each point is the mean of 5–40 experiments and the bars represent ±1 SEM; * indicates that $p<0.05$ compared with control values. The arrows indicate the dose required to inhibit carrageenin induced oedema by 50% in separate experiments. Data taken from Eakins, Higgs, Moncada, Mugridge and Vane, reference (73).

ported by the observation that a lipoxygenase inhibitor reverses the indomethacin induced elevation of leukocyte numbers in inflammatory exudates[73].

Indomethacin and aspirin inhibit rat PMN leukocyte cyclo-oxygenase at doses which also prevent the formation[77] of 11-HETE and 15-HETE. This indicates a common pathway in the formation of these products. The removal of 11-HETE and 15-HETE is unlikely, however, to contribute to anti-inflammatory activity as these hydroxy acids have relatively weak effects on leukocyte function[70].

The demonstration that some non-steroidal anti-inflammatory drugs have a differential effect on leukocyte migration may explain some anomalies arising from their use in the clinic. The aspirin-like drugs give good symptomatic relief in chronic inflammation but it is often stated that they do little to avert the underlying progress of the disease. Symptomatic relief such as analgesia and reduced swelling would result from the removal of cyclo-oxygenase derived mediators, but failure to inhibit lipoxygenase at comparable doses may allow the more chronic, leukocyte-mediated components of inflammation to proceed unchecked.

*Steroids*

Anti-inflammatory corticosteroids do not inhibit oxygenation of arachidonic acid[78] but they do prevent prostaglandin synthesis in a number of different tissues[7–10]. Steroids prevent the release of arachidonic acid from perfused guinea-pig lungs[7] and such an activity would result in reduced cyclo-oxygenase and lipoxygenase activity. It is now thought that anti-inflammatory steroids induce the formation of a substance which inhibits phospholipase $A_2$ which may explain their 'membrane stabilization' effects[10]. The indirect inhibition of arachidonate peroxidation could account for the steroid-induced reduction in prostaglandin concentrations and total leukocyte numbers in inflammatory exudates[78].

*Dual cyclo-oxygenase and lipoxygenase inhibitors*

The anti-inflammatory compound BW755C is equi-active in preventing cyclo-oxygenase and lipoxygenase activity[78,79]. Unlike indomethacin and the salicylates, BW775C does not enhance leukocyte migration at any dose and reduces oedema, prostaglandin concentrations and total leukocyte numbers in inflammation at similar doses[78]. Benoxaprofen has also been shown to inhibit lipoxygenase[80] and this may account for its effects on leukocyte function in inflammation[81].

Dual inhibitors of arachidonic peroxidation are likely to have advantages over selective cyclo-oxygenase inhibitors, by having a greater effect on leukocyte mediated responses in chronic inflammation. It is also possible that compounds such as BW755C will have a steroid-like profile of anti-inflammatory activity without the systemic side effects normally associated with steroid treatment.

**References**


1 Willis, A. L. (1969). Release of histamine, kinin and prostaglandins during carrageenin-induced inflammation of the rat. In Mantegazza, P. and Horton, E. (eds.) *Prostaglandins, Peptides and Amines*, p. 65. (London Academic Press)

2 Piper, P. J. and Vane, J. R. (1969). Release of additional factors in anaphylaxis and its antagonism by anti-inflammatory drugs. *Nature (London)*, **223,** 29

3 Ryan, G. B. and Majno, G. (1977). Acute inflammation. *Am. J. Pathol.*, **86,** 184

4 Vane, J. R. (1971). Inhibition of prostaglandin synthesis as a mechanism of action for the aspirin-like drugs. *Nature (London)*, **231,** 232

5 Smith, J. B. and Willis, A. L. (1971). Aspirin selectively inhibits prostaglandin production in human platelets. *Nature (London)*, **231,** 235

6 Ferreira, S. H., Moncada, S. and Vane, J. R. (1971). Indomethacin and aspirin abolish prostaglandin release from the spleen. *Nature (London)*, **231,** 237

7 Gryglewski, R. J., Panczenko, B., Korbut, R., Grodzinska, L. and Ocetkiewicz, A. (1975). Corticosteroids inhibit prostaglandin release from perfused lungs of sensitized guinea-pigs. *Prostaglandins*, **10,** 343

8 Hong, S. L. and Levine, L. (1976). Inhibition of arachidonic acid release from cells as the bio-

chemical action of anti-inflammatory corticosteroids. *Proc. Nat. Acad. Sci (USA)*., **73,** 1730
9 Nijkamp, F. P., Flower, R. J., Moncada, S. and Vane, J. R. (1976). Partial purification of RCS-RF (rabbit aorta contracting substance releasing factor) and inhibition of its activity by anti-inflammatory steroids. *Nature*, (London), **263,** 479
10 Flower, R. J. and Blackwell, G. J. (1979). Anti-inflammatory steroids induce biosynthesis of a phospholipase $A_2$ inhibitor which prevents prostaglandin generation. *Nature* (London), **278,** 456
11 Ferreira, S. H. and Vane, J. R. (1979). Mode of action of anti-inflammatory agents which are prostaglandin synthetase inhibitors. In Vane, J. R. and Ferreira, S. H. (eds.) *Anti-inflammatory drugs*. (50/II, 348) (Springer–Verlag)
12 Hamberg, M., Svensson, J., Wakabayashi, T. and Samuelsson, B. (1974). Isolation and structure of two prostaglandin endoperoxides that cause platelet aggregation. *Proc. Natl. Acad. Sci (USA)*, **71,** 345
13 Hamberg, M., Svensson, J. and Samuelsson, B. (1975). Thromboxanes: A new group of biologically active compounds derived from prostaglandin endoperoxides. *Proc. Natl. Acad. Sci. (USA)*, **72,** 2994
14 Moncada, S., Gryglewski, R. J., Bunting, S. and Vane, J. R. (1976). An enzyme isolated from arteries transforms prostaglandin endoperoxides to an unstable substance that inhibits platelet aggregation. *Nature (London)*, **263,** 663
15 Moncada, S. and Vane, J. R. (1979). Pharmacology and endogenous roles of prostaglandin endoperoxides, thromboxane $A_2$ and prostacyclin. *Pharm. Rev*., **30,** 293
16 Hamberg, M. and Samuelsson, B. (1974). Prostaglandin endoperoxides. Novel transformations of arachidonic acid in human platelets. *Proc. Natl. Acad. Sci. (USA)*., **71,** 3400
17 Nugteren, D. A. Arachidonate lipoxygenase in blood platelets. (1975). *Biochim. Biophys. Acta* **380,** 299
18 Hamberg, M. (1976). On the formation of thromboxane $B_2$ and 12L-hydroxy-5,8,10,14-eicosatetraenoic acid (12 ho - 20:4) in tissues from the guinea pig. *Biochim. Biphys. Acta*, **431,** 651
19 Borgeat, P., Hamberg, M. and Samuelsson, B. (1976). Transformation of arachidonic acid and dihomo-γ-linolenic acid by polymorphonuclear leukocytes. *J. Biol. Chem*., **251,** 7816
20 Murphy, R. C., Hammarstrom, S. and Samuelsson, B. Leukotriene C: A slow-reacting substance from murine mastocytoma cells. *Proc. Natl. Acad. Sci. (USA)*, **76,** 4275
21 Hamberg, M. and Samuelsson, B. (1967). On the mechanism of the biosynthesis of prostaglandins $E_1$ and $F_{1\alpha}$. *J. Biol. Chem*., **242,** 5336
22 Nugteren, D. H., Beerthuis, R. K. and Dorp, D. A. van. (1966). The enzymatic conversion of all-cis 8,11,14-eicosatrienoic acid into prostaglandin $E_1$. *Rec. Trav. Chim. Pays-Bas*., **85,** 405
23 Higgs, G. A., Bunting, S., Moncada, S. and Vane, J. R. (1976). Polymorphonuclear leukocytes produce thromboxane $A_2$-like activity during phagocytosis. *Prostaglandins*, **12,** 749
24 Goldstein, I. M., Malmsten, C. L., Kaplan, H. B., Jindahl, H., Samuelsson, B. and Weissman, G. (1977). Thromboxane generation by stimulated human granulocytes. Inhibition by glucocorticoids and superoxide dismutase. *Clin. Res*., **25,** 518A
25 Davison, E. M., Ford–Hutchinson, A. W., Smith, M. J. H. and Walker, J. R. (1978). The release of thromboxane $B_2$ by rabbit peritoneal polymorphonuclear leukocytes. *Br. J. Pharmacol*., **63,** 407P
26 Brune, K., Glatt, M. and Kalin, H. (1978). Pharmacological control of prostaglandin and thromboxane release from macrophages. *Nature (London)*, **274,** 261
27 Murota, S–I., Kawamura, M. and Morita, I. (1978). Transformation of arachidonic acid into thromboxane $B_2$ by the homogenates of activated macrophages. *Biochim. Biophys. Acta*, **528,** 507
28 Chang, W. C., Murota, S–I. and Tsurufuji, S. (1977). Thromboxane $B_2$ transformed from arachidonic acid in carrageenin-induced granuloma. *Prostaglandins*, **13,** 17
29 Salmon, J. A., Smith, D. R., Flower, R. J., Moncada, S. and Vane, J. R. (1978). Further studies on the enzymatic conversion of prostaglandin endoperoxide into prostacyclin by porcine aorta microsomes. *Biochim. Biophys. Acta*, **523,** 250
30 Humes, J. L., Bonney, R. J., Pelus, L., Dahlgren, M. E., Sadowski, S. J., Kuehl, F. A. and Davies, P. (1977). Macrophages synthesise and release prostaglandins in response to inflammatory stimuli. *Nature (London)*, **269,** 149

31 Chang, W. C., Murota, S–I., Matuso, M. and Tsurufuji, S. (1976). A new prostaglandin transformed from arachidonic acid in carrageenin-induced granuloma. *Biochem. Biophys. Res. Commun.*, **72,** 1259
32 Johnson, R. A., Morton, D. R., Kinner, J. H., Gorman, R. R., McGuire, J. C., Sun, F. F., Whittaker, N., Bunting, S., Salmon, J. A., Moncada, S. and Vane, J. R. (1976). The chemical structure of prostaglandin X (prostacyclin). *Prostaglandins*, **12,** 915
33 Higgs, G. A. and Salmon, J. A. (1979). Cyclo-oxygenase products in carrageenin-induced inflammation. *Prostaglandins*, **17,** 737
34 Trang, L. E., Granstrom, E. and Lovgren, O. (1977). Levels of prostaglandin $F_{2\alpha}$ and $E_2$ and thromboxane $B_2$ in joint fluid in rheumatoid arthritis. *Scand. J. Rheum.*, **6,** 151
35 Dusting, G. J., Moncada, S. and Vane, J. R. (1978). Vascular actions of arachidonic acid and its metabolites in perfused mesenteric and femoral beds of the dog. *Eur. J. Pharmacol.*, **49,** 65
36 Armstrong, J. M., Lattimer, N., Moncada, S. and Vane, J. R. (1978). Comparison of the vasodepressor effects of prostacyclin and 6-oxo-prostaglandin $F_{1\alpha}$ with those of prostaglandin $E_2$ in rats and rabbits. *Br. J. Pharmacol.*, **62,** 125
37 Whittle, B. J. R., Boughton-Smith, N. K., Moncada, S. and Vane, J. R. (1978). Actions of protacyclin ($PGI_2$) and its product, 6-oxo-$PGF_{1\alpha}$ on the rat gastric mucosa *in vivo* and *in vitro Prostaglandins*, **15,** 955
38 Williams, T. J. (1979). Prostaglandin $E_2$, prostaglandin $I_2$ and the vascular changes of inflammation. *Br. J. Pharmacol.*, **65,** 517
39 Higgs, G. A., Cardinal, D. C., Moncada, S. and Vane, J. R. (1979). Mircrocirculatory effects of prostacyclin ($PGI_2$) in the hamster cheek pouch. *Microvasc. Res.*, **18,** 245
40 Williams, T. J. and Peck, M. J. (1977). Role of prostaglandin-mediated vasodilation in inflammation. *Nature* (*London*), **270,** 530
41 Williams, T. J. and Morley, J. (1973). Prostaglandins as potentiators of increased vascular permeability in inflammation. *Nature* (*London*), **246,** 215
42 Moncada, S., Ferreira, S. H. and Vane, J. R. (1973). Prostaglandins, aspirin-like drugs and the oedema of inflammation. *Nature* (*London*), **246,** 217
43 Higgs, E. A., Moncada, S. and Vane, J. R. (1978). Inflammatory effects of prostacyclin ($PGI_2$) and 6-oxo-$PGF_{1\alpha}$ in the rat paw. *Prostaglandins,* **16,** 153
44 Komoriya, K., Ohmori, H., Azuma, A., Kurozumi, S., Hashimoto, Y., Nicolaou, K. C., Barnette, W. E. and Magolda, R. L. (1978). Prostaglandin $I_2$ as a potentiator of acute inflammation in rats. *Prostaglandins*, **15,** 557
45 Ferreira, S. H. (1972). Prostaglandins, aspirin-like drugs and analgesia. *Nature* (*London*), **240,** 200
46 Moncada, S., Ferreira, S. H. and Vane, J. R. (1974). Sensitization of pain receptors of dog knee joint by prostaglandins. In Robinson, H. J. and Vane, J. R. (eds.) *Prostagandin Synthetase Inhibitors*, p. 189. (New York: Raven Press)
47 Ferreira, S. H., Nakamura, M. and Abreu Castro, M. S. (1978). The hyperalgesic effects of protacyclin and $PGE_2$. *Prostaglandins*, **16,** 31
48 Rivkin, I., Rosenblatt, J. and Becker, E. L. (1974). The role of cyclic AMP in the chemotactic responsiveness and spontaneous motility of rabbit peritoneal neutrophils. *J. Immunol.*, **115,** 1126
49 Tateson, J. E., Moncada, S. and Vane, J. R. (1977). Effects of prostacyclin (PGX) on cyclic AMP concentrations in human platelets. *Prostaglandins*, **13,** 389
50 Gorman, R. R., Bunting, S. and Miller, O. V. (1977). Modulation of human platelet adenylate cyclase by prostacyclin (PGX). *Prostaglandins*, **13,** 377
51 Weksler, B. B., Knapp, J. M., and Jaffe, E. A. (1977). Prostacyclin ($PGI_2$) synthesised by cultured endothelial cells modulates polymorphonuclear leukocyte function. *Blood,* **50,** (Suppl. 1), 287
52 Higgs, G. A., Moncada, S. and Vane, J. R. (1978). Prostacyclin reduces the number of 'slow moving' leukocytes in hamster cheek pouch venules. *J. Physiol.*, **280,** 55P
53 Moncada, S. and Vane, J. R. (1978). Unstable metabolites of arachidonic acid and their role in haemostasis and thrombosis. *Br. Med. Bull*, **34,** 129
54 Moncada, S., Needleman, P., Bunting, S. and Vane, J. R. (1976). Prostaglandin endoperoxide and thromboxane generating systems and their selective inhibition. *Prostaglandins*, **12,** 323
55 Kitchen, E. A., Boot, J. R. and Dawson, W. (1978). Chemotactic activity of thromboxane

$B_2$, prostaglandins and their metabolites for polymorphonuclear leukocytes. *Prostaglandins*, **16**, 239
56 Goetzl, E. J. and Gorman, R. R. (1978). Chemotactic and chemokinetic stimulation of human eosinophil and neutrophil polymorphonuclear leukocytes by 12-L-hydroxy-5,8,10-heptadecatrienoic acid (HHT). *J. Immunol.*, **120**, 526
57 Kuehl, F. A., Humes, J. L., Egan, R. W., Ham, E. A., Beveridge, G. C. and Van Arman, C. G. (1977). Role of prostaglandin endoperoxide $PGG_2$ in inflammatory processes. *Nature (London)*, **265**, 170
58 Moncada, S. (1979). New developments in the knowledge of arachidonic acid metabolic products in inflammation. *Eur. J. Rheum. Inflam.*, **2**, 90
59 McCarty, J. and Goetzl, E. J. (1979). Stimulation of human T-lymphocyte chemokinesis by arachidonic acid. *Cell Immunol.*, **43**, 103
60 Ubatuba, F. B., Harvey, E. A. and Ferreira, S. H. (1975). Are platelets important in inflammation? *Agents Actions*, **5**, 31
61 Samuelsson, B., Borgeat, P., Hammarstrom, S. and Murphy, R. C. (1979). Introduction of a nomenclature: Leukotrienes. *Prostaglandins*, **17**, 785
62 Hammarstrom, S., Murphy, R. C., Samuelsson, B., Clark, D. A., Mioskowski, C. and Corey, E. J. (1979). Structure of Leukotriene C: Identification of the amino acid part. *Biochem. Biophys. Res. Commun*, **91**, 1266
63 Bragt, P. C. and Bonta, I. L. (1979). *In vivo* metabolism of $[1-{}^{14}C]$ arachidonic acid during different phases of granuloma development in the rat. *Biochem. Pharmacol.*, **28**, 1581
64 Hammarstrom, S., Hamberg, M., Samuelsson, B., Duell, E. A., Stawiski, M. and Voorhees, J. J. (1975), Increased concentrations of non-esterified arachidonic acid, 12L-hydroxy 5,8,10,14-eicosatetraenoic acid, prostaglandin $E_2$ and prostaglandin $F_{2\alpha}$ in epidermis of psoriasis. *Proc. Natl. Acad. Sci. (USA)*, **72**, 5130
65 Voorhees, J. J., Duell, E. A., Anderson, T. and Stawiski, M. Glucocorticoid reduces the elevated arachidonic acid and 12L-hydroxy-5,8,10,14-eicosatetraenoic acid levels in involved psoriasis epidermis. *Fed. Proc.*, (In press)
66 Borgeat, P. and Samuelsson, B. (1979). Arachidonic acid metabolism in polymorphonuclear leukocytes: Effects of ionophore A23187. *Proc. Natl. Acad. Sci (USA)*, **76**, 2148
67 Turner, S. R., Tainer, J. A. and Lynn, W. S. (1975). Biogenesis of chemotactic molecules by the arachidonate lipoxygenase system of platelets. *Nature (London)*, **257**, 680
68 Goetzl, E. J., Woods, J. M. and Gorman, R. R. (1977). Stimulation of human eosinophil and neutrophil polymorphonoclear leukocyte chemotaxis and random migration by 12-L-Hydroxy-5,8,10,14-eicosatetraenoic acid. *J. Clin. Invest.*, **59**, 179
69 Goetzl, E. J., Brash, A. R., Oates, J. A. and Hubbard, W. C. (1979). Functional determinants of the monohydroxy eicosatetraenoic acids (HETEs) which stimulate human neutrophil and eosinophil chemotaxis. *Fed. Proc.*, **38**, 1085
70 Palmer, R. M. J., Salmon, J. A., Narumiya, S., Higgs, G. A. and Eakins, K. E. (1980). Arachidonic acid metabolism by lipoxygenase in leukocytes of different species and the chemokinetic activity of some products. This volume, Chap. 35
71 Ford-Hutchinson, A. W., Bray, M. A. and Smith, M. J. H. (1980). Are there biologically active products of lipoxygenase pathways produced by polymorphonuclear leucocytes? This volume, Chap. 34
72 Austen, K. (1978). Homeostasis of effector systems which can also be recruited for imunologic reactions. *J. Immunol.* **121**, 793
73 Eakins, K. E., Higgs, G. A., Moncada, S., Mugridge, K. G. and Vane, J. R. (1980). The effects of indomethacin and BW755C on leukocyte migration and prostaglandin production in carrageenin-induced inflammation. *Br. J. Pharmacol.* **69**, 270
74 Eakins, K. E., Higgs, G. A., Moncada, S. and Mugridge, K. G. (1980). Non-steroid anti-inflammatory drugs which potentiate leukocyte migration in carrageenin-induced inflammation. *Br. J. Pharmacol.* **70**, 182
75 Adams, S. S., Burrows, C. A., Skeldon, N. and Yates, D. B. (1977). Inhibition of prostaglandin synthesis and leukocyte migration by flurbiprofen. *Cur. Med. Res.*, **5**, 11
76 Siegel, M. I., McConnel, R. T. and Cuatrecasas, P. (1979). Aspirin-like drugs interfere with arachidonate metabolism by inhibition of the HPETE peroxidase activity of the lipoxygenase pathway. *Proc. Natl. Acad. Sci. (USA).*, **76**, 3774
77 Siegel, M. I., McConnell, R. T., Porter, N. A., Selph, J. L., Truax, J. D., Vinegar, R. and

Cuatrecasas, P. (1980). Aspirin-like drugs inhibit arachidonic acid metabolism via lipoxygenase and cyclo-oxygenase in rat neutrophils from carrageenin pleural exudates. This volume, Chap. 36

78 Higgs, G. A., Flower, R. J. and Vane, J. R. (1979). A new approach to anti-inflammatory drugs. *Biochem. Pharmacol.*, **28,** 1959

79 Radmark, O., Malmsten, C. and Samuelsson, B. (1980). The inhibitory effects of BW755C on arachidonic acid metabolism in human polymorphonuclear leukocytes. *FEBS Lett* **110,** 213

80 Walker, J. R. and Dawson, W. (1980). Inhibitory effect of benoxaprofen and BW755C on rabbit PMN leucocyte lipoxygenase. This volume, Chap. 38

81 Meacock, S. C. R. and Kitchen, E. A. (1979). Effects of the non-steroid anti-inflammatory drug benoxaprofen on leukocyte migration. *J. Pharm. Pharmacol.*, **31,** 366

# 12

# General Discussion

**Dr R. McMillan (USA)** asked if any information existed on the presence of lipoxygenase products of thromboxanes in rheumatoid synovial fluid. His own studies suggested that in rheumatoid synovial fluid and synovial cells stable prostaglandins, particularly prostaglandin $E_2$ was the main product.

**Dr Higgs** said that the cyclo-oxygenase products should be considered first because they were relatively easy to measure. There was a report in the literature showing the presence of thromboxane $B_2$ in synovial fluid in patients with rheumatoid arthritis and the levels of $TXB_2$ were higher than in other types of chronic inflammation like osteoarthritis. He knew of no reports on prostacyclin or its breakdown products in human inflammatory exudate but he did believe that quite high levels of prostacyclin were generated in chronic inflammation. The methodology to measure lipoxygenase products was at present less sensitive but Dr J. A. Salmon had detected lipoxygenase products in inflammatory exudates from experimental animals although there were so far no reports in man.

**Mr M. A. Bray (UK)** drew attention to the indomethacin results. His own group obtained a similar enhancement of leukocyte chemokinesis and adherence in the middle dose range and he wondered whether this was due to indomethacin causing a switching of pathways towards lipoxygenase. If so, indomethacin could be unique because a similar enhancement was not seen with cyclo-oxygenase inhibitors.

**Dr Higgs** said that a number of theories were currently under consideration. Initially they believed it to be a diversionary pathway, but they then studied the action of other drugs. They saw potentiation with sodium salicylate, flurbiprofen and phenylbutazone. But they did not see it with naproxen or ibuprofen. It was of interest that those drugs which potentiated migration in low doses (indomethacin, aspirin and flurbiprofen) did so at a dose which significantly reduced cyclo-oxygenase. Sodium salicylate and phenylbutazone potentiated at doses which had no effect on cyclo-oxygenase. Another mechanism therefore appeared to be involved. Further interesting data were coming to light on the inhibition by these drugs of the peroxidase enzyme which converted hydroperoxy acid to the stable hydroxy acid. If it were the unstable intermediate which was enhancing chemotaxis then an effect on its breakdown would cause potentiation independent on a shift in pathways.

**Professor P. Gordon (USA)** on the structure-activity aspect wished to point out that the compound which he had studied, therafectin, which was a glucofuranose derivative, exerted a similar biphasic effect despite having a radically different (non-aromatic) chemical structure and a very different spectrum of toxicity (low or absent).

**Dr Higgs** said that there were obviously going to be several approaches to the problem of blanket inhibition of arachadonic acid peroxidation. A covalent inhibitor binding with the substrate was obviously one approach but it was likely to be highly selective. Removal of molecular oxygen by anti-oxidants or perhaps even a radical scavenger represented other possibilities.

**Professor A. Bennett (UK)** said that some years previously Dr Salmon had performed radio-immunoassay on six samples of human inflamed joint exudates and found immunoreactivity due to the presence of 6-keto-$PGF_{1\alpha}$.

**Dr Higgs** said that this was consistent with his own findings in association with workers at the Institute of Rheumatology, using an *in vitro* culture system for synovial tissue. Such tissue preparations had been shown to produce large quantities of prostacyclin.

**Dr Munthe (Norway)** enquired further about Dr Higgs' suggestion on the clinical implications of enhanced mononuclear infiltration by indomethacin and the possible effect of the doses currently being given on the inflammatory process.

**Dr Higgs** said that he had only been making suggestions for which there was as yet no evidence. It did seem that such experiments might explain a number of anomalies about the therapeutic activity of indomethacin and other aspirin-type drugs. Their lack of effect on the cellular component of inflammation might explain why they did very little to alter the course of the disease, while giving good symptomatic relief. In addition, if the clinician were titrating his patient to give a good analgesic effect and were administering a low dose to avoid gastrointestinal side effects then the possibility existed that he might enhance the leukocyte mediated side of the inflammation rather than suppressing it. This would explain why such drugs were not truly anti-inflammatory. Although it was true that there were usually very few leukocytes in the synovial membrane during rheumatoid inflammation, during relapse in chronic inflammation very large numbers of leukocytes were seen in the synovial fluid, if not in the tissue itself.

# Section III
# Anti-inflammatory and Anti-rheumatic Agents

CHAIRMAN: D. A. Willoughby
CO-CHAIRMAN: C. J. Dunn

# 13

# Review of pathogenesis of adjuvant arthritis and its relation to rheumatoid arthritis (Abstract)

C. M. PEARSON AND Y.-H. CHANG (USA)

Induced arthritis in rats has been utilized as an experimental model of rheumatoid arthritis and/or Reiter's syndrome for more than two decades. It seems to be the best available model of human inflammatory joint diseases. In addition to the usual technique of inducing this disease in rats by complete Freund's adjuvant it has recently been observed that a similar type of polyarthritis can be induced in rats with incomplete Freund's adjuvant (IFA) plus (a) bacterial cell wall structures (usually made up of a disaccaride and an hexapeptide) (b) Type II collagen (c) a synthetic compound, MDP, (muramyl-dipeptide) or (d) a totally unrelated compound, a alkadimamine (molecular weight 714). It has also recently been shown that antibodies to Type II collagen appear in 40% of rats injected with Type II collagen in IFA. Furthermore, antibodies to both Type I and Type II collagen will soon be reported in traditional adjuvant arthritis. This animal disease can be inhibited or minimized by the early administration of immunosuppressive agents, or antiviral agents such as interferon. Later modifications of these forms of arthritis occur when anti-inflammatory compounds such as corticosteroids, butazoladine or a number of NSAIDs are given soon before the arthritis is to appear. There is pathological evidence that the latter compounds reduce the inflammatory synovitis and bony proliferation by about 50% when administered at sufficient dosage levels. Many of these observations in the experimental setting appear to have significant implications in our understanding of human rheumatoid arthritis.

# 14

# The anti-inflammatory activity of aspirin: the active metabolite

M. J. H. SMITH (UK)

## INTRODUCTION

It was suggested by Vane[1] in 1971 that the major therapeutic effects of aspirin and of other non-steroidal acidic drugs were explicable in terms of an interference with the biosynthesis of prostaglandins. The basis of the idea was the finding that aspirin could inhibit the activity of the so-called prostaglandin synthetase enzyme system under *in vitro* conditions. The hypothesis has been restated in later years in a more explicit fashion. Thus, Gryglewski[2] concluded that the target biomolecule for NSAID is fatty acid cyclo-oxygenase and that inhibition of prostaglandin generation *in vivo* accounts for the therapeutic effectiveness of acidic NSAID. The evidence supporting this mechanism of action has been largely concerned with the analgesic and antipyretic effects of aspirin. It is, however, less acceptable as an exclusive mode of action for the anti-inflammatory and anti-rheumatic actions of aspirin and similar drugs[3–5]. Nevertheless, some authors such as Katler and Weissman[6] adhere to the view that the anti-inflammatory effects of aspirin and indomethacin can be explained almost entirely by virtue of their ability to inhibit cyclo-oxygenase, thus preventing the transformation of arachidonic acid to both prostaglandins and thromboxanes. The aims of the present communication are, first, to review the evidence that aspirin and salicylic acid inhibit the enzyme activity *in vitro*. Secondly, to examine the mechanisms by which aspirin interferes with prostaglandin biosynthesis *in vivo*. Finally, to consider whether such an interference should be regarded as an exclusive mode of action for the anti-inflammatory and anti-rheumatic effects of the drug.

### Inhibition of fatty acid cyclo-oxygenase activity *in vitro*

There is no dispute that aspirin inhibits the biosynthesis in a variety of preparations *in vitro*. However, there is very considerable variation in the $IC_{50}$ values between tissues and species (Table 14.1).

**Table 14.1** Inhibition of PG biosynthesis *in vitro* by aspirin

| *Source of enzyme activity* | $IC_{50}$ ($\mu$ mol/l) | *Reference number* |
|---|---|---|
| Rat platelets | 16 | 7 |
| Dog spleen | 37 | 8 |
| Rabbit brain | 61 | 9 |
| Guinea pig macrophages | 280 | 10 |
| Sheep seminal vesicles | 230 | 11 |
| | 9000 | 12 |
| Bovine seminal vesicles | 162 | 13 |
| | 15 000 | 14 |

This variation may arise, at least in part, from the existence of multiple molecular forms of the enzyme, each of which exhibits different biochemical and pharmacological profiles[15]. It may also be due to the mechanism of inhibition coupled with the assay technique used. Aspirin inhibits the enzyme (fatty acid cyclo-oxygenase; 8, 11, 14-eicosatrienoate hydrogen-donor; oxygen oxidoreductase EC.1.14.99.1) by an irreversible mechanism involving a non-enzymatic transfer of the acetyl group from the aspirin to a group or groups either at or near the active site of the enzyme[16]. Thus different results for the $IC_{50}$ may be obtained if the enzyme preparation is pre-incubated with the aspirin before addition of substrate rather than if the reactants are added in the reverse order.

Salicylic acid, the immediate metabolite of aspirin *in vivo*, also inhibits the biosynthesis of prostaglandins *in vitro*. It is, however, a much weaker inhibitor of the cyclo-oxygenase enzyme and when the two acids have been compared directly in the same investigation then the ratio of the $IC_{50}$ is of the order of 1:20 in favour of aspirin (Table 14.2). The mechanism of inhibition differs from that caused by aspirin in that it is reversible and cannot involve a trans-acetylation.

### Inhibition of prostaglandin formation *in vivo*

Some interesting questions may be posed. First, does aspirin exert its inhibitory action on fatty acid cyclo-oxygenase *in vivo* as the intact molecule? The drug is very rapidly hydrolysed to salicylic acid after its absorption in mammalian species and in man this process is complete within minutes[5]. Secondly, if the irreversible inhibition of the enzyme activity by the intact aspirin molecule occurs *in vivo*, is it restricted to a limited environment, i.e. only to readily accessible tissues, and an effect in more remote sites is due to a separate mechanism of inhibition?

**Table 14.2** Inhibition of PG biosynthesis *in vitro* by salicylic acid

| *Test system* | *Relative potency (aspirin = 1)* | *Reference number* |
|---|---|---|
| Bovine seminal vesicles | <0.5 | 17 |
| Dog spleen | 0.06 | 8 |
| Rabbit macrophages | 0.05 | 10 |
| Guinea pig lung | 0.05 | 1 |
| Rabbit kidney | 0.04 | 18 |
| Rat air bleb exudate | inactive | 19 |

There are two situations which are relevant to these queries. One is the circulating platelets, where there is ample evidence in man and animals not only that aspirin, after either oral or parenteral administration, inhibits the enzyme activity in this cellular component but also that the inhibition is irreversible[2,20]. Furthermore, the generation of thromboxane $B_2$ by circulating rat platelets is inhibited by the administration of aspirin but not by larger doses of salicylic acid[21]. This must represent the effect of the aspirin present in the circulation as acetyl salicylic acid.

The second area concerns the prostaglandin content of developing inflammatory exudates of one kind or another. Typical examples are those formed in implanted sponges[22] and in skin blebs[19]. Here, there is no evidence that the intact aspirin molecule penetrates into the exudates and aspirin and salicylic acid are equipotent in reducing the prostaglandin content of the fluid exudates[23]. It has been shown that salicylic acid, after oral administration, accumulates very rapidly in such exudates[24], as indeed it does in any body compartment either surrounded or bordered by acidic fluids[25]. The concentrations of salicylic acid which accumulate in the sponge exudates are more than sufficient to inhibit cyclo-oxygenase activity at the local site[23]. The actual inhibitor at inflammatory sites is therefore salicylic acid, which accumulates either after administration as such or indirectly after its formation from the hydrolysis of aspirin[23]. The hypothesis that a further metabolite of salicylic acid, gentisic acid (2,5-dihydroxybenzoic acid), is involved as an active metabolite is no longer tenable since the substance has been shown to be completely ineffective *in vivo* either as an inhibitor of prostaglandin production or as an anti-inflammatory agent[23]. There must also be intermediary situations in which both types of inhibition may occur. One of these could be the kidney[26]. However, the reduction in urinary prostaglandin content occurring during the clinical administration of NSAID can neither be interpreted as a reduction in total body prostaglandin[27] nor as evidence that the intact aspirin molecule has both reached and acted in the kidney.

It is more likely that after the administration of aspirin, intact acetyl salicylic acid irreversibly inhibits fatty acid cyclo-oxygenase activity in a relatively small number of accessible sites such as cellular components in the blood, vascular endothelium and those tissues immediately adjacent to local injection sites. Thus the direct administration of small amounts of aspirin, of the order of 1 mg, reduce the prostaglandin content of sponge exudates[23]. The rapid hydrolysis of aspirin *in vivo* infers that the intact molecule fails to penetrate more remote sites such as inflammatory exudates in the skin and joints. However, the immediate metabolic product, salicylic acid, preferentially accumulates on such sites in concentrations sufficient to exert a local blockade of prostaglandin biosynthesis.

**Relation between cyclo-oxygenase inhibition and anti-inflammatory activity**

If there is inhibition of cyclo-oxygenase activity in inflammatory exudates after the oral administration of aspirin, even if this is mediated by a metabolic transformation to salicylic acid, is this acceptable as an exclusive mechanism to explain the anti-inflammatory and anti-rheumatic properties of the drugs? There is experimental evidence that prostaglandins of the E series and $PGI_2$ are concerned in the early vascular events of acute inflammation[28,29]. Their major effects at local sites of inflammation are to increase vasodilatation and blood flow and to potentiate the actions of other mediators, histamine and the kinins, in promoting plasma exudation. An interference with their biosynthesis *in vivo* by salicylic acid and other NSAID, would therefore be expected to reduce heat, redness and swelling. However, there are many other phases in the development of acute and chronic inflammatory responses which are not mediated by prostaglandins. The best known is the accumulation of leukocytes at inflammatory sites and there is convincing evidence that indomethacin affects prostaglandin formation and leukocyte infiltration in sponge exudates by different mechanisms[30]. Several authors have commented that much larger doses of aspirin and indomethacin are required to produce effective anti-inflammatory and anti-rheumatic effects than are necessary for either analgesia or for inhibition of prostaglandin biosynthesis *in vivo*[31–34]. These observations do not support an exclusive role in inhibiting fatty acid cyclo-oxygenase as a site of action for salicylic acid and other non-steroidal acidic anti-inflammatory drugs[4,35].

A simple unifying mechanism of action is therefore inadequate to explain the effects of agents, such as the aspirin-like drugs, which modify the complex sequence of events occurring in acute and chronic inflammation. Interference with fatty acid cyclo-oxygenase activity at local areas of inflammation plays a part but the overall anti-inflammatory and anti-rheumatic activities of this group of drugs is due to multiple interactions with several components of inflammatory responses[36]. Aspirin only inhibits the cyclo-oxygenase enzyme activity *in vivo* as the intact molecule in a limited number of readily accessible tissues. After its oral administration it undergoes metabolic transformation to salicylic acid which is the active metabolite both with respect to inhibition of cyclo-oxygenase and anti-inflammatory activity at local sites of inflammation.

## References


1 Vane, J. R. (1971). Inhibition of prostaglandin synthesis as a mechanism of action for aspirin-like drugs. *Nature (London), New Biol.*, **231**, 232

2 Gryglewski, R. J. (1978). Screening and assessment of the potency of anti-inflammatory drugs *in vitro*. In *Anti-Inflammatory Drugs*, Vane, J. R. and Ferreira, S. H. (eds.), pp. 3–43. (Berlin: Springer-Verlag)

3 Smith, M. J. H. (1978). Aspirin and prostaglandins: some recent developments. *Agents Actions*, **8**, 427

4 Glenn, E. M. Bowman, B. J. and Rohloff, N. A. (1979). Anomalous biological effects of salicylates and prostaglandins. *Agents Actions*, **9**, 257

5 Siegel, M. I., McConnell, R. T. and Cuatrecasas, P. (1979). Aspirin-like drugs interfere with arachidonic acid metabolism by inhibition of the 12-hydroperoxy-5, 8, 10, 14-eicosatetraenoic acid peroxidase activity of the lipoxygenase pathway. *Proc. Natl. Acad. Sci. (USA)*, **76**, 3774

6 Katler E. and Weissmann, G. (1977). Steroids, aspirin and inflammation. *Inflammation*, **2**, 295

7 Patrono, C., Ciabattoni, G. and Grossi, D. (1975). Release of prostaglandin $F_{1\alpha}$ and $F_{2\alpha}$ from superfused platelets: quantitative evaluation of the inhibitory effects of some aspirin-like drugs. *Prostaglandins*, **9**, 557

8 Flower, R. J., Gryglewski, R., Herbaczynskia-Cedro, K. and Vane, J. R. (1972). The effect of anti-inflammatory drugs on prostaglandin bio-synthesis. *Nature (London), New Biol.*, **238**, 104

9 Flower, R. J. and Vane, J. R. (1972). Inhibition of prostaglandin synthetase in brain explains the antipyretic activity of paracetamol. *Nature (London)*, **240**, 410

10 Bray, M. A. and Gordon, D. (1978). Prostaglandin production by macrophages and the effects of anti-inflammatory drugs. *Br. J. Pharmacol.*, **63**, 635

11 Young, P. R., Dodge, D. W., Carter, G. W. and Kimura, E. T. (1974). Experimental anti-inflammatory and analgesic studies with 3-trifluoromethyl-5-triazolo (3,4-α)-isoquinoline. *Arch. Int. Pharmacodyn. Ther.* **212**, 205

12 Smith, W. L. and Lands, W. E. M. (1971). Stimulation and blockade of prostaglandin biosynthesis. *J. Biol. Chem.*, **246**, 6700

13 Gryglewski, R. (1974). Structure-activity relationships of some prostaglandin synthetase inhibitors. In *Prostaglandin Synthetase Inhibitors*, Robinson, H. J. and Vane, J. R. (eds.), pp. 33–52. (New York: Raven Press)

14 Tomlinson, R. V., Ringold, H. J., Quershi, M. C. and Forchielli, E. (1972). Relationship between inhibition of prostaglandin synthesis and drug efficacy. *Biochem. Biophys. Res. Commun.*, **46**, 552

15 Flower, R. J. and Vane, J. R. (1974). Some pharmacologic and biochemical aspects of prostaglandin biosynthesis and its inhibition. In Robinson, H. J. and Vane, J. R. (eds.) *Prostaglandin Synthetase Inhibitors*, (1977). pp. 9–18. (New York: Plenum Press)

16 Shen, T. Y. (1977). Prostaglandin synthetase inhibitors. In Berti, F., Samuelsson, B. and Velo, G. P. (eds.) *Prostaglandins and Thromboxanes*, pp. 111–136. (New York: Plenum Press)

17 Flower, R. J., Cheung, H. S. and Cashman, D. W. (1973). Quantitative determination of prostaglandins and malonyldialdehyde formed by arachidonate oxygenase system in bovine seminal vesicles. *Prostaglandins*, **4**, 325

18 Blackwell, G. L., Flower, R. J. and Vane, J. R. (1975). Some characteristics of the prostaglandin synthetase system in rabbit kidney microsomes. *Biochem. Biophys. Acta*, **398**, 178

19 Willis, A. L., Davison, P., Ramwell, P. W., Brocklehurst, W. E. and Smith, B. (1972). Release and actions of prostaglandins in inflammation and fever: inhibition by anti-inflammatory and antipyretic drugs. In *Prostaglandins in Cellular Biology*, Ramwell, P. W. and Pharris, B. B. (eds.), pp. 227–259. (New York: Plenum Press)

20 Roth, G. J. and Majerus, P. W. (1975). The mechanism of the effect of aspirin in human platelets. *J. Clin. Invest.*, **56**, 624

21 Vargaftig, B. B. Salicylic acid fails to inhibit generation of thromboxane $A_2$ activity after *in vivo* administration to the rat *J. Pharm. Pharmacol.*, **30**, 101

22 Higgs, G. A., Harvey, E. A., Ferreira, S. H. and Vane, J. R. (1976). The effects of anti-

inflammatory drugs on the production of prostaglandins *in vivo*. In Samuelson, B. and Paoletti, R. (eds.) Advances in Prostaglandin and Thromboxane Research. Vol. 1, pp. 105–110. (New York: Raven Press)

23 Smith, M. J. H. Ford-Hutchinson, A. W., Walker, J. R. and Slack, J. A. (1979) Aspirin, salicylate and prostaglandins. *Agents Actions*, **9** (In press)

24 Doherty, N. S., Anttila, M. and Dean, P. B. (1977). Penetration of naproxen and salicylate into inflammatory exudates in the rat. *Ann. Rheum. Dis.*, **36**, 244

25 Brune, K., Graf, P. and Rainsford, K. D. (1977). Biodistribution of acid anti-inflammatory drugs. *Drugs Exp. Clin. Res.*, **2**, 155

26 Flower, R. J. (1974). Drugs which inhibit prostaglandin biosynthesis. *Pharm. Rev.*, **26**, 33

27 Dawson, W. (1979). Mediators of inflammation, particularly prostaglandins and their relative importance *Eur. J. Rheumatol. Inflammation*, **3**, 17

28 Bonta, I. L. and Parnham, M. J. (1979). Time-dependent stimulatory and inhibitory effects of prostaglandin $E_1$ on exudative and tissue components of granulomatous inflammation in rats. *Br. J. Pharmacol.*, **65**, 465

29 Williams, T. J. (1979). Prostaglandin $E_2$, prostaglandin $I_2$ and the vascular changes in inflammation. *Br. J. Pharmacol.*, **65**, 517

30 Walker, J. R., Smith, M. J. H. and Ford-Hutchinson, A. W. (1976). Anti-inflammatory drugs, prostaglandins and leucocyte migration. *Agents Actions*, **6**, 602

31 Boardman, P. L. and Hart, F. D. (1967). Clinical measurement of the anti-inflammatory effects of salicylate in rheumatoid arthritis. *Br. Med. J.*, **4**, 264

32 Crook, D., Collins, A. J., Bacon, P. A. and Chan, R. (1976). Prostaglandin synthetase activity from human rheumatoid synovial microsomes. *Ann. Rheum. Dis.*, **35**, 327

33 Blackham, A. and Radziwonik, H. (1977). The effect of drugs in established rabbit monoarticular arthritis. *Agents Actions*, **7**, 473

34 Blackham, A., Farmer, J. B., Radziwonik, H. and Westwick, J. (1974). The role of prostaglandins in rabbit monoarticular arthritis. *Br. J. Pharmacol.*, **51**, 35

35 Whitehouse, M. W. and Rainsford, K. D. (1977). Side-effects of anti-inflammatory drugs. In Bonta, I. L., Thompson, J. and Brune, K. (eds.) *Inflammation: Mechanisms and their impact on therapy. Agents Actions Suppl. 3*, pp. 171–187. (Basel: Birkhauser Verlag)

36 Smith, M. J. H. (1975). Prostaglandins and aspirin: an alternative view, *Agents Actions*, **5**, 315

15

# Indomethacin–sodium salicylate combination/RGH-6705 as a new possibility in the treatment of inflammation (Abstract)

E. EZER, G. T. HAJOS AND L. SZPORNY (HUNGARY)

Animal studies indicated that if indomethacin treatment were combined with sodium salicylate the gastrointestinal side effects were very markedly diminished. The antagonism of ulceration of stomach and intestines could be optimalized using a certain indomethacin-sodium salicylate ratio. In human studies, gastrointestinal blood loss provoked by indomethacin was significantly reduced by concomitant dosage of sodium salicylate, show by $^{51}Cr$-labelled erythrocytes. In rheumatic patients the anti-inflammatory action of the combination was demonstrated, and the incidence of side effects was diminished.

# 16

# Tropesin: a new potential anti-rheumatic ester of indometacin

J. GRIMOVÁ, L. FIŠNEROVÁ, Z. ROUBAL, J. NĚMEC, Z. TRNAVSKÁ AND O. NĚMEČEK (CZECHOSLOVAKIA)

Indometacin is one of the most widely used non-steroidal anti-inflammatory drugs. Its excellent anti-inflammatory efficacy on the one hand, but its relatively high toxicity on the other hand, have initiated several working teams to search for derivatives of indometacin with more advantageous therapeutic properties. In the course of many years a great variety of analogues of indometacin have been synthesized, and esters doubtlessly belong among the most interesting compounds studied. During our work in this sphere, other working teams have applied for patents for glycollic acid ester[1] and trichloroethyl ester of indometacin[2]. From papers published so far it is evident that no new therapeutically usable derivative has been synthesized as yet that would retain the efficacy of indometacin and have a lower toxicity. Our research, therefore, has been mainly focused on this aspect. At the Research Institute for Pharmacy and Biochemistry, Prague, a series of indometacin esters with two types of hydroxy compounds, namely primary alcohols and phenols, was synthesized. The products were assessed using a method based on measuring the rate of cleavage of esters to the parent indometacin and the appropriate alcohol by action of serum esterases *in vitro*. Our requirement for the slowest possible rate of cleavage by animal and human serum esterases *in vitro* was best complied with by the ester of indometacin with tropic acid, 2-phenyl-3-(1-*p*-chlorbenzoyl-2-methyl-5-methoxy-3-indolyl) acetoxypropionic acid in racemic form, given the provisional name tropesin[3,4](Figure 16.1).

In experiments *in vivo* (Figure 16.2) in rats, after oral administration of a tropesin dose of 50 mg/kg, esterolysis was observed between 2–3, with a peak

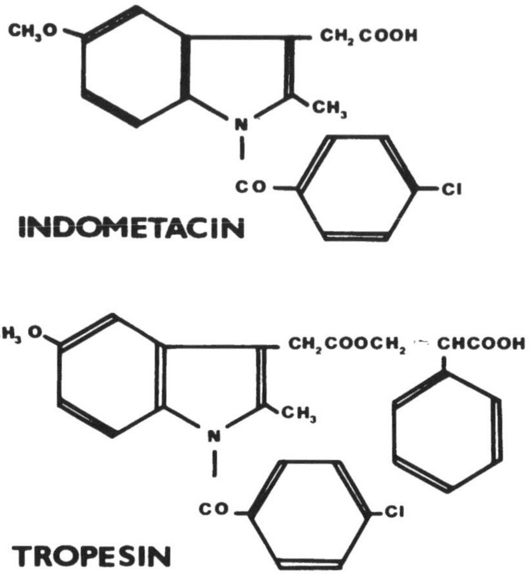


**Figure 16.1** Structural formulae of indometacin and tropesin

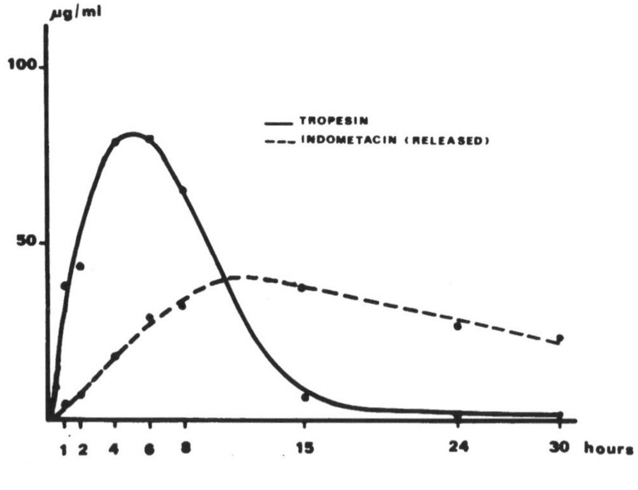


**Figure 16.2** Serum levels of tropesin and released indometacin in rats (50 mg/kg p.o.)

level of liberated indometacin between 10–13 h after ingestion.

Animal studies proved that the acute oral toxicity of tropesin was a fraction of that of indometacin (Figure 16.3). Tropesin was administered orally to rats and dogs in the daily therapeutic dose, triple the dose and ten times the dose for 3 months. After the highest dosage, in isolated cases some dogs were found to have superficial erosions of the gastric mucosa and dystrophic lesions of renal tubules without biochemical correlations. Indometacin, administered in parallel doses, caused severe lesions of the gastrointestinal tract with melaena and subsequent anaemia, as well as severe degenerative changes in renal tubules, in all dosage groups. From the toxicological aspect, tropesin is substantially more acceptable than indometacin.

| | $LD_{50}$ in mg/kg p.o. | |
|---|---|---|
| | MICE | RATS |
| TROPESIN | 190 (170; 213) | 140 (125;157) |
| INDOMETACIN | 46 (33; 63) | 39 (27; 54) |

**Figure 16.3** The medium lethal doses

The anti-inflammatory and anti-arthritic activities of tropesin, in comparison with indometacin, were studied in various models of both acute and chronic inflammatory reactions; kaolin, carrageenin, and adjuvant induced oedema, implanted pellets (Figure 16.4); adjuvant disease (Figure 16.5). Both compounds exhibited significant therapeutic activities without substantial quantitative differences.

The effects of tropesin and indometacin on the digestive tract mucosae were compared in several experiments on rats in relation to the dosage as well as the time and duration of administration. Figure 16.6 shows the therapeutic and ulcerogenic medium doses of both agents; their mutual relationships are essentially more favourable in the case of tropesin than of indometacin.

The advantageous pharmacological properties of tropesin have been also verified in present clinical trials. Repetitive administration of tropesin in daily doses up to 210 mg has not produced any clinical symptoms of intolerance; its therapeutic efficacy has also been very good. The programme of clinical trials also included pharmacokinetical analysis of tropesin in healthy volunteers. Figure. 16.7 shows the courses of the serum levels of tropesin and of indometacin liberated from tropesin, both after a single dose (70 mg) and

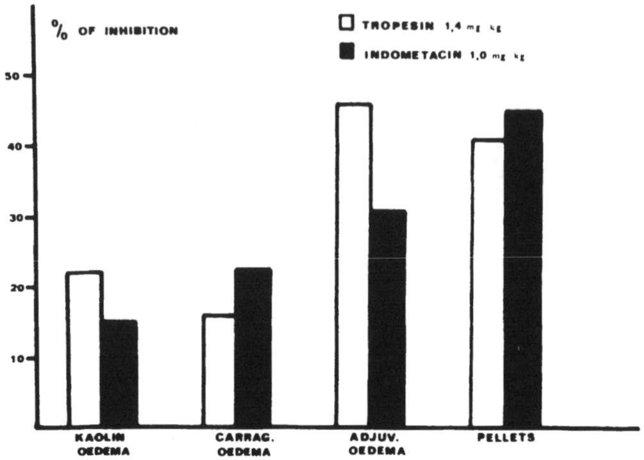


**Figure 16.4** Anti-inflammatory effect of tropesin

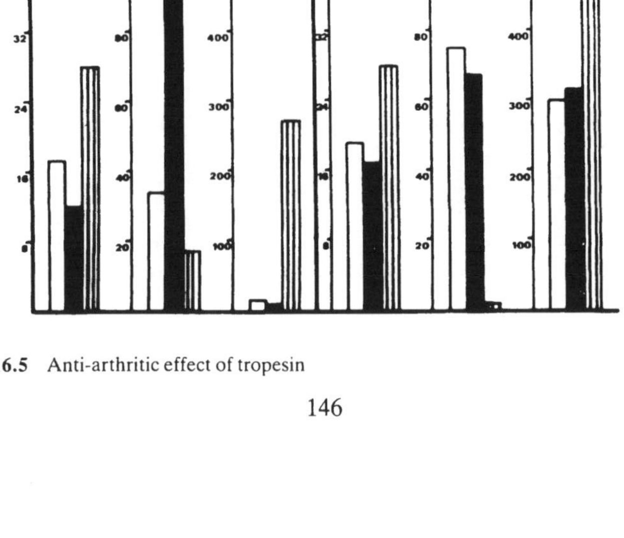


**Figure 16.5** Anti-arthritic effect of tropesin

| | Therap. dose mg/kg | $UD_{50}$ mg/kg |
|---|---|---|
| TROPESIN | 1,4 | 50 (36;70) |
| INDOMETACIN | 1,0 | 1,0 (0,7;1,6) |

**Figure 16.6** Therapeutic and ulcerogenic doses of tropesin and indometacin in rats

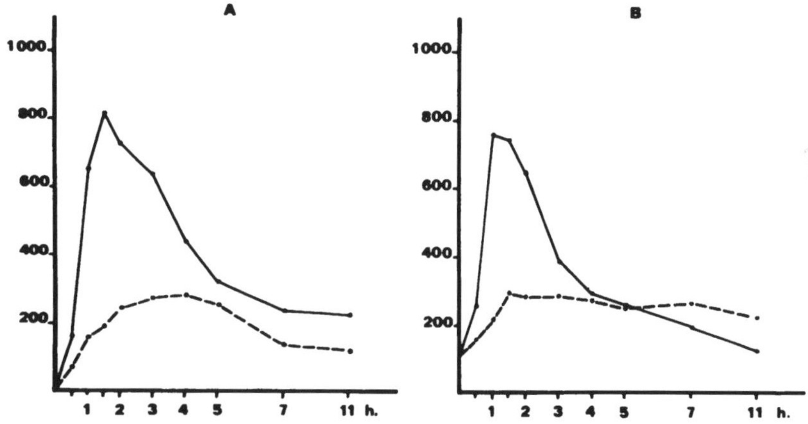


**Figure 16.7** Serum levels of tropesin (●——●) and released indometacin (●-●-●) in man (A single dose, B repeated dose)

during repetitive 5-day administration.

In view of the excellent results of the pre-clinical tests and clinical trials performed so far, tropesin might substantially enrich the therapeutic facilities in chronic musculoskeletal diseases which require long-term administration of an effective remedy with minimal toxic effects.

## References

1 BRD patent (1974) 2.234 651, CA 81, 3765m
2 BRD patent (1970) 2.342 303; US patent 3 488 731, CA 72, 66 817q
3 Fišnerová, L., Grimová, J., Rábek, V. and Roubal, Z. (1977). Pharmacologically interesting indometacin derivatives I. *Cs. Farmacie*, **26**, 227
4 Grimová, J., Fišnerová, L., Koruna, I., Mňouček, K., Rejholec V. and Roubal, Z. (1977). Pharmacologically interesting indometacin derivatives II. *Cs. Farmacie*, **26**, 232

# 17

# Development of an Arthus-like model of induced inflammation and its use in the anti-inflammatory characterization of orgotein (bovine Cu–Zn superoxide dismutase)

L. D. WILLIAMS, M. G. SAIFER, P. H.-C. DANG AND W. HUBER (USA)

## INTRODUCTION

The procedure of Ungar *et al.*[1] of gravimetrically measuring skin oedema, especially as induced by intradermal injection of anti-serum (reverse Arthus reaction), is a common model for assaying anti-inflammatory activity. We have found that the large number of subjective factors involved in the skin dissection and punching can be controlled by randomly blinding drug dosing and other parameters. However, variations in anti-serum from lot to lot may also influence the results, making it desirable to find a more uniform and less expensive inflammant.

Since Arthus-like reactions can be produced by chemically aggregated gamma-globulin[2] as well as by antigen–antibody soluble complex[3], the suggestion arose that protein A, an IgG binding cell wall peptide from *S. aureus*, would cause a similar Arthus-like inflammation.

## MATERIALS AND METHODS

Sprague–Dawley derived rats, usually 150–180 g, were purchased from

Simonsen Laboratories, Gilroy, CA. The inflammant used was IgGSORB, heat killed, formalin fixed, *Staphylococcus aureus* (Cowan strain) obtained from the Enzyme Center, Boston, Mass. The stock 10% suspension was diluted 1:1 with sterile saline for a 5% suspension and sonicated briefly before use. Anti-rat serum (rabbit) was obtained from Miles Laboratories, Elkart, Indiana.

**Procedure**

The rats were apportioned into balanced treatment groups. The hair was clipped evenly from the rats' backs with a pair of Oster small animal clippers. The rats were then numbered by a third party so that the experimenter did not know their drug treatment, and were then dosed with the blinded medications, consisting of investigational drug or placebo.

At zero time, eight 13 mm diameter circles were rubber stamped on the skin (Figure 17.1) and intradermal injections of 0.05 ml saline (four, left dorsal) and 0.05 ml inflammant (four, right dorsal) made in the centre of the circles.

At a set time after the intradermals, usually 4 h, each rat was killed with chloroform and the shaved area excised and stripped of fat and connective tissue, using dissecting scissors. The skin was laid inside-up, without stretching, on a sheet of tempered pressed wood and the eight injection sites were cut out with a 13 mm diameter steel hole punch and a mallet. The four saline sites were weighed and the four inflamed sites were weighed.

After the skin-punch weights from all the rats had been measured, the dose code was broken and the averages and standard deviations calculated from each dosing group. Inflammation was measured either directly as oedema weight, or indirectly as inflammatory index. Statistical significance of differences between groups was tested using Student's t test.

oedema weight = (average inflamed site weight) – (average saline site weight)

inflammatory index (II) = 100% × (oedema site weight)/(saline site weight)

% inhibition (weight) = 100% − 100% × (oedema weight average drug group)/(oedema weight average saline group)

% inhibition (II) = 100% − 100% × (II average drug group)/(II average saline group)

## RESULTS

Our data show that a killed, fixed preparation of *S. aureus* can, in fact, be substituted for anti-rat serum as inflammant in the reverse Arthus type bioassay of Ungar *et al.* Table 17.1 demonstrates this for two typical, representative

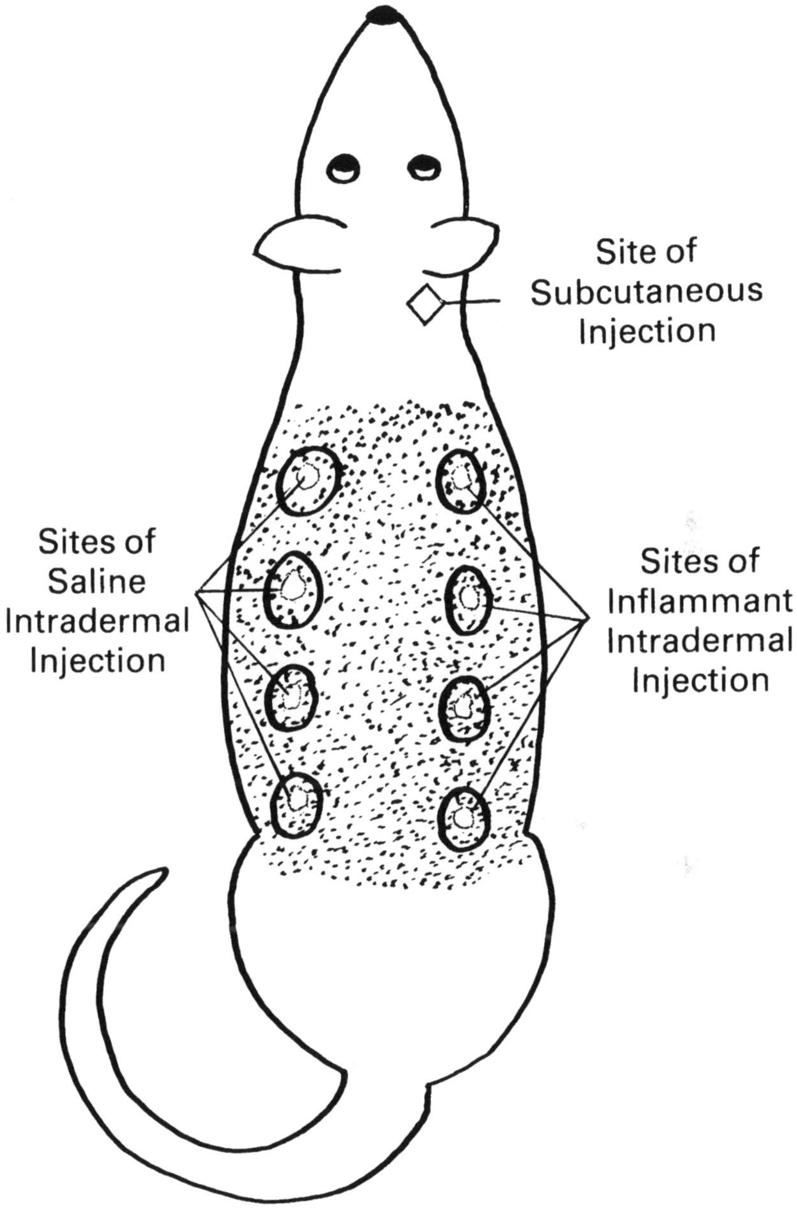


**Figure 17.1** Injection sites for skin odema in the rat

**Table 17.1** Comparison of inflammants in rat skin oedema

| | | | |
|---|---|---|---|
| *Experiment 103* | | *3.3% IgGSORB* | *Anti-rat serum* |
| Saline | weight difference | 653±142 | 584±174 |
| | II% | 74.5±17.6% | 62.5±17.5% |
| Orgotein | weight difference | 404±50 | 350±52 |
| (1 mg/rat) | II% | 47.1±12.2% | 35.3±5.6% |
| % Inhibition | weight difference | 38.1% | 40.0% |
| | II% | 36.8% | 43.5% |
| *Experiment 125* | | *5% IgGSORB* | *Anti-rat serum* |
| Saline | weight difference | 1019±68 | 1036±27 |
| | II% | 109.2±13.9% | 105.9±6.0% |
| Orgotein | weight difference | 642±176 | 626±31 |
| (1 mg/rat) | II% | 71.1±15.9% | 68.9±8.5% |
| % Inhibition | weight difference | 36.9% | 39.6% |
| | II% | 34.9% | 35.0% |

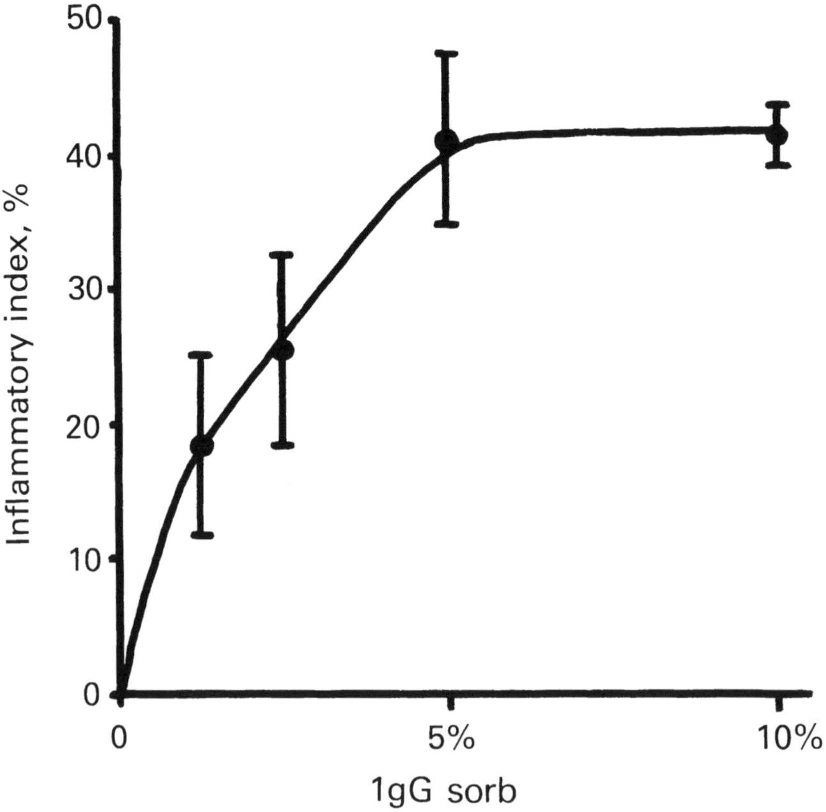


**Figure 17.2** Effect of IgGSORB concentration on skin oedema in the rat: average inflammation ± S.E. 3 or 4 rats per point; 0.05 ml per site; + 2 h sacrifice

experiments. The effect of IgGSORB concentration on skin oedema weight is shown in Figure 17.2 and relevant oedema kinetics in Figure 17.3.

Efficacy of orgotein (bovine Cu–Zn superoxide dismutase) in terms of dose and of dosing time before inflammant administration is presented in Table 17.2. Table 17.3 presents the same type data for other anti-inflammatory drugs such as dexamethasone, indomethacin, naproxen, plaquenil and prednisolone.

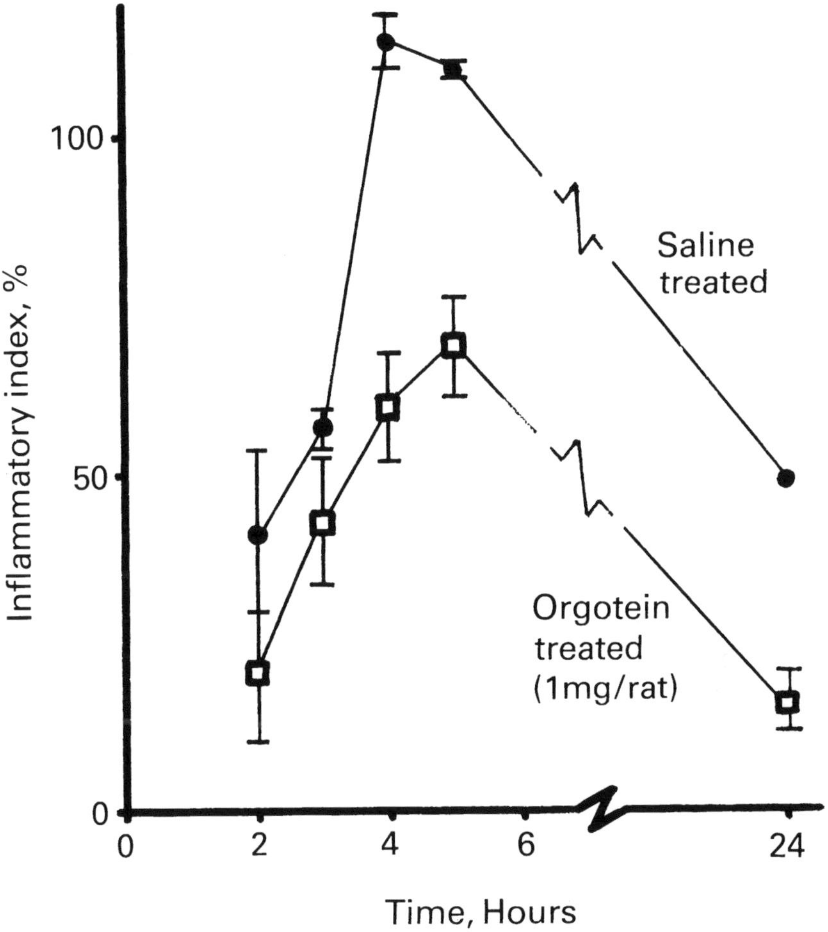


**Figure 17.3** Kinetics of IgGSORB-induced skin oedema in the rat: orgotein versus saline, 43 day old female rats dosed with 0.5 ml, s.c. at −2 h; 5% IgGSORB intradermally; average ± SE for 2 rats per point

Oedema response to a range of orgotein doses is shown in Figure 17.4 for four representative experiments. The day to day variation in orgotein induced oedema inhibition is shown in Table 17.4.

**Table 17.2** Effect of orgotein predosing time in the IgGSORB-induced rat skin oedema model

| *Experiment* | *Orgotein Dose/rat (mg)* | *Number of rats* | *% Inhibition (dose times)* | | *Saline 2p< (dose times)* | |
|---|---|---|---|---|---|---|
| 126 | mg | 4 | (−92 h) | (−24 h) | (−92 h) | (−24 h) |
| | 0.25 | 4 | 28% | 39% | 0.1 | 0.005 |
| | 2.5 | 4 | 43% | 38% | 0.005 | 0.01 |
| 127 | | 3 | (−113) | (−23) | (−113) | (−23) |
| | 0.025 | 3 | 20% | 27% | 0.05 | 0.01 |
| | 0.25 | 3 | *24% | 38% | 0.02 | 0.005 |
| | 2.5 | 3 | 37% | 48% | 0.005 | 0.005 |
| 131 | | 2 | (−92) | (−2) | (−92) | (−2) |
| | 0.025 | 2 | 16% | 10% | 0.05 | 0.02 |
| | 0.063 | 2 | 27% | 20% | 0.001 | 0.005 |
| | 0.125 | 2 | *28% | 14% | 0.001 | 0.001 |
| | 2 × 0.25 | 2 | 43% | | 0.001 | |
| 132 | | 2 | (−69) | (−24) | (−69) | (−24) |
| | 0.075 | 2 | 16% | 38% | 0.05 | 0.001 |
| | 0.25 | 2 | 43% | 34% | 0.001 | 0.001 |

* Significantly different from later dose, $2p<0.05$

**Table 17.3** Effect of standard anti-inflammatory drugs in the IgGSORB-induced rat skin oedema model

| *Drug* | *Dose/rat (mg)* | *Dose Time (h)* | *Number of rats* | *Inhibition %* | *significant 2p<* |
|---|---|---|---|---|---|
| Dexamethasone (SC) | 0.04 | −1.5 | 5 | 31% | 0.02 |
| Dexamethasone (SC) | 0.04 | −3 | 4 | 24% | 0.1 |
| Dexamethasone (SC) | 0.08 | −1.5 | 5 | 49% | 0.001 |
| Dexamethasone (SC) | 0.08 | −0.8 | 5 | 42% | 0.01 |
| Dexamethasone (SC) | 0.1 | −1 | 4 | 31% | 0.01 |
| Dexamethasone (SC) | 0.1 | −19 | 4 | 41% | 0.01 |
| Indomethacin (SC) | 0.5 | −1 | 4 | 52% | 0.001 |
| Indomethacin (SC) | 0.5 | −19.5 | 4 | 27% | 0.02 |
| Indomethacin (SC) | 0.6 | −1 | 5 | 12% | 0.2 |
| Indomethacin (SC) | 0.75 | −19 | 4 | 28% | 0.1 |
| Indomethacin (PO) | 0.8 | −72 | 5 | 3% | 0.9 |
| Naproxen (PO) | 0.2 | −1.4 | 5 | −13% | 0.2 |
| Naproxen (SC) | 1.0 | −1.7 | 5 | 11% | 0.2 |
| Naproxen (SC) | 1.25 | −1 | 4 | 14% | 0.4 |
| Naproxen (SC) | 2.0 | −2 | 5 | 2% | 0.9 |
| Plaquenil (PO) | 0.075 | −1 | 4 | 34% | 0.05 |
| Plaquenil (PO) | 0.25 | −1 | 4 | 42% | 0.005 |
| Plaquenil (PO) | 0.75 | −1 | 4 | 66% | 0.001 |
| Prednisolone-succ. (SC) | 0.375 | −1 | 4 | −11% | 0.3 |
| Prednisolone-succ. (SC) | 0.375 | −2 | 4 | 0% | 0.9 |
| Prednisolone-succ. (SC) | 1.0 | −1.4 | 4 | 41% | 0.005 |
| Prednisolone-succ. (SC) | 1.0 | −1.5 | 2 | 50% | 0.02 |

**Table 17.4** Day to day variation in measured inhibition by orgotein of IgGSORB-induced rat skin oedema

| *Orgotein mg/rat* | *Number of Experiments* | *% Inhibition ± SD* |
|---|---|---|
| 0.025 | 4 | 22±6 |
| 0.05 | 3 | 17±9 |
| 0.063 | 2 | 23±6 |
| 0.075 | 6 | 6±21 |
| 0.125 | 5 | 10±21 |
| 0.15 | 4 | 9±14 |
| 0.2 | 12 | 14±21 |
| 0.25 | 18 | 24±21 |
| 0.3 | 3 | −18±5 |
| 0.5 | 3 | 45±3 |
| 0.6 | 3 | 26±29 |
| 0.75 | 2 | −10±17 |
| 1. | 17 | 36±21 |
| 1.25 | 2 | 5±3 |
| 2. | 10 | 15±24 |
| 2.5 | 10 | 32±28 |

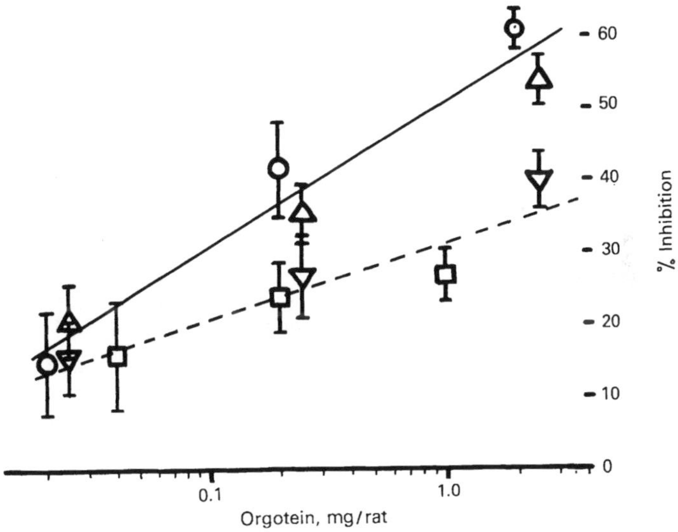


**Figure 17.4** Orgotein dose response in IgGSORB-induced skin oedema in the rat. Average inhibition ± SE for four experiments. Dose time, sacrifice time, number of rats per point, as follows:

0 −2 h; + 2 h; 5

□ −1 h; + 4 h; 5

△ − 19 h; + 4 h; 4

▽ − 19 h; + 4 h; 4

## DISCUSSION

A model of induced inflammation in rat skin, based on a reverse Arthus type reaction, has been tested using an IgG binding preparation of killed, fixed *S. aureus* and was found fully equivalent to and more manageable than rabbit anti-rat serum as inflammant. Inflammation, measured as oedema weight, peaks at 4–6 h. Statistically significant inhibitions of inflammation can be produced by orgotéin and by standard steroidal and non-steroidal anti-inflammatory drugs. Orgotein doses given up to 5 days before injection of inflammant still produced significant inhibition of oedema formation.

This is of particular interest since the last trace of superoxide dismutase enzyme activity in serum has disappeared by 24 h, as monitored by enzyme specific assays sensitive to $< 0.5\ \mu g/ml$[4]. The prolonged maintenance of orgotein efficacy in this model is in good agreement with clinical observations in man[5]. In addition, these data support prior findings showing that the anti-inflammatory efficacy of orgotein does not depend on the continuous presence of bovine Cu–Zn superoxide dismutase enzyme activity[6]. It also appears that orgotein in this model can affect some yet unknown *in vivo* processes, which in turn may be responsible for the maintenance of the anti-inflammatory effect long after demonstrable bovine Cu–Zn superoxide dismutase activity has disappeared from the circulation and the tissues.

Although the model suffers from the same sort of day to day variability as we have seen in other animal models of induced inflammation, the use of what should be a constant strength inflammant, along with the use of blind dosing and sacrifice, at least reduces the sources of non-random variation.

### References


1 Ungar, G., Kobrin, S. and Sezesny, B. (1959). Measurement of inflammation and evaluation of anti-inflammatory agents. *Arch. Int. Pharmacodyn. Ther.*, **123**, 71

2 Ishizaka, K., Ishizaka, T. and Sugahara, T. (1961). Biological activities of aggregated gamma globulin. III. Production of Arthus-like reactions. *J. Immunol.*, **86**, 220

3 Cochrane, C. G. and Weigle, W. O. (1958). The cutaneous reaction to soluble antigen-antibody complexes: a comparison with the Arthus phenomenon. *J. Exp. Med.*, **108**, 591

4 Huber, W. and Saifer, M. G. P. (1977). Orgotein the drug version of bovine Cu–Zn superoxide dismutase. I. A summary account of safety and pharmacology in laboratory animals. *In* Michelson, A. M., McCord, J. M. and Fridovich, I. (eds.). *Superoxide and Superoxide Dismutases*, 517–536. (New York: Academic Press)

5 Menander-Huber, K. B. (1979). Double-blind controlled clinical trials in man with bovine Cu–Zn superoxide dismutase (orgotein). In Bannister, W. H. and Bannister, J. V. (eds.) *The Significance of Superoxide and Superoxide Dismutase. Vol. II. Biological and Clinical Aspects*. (New York: Elsevier)

6 Huber, W., Menander-Huber, K. B., Saifer, M. G. P. and Williams, L. D. (1979). Bioavailability of superoxide dismutase: Implications for the anti-inflammatory action mechanism of orgotein. *Agents Actions Suppl.* (In press)

# 18

# The inhibition of macrophage accumulation in rats following injection of complete Freund's adjuvant (Abstract)

M. THOMSON, A. P. GREEN AND F. R. MANGAN (UK)

The accumulation of macrophages onto subcutaneously implanted nitrocellulose discs has been investigated in rats and mice, following the footpad injection of complete Freund's adjuvant and brewers yeast. The results show that only complete Freund's adjuvant injection in rats inhibited macrophage accumulation although all treatments caused a local inflammation. This property may be linked to the ability of complete Freund's adjuvant to induce a polyarthritis in rats.

# 19

# Possible synergism between ovariectomy and oestradiol in preventing Freund's adjuvant arthritis in the rat

A. SFIKAKIS, K. KARAMANIS, CH. LAIOU,
P. SFIKAKIS AND D. VARONOS (GREECE)

In a previous study[1] we noticed that long-term ovariectomy (50–70 days) resulted in (a) a significant increase of the weight of the thymus, both absolute and relative, and (b) in a decrease of the relative adrenal weight when compared to intact rats of similar age. On the other hand, the administration of oestradiol benzoate (300 $\mu$g/kg) for three consecutive days and a three day interval was followed by a significant decrease of the thymus weight, both absolute and relative and an increase of the relative adrenal weight reaching the level of thymus and adrenals found in intact rats.

The two purposes of the present study were first to determine the effect of ovariectomy and oestradiol administration on Freund's adjuvant arthritis in rats, and secondly to find, if any, a relationship between the degree of the primary and secondary inflammation and the weight of thymus and adrenals under the different experimental conditions of this study, in view of the well established role of thymus in cellular immunity and the role of the adrenocortical secretion in immunosuppression and inflammation[2].

## MATERIAL AND METHODS

The study was conducted on a strain of Wistar rats, susceptible to Freund's adjuvant arthritis, provided by the Hoechst Laboratories. These rats were subsequently raised in our laboratory.

The age of the rats at ovariectomy was 2 or 4 months. In each series of experiments the rats were matched in age and weight before ovariectomy and inoculated 35–40 days post ovariectomy, at the same time as the intact rats, with freshly prepared Freund's adjuvant (bacto-*M.tuberculosis* killed H 37 RA dessicated; Difco, 100 mg homogenized in 20 ml liquid paraffin).

Each rat received i.d. in the subplantar region of the right footpad 0.5 mg *Mycobacterium tuberculosis* in 0.1 ml liquid paraffin. Oestradiol benzoate, 250–300 $\mu$g per kg body weight from a 25 mg/100 ml olive oil solution, always freshly prepared, was administered s.c. on three consecutive days followed by a 3 day interval. This treatment, carried out in parallel with the vehicle (olive oil) treatment in the corresponding control rats, started 3 days post FA inoculation and was repeated two other times until the day of autopsy (21 day post-inoculation).

In one series of experiments one group of intact rats and one group of ovariectomized rats matched in age and weight with the FA inoculated rats were injected intradermally with saline instead of FA and were subsequently treated with the vehicle in the same schedule as FA treated controls.

Body weight and the diameter of the ankle joint of the inoculated footpad were measured with a micrometer before FA inoculation and on days 4, 8, 12 and 21. An increase in the diameter of the ankle joint of the opposite or uninjected hind paw, which was measured before inoculation and on days 12, 15, 17 and 21, was used as an index of secondary inflammation and induced arthritis. The scoring of joint involvement as described by Currey and Ziff[3] was also taken into account.

At autopsy, the thymus, adrenals and spleen, after being freed from adhering tissues, were weighed on a high precision electric balance of sensitivity 0.01 mg. For statistical evaluation of the results the $\chi^2$ test was used and the Student's t test. Whenever the SD between groups differed above 2 the Student's t test was performed after logarithmic transformation of the values.

## RESULTS

Table 19.1 gives the incidence of arthritis in the four studied groups of rats. It should be noticed that in intact rats in 3 out of 13 cases there was a regression of arthritis on day 21, while in oestradiol treated intact rats a regression was observed in 5 out of 7 rats with induced arthritis. The primary and secondary inflammation of the inoculated footpad in the studied rats (Table 19.1) are presented in Figure 19.1. This inflammation was calculated as the difference in the diameter of the ankle joint from its own control value in each rat, before inoculation. According to the results (Figure 19.1), ovariectomy alone under vehicle treatment had a favourable effect upon primary inflammation, since

**Table 19.1** Incidence of adjuvant arthritis in intact and ovariectomized rats

| *Group* | *Treatment* | *Number treated* | *Number with arthritis* | *Arthritis %* | *Difference from intact rats $\chi^2$-test* |
|---|---|---|---|---|---|
| Intact | olive oil | 18 | 13 | 72 | |
| Intact | oestradiol | 18 | 7 | 38.8* | $p<0.05$ |
| Ovariectomized | olive oil | 15 | 5 | 33† | $p<0.05$ |
| Ovariectomized | oestradiol | 15 | 1 | 6.6 | $p<0.001$ |

* Significance of difference from ovariectomized oestradiol treated $p<0.05$
† Significance of difference from ovariectomized oestradiol treated $p\simeq0.05$

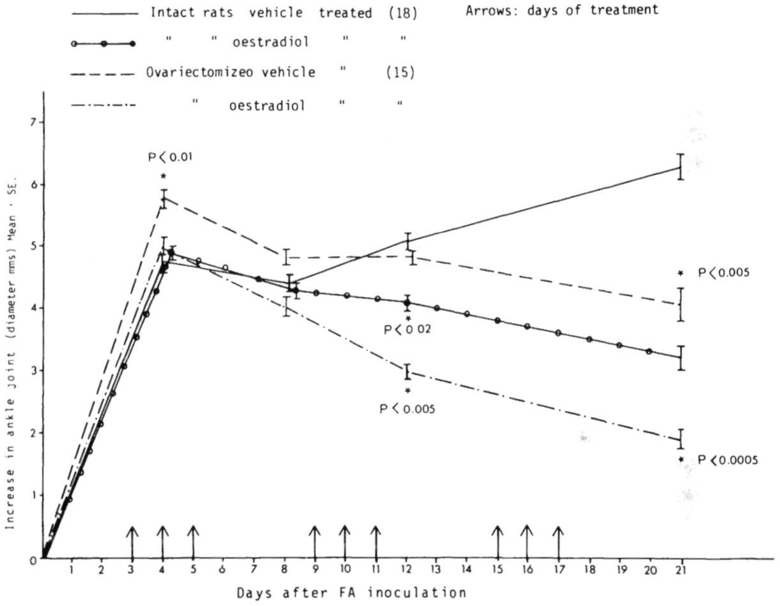


**Figure 19.1** Effect of ovariectomy and oestradiol treatment on primary and secondary inflamation in the Freund adjuvant inoculated footpad. Number of rats in parentheses. *p* values demonstrate significance between the value indicated by the asterisk versus corresponding controls

there was an increase on day 4 compared with intact rats and ovariectomized oestradiol treated rats. On the contrary, ovariectomy had a suppressive effect on secondary inflammation when compared to intact rats, the regression being highly significant on day 21. Oestradiol treatment enhanced the suppressive effect of ovariectomy upon secondary inflammation on day 12, the decrease in inflammation after oestradiol being highly significant ($p<0.0005$) and on day 21 the inflammation reached half the value of that observed in ovariectomized vehicle treated rats. Oestradiol treatment in non-ovariectomized rats suppressed secondary inflammation but at a much lower extent to that observed in ovariectomized rats.

**Table 19.2** Body weight in rats matched in age and weight before ovariectomy

| | *Intact* | *Ovariectomized* | *Significance of difference between intact and ovariectomized* |
|---|---|---|---|
| Saline inoculated | | | |
| Vehicle treated | (8) 254.5±8.62* | (8) 299.1±4.98 | $p<0.001$ |
| FA inoculated | | | |
| Vehicle treated | (8) 226.4±8.9 | (8) 266.1±10.40† | $p<0.02$ |
| FA inoculated | | | |
| Oestradiol benzoate treated | (8) 203.7±5.35* 15.129 | (8) 237.5±11.08 31.334 | $t=2.80=p<0.02$ |

* Significance of difference from corresponding controls: $p<0.05$
† Significance of difference from ovariectomized saline inoculated $p<0.01$
Figure in parentheses is the number of rats

Table 19.2 gives the effect of avariectomy upon body weight. It is clear that under the experimental conditions of this study the 56–60 days absence of the ovaries resulted in increase of body weight. On the other hand, FA inoculation decreased body weight in both intact and ovariectomized rats.

The effect of ovariectomy upon organ weight is illustrated on Figure 19.2. According to the results, the increase in thymus weight after ovariectomy ($p<0.001$) in comparison with corresponding controls cannot be attributed only to the increase of body weight (Table 19.2), since this increase persisted also when the results were expressed in relation to body weight ($p<0.005$), (Figure 19.2).

Adrenal weight did not follow the increase of body weight observed after ovariectomy and the decrease in the adrenal weight (Figure 19.2), became highly significant when expressed as relative weight both in SA and FA treated rats ($p<0.005$). With respect to FA effect in comparison with corresponding saline inoculated controls, the observed decrease in thymus weight after FA in intact animals was not as significant as the increase in absolute adrenal weight. On the other hand, the increase in the relative adrenal weight after FA (Figure 19.2) was significant in intact ($p<0.05$) as well as in ovariectomized rats ($p<0.005$). Concerning spleen weight, FA inoculation was followed by an increase in comparison with SA corresponding controls, but this increase was significant only in intact rats with respect to the relative weight ($p<0.05$). The effect of oestradiol treatment on the organ weights of FA inoculated intact and ovariectomized rats, which had lower incidence of FA arthritis from corresponding vehicle treated controls (Table 19.1), is illustrated in Figure 19.3.

The decrease in thymus weight after oestradiol (Figure 19.3) in comparison

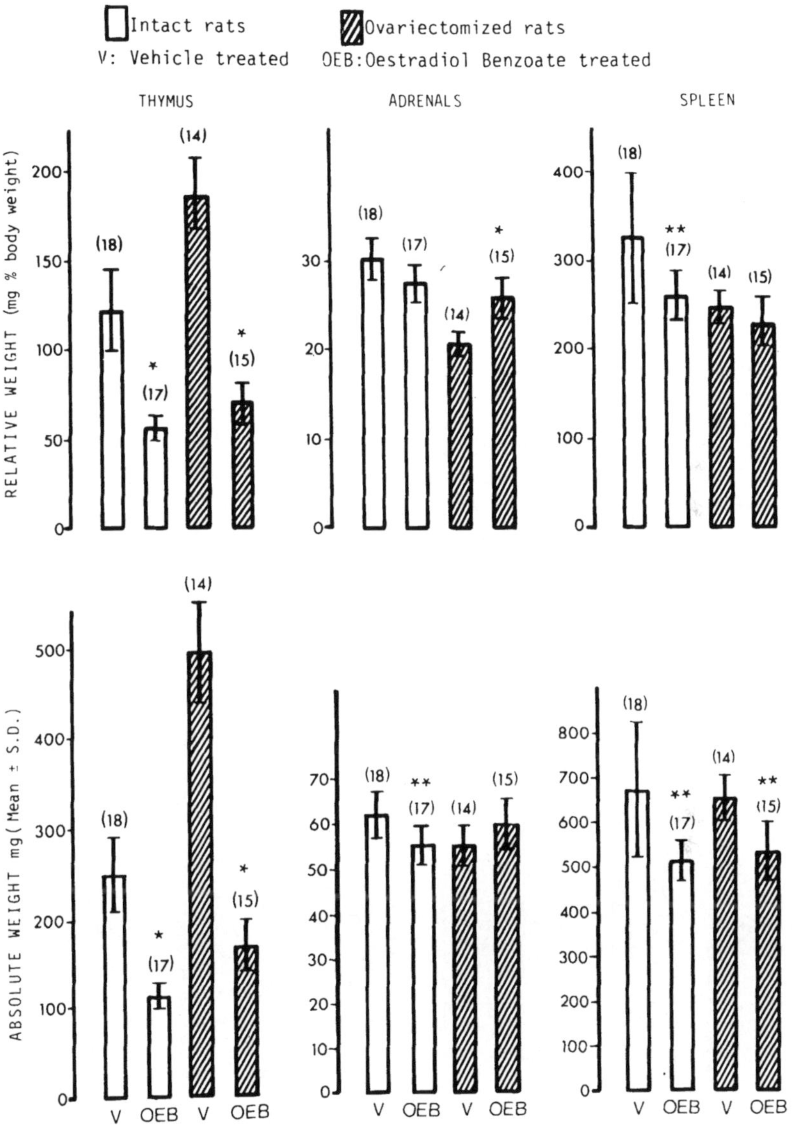


**Figure 19.2** Effect of oestradiol treatment on organ weights of intact and ovariectomized rats 21 days post Freund adjuvant inoculation. Number of organ weights in parenthesis. Significance of difference versus corresponding controls: * = $p < 0.005$–$0.0005$, ** = $p < 0.05$–$0.02$

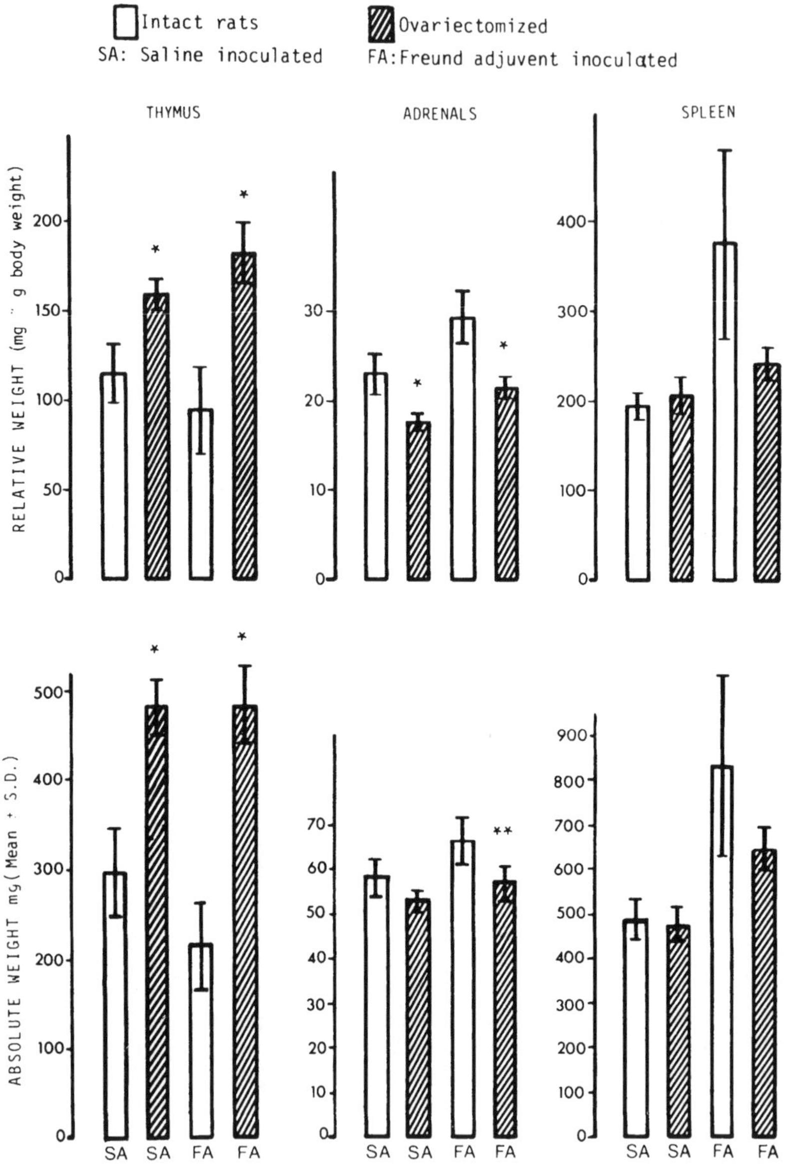


**Figure 19.3** Effect of ovariectomy on organ weights in rats matched in age and weight before ovariectomy, 21 days post inoculation with saline or Freund adjuvant and 60 days post ovariectomy. Significance of difference versus corresponding controls: * = $p < 0.001$–$0.0005$, ** = $p < 0.05$–$0.02$ (8 rats per group)

with corresponding controls was very impressive ($p<0.0005$) both in intact and ovariectomized rats. Oestradiol also suppressed spleen weight but to a lesser extent ($p<0.02$ or $p<0.05$). The effect of oestradiol on the adrenals of the ovariectomized rats in which the greatest suppression of FA arthritis (Table 19.1) and inflammation (Figure 19.1) was noticed, was stimulative, the increase in the relative adrenal weight being highly significant. Figure 19.3 also shows the effect of ovariectomy in vehicle treated oestradiol treated rats. The increase in thymus weight in vehicle treated ovariectomized rats when compared to vehicle treated intact rats was highly significant both in absolute ($p<0.0005$) and in relative values ($p<0.001$). The increase in thymus weight in oestradiol treated ovariectomized rats, when compared to oestradiol treated intact rats, was also significant but of a lower order ($p<0.005$) with respect to the absolute and ($p<0.05$) with respect to the relative weight. The decrease in the absolute weight of the adrenals in vehicle treated ovariectomized animals in comparison with vehicle treated intact rats was not significant; however, the decrease in the relative adrenal weight was highly significant ($p<0.0005$). In this group of rats primary inflammation (Figure 19.1) was significantly higher than the inflammation of the vehicle treated intact rats. In oestradiol treated rats, ovariectomy did not seem to significantly modify adrenal weight or spleen weight, which did not differ between vehicle treated intact and ovariectomized rats.

As the secondary inflammation of the inoculated footpad differed between oestradiol treated and vehicle treated ovariectomized rats more significantly in the group of younger rats (Table 19.3), organ weights were statistically evaluated separately in these rats of different age (Table 19.3). It is of interest that in the younger rats where oestradiol treatment caused a high suppression of inflammation compared with vehicle ovariectomized rats, adrenal weight was also significantly higher. On the contrary, in older rats where the difference in inflammation after oestradiol was not significant, no difference in adrenal weight was noticed.

## CONCLUSIONS AND DISCUSSION

The results of our study might be summarized as follows:

(1) Ovariectomy was shown to have a protective effect against FA arthritis ($p<0.05$).

(2) Administration of oestradiol benzoate three days post inoculation to intact rats was also shown to have a protective effect against FA arthritis.

(3) Oestradiol acted in synergism with ovariectomy, the incidence of arthritis being highly diminished ($p<0.001$) in oestradiol treated ovariectomized rats.

**Table 19.3** Secondary inflammation and organ weights in vehicle and oestradiol treated ovariectomized rats of different age

| Treatment | 4 months | | | 6 months | | |
|---|---|---|---|---|---|---|
| | *vehicle* | *significance of difference between groups* | *oestradiol* | *vehicle* | *significance of difference between groups* | *oestradiol* |
| Inflammation | | | | | | |
| day 12 | 5.07±0.366 | ($p$<0.001) | 2.85±0.241 | 4.62±0.38 | ($p$<0.02) | 3.08±0.418 |
| day 21 | 4.8±0.63 | ($p$<0.0005) | 1.65±0.121 | 3.41±0.846 | | 2.03±0.410 |
| Body weight | 262.2±7.25 | ($p$<0.01) | 233.3±5.48 | 266.1±10.4 | | 237.5±11.08 |
| Thymus weight | | | | | | |
| absolute | 511.3±61.56 | ($p$<0.001) | 175.2±13.46 | 483.3±30.04 | ($p$<0.005) | 161.7±26.56 |
| relative | 193.8±19.30 | ($p$<0.001) | 75.38±6.11 | 182.4±11.86 | ($p$<0.0005) | 66.2±8.71 |
| Adrenals weight | | | | | | |
| absolute | 52.0±4.38 | ($p$<0.02) | 66.60±2.97 | 57.2±2.69 | | 55.5±33.40 |
| relative | 19.7±1.28 | ($p$<0.0005) | 28.4±0.69 | 21.5±0.80 | | 23.5±1.48 |
| Spleen weight | | | | | | |
| absolute | 664.0±48.20 | | 544.1±62.91 | 646.1±31.97 | ($p$<0.05) | 527.2±35.55 |
| relative | 252.5±12.41 | | 234.4±28.60 | 243.8±11.39 | | 222.8±12.87 |

(4) The long-term ovarian absence in FA treated rats which protected against FA arthritis was followed by an increase in body weight, an increase in thymus weight both absolute and relative and a decrease in relative adrenal weight.

(5) The primary inflammation of the inoculated footpad was found to be significantly higher in ovariectomized rats in comparison with intact and oestradiol treated ovariectomized rats.

(6) Oestradiol treatment was followed by an impressive decrease in thymus weight in intact as well as in ovariectomized rats and a decrease in spleen weight of lower degree, the effect of oestradiol on the adrenals in ovariectomized rats where the lowest incidence of arthritis was noticed was of the opposite order

The results concerning the effect of ovariectomy and oestradiol on thymus and adrenal weights confirm our previous studies[1,4]. The reason for the decrease in the adrenal weight after ovariectomy should be attributed to hyposecretion of corticotrophic hormone (ACTH) due to decreased pituitary capacity to synthesize it and decreased responsiveness of pituitary corticotrophs to hypothalamic stimulation because of lack of oestrogens[5]. A decline in corticosterone output because of hyposecretion of ACTH might be partly responsible for the observed favourable effect of ovariectomy on primary inflammation. In contrast, as administration of oestradiol in ovariectomized rats was followed by increase in ACTH secretion as indicated by the increase in adrenal weight, an anti-inflammatory response through increased corticosterone output should be expected not only for the early phenomena of the inflammatory process but also for the later manifestations[2] which might explain in part the suppressive effect of oestradiol on inflammation of the inoculated footpad and its anti-arthritic effect. The corticosterone release might be considerably stimulated because oestradiol in ovariectomized rats increases the adrenocortical function[4], through ACTH secretion on one hand[5] and the synthesis and release of prolactin on the other[6]. Prolactin, according to recent data, potentiates the effect of ACTH on corticosterone secretion and plasma levels[7,8]. The finding of higher suppression of secondary inflammation after oestradiol in ovariectomized rats with higher adrenal response adds supportive evidence to the protective action of oestradiol through activation of the hypophyseal adrenal axis. The absence of increased adrenal weight after oestradiol in intact rats does not exclude an anti-inflammatory effect through activation of the hypophyseal adrenal axis because the presence of the ovaries might modify the homeostatic mechanism and obscure an effect upon the adrenals through stimulation of ACTH. On the other hand, as thymic involution is considered a representative sign of adrenocortical activation[9], it is difficult to answer to what extent the observed thymic involution after oestradiol should be attributed to a specific oestradiol effect and to what extent it should be considered as a secondary effect due to adrenocortical activation.

The protective effect of oestradiol against FA arthritis found in this study is in agreement with the data of Mueller and Kappas[10]. For the organ weights no comparison can be made because they were not studied in the mentioned work.

The results of the present study do not explain the mechanism by which ovariectomy protected against FA and had a synergistic effect with oestradiol. However, the finding of the impressive rise in the weight of the thymus after ovariectomy in vehicle as well as in oestradiol treated rats imposes a question that should be answered by further investigation with more elaborate methods: is the rise in thymic weight followed by an increase in the glandular secretion of the thymic hormone, due to thymosin, and to what extent thymosin, by modifying the immune response, might protect against FA arthritis?

## References

1 Sfikakis, A., Sfikakis, P. and Varonos, D. (1980). Oestradiol induced interaction between adrenals and thymus in the female rat. *Acta Endocrinol. Copenhagen), Suppl.* (In press)

2 Hayness, R. C. Jr. and Larner, J. (1975) Adrenocorticotropic hormone; adrenocortical steroids and their synthetic analogs. In Goodman, L. S. and Gilman, A. (eds.) *The Pharmacological Basis of Therapeutics*. 5th Edn, pp. 1472–1506. (New York: Macmillan)

3 Currey, H. L. F. and Ziff, M. (1968). Suppression of adjuvant disease in the rat by heterologous anti-lymphocyte globulin. *J. Exp. Med.*, **127,** 185

4 Sfikakis, A., Kyriakos, G., Messari, J. and Varonos, D. (1979). Effets de l'oestradiol sur les glandes préputiales, les surrenales et les androgènes sériques chez la rate castrée. *Ann. Endocrinol.* Comptes rendus de la 15e réunion des Endocrinologues de langue Française, **40,** 11

5 Coyne, M. D. and Kitay, J. (1963). Effects of ovariectomy on pituitary secretion of ACTH. *Endocrinology*, **85,** 1097

6 Blake, C. A., Norman, R. L. and Sawyer, C. H. (1972). Effects of oestrogen and/or progesterone on serum and pituitary gonadotropin levels in ovariectomized rats. *Proc. Soc. Exp. Biol. Med.*, **141,** 1100

7 Colby, H. D. (1979). Mechanism of action of prolactin on adrenocortical steroid secretion in hypophysectomized female rats. *Endocrinology,* **104,** 1299

8 Ogle, Th. F. and Kitay, J. I. (1979). Interaction of prolactin and adrenocorticotropin in the regulation of adrenocortical secretion in female rats. *Endocrinology*, **104,** 40

9 Cohen, H., Freedman, H. H., Kleinberg, W., Schechter, N. R. and Martin, G. J. (1954). Enhancement of corticotrophic activity: Effect on adrenal and thymus weights. *Endocrinology*, **54,** 81

10 Mueller, M. N. and Kappas, A. (1964) Estrogen Pharmacology II. Suppression of experimental immune polyarthritis (29715). *Proc. Soc. Exp. Biol. Med.*, **117,** 845

# 20

# Anti-inflammatory actions of an immunomodulator: therafectin 1,2-*O*-isopropylidene-3-*O*-3′-(*N*′,*N*′-dimethylamino n-propyl) -D-gluco-furanose, HCl

P. GORDON (USA)

---

Most of the non-steroidal anti-inflammatory agents in clinical use today are substituted aromatic organic acids. These agents are endowed with an unfortunately high incidence of toxicity[1] which may have to do with unavoidable unwanted side effects of their powerful influence on that pathway of arachidonic acid metabolism that leads to prostaglandin synthesis.

In this paper I present information on therafectin (SM-1213), representative of a new class of anti-inflammatory compounds apparently free of such toxicity.

The chemical structures exemplified by this class are relatively ethereal substitutions on glucose, as SM-1213, which is 1,2–*O*-isopropylidene-3-*O*-3′-(*N*′,*N*′-dimethylamino n-propyl)-D-gluco-furanose, HCl (see Figure 20.1). Interèsting laboratory effects of such compounds include, among others:

(1) Immunomodulation: immune responses can be enhanced or suppressed[2]. The number of immunocompetent cells increases, without regard as to whether they are facilitator or suppressor, in response to antigen, in the presence of the drug[3].

(2) Stimulation of antimicrobial action in phagocytes[4].

(3) Transient stimulation of an inflammatory response at very low dosage, as exerted by 0.075 (mg/kg)/24 h for 2 days per drinking water.

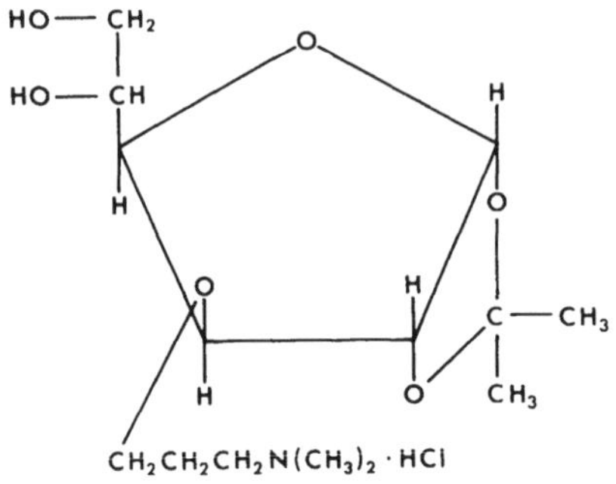


**Figure 20.1** Structure of therafectin or SM-1213

(4) Partial or complete inhibition of inflammatory responses, according to species and model, at higher dosage, as 1.0–20(mg/kg)/24 h for periods longer than 2 days.

(5) Apparent enhancement of the level of intracellular chemiluminescing active oxygens and inhibition of the release of such transients from inflammatory phagocytes.

(6) Magnification of drug effects when compound is added to drinking water, relative to dosage given once daily by oral gavage, a requirement dictated by the rapid rate of urinary excretion.

(7) Relative non-metabolizability due to the 3 position ethereal substitution and a hydrolysis-resistant substitution on the sugar reducing function[3].

(8) Absence of toxicity. 1.8(g/kg)/ 24 h for 30 days in rats and monkeys was without any gross or histological toxic effect[3].

In this presentation I will point in passing to the superficial diversity of such effects and focus principally on drug modification of animal inflammation models.

## GLYCOGEN INDUCTION OF PERITONEAL INFLAMMATION

20 mg glycogen was injected intraperitoneally into Ha/ICR or CD-1 mice and exudates were tapped and quantified 24 h later. Groups of 6 to 9 mice each were on different treatment regimens which continued up to cell harvest. Cells of each group were pooled for counting.

Results shown in Figure 20.2 reveal a stimulation of the inflammatory

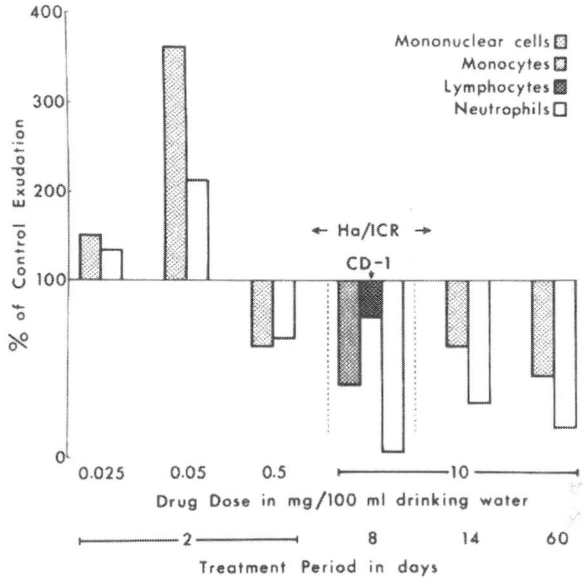


**Figure 20.2** Effect of dose regimens on peritoneal inflammatory exudates in Ha/ICR and CD-1 mice

response at low dosage given for two days to Ha/ICR mice. The stimulation peak occurs at or about 0.05 mg/100 ml drinking water, which results in an ingestion of about 0.075 mg/kg, and influences both mononuclear cells and neutrophils. At 10 times this dose, the drug generates an inflammation inhibition which becomes progressively greater as drug dose increases and administration is prolonged. The highest dose administered, 10 mg/100 ml drinking water, results in an injestion of about 15(mg/kg)/24 h, less than 1/100 the highest dose examined in the 30 day toxicity trials.

Anti-exudative effects are exerted against both mononuclear cells and neutrophils. In CD-1 mice (see Figure 20.2 and Table 20.1), drug effect is found to be directed equally against neutrophil, monocyte, and lymphocyte populations, when correction for the resident population is made, and to occur in the absence of a perturbation of the peripheral white blood cell counts, identifying the effect as principally a suppression of leukocyte migration.

## NEUTROPHIL CHEMILUMINESCENCE

Neutrophil-rich peritoneal cellular exudates were harvested 24 h following glycogen injection, as above, from control CD-1 mice and such mice given

**Table 20.1** Therafectin effect on peritoneal inflammatory exudate in male CD-1 mice

| | *Total WBC* | *Polymorpho-nuclear leukocytes* | *Monocytes* | *Lymphocytes* |
|---|---|---|---|---|
| Peripheral/mm$^3$ | | | | |
| control | $3.28 \pm 0.24 \times 10^3$ | $9.66 \pm 0.43 \times 10^2$ | $3.48 \pm 0.15 \times 10^2$ | $1.96 \pm 0.17 \times 10^3$ |
| therafectin | $3.36 \pm 0.15 \times 10^3$ | $7.72 \pm 0.86 \times 10^2$ | $2.35 \pm 0.36 \times 10^2$ | $2.35 \pm 0.13 \times 10^3$ |
| Peritoneal/mouse | | | | |
| basal | $8.51 \times 10^5$ | $2.00 \times 10^3$ | $1.04 \times 10^5$ | $7.45 \times 10^5$ |
| control exudate | $2.43 \pm 0.72 \times 10^6$ | $7.50 \pm 10^5$ | $6.20 \times 10^5$ | $1.10 \times 10^6$ |
| - basal | $1.58 \times 10^6$ | $7.48 \times 10^5$ | $5.16 \times 10^5$ | $3.55 \times 10^5$ |
| Therafectin | | | | |
| exudate | $1.39 \pm 0.24 \times 10^6$ | $2.70 \times 10^5$ | $2.60 \times 10^5$ | $8.50 \times 10^5$ |
| – basal | $5.39 \times 10^5$ | $2.68 \times 10^5$ | $1.56 \times 10^5$ | $1.05 \times 10^5$ |
| Drug effect on penetrance into peritoneal cavity | −66/ | −64/ | −70/ | −70/ |

In this study, therafectin was given in the drinking water at a concentration of 10 mg/100 ml (approximately 16 mg/kg) for 8 days. Exudates tapped 24 h following an injection of 20 mg glycogen/mouse.

drinking water containing 10 mg/100 ml therafectin for 8 days. Cells from eight animals in each group were pooled, washed, counted, and distributed as $1.5 \times 10^6$ neutrophils per plastic scintillation vial, in MEM, for assessment of active oxygen activity by chemiluminescence before and after addition to the system of $10^7$ heat-killed *Candida albicans*. The latter, of course, stimulated phagocytosis, and the attendant burst of oxidative metabolism. Chemiluminescence was examined by scintillation counting at ambient temperature, in the coincident mode, in the absence and presence of luminol, which amplifies light production produced by radical attack in the extracellular compartment. Counts were for 2 min. Before and in between assessments, vials were maintained at 37 °C.

Results shown in Table 20.2 are given in counts per minute. The data shows neutrophils harvested from treated animals to be different in two respects: in the absence of effect on rate of phagocytosis, (not shown), the chemiluminescence generated in the absence of luminol is increased, while the chemiluminescence generated in the presence of luminol is decreased. We have found these results repeatedly and consider them to be signature responses to the drug. We interpret them to indicate that therafectin modifies the manner of processing of active oxygens that are generated in response to the phagocytosis by neutrophils of a natural target (*C. albicans*). Specifically, the drug appears to enhance intracellular levels of these radicals, while inhibiting their release into the extra-cellular environment, where they exert tissue injuring and pro-inflammatory effects.

**Table 20.2** Therafectin modulation of active oxygen (superoxide etc.) production by glycogen-elicited peritoneal neutrophils in the mouse

| | *Phagocytosis-induced increased chemiluminescence (ct/min)* | | *Effect as compared to control (%)* |
|---|---|---|---|
| | *control* | *therafectin* | |
| Intracellular (- luminol) | | | |
| 30 min | 25 | 60 | + 140 |
| 60 min | 11 | 16 | + 45 |
| 90 min | 0 | 44 | + 1000 |
| Extracellular (+ luminol) | | | |
| 30 min | 817 | 401 | − 51 |
| 60 min | 132 | 13 | − 90 |
| 90 min | 297 | 214 | − 28 |

Therafectin given as 15 mg/kg/24 h in drinking water for 8 days. Scintillation vials contained cells in MEM plus 10% foetal calf serum (FCS) or 10% FCS containing luminol. Luminol-saturated FCS was diluted 1:100 with plain FCS and this solution was added at 10%.

## CARRAGEENAN FOOTPAD OEDEMA

Demonstration of therafectin's anti-inflammatory effect in this system requires adherence to certain conditions. The control increase in dorsoventral mouse or rat footpad diameter, as measured by a Schnelltaster caliper, as a general rule, must not exceed 40–45%. While indomethacin produces the same fractional decrease in swelling in the mouse, at all levels of carrageenan input, therafectin does not. At the doses of lambda, carrageenan often used to generate inflammation in the paw, producing a diameter increase of 70–100% or more; anti-inflammatory effects of SM-1213 are not observed.

Thus 250 mg per paw per 210 g rat, or 40 mg per paw per 28 g mouse, of Sigma Chemical Company Type 1 carrageenan (20% lambda, 80% kappa) has become our standard dose. Greater amounts of this inflammatory polyanion can suppress the drug effect, perhaps by successfully competing with cell-site receptors for the drug.

The second condition that one must observe to obtain optimum anti-inflammatory effects in the mouse or rat is to administer the drug for at least 6 days before assessment. As shown in Figure 20.2, anti-inflammatory effects augment with chronicity of treatment.

Thirdly, one must distribute the daily dosage rather than administer it in a single dose.

Results for carrageenan footpad oedema are shown in Figure 20.3 and Table 20.3. SM-1213 suppresses footpad oedema under the given conditions.

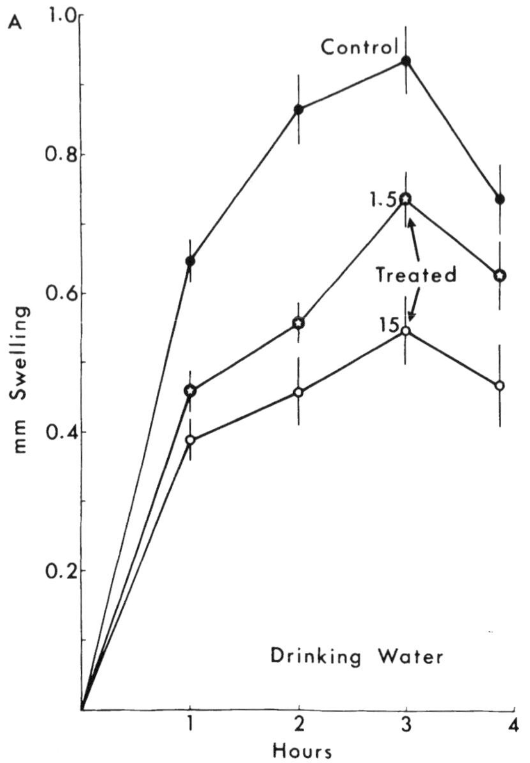


**Figure 20.3** Therafectin suppression of carrageenan footpad oedema in the Sprague-Dawley rat. Drug treatment was 1.5 mg or 15 (mg/kg)/24 h given in the drinking water for 8 days and carrageenan was 250$\mu$g Sigma Type I carrageenan per paw per 210 g rat. $n$ = 16. At peak, the high dose is significant at $p<0.001$ and the low dose at $p<0.01$

## MONOARTICULAR ARTHRITIS

Pathology was developed in rabbits by the subpatellar injection of $10^6$ heat-killed *E. coli* and quantified by caliper measurement of the dorsoventral diameter of the knee. Drug added to the drinking water on day 10 produces a striking suppression of inflammation developed by one injection of *E. coli* (Figure 20.4) and effects an essentially total suppression of inflammation, following injection and reinjection of the phlogistic agent (Figure 20.5). In the rabbit model, anti-inflammatory effects develop following a treatment period of 48 h; more rapidly than in the rat or mouse. We note other work indicating that rabbit monoarticular arthritis is generated largely by neutrophils[5],

**Table 20.3** Anti-inflammatory drug actions in carrageenan foot-pad oedema in CD–1 mice

| | *Increase in foot-pad diameter* (mm) | |
|---|---|---|
| Time post-carrageenan = | 3 h | 5 h |
| Control | 0.66 ± 0.04 | 0.43 ± 0.03 |
| SM-1213 (23.1 mg/kg/day) | 0.49 ± 0.04** | 0.38 ± 0.03 |
| Indomethacin (1 mg/kg) | 0.52 ± 0.04* | 0.35 ± 0.03 |
| Phenylbutazone (25 mg/kg) | 0.54 ± 0.04 | 0.40 ± 0.03 |

Measurements were made with the Schnelltaster caliper. For all groups, $n = 12$. SM-1213 was given in the drinking water for 10 days; phenylbutazone and indomethacin were given by gavage 1 h prior to carrageenan. Carrageenan concentration was 40 mg/foot-pad.
* $p < 0.05$
** $p < 0.01$

in contrast to carrageenan oedema which is heavily dependant on monocyte infiltration[6].

## ADJUVANT ARTHRITIS

Complete Freund's adjuvant was injected intracutaneously into the right hind paw of adult Sprague–Dawley and Lewis rats, and drug effect on established pathology that subsequently developed was assessed. Medication was added to the drinking water on day 11 for Sprague–Dawley rats and on day 14 for Lewis rats. Articular pathology was assessed by a scoring technique. Each paw received a score of 0, ½, 1, 2, 3, 4; 4 reflected total immobility of the limb. Non-articular lesions on the ears and tail were counted daily and scored separately.

Results for secondary lesions are shown in Figures 20.6 and 20.7. Results for primary scores, although not shown here, were similar. The results reveal a moderate suppression of the intensity of established adjuvant arthritis lesions, an effect which develops gradually. However, the drug strikingly suppresses the non-articular lesions of adjuvant arthritis (Figure 20.8). These are of necessity 'early' lesions in the animal model used. Ear lesions were typically swellings, while tail lesions were epidermal pustules. Both pathologies have been described by Pearson. The tail pustules were identified by him as being rich in neutrophils[7].

## DISCUSSION

Studies of this novel anti-inflammatory sugar reveal it to suppress both neutrophil and monocytic contributions to inflammation. The profound effect on monoarticular arthritis in the rabbit and on extra-articular lesions in adjuvant arthritis indicate that neutrophil effects may be suppressed most profoundly. It is apparent that inflammation in the rabbit was more profoundly inhibited than in the rat. While the basis for this difference is not yet specifically understood, I suggest that it may be due in part to the predominant role that neutrophils play in the rabbit model studied, and to the possibly particular status of rat arachidonic acid metabolism. By the latter I refer to a report also given at this meeting that the hydroxy fatty acids that are products of arachidonic acid metabolism are chemokinetic for human and rabbit leukocytes but not for the leukocytes of the rat[8]. If inhibition of the lipoxygenase pathway by which such chemoattractants are synthesized proves to be a prime mode by which therafectin exerts its anti-inflammatory effects, as I think will be the case, then this component of therafectin action might not be seen in the rat. Lipoxygenase activity generates oxidative radical transients and is associated with luminolamplified chemiluminescence that is quenched by superoxide dismutase[9]. Thus our observation of the suppression by drug treatment of this class of chemiluminescence is compatible with a drug inhibition of the pathway in question.

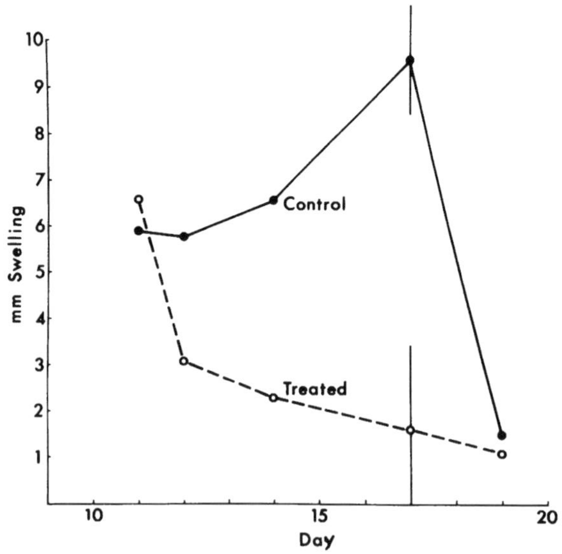


**Figure 20.4** Therafectin suppression of monoarticular arthritis in the rabbit. Drug at a level of 0.1 mg/ml was added to the drinking water on day 10 and treatment was maintained throughout the study. $n = 8$. On day 17 mean response of control and treated groups were significantly different, $p<0.01$

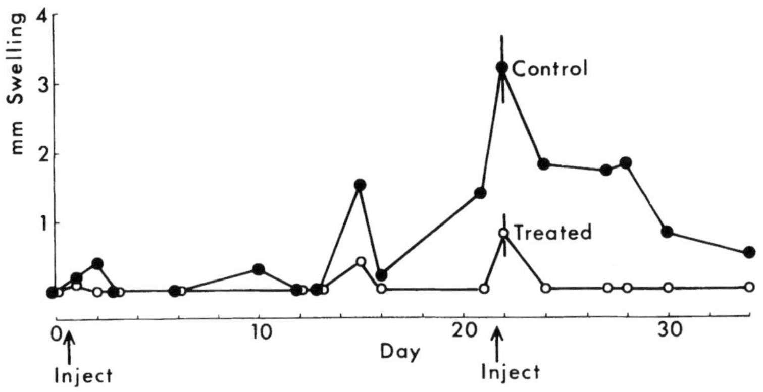


**Figure 20.5** Therafectin suppression of monoarticular arthritis in the rabbit given two injections of *E. coli* on day 0 and day 21. Drug was administered as 0.1 mg/ml in the drinking water on days 3–6, 12–16, and 22–28. $n = 4$. Mean responses of control and treated groups on day 22 were significantly different, $p<0.02$. Means of days 24, 27, and 28 were significantly different at $p<0.05$

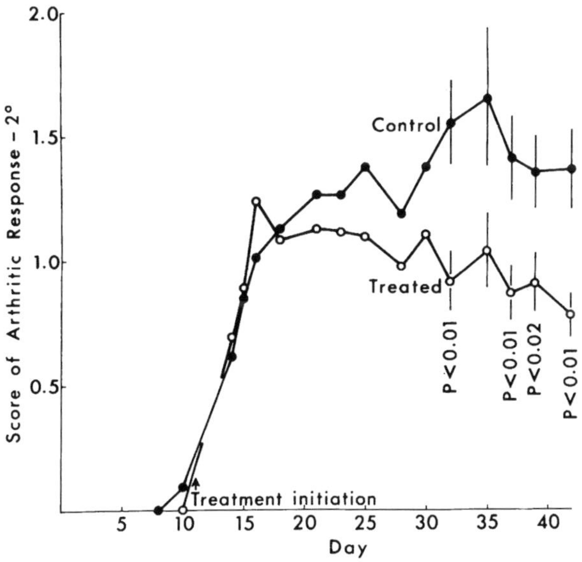


**Figure 20.6** Effect of therafectin on established adjuvant arthritis in the adult Sprague–Dawley rat. Drug treatment was initiated on day 11 as 0.1 mg/ml given in the drinking water. Drug consumption was approximately 15 (mg/kg)/24 h. Significance of differences obtained are given in the figure

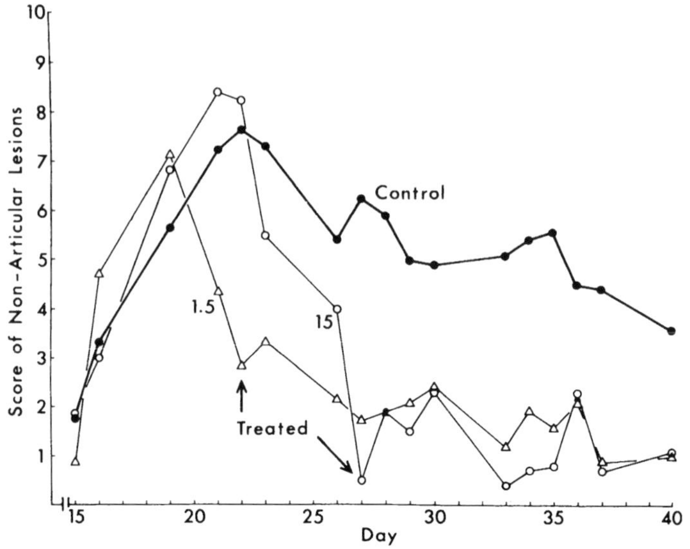


**Figure 20.7** Effect of therafectin on articular lesions of established adjuvant arthritis in the adult Lewis rat. Treatment was started on day 15; 2 doses were used, 0.1 mg and 0.01 mg/ml allowing consumption of approximately 15 mg and 1.5 (mg/kg)/24 h. $n = 12$. Mean differences between control and treated groups were significant on days 33, 34, 35, 37, and 40–47 at levels of $p<0.05$ and $p<0.01$

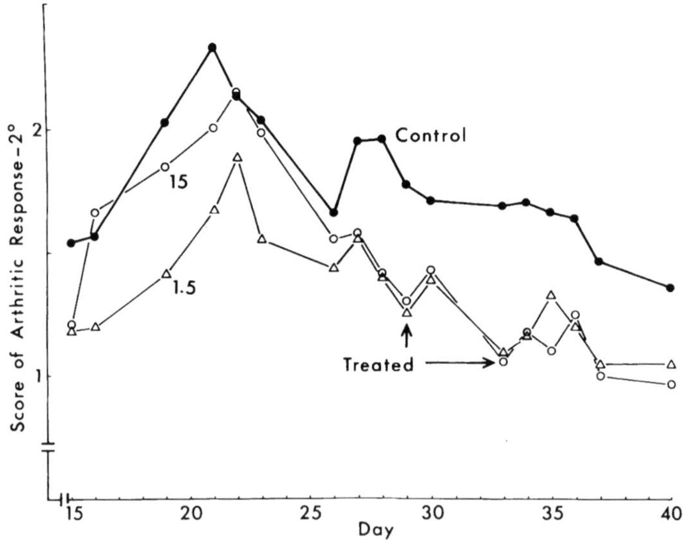


**Figure 20.8** Effect of therafectin on nonarticular lesions of tail and ears in established adjuvant arthritis in the adult Lewis Rat. Score differences reached significances of $p<0.02$ on days 27, 33, 34, and 35

That the anti-inflammatory effect requires several days of treatment to emerge suggests, on the other hand, that a component of the anti-inflammatory action may involve depletion and non-renewal of an inflammatory precursor or enzyme. While continuing to focus on the lipoxygenase system, we will have to rule in or rule out a contribution from bradykininogen[10].

That the effect of the drug on adjuvant arthritis, and especially the striking suppression of extra-articular lesions, at the supracellular level may have to do with the suppression of pathology produced by immune complexes, is suggested by a recent finding made in our laboratory. When hamsters are rendered hyperimmune to the double-strandedness of RNA by the repeated administration of Poly 1–Poly C-albumin complex in complete Freund's adjuvant, and are subsequently infected by a virus producing ds-RNA intermediates (Influenza $A_2$/Japan) they develop a much more severe systemic toxicity, as determined by weight loss and a reduction in reticulocyte count than do unhyperimmunized infected controls. In a manner analogous to effects of drug in adjuvant arthritis, therafectin, given 2 days post-infection, suppresses these consequences of hyperimmunization and generation of antigen.

This discussion is rich in speculations. Therafectin has only recently come under study as an anti-inflammatory agent and much remains to be learned about the basis of its actions in animal models and about the relationship of such actions to effects in man.

## References


1 Dodge, P. W., Brodie, D. and Mitchell, B. D. (1979). Evaluation of the toxicity of anti-inflammatory drugs. In Vane, J. R. and Ferreira, S. H. (eds.) *Anti-inflammatory Drugs*. Vol. 50/11, Chap. 29, p. 280. Berlin: Springer-Verlag.

2 Majde, J. A. and Gordon, P. (1976). Immunomodulation by 1,2-2-0-isopropylidene-3-0-3'-(N'N'-dimethyl-amino-n-propyl)-D-glucofuranose SM-1213, a drug with antiviral activity. In Sixteenth Interscience Conference on Antimicrobial Agents and Chemotherapy, Abstract, Chicago, Illinois

3 Files, Greenwich Pharmaceuticals Incorporated. 95 East Putnam Avenue, Greenwich, Connecticut, 06830

4 Hadden, J. W., Englard, A., Sadlik, J. R., and Hadden, E. M. (1979). The comparative effects of Isoprinosine, Levamisole, Muramyl Dipeptide, and SM-1213 on lymphocyte and macrophage proliferation and activation *in vitro*. *Int. J. Immunopharmacol.*, **1,** 17

5 Goldlust, M. G., Rich, L. C., and Brown, W. R. (1978). Immune synovitis in rabbits: Effects of differing schedules for intra-articular challenge with antigen. *Am. J. Pathol.*, **91,** 329

6 di Rosa, M., Papadimitriou, J. M., Willoughby, D. A. (1971). A histopathological and pharmacological analysis of the mode of action of nonsteroidal anti-inflammatory drugs. *J. Pathol.*, **105,** 239

7 Pearson, C. M. and Wood, F. E. (1959). Studies of polyarthritis and other lesions induced in rats by injection of Mycobacterial adjuvant. I. General clinical and pathologic characteristics and some modifying factors. *Arthritis Rheum.*, **2,** 440

8 Palmer, R. M. J., Salmon, J. A., Narumiya, S., Higgs, G. A., and Eakins, K. E. (1980). Arachadonic acid metabolism by lipoxygenase in leukocytes of different species and the chemokinetic activity of some products. This Volume, Chap. 35

9 Michelson, A. M. (1974). Is singlet oxygen a substrate for superoxide dismutase? No. *FEBS Lett.* **44,** 97

10 Ferreira, S. H. and Vane, J. R. (1979). Mode of action of anti-inflammatory agents which are prostaglandin synthetase inhibitors. In Vane, J. R. and Ferreira, S. H. (eds.) *Anti-inflammatory Drugs*. Vol. 50/11, Chap. 31, p. 348. Berlin: Springer-Verlag

# 21

# Effects of benoxaprofen on macrophage function (Abstract)

G. W. CIVIL, D. HILLMAN, E. A. KITCHEN,
S. C. R. MEACOCK AND W. DAWSON (UK)

Benoxaprofen is a new non-steroidal anti-inflammatory drug which has been shown to have little cyclo-oxygenase inhibitory activity[1] and to inhibit leucocyte migration (*in vivo* and *in vitro*)[2,3]. The effects of benoxaprofen *in vivo* on the chemotactic activity (CA) of inflammatory exudates have now been studied. In addition, the *in vitro* effects on phagocytosis by macrophages and on some of the accompanying biochemical events have been assessed. CA of 24 h pleural and peritoneal exudates from rats injected with glycogen or λ-carrageenin were evaluated. Oral administration of benoxaprofen reduced the levels of chemotaxins for macrophages in the exudates but had no significant effect on PMN migration. Phagocytosis by unelicited rat peritoneal macrophages of latex spheres was stimulated by benoxaprofen at low concentrations (1–10 μg/ml) but was reduced at 15 and 30 μg/ml by 20–25%. Stimulation of the hexose monophosphate (HMP) shunt during phagocytosis was inhibited by ~50% at 30 μg/ml and at lower concentrations in a dose related manner. Similar drug effects were seen on the HMP shunt stimulated by ascorbic acid. However, stimulation by Concanavalin A of the HMP shunt was potentiated by benoxaprofen at 30 μg/ml. Drug effects were partially reversed by washing the cultured cells. Benoxaprofen had no effect on the secretion or synthesis of β-glucuronidase by mouse macrophages after phagocytosis of serum treated zymosan particles. It is concluded that benoxaprofen can modify macrophage function and can also reduce the formation of chemotaxins for these mononuclear cells in inflammatory exudates.

## References

1 Cashin, C. H., Dawson, W. and Kitchen, E. A. (1977). *J. Pharm. Pharmacol.*, **29**, 330
2 Meacock, S. C. R., and Kitchen, E. A. (1979). *J. Pharm. Pharmacol.*, **31**, 366
3 Meacock, S. C. R., Kitchen, E. A. and Dawson, W. (1979). *Eur. J. Rheum. Inflam.*, **3**, 23

# 22

# Some 'anti-arthritic' properties of an oversulphated glycosaminoglycan in degenerative joint disease

G. VERBRUGGEN, E. M. VEYS, F. P. LUYTEN
AND S. SUYKENS (BELGIUM)

## INTRODUCTION

Normal human joints contain only a few milligrams of hyaluronate whereas in degenerative or in inflammatory conditions these joints may contain several hundreds of milligrams of this polysaccharide. The increase in total hyaluronate content in diseased joints reflects the higher synthesis of this polysaccharide by the synovial cell in pathology[1]. The intrinsic viscosity of these fluids (as a parameter of the mean hyaluronate molecular weight) however is decreased[2-3]. In view of the pH required for acid hydrolase activity we have some difficulties in accepting this lowering in hyaluronate molecular weight as a consequence of any extracellular acid hydrolase activity. In this way a disturbed synthesis seems more plausible and the overproduction of a less polymerized hyaluronate can be seen as a loss of quality control by the synovial cell under inflammatory stress[4].

In fact, an inverse correlation between intrinsic viscosities of synovial fluids of varying rheumatic conditions and their respective *N*-acetyl-β-glucosaminidase or β-glucuronidase levels was demonstrated[4] and the activities of these hydrolases reflect very well the inflammatory state[4].

This 'activation' of synovial cells was already demonstrated in the early seventies (connective tissue activating peptides)[5]. Synovial cells and chondrocytes present a remarkable parallelism in their polysaccharide metabolism. An enhanced radiosulphate incorporation (as a specific index of a higher glycosaminoglycan synthesis) in osteoarthritic cartilage[6] and a close correlation between this increased sulphate incorporation and the decreased hexosamine levels[6] has been reported elsewhere. The resulting proteoglycans however differ in their chemical composition (increased protein/uronic acid[7] and galactosamine/glucosamine ratios[8], shorter chondroitin sulphate chain lengths[6] are a constant finding). Furthermore, a defective aggregation of these proteoglycan sub-units into larger complexes[9-10] probably results in a higher extractability of these molecules from diseased cartilage[8].

Although these variables are sometimes ascribed to enzymatic auto-aggression[11-13], it remains plausible that some of these phenomena also reflect an enhanced but defective repair by the chondrocyte in an attempt to compensate for the loss of matrix constituents. The concept that an increased repair by connective tissue cells could result in the production of qualitatively unadapted proteinpolysaccharide complexes brought us to the study of some mediators which might be capable of regulating this disturbed synthesis.

*In vitro* studies on cultured fibroblasts, synoviocytes and chondrocytes showed that proteoglycan synthesis can be positively influenced by several glycosaminoglycans[14-19]. The glycosaminoglycan polysulphate we used* is one of these polysaccharides. In previous studies this substance was proven to stimulate hyaluronate synthesis by monolayer cultured synovial cells[18]. This effect was reproducible in *in vivo* conditions. When the drug was injected intra-articularly we could demonstrate an increased synthesis of better polymerized hyaluronic acid by the synovial lining cell[20]. In our *in vitro* system we went into more detail with regard to the specific effects upon proteinpolysaccharide metabolism of human articular chondrocytes.

## MATERIAL AND METHODS

### Cell culture techniques

Human articular chondrocytes were isolated as described by Green[21]. Briefly, the cells were freed from their matrix with clostridial collagenase after preliminary treatment with testicular hyaluronidase and trypsin in order to remove any adherent synovial cells. 5–10 × $10^5$ cells were inoculated into 25 $cm^2$ flasks containing 5 ml of Ham's F12 medium supplemented with 10% foetal calf serum. Penicillin (10 IU/ml), streptomycin (10 $\mu$g/ml) and L-glutamin (0.002 mol/l) were added to the media. After the cells became attached to the plastic surface of the flask, Ham's F12 medium was replaced by Dulbecco's modified Eagle's medium supplemented with 10% foetal calf serum and containing the same additives. Media were changed every 3 to 4 days. For assay of proteoglycan synthesis chondrocytes were exposed to one $\mu$Ci of [$^{14}$C]glucosamine per millilitre of fresh medium for two periods of 24 h. Glycosaminoglycan polysulphate (GAGPS) was added in a final concentration of 10 $\mu$g/ml during the second 24 h period. The first 24 h phase served as a control. These experiments were carried out after cells reached

* Arteparon, Luitpold-Werk München

confluency.

**Chemical analyses**

Study of labelled mucopolysaccharides was carried out by following procedures.

(1) Ion exchange chromatography was used to separate glucosaminoglycan (GAG) complexes from culture media. These GAG complexes were eluted from DEAE A50 Sephadex columns (1.5 × 12 cm), previously equilibrated with a 50 mol/l Tris–HCl buffer at pH 7.0. Media were used as such. After the sample was applied, 100 ml of buffer containing LiCl at a final concentration of 0.3 mol/l was passed through the column in order to wash out the non incorporated [$^{14}$C]glucosamine and the labelled glycoproteins. The GAG complexes were then eluted with a continuous salt gradient (0.3 → 2 mol/l). The flow rate was 0.5–3 ml/min and 50 drop fractions were collected. 0.25 ml aliquots of each fraction were mixed with 5 ml scintillation cocktail (Scintisol) and counted for radioactivity in an LKB liquid scintillation counter. The fractions containing hyaluronic acid, resp. proteoglycan complexes were pooled separately and used for particle sieve chromatography.

(2) Samples of the hyaluronate (HA), resp. proteoglycan (PG) pools were pumped through a Sepharose 2B column in an ascending direction. The Sepharose was packed in 0.1 mol/l sodium acetate at pH 6.0 containing NaCl at a 1 mol/l concentration. 60 drop fractions (3.8 ml) were collected with a cooled LKB automatic fraction collector. 1 ml aliquots of each fraction were mixed with 10 ml scintillation cocktail and counted for radioactivity in a liquid scintillation counter.

(3) For some experiments PG aggregates were dissociated into their subunits by adjusting the pH of the PG solution to 3.0[26]. Subsequently, the sample was applied to the same Sepharose 2B column.

**Analysis of synovial fluids**

Analysis of synovial fluids was done in a few patients suffering from osteoarthritis of the knee. They received intra-articular injections of 100 mg of GAGPS at 3 day intervals. 5 ml samples of synovial fluid were collected before treatment, during treatment and after discontinuation of treatment. The initial findings were compared with the data obtained from a control group consisting of 12 patients with hydrathrosis of the knee due to osteoarthritis. Evolution of HA concentration and of viscometric behaviour of these samples was studied.

(1) Estimation of HA concentrations in synovial fluid was done by analysis of terminal reducing *N*-acetyl-hexosamine groups from liberated oligosaccharides after hyaluronidase treatment[22].

(2) Determination of specific viscosities. To this end, synovial fluids were diluted 1/50 with a 0.067 mol/l phosphate–citrate buffer at pH 7.3 containing 0.15 mol/l NaCl. A vertical capillary viscometer[23] was used for the viscosity measurements.

(3) Calculation of the intrinsic viscosity $[\eta]$ as a parameter of the mean degree of polymerization of the HA molecules was performed with the empiric formula developed by Sundblad[1] $[\eta] = \eta_{sp}\, c(1 + 0.18\, (\eta_{sp})$

(4) The anomalous viscosity index ($\eta_{AN}$ = degree of viscous anomaly) is also related to the polymerization of the HA molecules, but is more sensitive to the presence of small amounts of high polymer fractions in pathological synovial fluids.[1]. It was calculated from viscosity measurements by means of an identical vertical capillary viscometer[23]. Undiluted fluids were used for the determination of this index.

## RESULTS AND DISCUSSION

The experiments were performed on monolayer cultured chondrocytes (± 2 months in culture). When about 10 μg/ml of GAGPS were added to the nutrient media, an increase of both HA and PG synthesis was noticed. Ion-exchange chromatography patterns are illustrative for these findings (Figure 22.1). On Sepharose 2B gel chromatography significantly larger amounts of HA and of these PG complexes were eluted in the void volume, indicating a larger hydrodynamic size for these respective mucopolysaccharides following GAGPS 'treatment' (Figures 22.2 and 22.3). The higher hydrodynamic sizes of the proteoglycans observed has to be explained both by an increase in molecular weight of the PG sub-units (Figure 22.4) and by an increased aggregation between these high molecular weight sub-units. Although after GAGPS addition PG sub-units show higher molecular weights, these sub-units are retarded by the gel. The significant increase in amount of material eluted in the void volume of a Sepharose 2B column could then hardly been explained by the increased size of the PG sub-units. So we postulated that GAGPS in some way affects the aggregation between these sub-units. In previous studies conducted on older monolayer cultures this increase in molecular weight of the PG sub-units was not that obvious, in spite of their moderately longer glycosaminoglycan chain lengths. The increased intermolecular aggregation into PG complexes which we observed in these experiments were not of the same magnitude as those described here. 'Young' monolayers thus seem to be more susceptible to that GAGPS stimulation.

With respect to hyaluronate metabolism these effects were perfectly

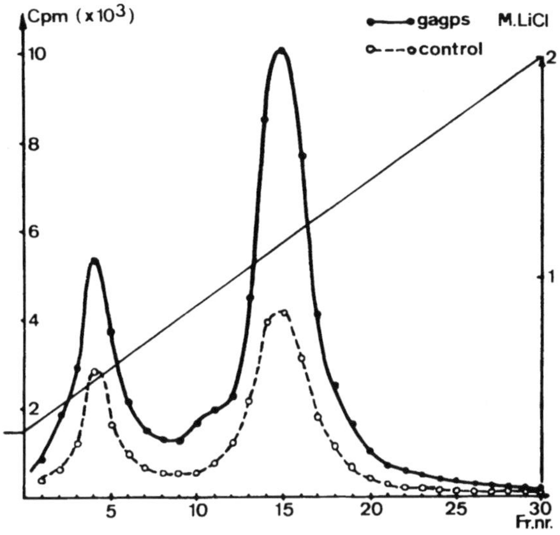


**Figure 22.1** Anion-exchange chromatography of [$^{14}$C]glucosamine mucopolysaccharides. First peak: HA; second peak: PG. Left ordinate: radioactivity incorporated in the hyaluronate and proteoglycan pool. Right ordinate: LiCl molar salt concentration. Abscissa: fraction number. ○ = controls; ● = GAGPS

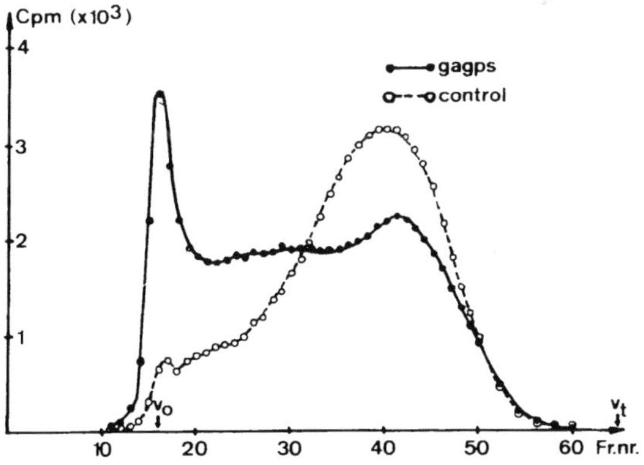


**Figure 22.2** Sepharose 2B gel chromatography of the hyaluronate pool. ○ = control; ● = GAGPS

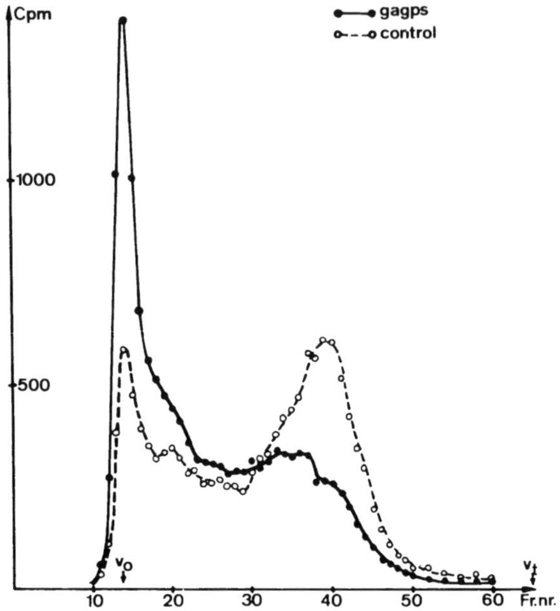


**Figure 22.3** Sepharose 2B gel chromatography of the proteoglycan pool. ○ = control; ● = GAGPS

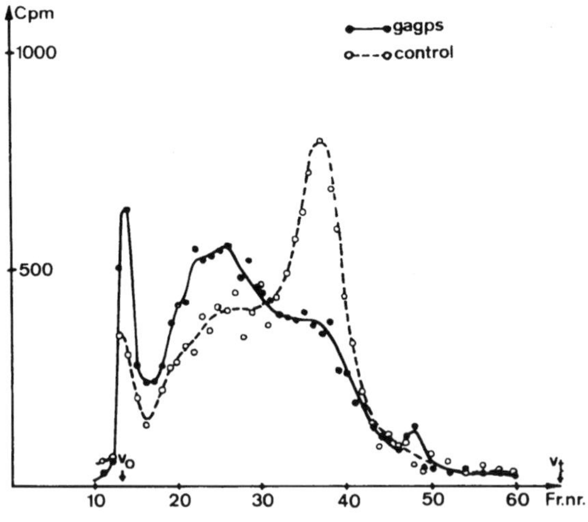


**Figure 22.4** Sepharose 2B gel chromatography of proteoglycan sub-units. ○ = control; ● = GAGPS

reproducible in *in vivo* conditions when a series of 100 mg of GAGPS were injected into the knees of patients suffering from osteoarthritis[20]. The intrinsic viscosity raised after repeated administration and whereas hyaluronate concentration in these fluids also increased constantly, a significant augmentation of the specific viscosity was the rule (Figures 22.5 and 22.6). In some cases under treatment, puncture revealed a gelatinous mass instead of a viscous fluid.

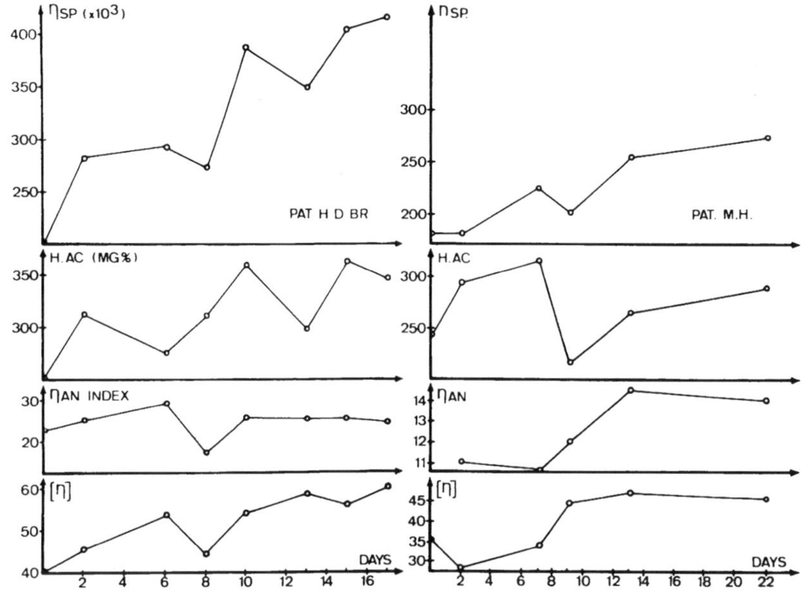


**Figure 22.5** Viscometric behaviour of synovial fluid after a series of intra-articular injections of 100 mg of GAGPS. The patient (osteoarthritis of the knee) received the drug at intervals of 2–3 days. $_{sp}$ = specific viscosity. h.ac = hyaluronate concentration in mg/100 ml. $\eta_{AN}$ index = index of anomalous viscosity. [η] = intrinsic viscosity as a parameter of mean molecular weight of the hyaluronate molecules.

We know that after intra-articular injection this glycosaminoglycan polysulphate is captured by subsynovial tissue and cartilage where it remains detectable for about two weeks[24]. Furthermore, it was shown that the drug is able to control degenerative evolution in experimentally induced osteoarthritis in dogs[25]. Finally, the beneficial effects of this drug in natural osteoarthritis in man is well documented.

The impact of the drug on some biochemical abnormalities thus far observed in proteoglycan and hyaluronic acid metabolism in resp. articular cartilage and the synovial membrane in osteoarthritic joints, strengthens our opinion that this glycosaminoglycan polysulphate (and possibly other glycosaminoglycans) interferes with a key function in the regulation of proteinpolysaccharide metabolism. This type of drug may offer us a

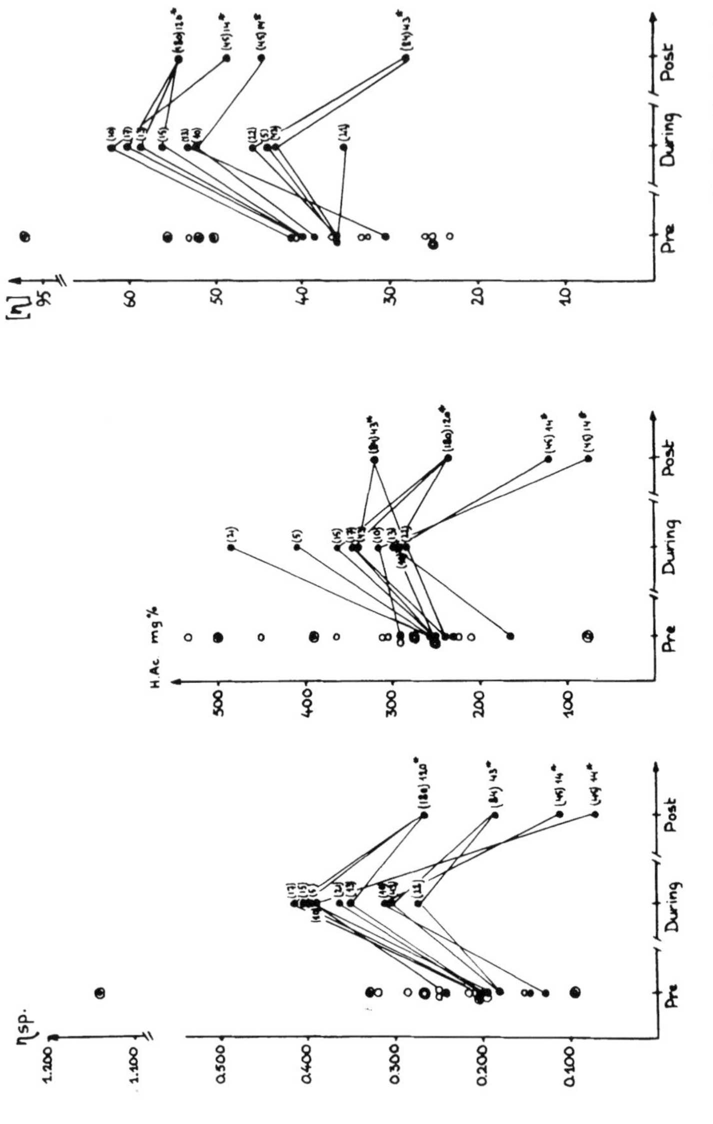


**Figure 22.6** Evolution of synovial fluid rheology. Specific viscosity ($\eta_{sp}$), hyaluronic acid concentration (h.ac mg/100 ml) and intrinsic viscosity numbers ([η]) are shown before, during and after discontinuation of treatment. The values before treatment are compared with those of a control group (○ = osteoarthritis; ⊙ = *degenerative joint disease following burnt-out rheumatoid arthritis*) ( ): days after onset of treatment, *: days after discontinuation of treatment

fundamental approach in the management of degenerative evolution in osteoarthritis and perhaps in other articular diseases.

## References


1 Sundblad, L. (1953). *Acta Soc. Med. Ups.*, **58,** 115
2 Balazs, E. A. *et al.* (1967). *Arthritis Rheum.*, **10,** 357
3 Castor, C. W. *et al.* (1966). *Arthritis Rheum.*, **9,** 783
4 Verbruggen, G. and Veys, E. M. (1980). *Acta Rheum. (Belgium)* (In press)
5 Castor, C. W. *et al.* (1971) *Arthritis Rheum.*, **14,** 41
6 Mankin, H. J. and Lipiello, L. (1970). *J. Bone Jt. Surg.*, **52A,** 424
7 Hardingham, T. E. *et al.* (1972). *Biochem. J.*, **129,** 101
8 McDevitt, C. A. *et al.* (1973). *Biochem. Soc. Trans.*, **1,** 287
9 Brandt, K. *et al.* (1976). *Arthritis Rheum.*, **19,** 1308
10 McDevitt, C. A. *et al.* (1978). *Ann. Rheum. Dis.*, **37,** 484
11 Greiling, *et al.* (1971). In Müller, W, Harwerth, H. G. and Fehr, K. (eds). *Rheumatoid Arthritis, Pathogenetic mechanism and consequences in therapeutics*, p. 173. (London: Academic Press)
12 Fell, H. B. and Dingle, J. T. (1963). *Biochem. J.*, **87,** 403
13 Sapolski, A. I. *et al.* (1974). *J. Clin. Invest.*, **53,** 1044
14 Nevo, Z. *et al.* (1972). *Dev. Biol.*, **28,** 219
15 Kosher, R. A. *et al.* (1973). *Dev. Biol.*, **35,** 210
16 Wiebkin, O. W. and Muir, H. (1973). In E, Kulonen, *Biology of fibroblast*, J. Pikkarainen, (eds.) p. 231. (New York: Academic Press)
17 Schwartz, N. B. and Dorfman, A. (1975). *Conn. Tiss. Res.*, **3,** 115
18 Verbruggen, G. and Veys, E. M. (1977). *Acta Rheum. (Belgium).*, **1,** 75
19 Verbruggen, G. and Veys, E. M. (1980). *J. Rheumatol.*, (In press)
20 Verbruggen, G. and Veys, E. M. (1979). *J. Rheumatol.*, **6,** 554
21 Green, W. T. (1971). *Clin. Orthop. Relat. Res.*, **75,** 248
22 Reissig, *et al.* (1955). *J. Biol. Chem.*, **217,** 959
23 Levine, M. G. and Kling, D. M. (1956). *J. Clin. Invest.*, **35,** 1419
24 Enislidis, A. C. (1972). *Med. Welt*, **23,** 733
25 Ueno, R. (1976). *Z. Orthop. Ihre Grenzgeb.*, **114,** 105
26 Muir, H. (personal communication)

# 23

# Anti-arthritic properties of ICI 55897 (Clozic) (Abstract)

M. E. J. BILLINGHAM (UK)

ICI 55897 has a novel spectrum of properties in experimental models of inflammation when compared with conventional non-steroidal anti-inflammatory drugs (NSAIDS). A chronic, persistent form of rat adjuvant arthritis is inhibited by ICI 55897, but otherwise the molecule possesses minimal activity in standard anti-inflammatory and analgesic tests. For example, ICI 55897 has little or no activity in the acute, carrageenin oedema test in the rat, at doses and serum levels which are many times higher than those necessary to inhibit the chronic model of adjuvant arthritis. In further contrast to the NSAIDS, ICI 55897 produces no gastrointestinal irritation in laboratory animals. This different spectrum of activity of ICI 55897, in comparison with the NSAIDS, may be explained by the very weak inhibitory activity of ICI 55897 against prostaglandin synthetase, i.e., the enzyme system which is the target of the NSAIDS. ICI 55897 inhibits a chronic form of arthritis in the rat, but not by an inhibition of the overlying acute symptoms of the inflammatory process. Clinical results, to date, have substantiated this view. ICI 55897 has demonstrated an effect against human rheumatoid arthritis which is similar to that produced by the disease modifying agents, gold and pencillamine, rather than the symptomatic effect produced by the NSAIDS. Treatment with ICI 55897 is associated with clinical improvement and a return of the ESR and acute phase proteins (i.e., the biochemical markers of disease activity) to normal values; this is in distinct contrast to the NSAIDS where an effect on ESR and acute phase proteins has yet to be demonstrated.

24

# Effect of ICI 55897 (Clozic), indomethacin and dexamethasone on collagenase and prostaglandin production by cultured rheumatoid synovial tissue (Abstract)

D. E. WOOLLEY; S. J. GADHER, S. J. FOSTER
AND M. E. J. BILLINGHAM (UK)

Explants of rheumatoid synovial tissue produce significant quantities of neutral collagenase and prostaglandins when cultured for 5–6 days at 37°C in serum-free Dulbecco's modified Eagle's medium (Dayer *et al.* (1976). *Proc. Natl. Acad. Sci. (USA)*, **73**, 945). Cultures which were supplemented with ICI55897 over the concentration range 20–400 $\mu$g/ml (all culture flasks contained 10 mg/ml human serum albumin) showed no significant change in the production of either total collagenase or prostaglandins. Total collagenase was measured using the $^{14}$C-labelled collagen fibril assay following trypsin activation of culture medium, and the prostaglandins $PGE_2$ and $PGF_{2\alpha}$ were measured by radio-immunassay. No change was detected in glucose depletion or lactate dehydrogenase activity of the culture medium, suggesting that viability over 5 days of culture was similar to that of the controls. Most experiments were carried out using a concentration of 150 $\mu$g/ml of ICI 55897 and no change was detected for levels of the prostaglandins $PGE_2$ and $PGF_{2\alpha}$ although a slight reduction in collagenase was occasionally observed. In contrast, indomethacin (5 $\mu$g/ml) inhibited all prostaglandin production, but had a variable effect on collagenase production which occasionally was slightly higher than control values. Dexamethasone ($10^{-7}$mol/l) was shown to inhibit both collagenase and prostaglandin production. Such comparative studies suggest that ICI 55897 has a different effect on rheumatoid tissue than indomethacin or dexamethasone. Clinical studies with ICI 55897 have demonstrated that it has an effect in rheumatoid arthritis which is similar to that produced by the disease-modifying agents, gold and pencillamine, rather than the symptomatic effect produced by the NSAIDS.

# 25

# The use of thymopoietin as an anti-inflammatory agent (Abstract)

A. SEDGWICK, P. A. THROWER, D. A. WILLOUGHBY AND E. C. HUSKISSON (UK)

Following the use of levamisole as an anti-rheumatic drug and its postulated action via T suppressor cells, a study has been undertaken using thymopoietin. The preparation of thymopoietin used has been a synthetic pentapeptide. This has been found to have a significant effect on acute carrageenin pleurisy in that it caused a significant reduction in cell migration but had no effect on exudate volume. Thymopoietin also caused a reduction of the cotton pellet granuloma model. Preliminary results of a clinical trial in man show promising results.

# 26

# Production of hydrogen peroxide from neutrophils of rats (Abstract)

E. M. GLENN, BARBARA J. BOWMAN AND
N. A. ROHLOFF (USA)

The production–release of hydrogen peroxide ($H_2O_2$) from peritoneal neutrophils of rats has been investigated. Cells are elicited by intraperitoneal injections of *Mycobacterium butyricum* in saline 24 h before cell harvest. Among many other possibilities, phorbol myristate acetate, *M. butyricum* and *Agkistrodon piscivorus* venom are the most effective stimulators of $H_2O_2$ production. The various routine kinetic parameters of these reactions have been studied and some will be presented here. Various non-steroidal anti-inflammatory drugs have been examined for their effects on $H_2O_2$ production and, among these, phenylbutazone is the most potent inhibitor. $C_{21}$ steroidal anti-inflammatory drugs (6 alpha-methylprednisolone succinate and cortisol succinate, especially) are potent inhibitors of $H_2O_2$ production by stimulated and non-stimulated cells. Arachidonic acid and linolenic acid, among others, are extremely potent inhibitors of $H_2O_2$ production–release from stimulated neutrophils and these effects do not appear to be related either to the cyclo-oxygenase initiated or the lipoxygenase initiated 'cascade'. These and other studies, as well as their probable significance, if any, will be discussed.

# 27

# Effects of D-penicillamine on granulation tissue and connective tissue of skin, aorta and bone in rats (Abstract)

I. LORENZEN AND P. JUNKER (DENMARK)

Granulation tissue was produced in rats by subcutaneous implantation of viscose-cellulose sponges. After 52 days treatment with D-penicillamine 100 or 500 (mg/kg)/day half of the animals were killed, the rest after an additional 29 days without treatment. Each treatment group had a paired control group. D-penicillamine caused a substantial and dose dependent inhibition of the collagen crosslinking in all tissues as reflected by increased proportions of soluble collagen fractions and aldehyde crosslink precursors in purified collagen. The most marked changes occurred in skin and aorta, in the latter associated with increased tissue weight and water percentage. In purified acid soluble and 60 °C soluble skin collagen the hdroxyproline/proline ratio was increased after D-penicillamine treatment indicating that the degree of proline hydroxylation in these fractions was increased. The amount of granulation tissue was not affected by the treatment, whereas a reduction of the total amount of collagen and DNA in skin was observed. The collagen profile in granulation tissue, skin and bone was not normalized at the end of the experiment, and in aorta excess deposition of collagen and DNA was observed. These findings indicate that D-penicillamine induces qualitative alterations of the granulation tissue of possible significance to its anti-rheumatic efficacy, but that the amount of fibrotic tissue not was influenced. The effect on normal tissues was far more pronounced, and in vascular tissue even progressive. Formation of crosslink deficient interstitial collagen in normal tissues may severely reduce its supportive capacity and imply side effects from long-term treatment with penicillamine.

# 28

# D-penicillamine in rheumatoid arthritis: fixed versus variable regimes

D. R. BLAKE, E. F. J. RING, R. C. BUCKNALL AND P. A. BACON (UK)

## INTRODUCTION

D-penicillamine is of proven therapeutic value in the treatment of rheumatoid arthritis[1], although the increased incidence of side effects associated with high dose regimes (greater than 1 g/per day) has encouraged clinicians to examine the response to lower doses.

A comparison of two dose regimes, 1200 mg with 600 mg, suggested that the latter was equally effective with fewer side effects[2]. A low dose regime of 125 mg/per day has been reported to be effective in certain cases[3].

These and other studies imply that individual response is both wide and apparently unpredictable. We have therefore examined a more flexible approach to prescribing penicillamine, using quantitative thermography as an objective index of inflammatory activity[4]. This paper reports the results of a trial designed to compare a variable prescribing method with two fixed regimes (750 mg and 125 mg).

## PATIENTS AND METHODS

### Criteria for admission to trial

Patients fulfilling the American Rheumatism Association's criteria for the diagnosis of definite or classical rheumatoid arthritis[5] were considered for the study. All had definite rheumatoid arthritis for a minimum period of 6 months, and had failed to respond to a full therapeutic dose of at least one non-steroidal anti-inflammatory drug taken consistently for 3 months. Patients who had previously received gold or penicillamine, or had taken immunosuppressive drugs or cloroquine within the previous 6 months were excluded. Concurrent administration of prednisolone was permitted provided the dose was below 5 mg and had been so in the previous 3 months.

### Treatment groups

Patients were consecutively allocated to one of the following three schedules:

(1) Standard dose fixed regime – penicillamine 750 mg/day. Initial dose 125 mg/day and dose adjusted by 125 mg at no less than 2 weekly intervals.

(2) Low dose fixed regime – 125 mg/day.

(3) Variable dose regime – the dosage was increased at 2 weekly intervals until a dosage of 500 mg was established, and thereafter adjusted according to the results of quantitative thermography, with a compound index measuring six joint areas. If the thermographic index was stable or had increased, penicillamine dose was increased by 125 mg; when the thermographic index had fallen on two consecutive months, the dose of penicillamine was decreased by 125 mg.

### Assessment

Assessments were carried out at monthly intervals. In addition to the quantitative thermographic index measurements, progress was assessed by the following indices: (1) plasma viscosity, (2) haemaglobin, (3) sheep cell agglutination test and latex fixation test, (4) duration of morning stiffness, (5) the grip strength of both hands, and (6) a joint pain index (Ritchie articular index[6]). All clinical assessments were made by the same observer.

## RESULTS

To date, 40 patients have entered the trial, 15 patients in both fixed regimes and 10 in the variable regime. The three groups were comparable in terms of duration of disease, age and sex. There was no significant difference in disease activity between the three groups at the commencement of the study. The mean daily dose of penicillamine taken by patients in the variable group at one year was 500 mg (range 250 – 1000 mg).

### Withdrawals

Six patients did not complete the study due to the adverse side effects of penicillamine – five from the 750 mg regime and one from the variable regime. There were no withdrawals from the low dose regime. All side effects occurred after the third month of therapy when the dosage was fully established. In five of the six cases, the drug was withdrawn at the request of the general practitioner or the patient, and all were from the 750 mg fixed regime. Two were for mild thrombocytopenia and one for proteinuria, and in each case recovery was rapid on discontinuing the drug. Two patients discontinued their medication themselves, one for severe nausea and the other because of a rash.

The patient withdrawn from the variable regime developed signifcant proteinuria (3 g/1) while taking 750 mg penicillamine during the seventh month of treatment, which again rapidly improved on discontinuing the drug. The high fixed regime was discontinued at 6 months because of the incidence of side effects and the poor patient acceptability (33%).

**Response**

*1 By clinical assessment*

Three clinical assessments were made: (1) the grip strength in both hands, (2) a cumulative articular pain index (Ritchie Index), and (3) the duration of morning stiffness.

In all groups these three parameters significantly improved. However, there was no significant difference in response at 1 year between our variable prescribing method and the low fixed regime. Patients in the low dose regime showed a significant improvement in these three parameters from the 6 month of therapy [(1) $p = 0.05$, (2) $p = 0.01$, (3) $p = 0.025$], while in the variable regime, a significant improvement in the articular index occurred from the third month of treatment ($p = 0.025$).

*2 By objective indices of inflammatory activity*

The haemaglobin and plasma viscosity improved in all groups, but no significant difference was shown between the low dose and variable regime at 9 months or 1 year. Similarly, patients in the low dose regime showed a significant rise in haemaglobin and fall in plasma viscosity only from the sixth month of treatment ($p = 0.025$; $p = 0.0025$). The rheumatoid factor titre showed a tendency to fall in all groups, but failed to reach statistical significance in any.

*3 By quantitative thermography*

Figure 28.1 shows the changes at 3 monthly intervals in the mean thermographic index of each group. Patients in the low dose regime showed no significant response until the sixth month, and thereafter showed continued improvement. The variable regime improved significantly from the third month although the response failed to reach significance at 1 year. This lack of response is accounted for by two patients who at 9 months reduced their penicillamine dose inappropriately, but have subsequently responded.

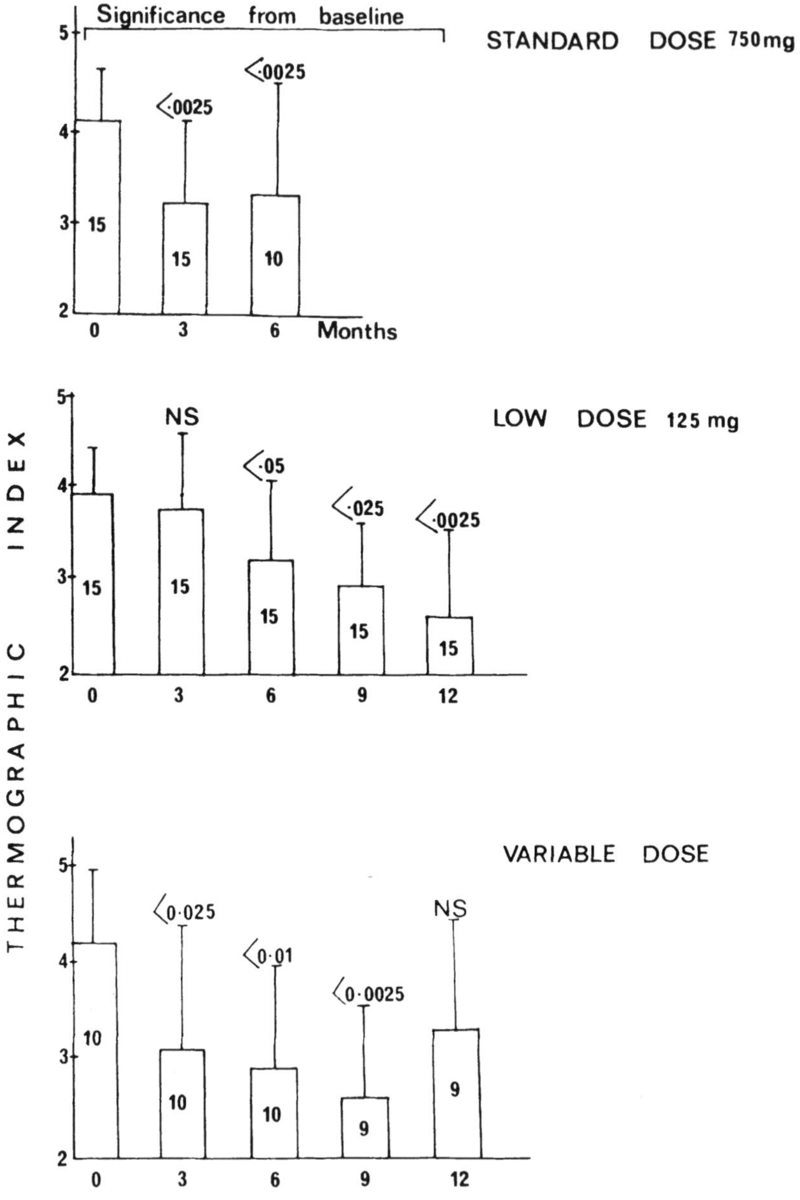


**Figure 28.1** The effect of different dose regimes on the mean thermographic index at 3 monthly intervals

## DISCUSSION

This study has confirmed the suggestion that lower doses of penicillamine may be used for patients with active rheumatoid arthritis with considerable benefit. A low dose was associated with remarkably little toxicity. The numbers in the groups were too small to make any significant assessment of the rate of toxicity but nevertheless no patient had to be withdrawn from this group as compared with the fixed high dose regime. The drawback to the low dose regime is the slow rate of response. Until 6 months, the patients did not appear to have responded at all. This is a slower rate of response than the higher doses of penicillamine or alternative drugs, such as gold. Interestingly, within the low dosage regime all parameters, both objective and subjective, demonstrated improvement at the same time, although the thermographic assessment appeared to be the most sensitive index.

The problem of slow response may be overcome by the variable dose regime. In this case, the rate of response was more rapid with obvious advantages to the patient. It may well be that the dose should have been reduced more rapidly in those patients who responded early. Nevertheless, the group on a variable dose regime did not show a significant number of toxicity problems either.

Penicillamine has been in widespread clinical use for nearly a decade. During this time the suggested doses have fallen steadily, with a reduction in the dose related group of side effects, such as loss of taste and gastrointestinal problems. However, there has been little obvious change in the later complications, i.e., nephropathy and leg rash. The ideal dose is still not known. In these circumstances it seems sensible to tailor the dose to the requirement of the individual patient. Rheumatoid disease contains a very wide spectrum of disease activity and it is most unlikely that any fixed dose regime will suit every patient. A more flexible approach to penicillamine dosing could be adopted more widely with benefit to the patient but without loss of efficacy.

### References


1 Multicenter Trial Group (1973). Controlled trial of D-pencillamine in severe rheumatoid arthritis. *Lancet*, **1**, 275

2 Dixon, A. S. J., Davies, J., Dormandy, T. L., Hamilton, E. B. D., Holt, P. J. L., Mason, R. M., Thompson, M., Weber, J. C. P. and Zutshi, D. W. (1975). Synthetic D-penicillamine in rheumatoid arthritis: double-blind controlled study of a high and low dosage regimen. *Ann. Rheum. Dis.*, **34**, 416

3 Day, A. T., Golding, J. R., Lee, P. N. and Butterworth, A. (1974). Pencillamine in rheumatoid disease: a long-term study. *Br. Med. J.*, **1**, 180

4 Collins, A. J., Ring, E. F. J., Cosh, J. A. and Bacon, P. A. (1974). Quantitation of thermography in arthritis using multi-isothermal analysis. I. The thermographic index. *Ann. Rheum. Dis.*, **33**, 113

5 Ropes, M. W., Bennett, G. A., Cobb, S., Jacox, R. and Jessar, R. (1958). Revision of diagnostic criteria for rheumatoid arthritis. *Bull. Rheum. Dis.*, **9**, 175

6 Ritchie, D. M., Boyle, J. A., McInnes, J. R., Jasani, K. M., Dalabos, T. C., Grieveson, P. and Buchanan, W. W. (1968). Clinical studies with an articular index for the assessment of joint tenderness in patients with rheumatoid arthritis. *Q. J. Med.*, **147**, 393

# 29

# Effects of anti-inflammatory drugs on polymorphonuclear leukocyte aggregation (Abstract)

F. M. CUNNINGHAM AND M. J. H. SMITH (UK)

Rat peritoneal leukocytes (84 ± 4% neutrophils) have been shown to aggregate *in vitro* after addition of zymosan activated plasma (ZAP) or formylmethionyl-leucyl-phenylalanine (FMLP). Aggregation, caused by high circulating levels of activated complement products, plays a role in the transient neutropenia associated with certain clinical conditions and the effects of some anti-inflammatory drugs on FMLP and ZAP induced aggregation have therefore been examined. PMN suspensions (0.5 ml of $1 \times 10^7$ cells $ml^{-1}$) were stirred at 900 rev/min for 5 min at 37 °C in a Payton aggregometer, an aliquot of drug was then added to the cuvette 1 min prior to the addition of either $5 \times 10^{-7}$ mol/l FMLP or 2% ZAP. Aggregation was measured as a change in optical density and results expressed as the percentage reduction of the response in the presence of the drug compared to that observed with vehicle alone. Methyl prednisolone (0.03–2 mg $ml^{-1}$), hydrocortisone sodium succinate (0.1–4 mg $ml^{-1}$) and colchicine ($10^{-5}$–$10^{-3}$ mol/l) caused a dose related reduction in the aggregation response to both FMLP and ZAP. Indomethacin ($10^{-6}$–$10^{-4}$ mol/l) and aspirin ($2.5 \times 10^{-3}$ mol/l) significantly reduced the aggregation response to FMLP without altering the response to ZAP. The mechanism of these effects may involve blockade of the receptor sites on the PMN to the aggregating agents and inhibitory activity on pathways of arachidonic acid metabolism.

# 30

# Aggregation of rat polymorphonuclear leukocytes *in vitro* by chemotactic factors (Abstract)

**M. E. SHIPLEY, F. M. CUNNINGHAM AND M. J. H. SMITH (UK)**

Rat leukocytes containing 84 ± 4% polymorphonuclear leukocytes (PMNs) were obtained by peritoneal lavage 24 h after the injection of 6 ml of 12% sodium caseinate. The cells were washed and resuspended at a concentration of 1–1.3 × $10^7$ cells/ml in Eagle's minimum essential medium buffered to pH 7.4 with 30 mmol/l HEPES. The change in particle numbers reflecting aggregation was measured by the decrease in optical density in a Payton aggregometer (37 °C, 900 rev/min stirring speed). Both formyl-methionyl-leucyl-phenylalanine (FMLP), over the range $10^{-5}$–$10^{-8}$ mol/l and zymosan activated serum or plasma, over the range 0.5–10% v/v, produced dose related aggregation responses. The reaction was diminished in the presence of 0.5% human serum albumin and potentiated in the presence of cytochalasin B (optimal concentration 250 ng $ml^{-1}$). The optimal cell concentration was found to be 1.2 × $10^7$ cells/ml and the technique was highly reproducible (coefficient of variation <8.5%). The aggregation of peripheral rat PMNs in response to FMLP was significantly reduced when compared to that of elicited peritoneal cells.

Aggregation of PMNs has been shown to be important in certain clinical conditions which are characterized by high circulating levels of activated complement components, e.g. shock lung and endotoxin shock. Aggregation responses may also play a role in the adherence of PMNs locally to the vascular endothelium around inflammatory sites where high levels of chemotactic factors may be present. As a means of investigating both the phenomenon of aggregation and its possible modification by drugs and as a sensitive detector of chemotactic factors the system described has the advantage of reproducibility and ease of production of large numbers of cells in the rat.

# 31

# Preliminary report on the effect of a new derivative of acetyl salicylic acid on tissue-algogen component due to damaging stimulation of cutis

L. VECCHIET, O. PONTANO, G. OBLETTER AND L. CARRATELLI (ITALY)

## INTRODUCTION

A derivative of acetyl salicylic acid recently synthesized, acid 5-(2,4-difluorenil)-salicylate (diflunisal), seems to be endowed with an elevated anti-phlogistic and analgesic activity[1–4].

To study such activity in the clinical situation, we adopted a test developed by the Scuola Fiorentina (carbonic snow test) consisting of provoking a standard damaging stimulation on the skin and in reporting and analysing the consequent tissue-algogen reactions[5].

## TEST DESCRIPTION

A round 1 cm diameter block of carbonic snow with a plane surface was applied three times on the flexorial surface of the forearm with a pressure of 60 g for 5 s each time, with intervals between contact of 10 s. In order to produce a constant force we used an instrument fitted to the delimitation of the carbonic snow surface to modulate its pressure on the cutis.

Subjective and objective cutaneous phenomena induced by the

stimulation with carbonic snow are as follows:

(1) Immediate pain was felt at a maximum intensity by all the subjects and was attributed to direct stimulation of peripheral nociceptors leading to quick conduction fibres.

(2) Reflex erythema appeared in 6 and 26 s ($x = 13 \pm 6$; $\varepsilon = 44\%$) and its tonality varied from fiery red to pale red and pink and the major and minor diameters varied, respectively, from $5 \times 4$ to $3.5 \times 3$ cm. It is caused by secondary arteriolar vasodilatation, due to a reflex mechanism to pain receptor stimulation.

(3) Fixed erythema appeared in all the subjects, in a time varying from 40 to 53 min from the beginning of the stimulation, as a peripheral ring of reddening ($x = 48\text{s} \pm 5$; $\varepsilon = 10.4\%$). It appeared in the zone stimulated from 1 min 10 s to 1 min 30 s ($x = 1$ min 21 s $\pm$ 7 s; $\varepsilon = 9\%$). It spread in all the subjects in a period varying from 1 min 35 s to 2 min 07 s ($x = 1$ min 52 s $\pm$ 10 s; $\varepsilon = 8\%$). The spread was from 1–3 mm. In this phase 1–3 pseudopodis also generally appear. Successively, the zone of skin corresponding to fixed erythema rose and formed a protruding pomphus; this started from 3 min 40 s to 4 min 20 s = ($x = 4$ min 03 s $\pm$ 14 s; $\varepsilon = 11\%$). Fixed erythema and pomphus are attributed to the release of vasoactive and permeabilizing substances[6,7].

(4) Erytralgic halo included a zone surrounding the lesion and 15 s after the stimulation it assumed dimensions of $4 \times 5$–$2 \times 1$ mm. It is attributed to the diffusion of substances endowed with algogen vasoactive effects from the middle of the stimulated zone to the periphery[8].

(5) Recurring pain was felt by all the subjects after a period of 1 min 50 s to 2 min 20 s ($x = 2$ min 07 s $\pm$ 11 s; $\varepsilon = 8\%$) and was perceived as a burning pain. It is considered to be caused by the action of substances with an algogen effect releasing themselves because of tissue damage[9].

(6) Diffused hyperalgesia rose in a period from 3 min 50 s to 5 min 10 s ($x = 5$ min 26 s $\pm$ 27 s; $\varepsilon = 8\%$) and spread in a zone from 6.8 to 8.3 cm. This phenomenon is interpreted on a humoral and nervous basis[6,7,10–12].

## PERSONAL ENUMERATION OF CASES

In a preliminary way we carried out the cutaneous test with carbonic snow on some voluntary undergraduates and medical students: five male subjects from 23 to 27. In three of them we carried out a stimulation in base conditions and a stimulation after the assumption of 500 mg of diflunisal every 12 h for 24 h. In two subjects we evaluated only the blistered reaction, giving the drug in the same dosage in the 24 h preceding and following the stimulation. We then performed a comparative study on the tissue-algogen phenomena with the aid of photographs taken at prefixed times, i.e. immediately after, 2 min, 4 min, 15 min and 24 h after the stimulation.

## SYNTHESIS OF RESULTS

In the first three subjects the stimulation, after assumption of diflunisal, demonstrated:

(a) An intense immediate pain. (Figure 31.1)
(b) A reflex erythema without particular modifications
(c) A fixed erythema usually of a pale tone and with a clear border (Figures 31.2 and 31.3)
(d) A burning recurring pain appearing after a longer period of latency, not very intense and lasting a short while (Figure 31.1).
(e) A pomphoid raising appearing after a longer period of latency but of a small diameter (Figures 31.4 and 31.5).
(f) An erytralgic halo scarcely distinguishable with secondary hyperalgesia appearing after a much longer latency and less diffusion (Figure 31.1).
(g) A blister small in both expansion and liquid content (Figure 31.6).

In the other two subjects where the stimulation was preceded and followed by the assumption of the drug, tissue reactions were remarkably reduced and the raising of the blister is nearly totally lacking (Figures 31.7 and 31.8).

## CONCLUSIONS

The identification of immediate pain before and after diflunisal confirms that the drug does not act on receptors and centres of pain. The absence of modifications in the reflex erythema as above, attributable to neurovegetative phenomena induced by painful stimulation, is another confirmation of it.

The clear lessening of burning pain either in intensity or duration, together with the minor expansion of secondary hyperalgesia on the base of the physiopathogenetic interpretation attributed to the phenomenon, must be attributed to the minor presence of algogen substances in the active state.

The decrease of the size of the pomphoid and, principally, the nearly total lacking of a blister must be attributed to a decreased presence in the active state of the substances acting on the permeability of microvessels.

From this test, even though preliminary, we can advance the hypothesis that diflunisal, besides its capacity of inhibiting prostaglandins[3,13,14], has also a well identifiable activity of inhibiting chemical mediators with a permeability activity.

The application of the test offers useful starting points for the

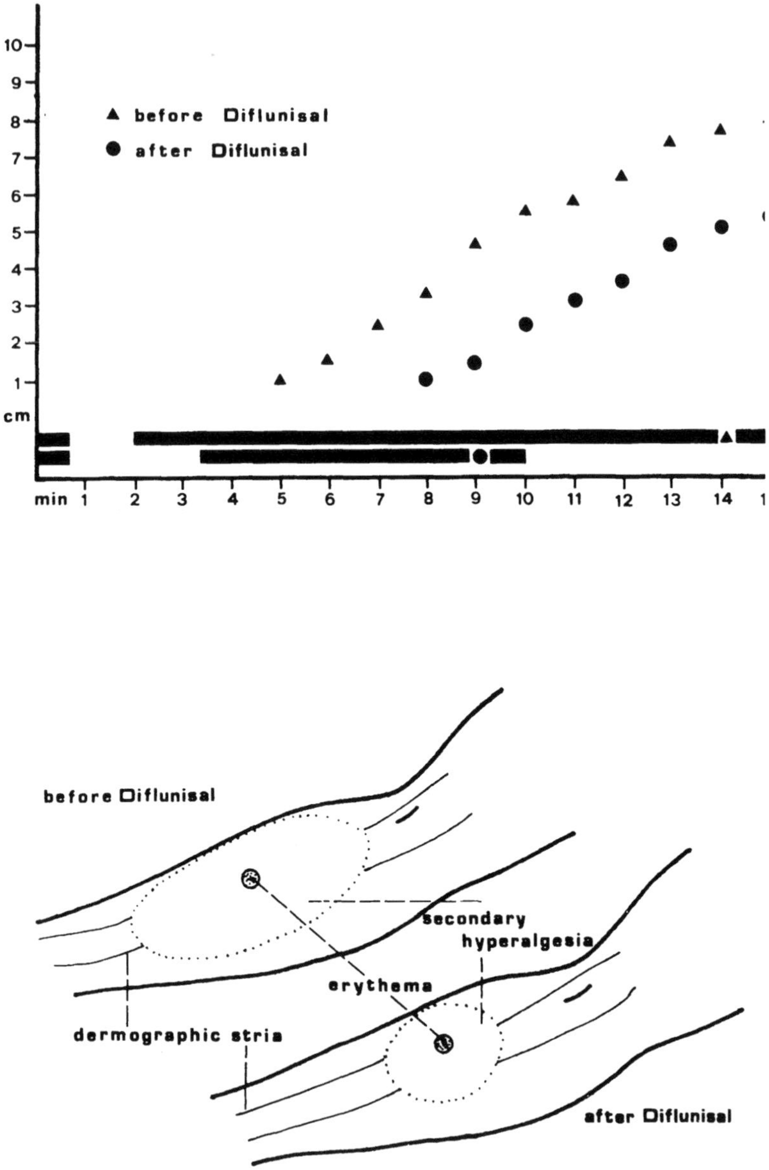


**Figure 31.1** Graphic representation of immediate, recurring pain and of secondary hyperalgesia in base conditions and after administration of diflunisal. The continuous lines on the abscissa show the time of appearance and duration of immediate and recurring pain. On the ordinate are the dimensions of the secondary hyperalgesia zones during the first 15 min

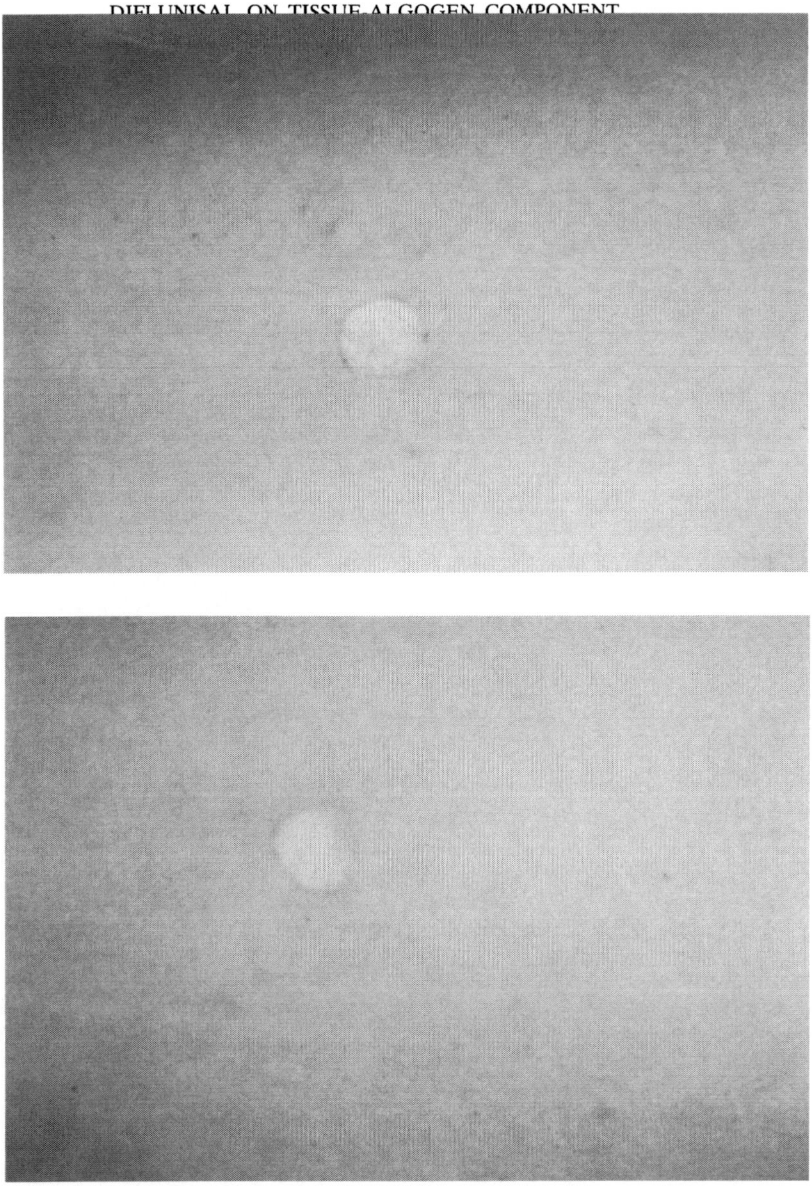

(a)

(b)

**Figure 31.2** Effects of cutaneous stimulation due to carbonic snow. Pictures obtained immediately after stimulation (a) in base conditions, (b) after diflunisal

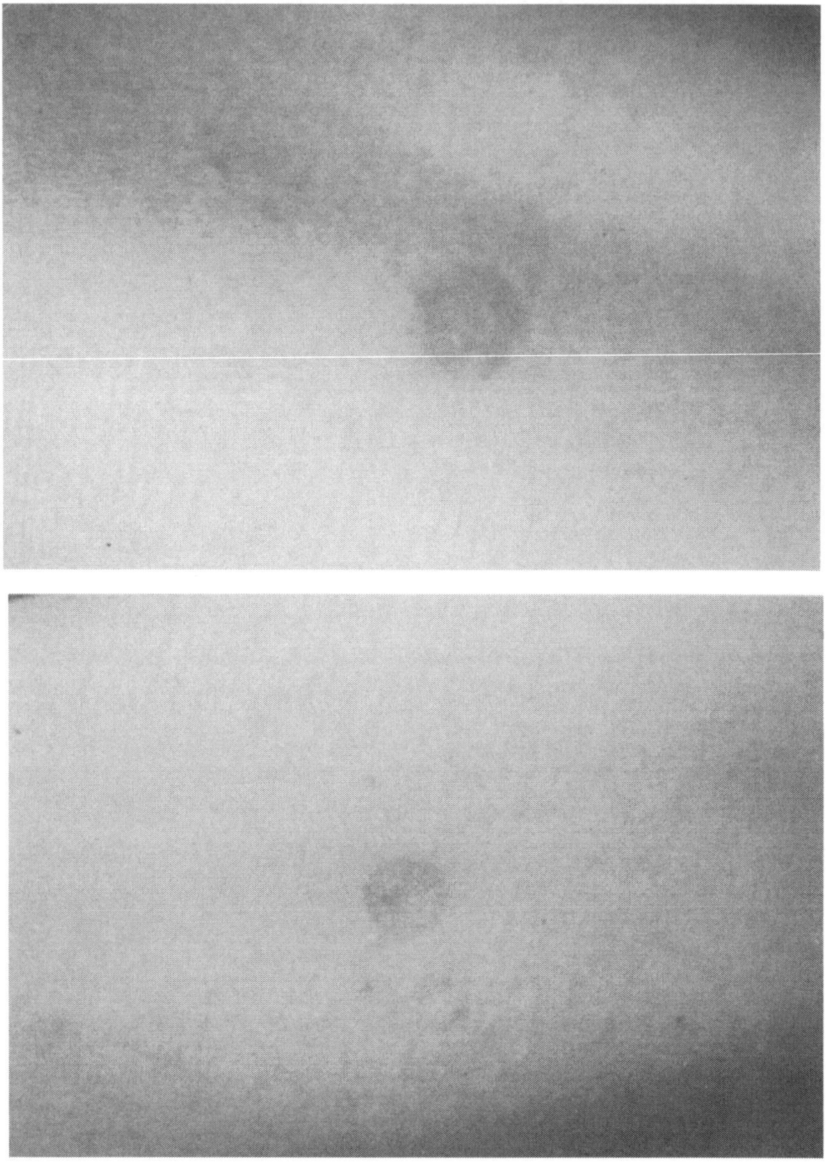

**Figure 31.3** Effects of cutaneous stimulation due to carbonic snow. Pictures obtained 2 min after stimulation (a) in base conditions, (b) after diflunisal

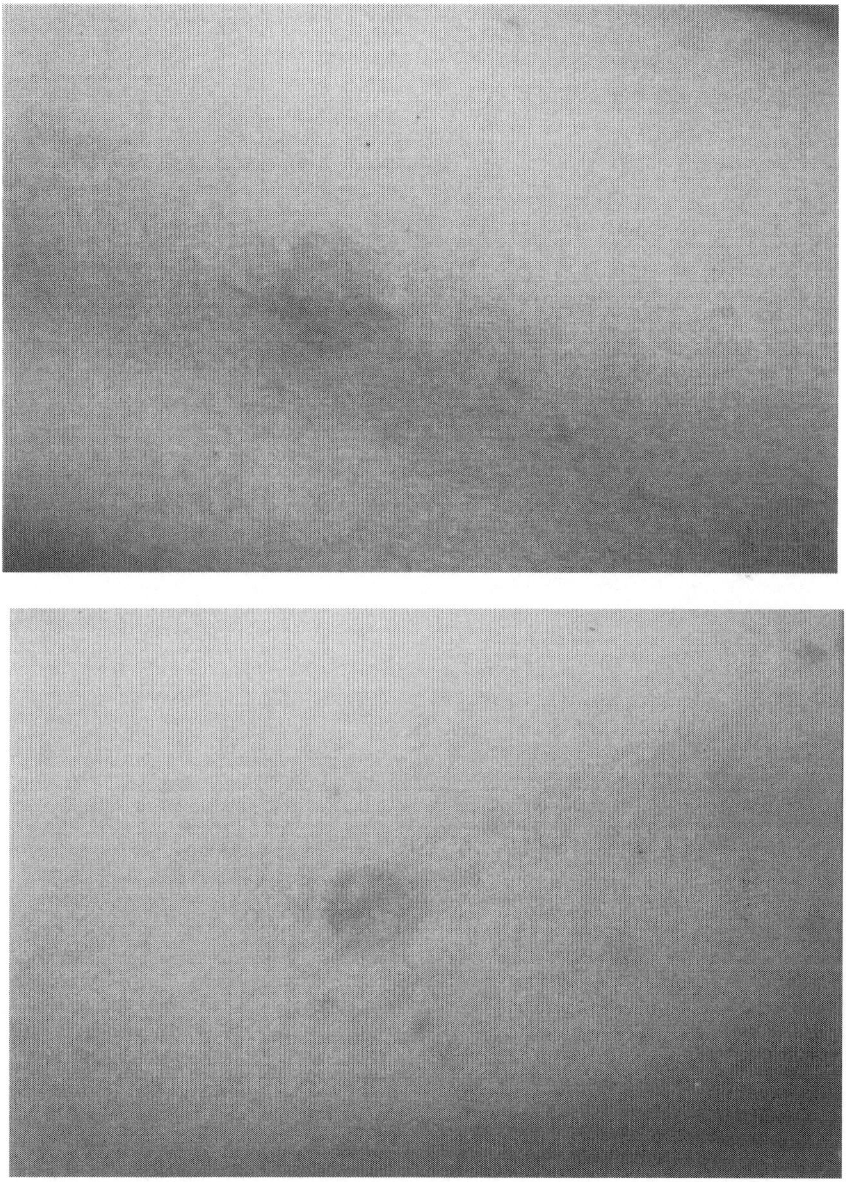

**Figure 31.4** Effects of cutaneous stimulation due to carbonic snow. Pictures obtained 4 min after stimulation (a) in base conditions, (b) after diflunisal

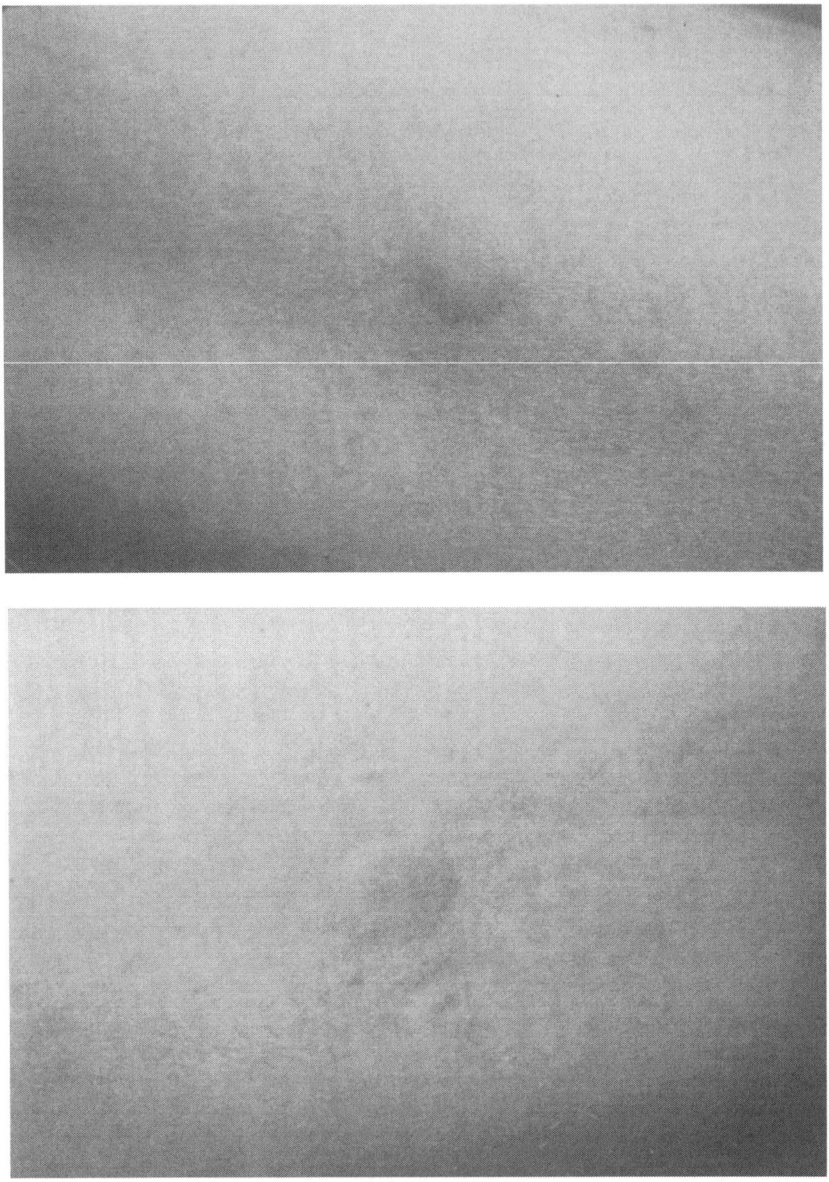

**Figure 31.5** Effects of cutaneous stimulation due to carbonic snow. Pictures obtained 15 min after stimulation (a) in base conditions, (b) after diflunisal

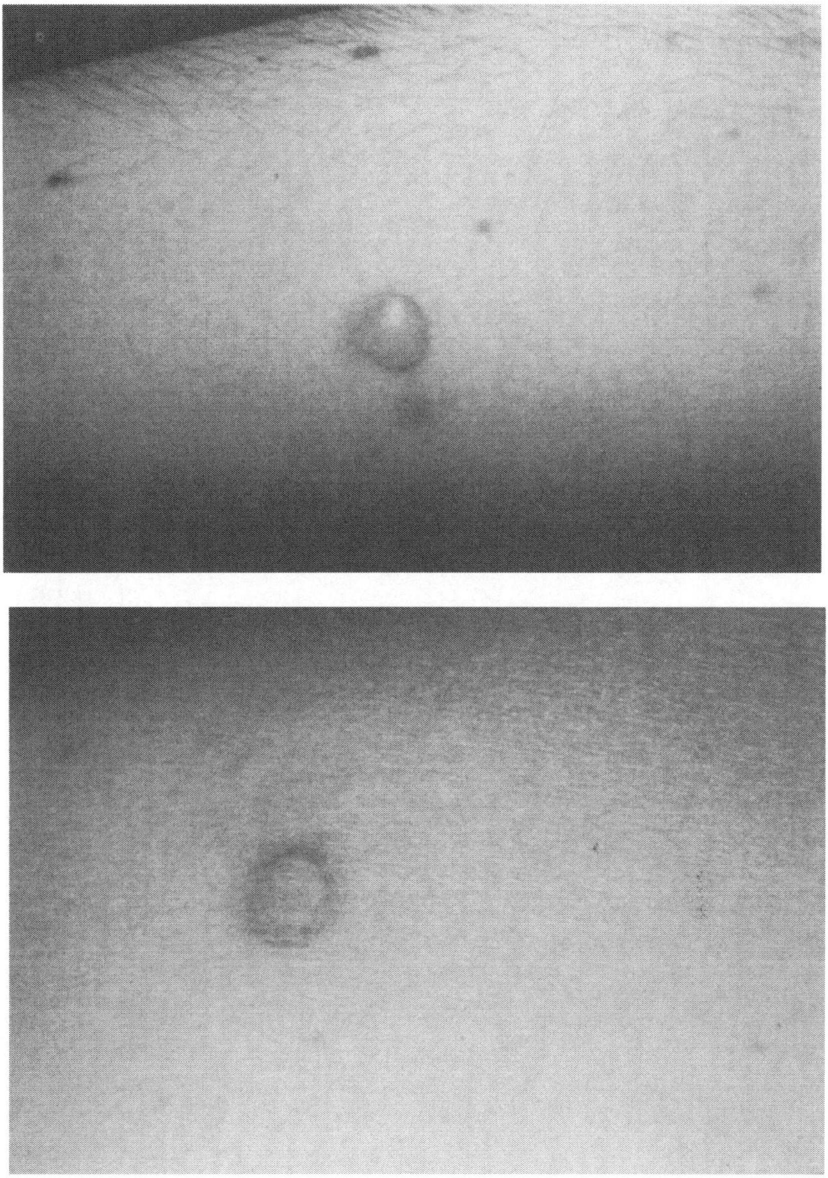

**Figure 31.6** Effects of cutaneous stimulation due to carbonic snow. Pictures obtained 24 h after stimulation (a) in base conditions, (b) after assumption of diflunisal

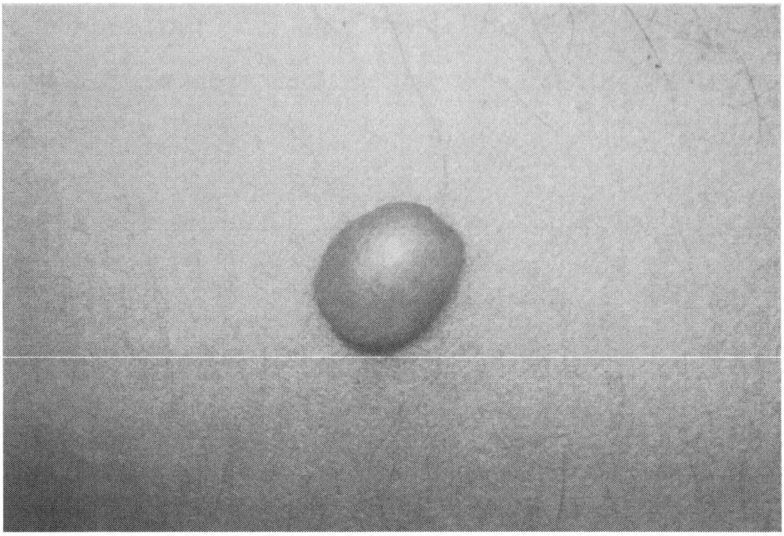

Figure 31.7 (a)

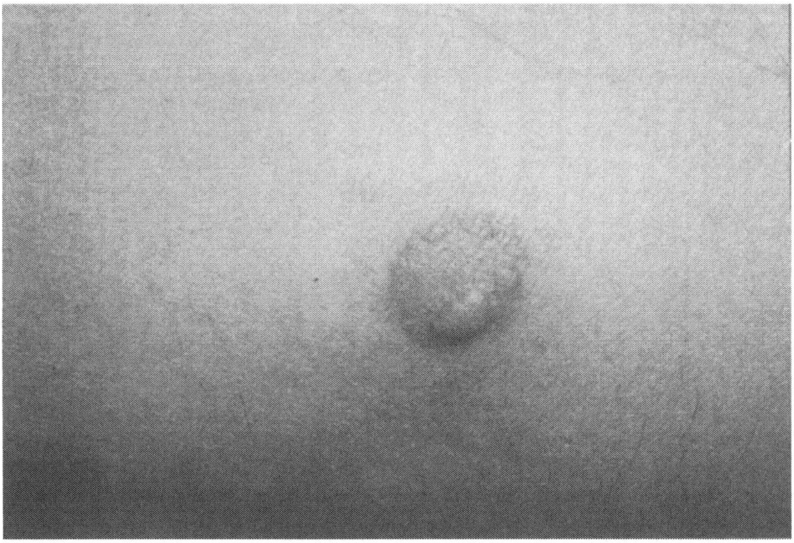

Figure 31.7 (b)

(c)
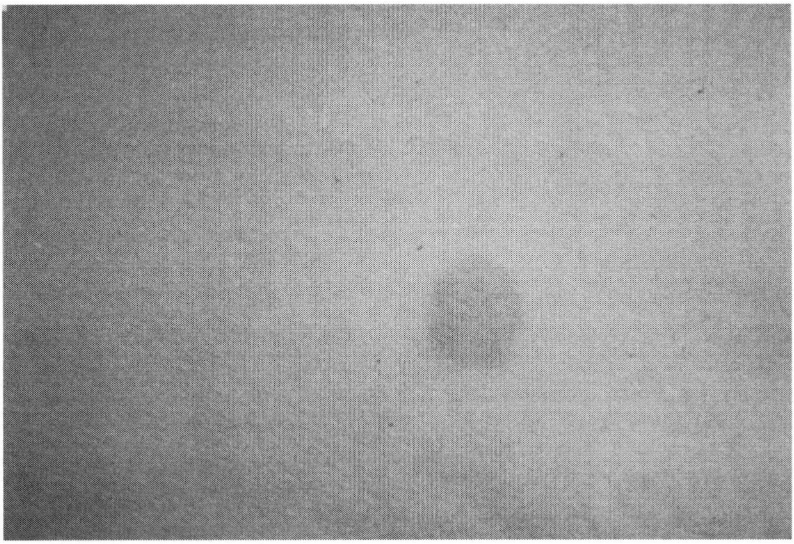

**Figure 31.7** Effects of cutaneous stimulation due to carbonic snow. Pictures obtained 24 h after stimulation (a) in base conditions, (b) administration of diflunisal for 24 h before stimulation, (c) administration of diflunisal for 24 h before and after stimulation

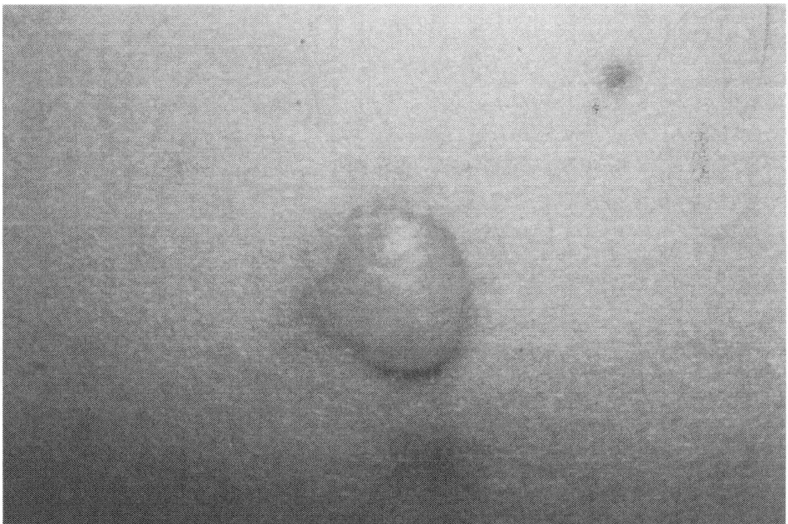

**Figure 31.8 (a)**

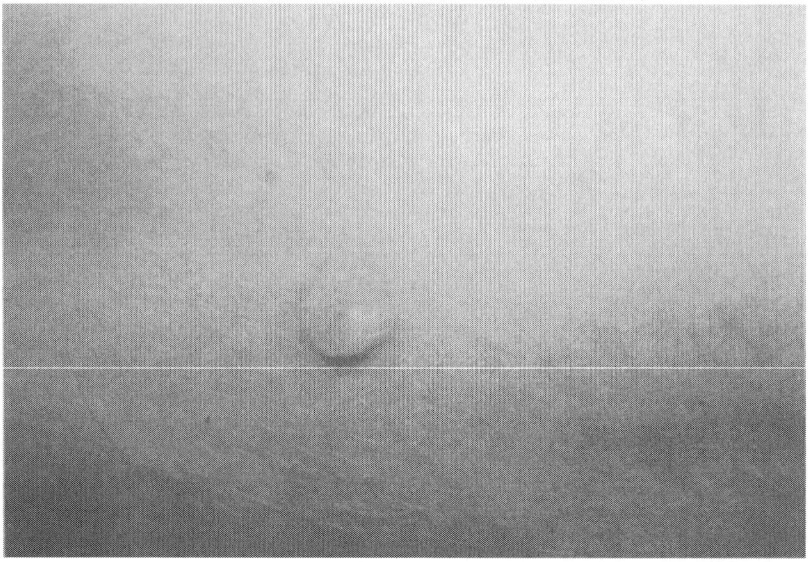

**Figure 31.8** (b)

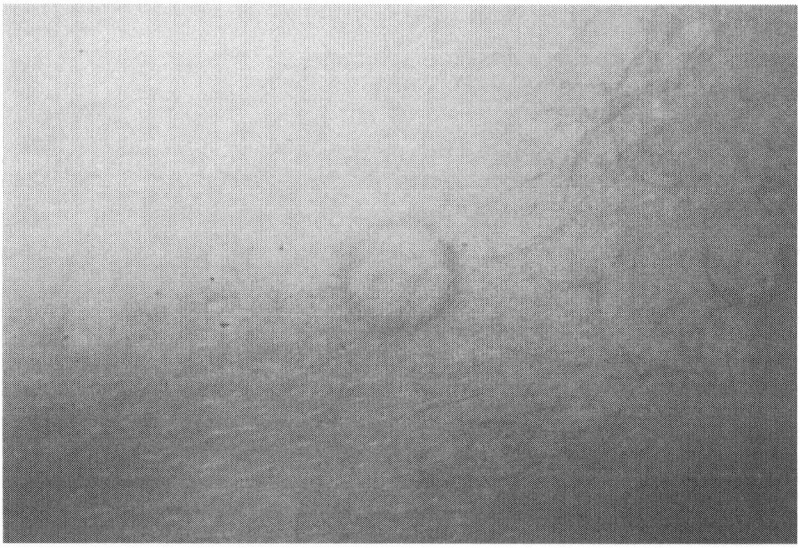

**Figure 31.8** (c) For details see Figure 31.7

demonstration and the interpretation of the analgesic and anti-inflammatory activity of diflunisal in the clinical aspect.

## References


1 Hannah, J., Ruyle, W. V., Kelly, K., Matzuk, A. R., Holtz, W. J., Witzel, B. E., Winter, C. A., Silber, C. A. and Shen, T. Y. (1970). Flufenisal, a novel salicylate. *Joint Conf. Chem. Inst. Can. Am. Chem. Soc.*, **18**

2 Shen, T. Y. (1972). Perspectives in non-steroidal anti inflammatory agents. *Agnew. Chem.* **II**, 460

3 Patrono, C., Ciabattoni, G., Grego, F. and Grossi Belloni, D. (1976). Comparative evaluation of the inhibitory effects of aspirin-like drugs on prostaglandin production by human platelets and synovial tissue. In Samuelsson, B. and Paoletti, R. (eds.) *Advances in Prostaglandin and Thromboxane Research*, p. 125

4 Tempero, K. F., Cirillo, V. J. and Steelman, S. L. (1977). Diflunisal: a review of the pharmacokinetic and pharmacodynamic properties, drug interaction and special tolerability studies in humans. *Br. J. Clin. Pharmacol.*, **4,** 31S

5 Galletti, R., Marra, N. and Vecchiet, L. (1960). Studio analitico dei fenomeni reattivi cutanei conseguenti a stimolazione con neve carbonica in soggetti normali. Estratto da "Lo Sperimentale"

6 Lewis, T. (1942). *Pain.* (New York: Macmillan)

7 Lunedei, A. (1948). *Relazione 49 Cong. Soc. It. Med. Int.*, Pozzi, L. (ed.) Roma

8 Arcangeli, P. and Galletti, R. (1974). Endogenous pain producing substances. In Bonica, J. J., Procacci, P. and Pagni, C. A. (eds.) *Recent advances in pain*. (Springfield C.C. Thomas)

9 Vecchiet, L., Matassi, L., Buzzelli, G., Fini, F. and Branzi, G. C. (1968). Rilievi sull'attività tissulo-algogena del plasma dopo la voro muscolare. *La Set. Medica*, **56,** 823

10 Keele, C. A. and Armstrong, D. (1964). *Substances producing pain and itch.* (London: Arnold)

11 Vecchiet, L., Galletti, R., Matassi, L., Chiarini, P. and Buzzelli, G. (1973). Il ruolo del kininogeno nella riattivazione della flogosi sperimentale da cantaridina. *Clin. Ter.*, **67,** 339

12 Vecchiet, L., Galletti, R., Chiarini, P. and Fabrizi, L. (1973). Rapporti tra dolore ed aumento della permeabilità dei microvasi nel quadro della flogosi sperimentale da cantaridina. *Clin. Ter.*, **667,** 521

13 Roth, G. J., Stanford, N. and Majerus, P. W. (1975). Acetylation of prostaglandin-synthetase by aspirin. *Proc. Natl. Acad. Sci (USA)*., **72,** 3073

14 Majerus, P. W. and Stanford, N. (1977). Comparative effects of aspirin and diflunisal on prostaglandin-synthetase from human platelets and sheep seminal vesicles. *Br. J. Clin. Pharmacol.*, **4,** 15S

# Discussion

**Professor D. A. Willoughby (Chairman)** in opening the discussion of the session devoted to anti-inflammatory drugs, noted that Professor Smith had put forward the concept that the active metabolite of aspirin was salicylic acid and that this active metabolite inhibited cyclo-oxygenase. He asked whether the inhibition of the cyclo-oxygenase was a desirable feature and how salicylic acid could interfere with the accumulation of leukocytes at an inflammatory site.

**Professor M. J. H. Smith (UK)** said that it was irrelevant whether the inhibition of cyclo-oxygenase was a desirable feature. The answer to the second question was that salicylic acid, which was the immediate metabolite of aspirin *in vivo*, caused anti-inflammatory actions by multiple mechanisms, of which one might well be the inhibition of the accumulation of leukocytes at anti-inflammatory sites. This was perhaps a relatively minor feature but it had interest because of the apparent anomaly between the equipotence of aspirin and salicylic acid as anti-inflammatory agents, in several acute inflammatory models and in some of the more chronic inflammatory diseases in man. He believed that aspirin was being absorbed and very rapidly hydrolysed and that salicylic acid accumulated in inflammatory exudates at concentrations sufficient to inhibit cyclo-oxygenase. The same occurred when salicylic acid itself was given and there was no acceptable evidence that a further metabolite of salicylic acid, gentisic acid, was concerned either in inhibiting the enzyme or any aspect of the anti-inflammatory action.

**Dr R. Vinegar (USA)** did not agree. His own *in vivo* qualitative studies had shown that salicylates did not work locally. Inhibition of cells in an animal model at doses that did not kill the animal were obtained only in the presenceof the adrenal glands. In other words, the only time when sodium aspirin was able to affect cells was.when it was working through the adrenal glands.

**Professor Smith** said that they had evidence for their suggestion stretching over 25 years in various inflammatory models. In the most recent, the implanted sponge system, there was unequivocal evidence that doses of salicylic acid and indeed aspirin below those which could cause adrenocortical stimulation, could significantly and reproducibly inhibit cellular accumulation. The sponge was a very mild inflammatory model and there was no doubt that drugs worked in it at doses far lower than those necessary to invoke adrenocortical stimulation. In fact, they worked in adrenelectomized animals.

**Dr Vinegar** asked why aspirin was extremely reactive when injected locally in the pleurisy model of inflammation while sodium salicylate was completely inactive when injected locally, irrespective of the concentration.

**Professor Smith** agreed that if a small dose of aspirin were added locally in the sponge model one could produce an almost complete inhibition of prostaglandin production with no effect whatever on the leukocytes. On adding the aspirin systemically there was a comparable effect on prostaglandin accumulation and a very significant effect on leukocytes. Sodium salicylate was therefore equipotent with aspirin when given systemically, and this was beyond dispute. However, he wished to stress that there was no need to invoke any extra metabolic product of either aspirin or salicylate in this model. In addition, there was distinct evidence from other workers that salicylic acid given systemically would preferentially accumulate in inflammatory exudate. He did not think that this was an exclusive model of action of aspirin inhibition of the enzyme. The situations in which aspirin would act as an intact molecule to cause irreversible inhibition of cyclo-oxygenase were very limited. They were limited to the circulation, where acetyl salicylate ion persisted for some time to affect blood platelets, and they were also limited when the drug was given directly by injection into a developing inflammatory exudate. He certainly agreed that it was very unlikely that the intact acetyl salicylate molecule entered the developing exudate itself.

**Dr P. Bacon (UK)** wished to know whether, now that the inhibition of leukocyte accumulation seemed another likely action for aspirin, this made it a better drug or whether the accumulation of leukocytes was as unimportant in chronic inflammation as was the inhibition of prostaglandin synthetase.

**Professor Smith** said that these mechanisms did not make it a better drug. Indeed it was quite a poor drug and no one should think of treating a developing case of rheumatoid arthritis for a long period of time with salicylates. In the past there had been nothing better and the reason that aspirin had come into prominence was that it was more palatable and more easily administered but it had no real advantages over the older mixtures containing sodium salicylate. Such mixtures were of course liquid preparations which deteriorated on storage.

**Professor Willoughby** next directed the discussion to the work of Dr Ezer and his colleagues from Budapest who had used combined therapy with indomethacin and sodium salicylate and reported a reduction in gastrointestinal side effects resulting from the combination. He wondered why the combination should produce this fortunate effect.

**Dr E. Ezer (Hungary)** said that the question was not fully resolved. The effect of sodium salicylate in reducing the side effects of indomethacin was accidentally discovered in 1947. One possible explanation was that while indomethacin reduced prostacyclin synthesis in the stomach, sodium salicylate might exert a compensatory effect on this synthesis and thus protect the stomach wall against ulceration. Whatever the explanation, they had very good clinical results from this combination and they hoped next year to introduce it in Hungary.

On being asked whether serum levels of indomethacin were reduced by the addition of aspirin or salicylate he said that reports to this effect in the literature were contradictory. In animal experiments using large doses of indomethacin and sodium salicylate the serum level of the former had indeed been decreased by some 30%. However, using therapeutic doses in man, there were no differences in serum levels following administration of indomethacin alone or in combination.

On being asked about his use of gastrointestinal bleeding rather than some more direct assay for estimation of inhibition of prostaglandin biosynthesis, he said that this castor oil diarrhoea test was both simple and effective. The anti-inflammatory effects of various drugs and their capacity to inhibit prostaglandin synthesis had been shown reliably to parallel the delay in the appearance of diarrhoea seen in the castor oil test.

**Professor Willoughby**, in directing discussion towards Dr Huber's contribution, noted that he had used the Arthus model for testing the effect of orgotein. In his view, it was much better to use the Arthus model in the pleural cavity rather than following subcutaneous or intradermal administration, if one wished to study the movement of cells into the inflamed site and the actual oedema.

**Dr S. C. R. Meacock (UK)** asked Dr Huber whether orgotein inhibited the complement system because the Arthus reaction depended upon complement activation.

**Dr W. Huber (USA)** said that he had looked *in vitro* and not found any such complement inhibition, although the effect might occur *in vivo*. He wished to make a general point about bioassays for the evaluation of anti-inflammatory and other drugs, which was that an assay system after working satisfactorily for some time, might suddenly cease to work. They had come to the point where they performed each assay completely blind and where they incorporated not only a negative but also a positive control. After many trials they had decided that prednisolone was probably an adequate positive control and if the assay showed no prednisolone response it was discarded.

On being asked about the half life of orgotein (bovine Cu–Zn superoxide dismutase) he said that this was a function of the route of administration. When given intravenously it was no more than 6–12 min in all species. However, it could be given intramuscularly or subcutaneously, since it had no tissue toxicity, and in these circumstances the half-life was in the order of 1.5–2.5 h. However, the anti-inflammatory efficacy was much longer lasting than the chemically demonstrable half-life. It was thus necessary to conclude that at least part of the anti-inflammatory activity was not related to the presence of circulating enzymes.

**Dr P. Gordon (USA)** agreed that the anti-inflammatory effect could be separated from the dismutase activity. He had been examining the chemiluminescence of phagocytozing human neutrophils, a phenomenon apparently closely related to the dismutase activity. Heat treatment produced a striking suppression of chemiluminescence but even preparations inactivated by this means retained activity against the release or attack on substrate of so-called active oxygens.

**Dr D. F. Horrobin (Canada)** asked whether there was any evidence that the variability in the assays referred to by Professor Huber were related to the season. His own group had followed the effect of zinc on prostaglandin biosynthesis over 3 successive years and had shown dramatic seasonal variations, particularly between March and May and September and November. These variations could be abolished by pinealectomy. Recent work from other centres also suggested that antigen–antibody reactions showed seasonal variations which could only be blocked by thick lead shielding.

**Dr Huber** agreed that they too had seen seasonal variation. Despite strict environment control in the animal quarters they had been forced to conclude that the source of the variation was within the animals themselves.

**Dr C. J. Dunn (Co-Chairman)** noting the paradoxical effects of stimulation and inhibition obtained by Dr Gordon with therafectin, asked whether this sugar compound might be incorporated into the membrane of the leukocyte.

**Dr Gordon** said that therafectin was essentially non-metabolizable. They had specifically designed it so as not to be incorporated by hexokinase into sugar pathways and they developed a compound 75–95% of which passed through the system and appeared in the urine within 24 h. Thus, it was not incorporated into any system. As to the paradoxical effects of the drug, they were certainly real. A number of different centres were working on the inflammation enhancing effect that occurred at low levels of the drug, of the order of 0.5–2 ng/ml which could be generated *in vivo* by administering 0.05–0.1 mg/kg/day. But one could override these pro-inflammatory effects simply by administering more than 1 mg/kg/day. What was seen in very low dosages was the enhancement of the microbicidal activity of leukocytes. Indeed, some groups were examining therafectin as a possible anti-microbial agent. This anti-microbial activity was preserved at all dosage levels, even those that were profoundly anti-inflammatory and which profoundly inhibited the transfer of cells from the bloodstream to inflammatory sites. At maximum dosage one could suppress neutrophil transfer by 85% and monocyte transfer by 60%. The cells which did transfer were modified in two ways. They were more microbicidal than control cells, but on the other hand they were much less likely to release chemiluminescent material to the intracellular space, which he felt was a phenomenon related to their anti-inflammatory action. In addition, there was now evidence than 1 ng/ml of the drug modified the response of macrophages from BCG activated animals. In the absence of the drug, control macrophages from activated animals were inclined to die when they phagocytosed their targets, unlike macrophages from non-affected individuals. Control macrophages phagocytozed safely; activated macrophages phagocytozed at their own risk. One could suppress this risk factor by adding anti-oxidants such as catalase, very large amounts of vitamin C or cytochrome C and apparently therafectin was also very effective in suppressing this disorderly self-destruction.

On being asked what evidence there was to describe therafectin as an immunomodulator, Professor Gordon said that if doses of the order of 0.1 mg/kg were given to animals during days 3–5 of an immunization with human red blood cells, a striking enhancement in the cellular immune response was found at days 14 or 28. A similar result could be obtained with candidal infection. On giving 0.1–0.4 mg/kg of therafectin from days 5–11 after administration of a candidal infection one found that at day 18, the time of primary peak in the antibody response, the kidneys of treated animals were sterile. Thus metastatic candidal infection had resolved, whereas in over 50% of controls the infection persisted. On re-challenging the animals with *Candida* 3 months later, one found that those which experienced the first infection under the drug, the second infection was practically absent. In the controls, the second infection was smaller, but quite evident. Japanese workers had also shown immunopotentiation *in vitro*. Using human mononuclear cells and zymosan as a mitogen they had shown that the mitogenic response was increased by 150% by the addition of 1 ng/ml of the drug. Finally, it was possible to perform the reverse experiment in a system where the drug decreased immune responses. Prolonged ether anaesthesia in mice created a very powerful immune response. In this model, with control levels of the cellular immune response 2–3 times higher than normal for the strain, they had found that administration of therafectin or levamisole produced a striking reduction in this augmented response when it was assessed at 14 days. Finally, in immature rats, presumably with immature macrophages, therafectin strikingly enhanced adjuvant arthritis. In the adult strain, therafectin slightly suppressed it, which he also regarded as evidence for immunomodulation.

**Professor Willoughby** said that therafectin and benoxaprofen showed a similar biphasic response and together with Clozic they seemed to be primarily drugs which were exerting their action via cells.

**Dr. G. W. Civil (UK)** said that they had some evidence that benoxaprofen acted at the cell membrane and he wondered whether therafectin was similarly localized at membranes or whether it could penetrate the cell. Therafectin apparently influenced neutrophils more than macrophages but they felt that benoxaprofen exerted a greater effect on the mononuclear cells than on the polymorphonuclear.

**Dr Gordon** said that there was some suggestion that therafectin reacted with cyclic nucleotides but there existed an interlinking chain of events which could make this effect indirect. They also saw effects on nuclear RNA and protein synthesis in brain and macrophages.

**Dr M. E. J. Billingham (UK)** said that they had not yet attempted to establish whether Clozic worked on cells. So far they had only looked at effects on collagenase production in isolated rheumatoid tissue in culture. In response to the Chairman, he said that it might have some cellular effects but he would not speculate on what cell type.

**Dr Huber,** agreeing with Dr Gordon, said that if toxicity permitted, it was very important to establish whether any drug had a pro-inflammatory as well as an anti-inflammatory phase. They had done so for orgotein. Small doses given into the paw of the rat or mouse in the carrageenin induced inflammatory system would reduce the inflammation, but on increasing these doses by a factor of 100 there was a very pronounced pro-inflammatory effect. Even without the carrageenin, SOD injected alone directly into the paw would increase its volume by 400–500% over a period of 24 h.

**Dr A. W. Ford-Hutchinson (UK)** asked whether Clozic had any effects on the prevention of bone erosion in tertiary adjuvant arthritis.

**Dr Billingham** said that they had examined several strains of rat for adjuvant disease, and had found that in some strains about 10–15% developed a very long-term arthritis, persisting for weeks or months. Their earlier work indicated that Clozic allowed the bone to remodel back towards its original state from a condition of hyperplasia with a cotton-wool like appearance. However, recent work had shown that in this late stage of arthritis, remodelling of bone occurred with non-steroidal anti-inflammatory drugs as well.

**Dr G. Faure (France)** said that benoxaprofen appeared to interfere with the generation of chemotactic peptides. This suggested an interference with complement activation and he wondered whether anyone had found direct evidence of such inhibition.

**Dr S. C. R. Meacock (UK)** had found no direct evidence of inhibition of complement activation *in vitro*. The chemotactic factors were generated even in the presence of benoxaprofen. He believed that the drug was acting in two ways. Its action on the cell surface prevented the cell from recognizing the chemotaxin. It also seemed to be preventing the formation of chemotaxins, but these were not the ones derived from the complement system, despite the fact that they were macromolecules.

**Dr N. R. Ackerman (USA)** had studied adjuvant arthritis in the rat and had seen evidence of loss of cartilage as well as loss of bone. Non-steroidal agents had activity especially in preventing the bone erosion changes as well as the subsequent fibrotic reaction. He wondered whether Clozic too was effective in preventing such erosion.

**Dr Billingham** said that the work he had described earlier was in established disease and osteoporotic and erosive changes had occurred. However, giving 10–20 mg/kg of Clozic on a prophylactic basis would prevent the changes from occurring, a very similar effect to that seen with non-steroidal drugs.

**Dr Dunn** drew the distinction between a therapeutic approach which involves trying to protect the damaged connective tissue and a more attacking approach intended to influence the inflammatory reaction which caused tissue damage.

**Dr A. Verbruggen (Belgium)** said that their ideas were very much in line with a new approach which aimed to influence the synthesis of proteoglycan and hyaluronic acid by chondrocytes and synovial cells. That indeed was becoming their policy.

**Dr Billingham** said that it would be very difficult to establish whether one was protecting cartilage. In osteoarthrosis for example, the chondrocytes, whether through a degenerative or inflammatory process, were stimulated to release a number of enzymes which dissolved the matrix which was then replaced with a somewhat altered matrix. But it would be difficult to establish whether a drug were directly affecting that process, and certainly no such conclusion could be drawn as yet for Clozic. In his view, in chronic inflammatory processes such as those in rheumatoid arthritis or connective tissue disease, a sequence of events activated the chondrocytes and this process was later continued by pannus formation. If that sequence of events could be broken then the lesions gradually came under control and the natural reparative processes took over. He did not believe that non-steroidal drugs could break the cycle of events.

**Dr I. F. Skidmore (UK)** believed that certain non-steroidal anti-inflammatory drugs would inhibit both bone remodelling and cartilage destruction in adjuvant arthritis. Yet they did not do so in rheumatoid arthritis.

**Professor Willoughby** said that all of these findings emphasized the fact that there was no adequate animal model of rheumatoid arthritis. The complete Freund's adjuvant was a very good model for anti-inflammatory activity but no one would pretend that it completely resembled rheumatic disease in man.

**Dr Ackerman** said that many clinicians believed that non-steroidal agents had little effect on erosive changes, but there appeared to be no well-controlled long-term studies against placebo demonstrating that this was so.

## DISCUSSION

**Dr Skidmore** said that the Nuffield Foundation Arthritis and Rheumatism Council mounted a 3 year study comparing prednisone with phenylbutazone, in which clinical external manifestations, biochemical parameters and radiological changes were examined. There was no evidence of any diminution in the progress of the disease with phenylbutazone. For 2 of the 3 years there was clear evidence of retardation of radiological changes with the steroid but at the end of the period the groups were indistinguishable. That might perhaps be an indication that steroids could slow down the erosive process.

**Dr Bacon** said that there was no real evidence that non-steroidal agents did anything but give symptomatic relief in rheumatoid arthritis and the pre-occupation with designing other drugs which worked in the same way was counterproductive. Clinicians like him wished to see more drugs working on a different basis which could be shown to influence the human disease. It was then up to the pharmacologists to establish how they worked.

**Mr S. J. Hopkins (UK)** although agreeing that there was no good model for RA said that he understood that ICI were using the collagen induced arthritis model and he asked whether Clozic had any effect on that model.

**Dr Billingham** said that they had used collagen induced arthritis and that both indomethacin and Clozic had inhibitory effects.

**Dr P. A. Thrower (UK)**, on being asked about her work with the Chairman on intravenous thymopoietin, said that a group of 12 patients had been treated at a dose of 50 mg weekly and that they were in the process of comparing that group with a control group on levamisole. Some patients had improved and others had not but the data was not yet ready to report. On being asked about the half-life of a single intravenous injection, it was said to be in the order of 5 s. She did not feel that a single injection had any effect, and she hoped that the action would be more like that of penicillamine-like drugs.

**Professor A. Sfikakis (Greece)** had found that ovariectomy resulted in a significant suppression of adjuvant arthritis. Oestradiol administration also suppressed it, and the combination of ovariectomy and oestradiol had a highly significant suppressive effect. Oestradiol stimulated the pituitary adrenocortical axis to increase corticosteroid secretion. The difference was that ovariectomy produced a highly significant increase in thymus weight, although oestradiol did not. The increase in weight might lead to increased thymopoietin production which, together with activation by oestradiol, would help to explain the highly significant suppression of adjuvant arthritis in this rat model. The parallels in human beings were pregnancy, with increased oestradiol, and the menopause, which was analogous to ovariectomy and in which the incidence of rheumatoid arthritis was also known to be decreased.

**Professor Willoughby** agreed that the thymus undoubtedly played a major role. Some years previously they had performed neonatal thymectomies and shown a striking suppression of granulation tissue around a cotton pellet. Subsequently they had obtained similar results following adult thymectomy. Their basic thinking was that thymopoietin might have levamisole-type activity. He wished then to turn the discussion towards the action of penicillamine.

**Professor Trnavsky (Czechoslovakia)** asked Dr Lorenzen if there were any clinical evidence of effects of long term administration of penicillamine on the vascular system.

**Professor I. Lorenzen (Denmark)** had investigated whether penicillamine had any influence on the later stages of inflammation by studying its influence on the collagen of granulation tissue. Such collagen was indeed accessible to catabolism, implying an inhibition of fibrosis, but unfortunately the collagen of normal skin, bone and aorta was more sensitive still. In considering whether this was also true in treating patients with rheumatoid arthritis it had to be made clear that the doses which he had been using in animal experiments were 10–15 times higher than those normally used in treating patients. On the other hand, the animal study was short-term whereas patients were treated for years. The additional fact that penicillamine was eliminated from the body very slowly gave grounds for believing that following years of treatment it might influence collagen in other tissues. Studies which he had performed on the effects of penicillamine on the collagen of skin in RA patients showed similar alterations to those observed in rats.

**Dr Bacon** said that there was no clinical evidence that penicillamine exerted the same adverse effects on skin as long-term steroids did. And several studies on wound healing in patients on the drug had failed to show any biologically significant alteration.

**Professor Lorenzen** agreed that there were few, if any, studies showing early mechanical alteration in connective tissue and skin, but he thought that the time was not right to take these possibilities into consideration. In addition, the changes which he had described were only in part reversible and changes in the collagen of the aorta progressed after penicillamine treatment. He had investigated the effect of penicillamine on the aorta in some detail and actually seen an increase in aortic collagen as opposed to other tissues. This might be a reaction to the weakening of the aortic wall inducing secondary collagen formation. Following drug treatment there was also a decrease in the elastic property of the aorta which might be relevant to the sensitivity of the vascular wall to normal haemodynamic injury.

**Professor Willoughby** finally directed attention to methods for assessing aggregation by chemotactic factors *in vitro*. He suggested that aggregation by such factors was somewhat anomalous, but that if these factors caused cells to adhere it might be more difficult for them to pass through gaps.

**Dr M. E. Shipley (UK)** agreed. What they were measuring was one of the many changes in the membrane which might well occur only after the cells had undergone chemotaxis. Nonetheless, it was clear that in certain clinical conditions aggregation occurring in the vasculature did lead to damage, particularly after haemodialysis. They wished to know whether such changes were relevant in other inflammatory conditions. In certain conditions, increased amounts of activated complement were found in the circulation which could be of importance because aggregation and increased adherence, which seemed to go in parallel, might reduce the ability of the polymorphonuclear leukocyte to move to a site of inflammation and act there.

# Section IV
# Pharmacological Mediators

CHAIRMAN: G. P. Lewis
CO-CHAIRMAN: P. Bacon

# 32

# Changes in the inflammatory mediator content in the colonic mucosae of immune colitides in guinea pigs (Abstract)

I. J. ZEITLIN, A. A. NORRIS AND A. J. LEWIS (UK)

An immune colitis based on a delayed-type hypersensitivity reaction was induced in dinitrochlorobenzene (DNCB) sensitized guinea pigs by intrarectal challenge with DNCB in Orabase (Squibb Ltd.)[1]. A low challenge dose (0.25% DNCB), given once daily for 5 days induced mild inflammatory changes in the distal colon and rectum characterized by goblet cell depletion and mild cellular infiltration of the mucosa and submucosa. A higher challenge concentration (5% DNCB) given once daily for 3 days resulted in severe colonic ulceration with crypt abscess formation and a heavy cellular infiltrate in the mucosa and sub-mucosa. Diarrhoea, rectal bleeding and body weight loss were also prominent features. The inflammatory mediators, histamine, 5-HT, glandular kallikrein and $PGE_2$ were measured in freeze-dried colonic mucosae of the two colitides. Histamine content was 3 times control ($p< 0.01$) in 0.25% DNCB induced colitis, although no significant change was observed in 5% DNCB challenged animals. Mucosal 5-HT content was significantly reduced ($p < 0.01$) in both models. Glandular kallikrein content did not differ from control ($p > 0.05$) $PGE_2$ was significantly increased ($p < 0.05$) in both models. The possible significance of these changes with respect to severity of inflammation and aetiology of colitis is described.

### Acknowledgments

A. A. Norris was in receipt of a Science Research Council CASE studentship. We are grateful to Sandoz Ltd. and Upjohn Ltd. for gifts of bradykinin and prostaglandin, respectively.

### Reference

Lewis, A. J., Norris, A. A. and Zeitlin, I. J. (1979). *Br. J. Pharmac.*, **66**, 499P

# 33

# Simultaneous continuous monitoring of blood volume and permeability in rabbit synovium: action of histamine

H. A. AL-HABOUBI AND I. J. ZEITLIN* (UK)

## INTRODUCTION

We have recently reported that daily intraperitoneal (i.p.) injections of cimetidine hydrochloride (1 mg/kg) greatly suppressed the joint swelling occurring in the early and late phases of rat adjuvant arthritis[1]. This apparent anti-inflammatory effect of cimetidine was not due to non-specific actions. Injection of the same dose of cimetidine hydrochloride (i.p.) suppressed the swelling produced by injection into the paw pad of the specific $H_2$ agonist, Dimaprit, but not that due to the $H_1$ agonist, 2-pyridylethylamine. To learn more about the roles of histamine $H_1$ and $H_2$ receptors in the synovial microvasculature, we have devised a technique to simultaneously monitor blood volume and permeability in the rabbit synovium.

## METHODS

Male rabbits were anaesthetized with pentobarbitone. The skin overlying a stifle joint was deflected and a 'push–pull' needle cannula (outer diameter 1.4 mm) inserted into the synovial cavity[2]. Where relevant, the siting of the needle tip was ascertained by a dye infusion at the end of the experiment. The exposed joint was then coated with vaseline and covered with a gauze, moistened with Krebs solution and maintained at 37°C by a thermistor-controlled radiant heater. The synovial cavity perfused (0.1 ml/min) with

* Correspondence

warm Krebs solution which contained both agonists and/or antagonists when required.

**Permeability**

$^{125}$I-labelled albumin was injected i.v. The synovial perfusate was passed through a flow cell in a well crystal detector, set to detect $^{125}$I to permit semi-quantitative monitoring of albumin leakage into the synovium (Figure 33.1). The perfusate was finally collected for quantitative $^{125}$I counting for the construction of dose-response curves.

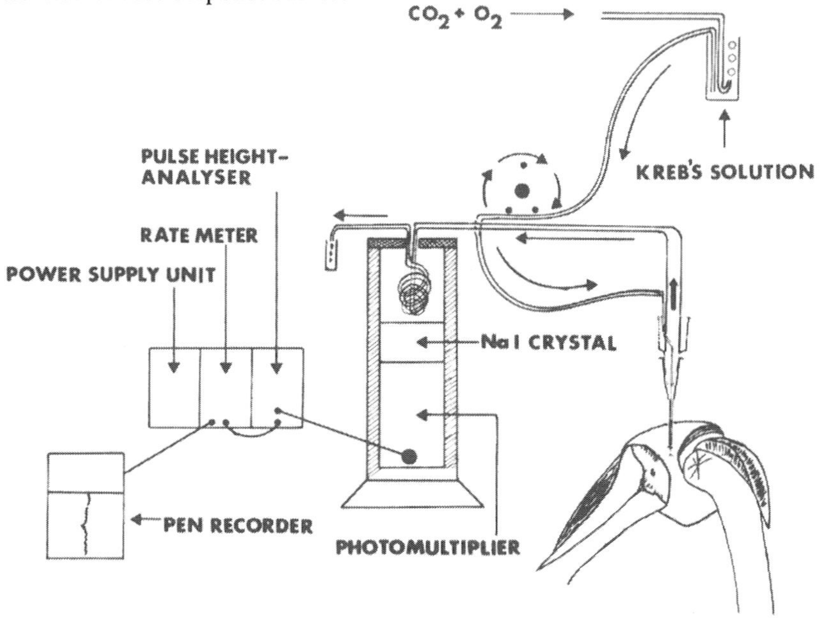


**Figure 33.1** Synovial perfusion technique

**Blood volume**

Labelling of erythrocytes was carried out *in vivo* using the method of Hamilton and Alderson[3]. The content of [$^{99m}$Tc] erythrocytes in the joint was monitored continuously using a collimated (15 mm diameter) thalium-activated NaI crystal detector placed 2–4 mm from the joint. Technetium counting was carried out for 10 s every 5 min and counts were corrected for decay and used to construct dose-response curves. At the end of each experiment, blood samples were taken to test for dissociation of the $^{99m}$Tc from the erythrocytes. Control experiments showed that changes in $^{99m}$Tc count were directly related to changes in blood volume within the joint.

## RESULTS

The simultaneous effect on synovial blood volume and permeability of infusing the rabbit synovium with increasing concentrations of histamine are shown in Figure 33.2. Low concentrations of histamine (0.1–1.0 ng/ml) produced an increase in synovial blood volume, but had little effect on the appearance of [125I] albumin in the synovial perfusate. Concentrations of histamine above 10 ng/ml both progressively reduced the synovial blood volume towards the basal value and caused the appearance of increasing concentrations of labelled albumin in the synovial perfusate.

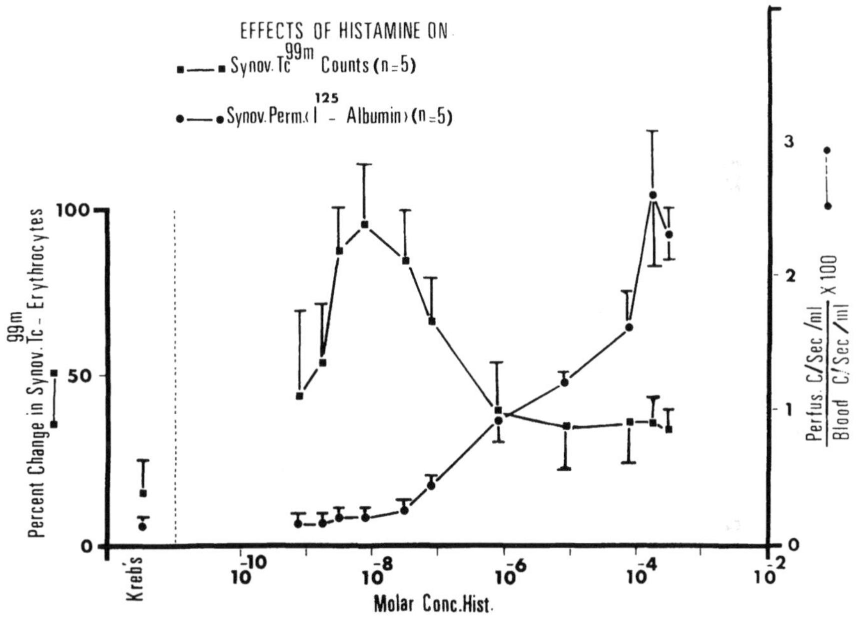


**Figure 33.2** Simultaneous monitoring of synovial [$^{99m}$Tc]erythrocyte content and extravasation of [$^{125}$I]albumin during intra-articular perfusion with histamine. Figure shows means and standard errors

When the synovium was infused with increasing concentrations of histamine in the presence of either mepyramine maleate (2.5 × $10^{-5}$ mol/l) or cimetidine hydrochloride (2.5 × $10^{-5}$ mol/l), the initial increase in synovial vascular blood volume was completely abolished. Neither antagonist alone caused a significant change in blood volume ($p$>0.05).

Cimetidine at this molar concentration also almost completely suppressed the increase in synovial permeability produced by concentrations of histamine of up to $5 \times 10^{-3}$mol/l ($n = 5$). Mepyramine ($2.5 \times 10^{-5}$ mol/l) suppressed the permeability increase produced by concentrations of histamine up to $10^{-4}$ mol/l, but not above this concentration.

## CONCLUSIONS

Intra-articular infusion of low histamine concentrations in the rabbit synovium caused an increase in synovial blood volume which disappeared at higher concentrations in parallel with an increase in synovial vascular permeability. The blood volume increase and the permeability increase were inhibited by both mepyramine maleate and cimetidine hydrochloride indicating the presences of both $H_1$ and $H_2$ histamine receptors in the rabbit synovial microvasculature. Grennan, Rooney, St. Onge, Brooks, Zeitlin and Dick[4] reported that in the dog synovium the vasodilator action of histamine was largely mediated by $H_2$ receptors. However, unlike the present finding with the rabbit, the dog synovial vasculature showed no evidence of the presence of $H_1$ receptors.

**Acknowledgments**
Part of this work was supported by a grant to I.J.Z from the Camilla Samuel Fund.

**References**

1 Al-Haboubi, H. A. and Zeitlin, I. J. (1979). *Br. J. Pharmacol*, **67**, 446P
2 Dudar, J. D. and Szerb, J. C. (1970). *Exp. Physiol. Biochem.*, **3**, 341
3 Hamilton, R. G. and Alderson, P. O. (1977). *J. Nucl. Med.*, **18**, 1008
4 Grennan, D. M., Rooney, P. J., St. Onge, R. A., Brooks, P. M., Zeitlin, I. J. and Dick, W. C. (1975). *Eur. J. Clin. Invest.*, **5**, 75

# 34

# Leukotriene B: a biologically active release product of polymorphonuclear leukocytes

A. W. FORD-HUTCHINSON, M. A. BRAY, M. E. SHIPLEY
M. V. DOIG AND M. J. H. SMITH (UK)

## INTRODUCTION

Arachidonic acid (AA) may be metabolized either by cyclo-oxygenase enzyme systems to form prostaglandins and thromboxanes or by lipoxygenase enzymes to produce mono-, di- and trihydroxy fatty acids via either hydroperoxy or epoxide intermediates[1]. The biological functions of the products of lipoxygenase pathways of AA metabolism are largely unknown. Activities which have been ascribed to these compounds include SRS-A activity[2]; chemotactic and chemokinetic activities towards polymorphonuclear leukocytes (PMNs) and eosinophils[3]; a possible involvement in T lymphocyte activation[4] and regulation of the biosynthesis[5] of $PGI_2$. PMNs have been shown to release a number of products of the lipoxygenase pathways of AA metabolism when exposed to stimuli[6,7] such as the calcium ionophore A23187. The present work describes the release of chemokinetic and aggregating activity from rat and human PMNs exposed to calcium ionophore A23187 and demonstrates that these activities are due to leukotriene B, a metabolite of AA produced by lipoxygenase enzymes.

## METHODS

Cell suspensions (>85% PMN) were prepared from rat peritoneal exudates obtained 24 h after injection of 12% sodium caseinate[8]. Human PMNs were obtained from peripheral blood following dextran sedimentation and purification on a Ficoll–Hypaque density gradient[9]. Release of lipoxygenase products was induced by incubating rat or human PMNs with calcium ionophore A23187 (10 mol/l) for 4 min[10]. Biological assay of lipoxygenase products was carried out by measuring production of either aggregating or chemokinetic activities[10]. Aggregation assays were carried out in a Payton aggregometer using rat PMNs[11], the stimuli for aggregation[12] being either 10 mol/l AA, 100–1000 fold dilutions of supernatants from PMNs treated with calcium ionophore A23187 or lipoxygenase products during stages of purification. Chemokinetic assays were carried out in an agarose micro-droplet assay system using human PMNs as the cell source[13]. The effects of drugs on aggregation induced by AA and the release of aggregating and chemokinetic activities from PMNs was assessed as described previously[10,12].

In order to characterize the products released following stimulation with ionophore A23187, the reaction was terminated after 4 min incubation by the addition of 1.5 volumes of methanol. The hydroxy fatty acids in the supernatant were extracted with diethyl ether and partially purified by chromatography on silicic acid as described by Borgeat and Samuelsson[6]. Resulting products were further separated by reverse phase high pressure liquid chromatography on a column (4.6 × 250 mm) packed with Spherisorb 50DS eluted at a flow rate of 1ml/min with a mixture of methanol/water, 75:25 (v/v) plus acetic acid[6] to 0.01%. The active peak was derivatized to form the methyl ester, trimethylsilyl ether and was chromatographed on a 20 m SE54 (WCOT) capillary column coupled to a VG Micromass 16F mass spectrometer.

## RESULTS

### Aggregation induced by arachidonic acid

Addition of AA to rat peritoneal PMNs produced a transient aggregation response. The optimal AA concentrations and the enhancing effect of cytochalasin B were very similar to those previously reported for human PMNs[14,15]. The effects of drugs on this reaction are shown in Table 34.1. Indomethacin, 5, 8, 11, 14–eicosatetraynoic acid (ETYA), nordihydroguaiaretic acid (NDGA) and benoxaprofen, drugs known to affect lipoxygenase pathways, all produced significant inhibition of the aggregation. In contrast, other anti-inflammatory agents which are known to affect cyclo-oxygenase enzyme systems were not inhibitory. Significant enhancement of the response was observed with $10^{-5}$ $-10^{-7}$ mol/l indomethacin and $10^{-4}$ mol/l phenylbutazone possibly via stimulation of lipoxygenase pathways, as has previously been observed for indomethacin[16]. There was no correlation between the inhibition of the aggregation response and inhibition of $TXB_2$ production by these cells in the presence of indomethacin, ETYA and NDGA[12].

**Table 34.1** Effects of drugs on the aggregation of rat PMNs induced by arachidonic acid

| | *% inhibition of aggregation response* | | | | |
|---|---|---|---|---|---|
| Drug concentration (mol/l) | $10^{-3}$ | $10^{-4}$ | $10^{-5}$ | $10^{-6}$ | $10^{-7}$ |
| Indomethacin | — | 95† | 23† | −21* | −19* |
| 5,8,11,14-eicosatetraynoic acid (ETYA) | — | 100† | 58* | 1 | −2 |
| Nordihydroguaiaretic acid (NDGA) | — | 100† | 100† | 53* | 12 |
| Benoxaprofen | — | 100† | 12 | 0 | — |
| Acetyl salicylic acid | −12 | — | 0 | — | — |
| Sodium salicylate | −7 | — | −6 | — | — |
| Phenylbutazone | — | −35* | −11 | — | — |
| Fenclofenac | — | −22 | 17 | — | — |

Cells were pretreated with cytochalasin B (10 μg/ml) and drugs for 4 min prior to addition of AA.
$^*p > 0.01$, $^\dagger p > 0.001$ from control response.

**Release of aggregating and chemokinetic activity from PMNs exposed to ionophore A23187**

When rat peritoneal or human peripheral PMNs were exposed to 10 μ mol/l calcium ionophore A23187 one or more substances were released into the supernatant which caused the aggregation of rat PMNs and the chemokinesis of human PMNs. With both rat and human cells maximal release occurred after 4 min incubation with ionophore. The optimal ionophore concentration was 10 μmol/l and both aggregating and chemokinetic activities could be detected in 1000 fold dilutions of the supernatant.

The effects of a number of drugs, which inhibit cyclo-oxygenase and lipoxygenase pathways of AA metabolism, on the generation of aggregating and chemokinetic activities are shown in Table 34.2. ETYA, NDGA, indomethacin, BW755C and benoxaprofen all inhibited the release of both activities. All of these compounds have been reported to inhibit the production of products of lipoxygenase pathways of AA metabolism[17-21]. In contrast, the conventional non-steroidal anti-inflammatory drugs, aspirin, naproxen, flurbiprofen and phenylbutazone, all of which are known to be potent inhibitors of cyclo-oxygenase enzyme systems, produced little or no inhibition. Using these assay systems ETYA, NDGA and indomethacin produced similar effects on human peripheral PMNs, as shown in Table 34.3.

**Table 34.2** Effect of drugs on the generation of aggregating and chemokinetic activities from rat PMNS exposed to ionophore A23187

| *Drug* | *Concentration* (mol/l) | *% inhibition of production of aggregating activity* | *% inhibition of production of chemokinetic activities* |
|---|---|---|---|
| ETYA | $10^{-4}$ | 98* | 95* |
| | $10^{-5}$ | 97* | 95* |
| | $10^{-6}$ | 12 | 54* |
| | $10^{-7}$ | 0 | 18 |
| NDGA | $10^{-4}$ | 100* | 100* |
| | $10^{-5}$ | 99* | 99* |
| | $10^{-6}$ | 90* | 90* |
| | $10^{-7}$ | 49* | 50* |
| Indomethacin | $10^{-4}$ | 71* | 51† |
| | $10^{-5}$ | 0 | 0 |
| | $10^{-6}$ | 0 | 11 |
| BW755C | $10^{-4}$ | 94* | 68† |
| | $10^{-5}$ | 15 | 5 |
| | $10^{-6}$ | 7 | 7 |
| Benoxaprofen | $10^{-4}$ | 97* | 100* |
| | $10^{-5}$ | 0 | 16 |
| Acetyl salicylic acid | $5 \times 10^{-4}$ | 0 | 36† |
| Phenylbutazone | $10^{-4}$ | 2 | 24 |
| Naproxen | $10^{-4}$ | 10 | 19 |
| Flurbiprofen | $10^{-4}$ | 12 | 21 |

* $p < 0.001$ † $p < 0.01$

**Characterization of the material responsible for the aggregating and chemokinetic activities**

Following acidification of the media, biological activity could be recovered in an ether extract. When the extract was dissolved in diethylether/hexane, 20:80, and applied to a column of silicic acid equilibrated with the same solvent, the biological activity was retained on the column. The aggregating and chemokinetic activities could be subsequently eluted from the column with ethyl acetate. The eluted ethyl acetate fraction was redissolved in a small volume of methanol and was chromatographed on a reverse phase high pressure liquid chromatography (HPLC) column under conditions identical to those described by Borgeat and Samuelsson[6]. The extract from 4 ml of cell suspension was applied to the column and fractions were collected at 1 min intervals. Each resulting fraction was evaporated to dryness and redissolved in 100 $\mu$l of medium which was subsequently diluted 1:1000 for biological assay. The results shown in Figure 34.1 using rat PMNs demonstrate that

**Table 34.3** Effects of ETYA, NDGA and indomethacin on the generation of aggregating and chemokinetic activities from human PMNs exposed to ionophore A23187

| *Drug* | *Concentration* (mol/l) | *% inhibition of production of aggregating activity* | *% inhibition of production of chemokinetic activity* |
|---|---|---|---|
| ETYA | $10^{-4}$ | 75* | 72* |
| | $10^{-5}$ | 15† | −20 |
| NDGA | $10^{-4}$ | 86* | 47* |
| | $10^{-5}$ | 13† | 22 |
| Indomethacin | $10^{-4}$ | 21* | 14 |
| | $10^{-5}$ | −5 | −17 |

* $p<0.005$ † $p<0.01$

>95% of the biological activity was recoverable from a single UV absorbent peak with an elution position the same as that reported for 5,12-dihydroxyeicosatetraenoic acid (leukotriene B)[6]. No aggregating or chemokinetic activity was recovered in the fractions where the monohydroxy eicosatetraenoic acids would be expected to elute. Identical results were obtained with human PMNs.

Ultraviolet spectra were obtained for the methyl ester of the compound which showed three major bands ($E_{\mathrm{Max}}^{\mathrm{MeOH}}$ 262 ± 2, 271 ± 2 and 282 ± 2 nm) indicating the presence of three conjugated double bonds[22]. Gas–liquid chromatographic (GLC) analysis of the active fraction following derivatization to the methyl ester, trimethylsilyl ether, showed a major peak with a C value of 23.6. Mass spectra were obtained for this peak which showed a characteristic mass fragmentation pattern as previously reported[22] for leukotriene B.

## DISCUSSION

The present results, utilising known inhibitors of lipoxygenase pathways, suggest that arachidonic acid induced aggregation of PMNs and release of aggregating and chemokinetic activities by rat and human PMNs exposed to ionophore A23187 are caused by products of lipoxygenase pathways of AA metabolism. The HPLC retention time suggested that the activity was due to the presence of leukotriene B (5,12-dihydroxyeicosatetraenoic acid). The presence of three conjugated double bonds was confirmed by the ultraviolet spectra and the GLC retention times also suggested that the compound was leukotriene B. The structural identification was confirmed by mass spectrometry, characteristic mass fragmentation patterns being obtained for the methyl ester, trimethylsilyl ether of leukotriene B from both rat and human PMNs.

The release of biologically active products of lipoxygenase pathways may

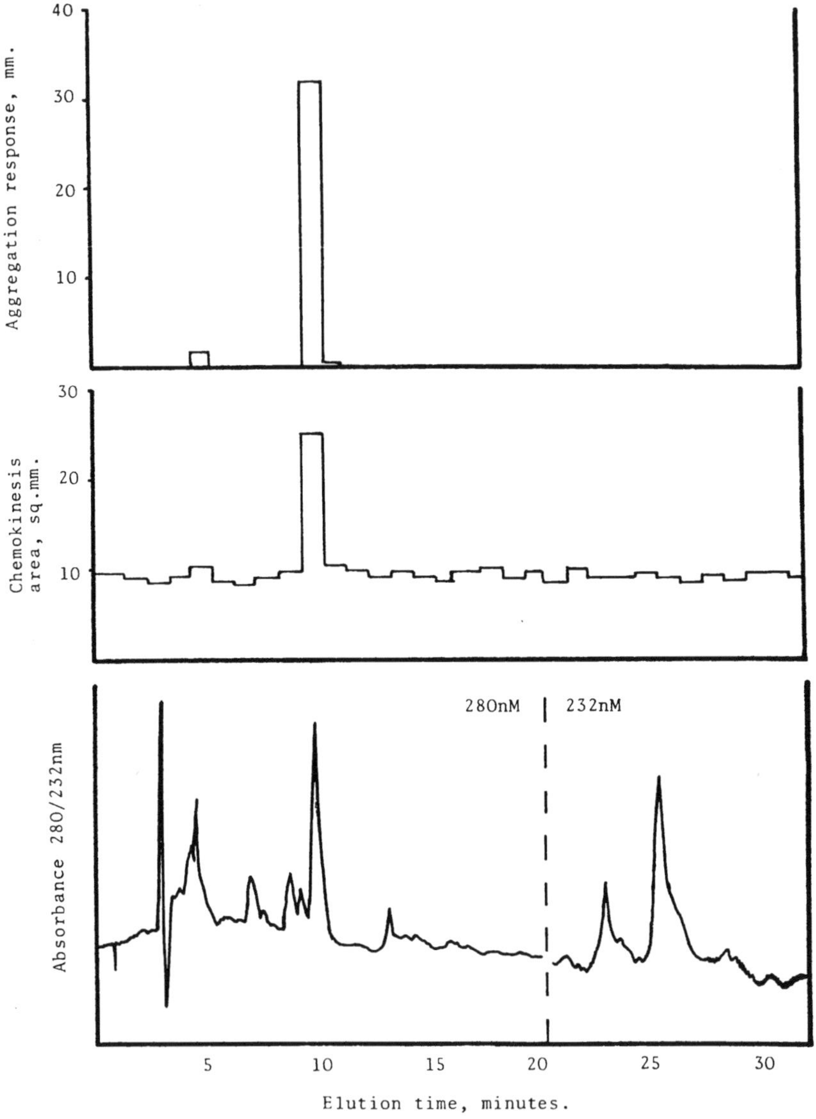


**Figure 34.1** Separation by HPLC of lipoxygenase products released by rat PMN exposed to ionophere A23187

be a common feature of exposure of PMNs to a variety of inflammatory and phagocytic stimuli[7]. Such release may be associated with $O_2$ uptake, $O_2$ production and stimulation of hexose monophosphate shunt activity that occurs following exposure to such stimuli[23] and may also be involved in neutrophil degranulation[24]. These substances could also be responsible for the release of chemotactic and chemokinetic activities in a number of situations, for example, the rat peritoneum following antigen challenge[25]. It will be of considerable importance to assess the role of leukotriene B and related compounds *in vivo* particularly in relationship to inflammation and PMN aggregation and chemokinesis provide useful *in vitro* bioassays for further studies on these compounds.

**Acknowledgments**

We are grateful to the Arthritis and Rheumatism Council (M.A.B.) the Science Research Council (M.V.D.) and Lilly Research. Ltd., for financial support.

**References**

1 Jones, R. L. (1979). Pathways of arachidonic acid metabolism. In Rainsford, K. D. and Ford-Hutchinson, A. W. (eds.) *Prostaglandins and Inflammation*. pp 19–26. (Basel: Birkhauser-Verlag)

2 Murphy, R. C. Hammarstrom, S. and Samuelsson, B. (1979). Leukotriene C: a slow-reacting substance from murine mastocytoma cells. *Proc. Natl. Acad. Sci. (USA)*, **76,** 4275

3 Goetzl, E. J. and Sun, F. F. (1979). Generation of unique monohydroxy-eicosatetraenoic acids from arachidonic acid by human neutrophils. *J. Exp. Med.*, **150,** 406

4 Kelly, J. P., Johnson, M. C. and Parker, C. W. (1979). Effect of inhibitors of arachidonic acid metabolism on mitogenesis in human lymphocytes: a possible role of thromboxanes and products of the lipoxygenase pathway. *J. Immunol.*, **122,** 156–3

5 Salmon, J. A. Smith, B. R., Flower, R. J., Moncada, S. and Vane, J. R. (1978). Further studies on the enzymatic conversion of prostaglandin endoperoxides into $PGI_2$. *Biochem. Biophys. Acta*, **523,** 252

6 Borgeat, P. and Samuelsson, B. (1979) Arachidonic acid metabolism in polymorphonuclear leukocytes: effects of ionophore A23187. *Proc. Natl. Acad. Sci (USA)*, **76,** 2148

7 Stenson, W. F. and Parker, C. W. (1979) Metabolism of arachidonic acid in ionophore-stimulated neutrophils. *J. Clin. Invest.*, **64,** 1457

8 Cunningham, F. M., Smith, M. J. H., Ford-Hutchinson, A. W. and Walker, J. R. (1979). Migration of peritoneal leucocytes in the rat. *J. Pathol.*, **128,** 15

9 Cunningham, F. M., Ford-Hutchinson, A. W., Oliver, A. M., Smith, M. J. H. and Walker, J. R. (1978). The effects of D-penicillamine and levamisole on leucocyte chemotaxis in the rat. *Br. J. Pharmacol.*, **63,** 119

10 Bray, M. A., Ford-Hutchinson, A. W., Shipley, M. E. and Smith, M. J. H. (1980). Calcium ionophore A23187 induces release of chemokinetic and aggregating factors from polymorphonuclear leucocytes. *Br. J. Pharmacol.* (In press)

11 Cunningham, F. M., Shipley, M. E. and Smith, M. J. H. (1980). Aggregation of rat polymorphonuclear leucocytes *in vitro*. *J. Pharm. Pharmacol.*, **32,** 377

12 Ford-Hutchinson, A. W., Bray, M. A. and Smith, M. J. H. (1979). The aggregation of rat neutrophils by arachidonic acid: a possible bioassay for lipoxygenase activity. *J. Pharm. Pharmacol.*, **12,** 868

13 Smith, M. J. H. and Walker, J. R. (1980). The effects of some anti-rheumatic drugs on an *in vitro* model of human polymorphonuclear leukocyte chemokinesis. *Br. J. Pharmacol.*, **69,** 473

14 O'Flaherty, J. T., Showell, H. J., Becker, E. L. and Ward, P. A. (1979). Neutrophil aggregation and degranulation: effect of arachidonic acid. *Am.J.Pathol.*, **95,** 433

15 O'Flaherty, J. T., Showell, H. J., Becker, E. L. and Ward, P. A. (1979). Role of arachi-

donic acid derivatives in neutrophil aggregation: a hypothesis. *Prostaglandins*, **17**, 915

16 Siegel, M. I., McConnell, R. T. and Cuatrecasas, P. (1979). Aspirin-like drugs interfere with arachidonate metabolism by inhibition of the 12-hydroperoxy-5, 8, 10, 14-eicosatetraenoic acid peroxidase activity of the lipoxygenase pathway. *Proc. Natl. Acad. Sci. (USA)*, **76**, 3774

17 Tobias, L. D. and Hamilton, J. G. (1979). The effect of 5,8,11,14–eicosatetraynoic acid on lipid metabolism. *Lipids*, **14**, 181

18 Tapell, A. L., Lundberg, W. and Boyer, P. D. (1953) Effects of temperature and antioxidants upon the lipoxidase-catalysed oxidation of sodium linoleate. *Arch. Biochem. Biophys.*, **42**, 293

19 Hamberg, M. and Samuelsson, B. (1974). Prostaglandin endoperoxides: novel transformation of arachidonic acid in human platelets. *Proc. Natl. Acad. Sci. (USA)*, **71**, 3400

20 Higgs, G. A. Flower, R. J. and Vane, J. R. (1979). A new approach to anti-inflammatory drugs. *Biochem. Pharmacol.*, **28**, 1959

21 Walker, J. R. and Dawson, W. (1979). Inhibition of rabbit PMN lipoxygenase activity by benoxaprofen. *J. Pharm. Pharmacol.*, **11**, 778

22 Borgeat, P. and Samuelsson, B. (1979). Metabolism of arachidonic acid in polymorphonuclear leucocytes. Structural analysis of novel hydroxylated compounds. *J. Biol. Chem.*, **254**, 7865

23 Bokoch, G. M. and Reed, P. W. (1979). Inhibition of the neutrophil oxidative response to a chemotactic peptide by inhibitors of arachidonic acid oxygenation. *Biochem. Biophys. Res. Commun.*, **90**, 481

24 Smolen, J. and Weissman, G. (1980). Lysosomal enzyme release from human granulocytes is inhibited by indomethacin and ETYA. *Advances in Prostaglandins and Thromboxanes Research*. (In press)

25 Valone, F. H. and Goetzl, E. J. (1978). Immunological release in the rat peritoneal cavity of lipid chemotactic and chemokinetic factors for polymorphonuclear leucocytes. *J. Immunol.*, **120**, 102

# 35

# Arachidonic acid metabolism by lipoxygenase in leukocytes of different species and the chemokinetic activity of some products (Abstract)

R. M. J. PALMER, J. A. SALMON, S. NARUMIYA, G. A. HIGGS AND K. E. EAKINS (UK)

Mono-hydroxy acids derived from arachidonic acid (AA) via the lipoxygenase pathway have been reported to be chemokinetic and chemotatic for human leukocytes, 5-hydroxyeicosatetraenoic acid (5-HETE) being the most potent[1]. In the present study we have investigated the metabolism of AA in rat and rabbit peritoneal exudate cells (PEC) and in human leukocytes together with the chemokinetic activity of the products for each species. Following extraction and purification, the metabolites formed during incubation of [$^{14}$C]AA with rat and rabbit PEC and human peripheral blood leukocytes were identified by UV spectrophotometry and gas chromatography mass spectrometry. Lipoxygenase activity was detected in the leukocytes of all three species but the end products varied. Normal rat PEC produced a mixture of 11- and 12-HETE while those of the rabbit formed predominantly 5-HETE and lesser amounts of 11- and 12-HETE. Human cells were also able to biosynthesize a mixture of 5-, 11- and 12-HETE. The relative chemokinetic potencies of 5-, 12- and 15-HETE and the analogous hydroperoxy acids were examined in an agarose micro-drop assay[2] using rat and rabbit PEC and human peripheral leukocytes. All the acids studied were active on rabbit PEC in concentrations between 0.1 and 3.2 $\mu$g/ml with a rank order of 12-HETE > 15-HPETE > 15-HETE > AA = 5-HPETE > 5-HETE. AA and the 5- and 12-substituted acids were chemokinetic between 0.32 and 3.2 $\mu$g/ml on human leukocytes, 5-HETE being most potent. Both 15-HPETE and 15-HETE were without effect at concentrations up to 10 $\mu$g/ml. In contrast, none of the acids showed activity on the rat PEC at concentrations up to 10 $\mu$g/ml. Thus, a major product is the most active on the human leukocyte but this does not appear to be true for rabbit and rat PEC. These results may reflect differences between circulating and exudate leukocytes or may suggest a more complex role for these products in recruitment or activation of other cell types.

## References

1 Goetzl, E. J. and Sun, F. F. (1979). Generations of unique mono-hydroxy eicosatetraenoic acids from arachidonic acid by human neutrophils. *J. Exp. Med.*, **150,** 406

2 Smith, M. J. H. and Walker, J. R. (1980). The effect of some antirheumatic drugs on an *in vitro* model of human polymorphonuclear leukocyte chemokinetics. *Br. J. Pharmacol.*, **69,** 433

# 36

# Aspirin-like drugs inhibit arachidonic acid metabolism via lipoxygenase and cyclo-oxygenase in rat neutrophils from carrageenin pleural exudates (Abstract)

M. I. SIEGEL, R. T. McCONNELL, N. A. PORTER,
J. L. SELPH, J. E. TRUAX, R. VINEGAR AND
P. CUATRECASAS (USA)

Aspirin-like drugs inhibit the metabolism of arachidonic acid via lipoxygenase and cyclo-oxygenase in rat neutrophils from carrageenin pleural exudates. These non-steroidal anti-inflammatory drugs inhibit the formation of 11-hydroxy- and 15-hydroxy-eicosatetraenoic acid (HETE) as well as prostaglandins. In addition, the concentration and time dependent irreversible inhibition of lipoxygenase by aspirin and indomethacin parallels closely the patterns observed for inhibition of cyclo-oxygenase. The results suggest that some common steps may exist for the synthesis of HETE and prostaglandins from arachidonic acid in rat neutrophils. The ability of aspirin-like drugs to inhibit the formation of the chemotactic hydroxy fatty acids may contribute to their anti-inflammatory activity.

# 37

# The possible role of divalent cations, microtubules and cyclic nucleotides in lymphokine induced macrophage aggregation

P. BADENOCH-JONES (UK), B. ROUVEIX (FRANCE) AND J. L. TURK (UK)

## INTRODUCTION

Lymphokines (LKY) are non-antibody-soluble products of activated lymphocytes, thought to be mediators of cell mediated immunity. They include putative inflammatory mediators of delayed hypersensitivity such as skin reactive factor. Although they have a number of *in vivo* and *in vitro* effects, the interaction of LKY with macrophages as their target cell has been best studied. The ability of migration inhibitory factor (MIF) reversibly to decrease the spontaneous migration of macrophages *in vitro* is the basis of the most widely used assay system for lymphokine activity. Despite much work the exact molecular mechanism of MIF action is not known, although recent work is encouraging. It has been known for some time that MIF containing lymphocyte culture supernatants will aggregate macrophages; this was first studied systematically by Lolekha *et al*[1]. These authors showed that macrophage aggregating factor (MAF) was produced by activated lymphocytes under the same conditions as was MIF. Both the aggregation of normal macrophages by preformed LKY (indirect) or the aggregation of sensitized PEC (peritoneal exudate cells, containing both macrophages and lymphocytes) by specific antigen (direct) was observed. The production of MAF and the direct aggregation of sensitized PEC was found to correlate with the state of delayed hypersensitivity in the guinea pig. It remains to be proven, however, that these two aggregations (direct and indirect) are mediated through the same mechanism. Despite the practical advantages of measuring macrophage aggregation compared with measuring migration inhibition, the assay of MAF for the detection of LKY activity has not received much attention in the literature. This is, no doubt, due to the subjective measurements of macrophage aggregation used compared with the semi-quantitative MIF assay. We have recently developed a method for the quantitative assay of lymphokine induced macrophage aggregation[2,3] by measuring the light absorbance of macrophage suspensions using a modified Born platelet aggregometer.

Measurement of aggregation has been found to be more sensitive than MIF measurement for the detection of LKY activity and is maximal at 30 min after addition of preformed LKY (Table 37.1). Thus, this is one of the earliest reported effects of LKY on macrophages. It is not unequivocally known whether the same molecular species is responsible for aggregation and migration inhibition. Because of this, and because aggregation is such a non-specific parameter, we have carried out preliminary studies on the mechanism of this aggregation and attempted to relate this to current ideas on the mechanism of action of MIF.

**Table 37.1** Time course of LKY induced macrophage aggregation

| *Time* (min) | *Aggregation test-control* (cm) |
|---|---|
| 0 | 0 |
| 5 | $^{-}0.5 \pm 1.2$ (3) |
| 15 | $4.6 \pm 1.9$ (3) |
| 30 | $10.9 \pm 2.0$ (6) |
| 45 | $7.9 \pm 1.6$ (3) |
| 60 | $6.1 \pm 0.9$ (3) |

For details of LKY and cell preparations and the assay method see reference 3. Results are means ± SE of one batch of LKY assayed on three separate cell preparations.

## STUDIES ON THE MECHANISM OF AGGREGATION

We have shown that LKY induced macrophage aggregation can be inhibited by the glycolytic inhibitors, 2-deoxyglucose and iodoacetamide. Thus, it appears that the aggregation is dependent on the metabolic integrity of the macrophages and is not a passive agglutination. In addition, colchicine ($10^{-5}$ mol/l) will completely inhibit this aggregation, thus suggesting a possible role for microtubules (Table 37.2). Colchicine is reported to stimulate spontaneous macrophage migration *in vitro*, at $10^{-8}$–$10^{-4}$ mol/l, and will overcome the inhibitory effects of MIF at concentrations[4] of $10^{-5}$–$10^{-7}$

mol/l). Recent work[5,6] has suggested a direct role of microtubules in the mechanism of action of MIF.

**Table 37.2** The effect of colchicine ($10^{-5}$ mol/l) on lymphokine and ionophore induced migration inhibition and aggregation of macrophages

| *Addition* | *% Migration inhibition* |
|---|---|
| Colchicine | $-78 \pm 21$ (5)[a] |
| Ionophore ($10^{-6}$ mol/l) | $78 \pm 5$ (5)[b] |
| Ionophore + colchicine | $1 \pm 8$ (5)[d] ($43 \pm 5$)[d] |
| Ionophore ($10^{-7}$ mol/l) | $21 \pm 2$ (5)[b] |
| Ionophore + colchicine | $-57 \pm 15$ (5)[d] ($12 \pm 2$)[f] |
| Lymphokine | $54 \pm 4$ (5)[b] |
| Lymphokine + colchicine | $-28 \pm 13$ (5)[d] ($28 \pm 7$)[e] |
| | *Aggregation, test-control* (cm) |
| Ionophore ($10^{-6}$ mol/l) | $9.2 \pm 1.9$ (4)[c] |
| Ionophore + colchicine | $0.2 \pm 0.9$ (4)[d] |
| Lymphokine | $12.3 \pm 1.3$ (4)[c] |
| Lymphokine + colchicine | $2.5 \pm 1.3$ (4)[d] |

Results are mean ± SEM. Migration inhibition is calculated as $100 - \frac{\text{test migration}}{\text{control migration}} \times 100$ this and aggregation were measured as described in reference 3. Note that the effect of colchicine on migration inhibition is presented either with colchicine added only to the test or added to both the test and control (data in brackets). For the ionophore the control was medium only; in the case of aggregation, colchicine was only added to both test and control. (*a*) Significant stimulation ($p<0.05$), (*b*), Significant inhibition of migration ($p<0.001$), (*c*) Significant aggregation ($p<0.001$), (*d*) Significant reversal by colchicine ($p<0.001$), (*e*) Significant reversal ($p<0.01$), (*f*) Significant reversal ($p<0.02$)

Convincing evidence has been presented that MIF actively promotes the polymerization of tubulin and thus, as a result of the constraints of macrophage movement by microtubules, inhibits their migration. If microtubules are involved in the rapid aggregation induced by LKY then this is likely to be mediated via changes in cell surface topography and this may alter cellular adhesiveness, which is probably the parameter being measured in the aggregation assay. Furthermore, McCarthy *et al.*[6] have shown that macrophages need only be in contact for 1 h with LKY (the shortest time period these authors measured) for subsequent tubulin polymerization to be increased. Thus, although aggregation is a rapid process (30 min), whereas migration inhibition is not usually measured before 6–8 h (because sufficient migration must occur before migration inhibition can be measured) it may well be that the initial reactions are the same.

Another similarity between the mechanism of migration inhibition and aggregation is the effect of the divalent cation ionophere A23187. We have found that A23187 causes a large aggregation of macrophages at $10^{-6}$ mol/l, which is $Ca^{2+}$ $Mg^{2+}$ dependent[8], and that this is inhibited by $10^{-5}$ mol/l colchicine (Table 37.2). A23187 has also been shown to inhibit macrophage migration at $10^{-6}$ to $10^{-7}$ mol/l and this was reversed in $Ca^{2+}/Mg^{2+}$ free media[9]. We have also found this and furthermore this inhibition of migration is fully reversed by $10^{-5}$ mol/l colchicine (Table 37.2). Previously, it had been shown that A23187 mimics some of the macrophage activating[10] effects of LKY and it was suggested that LKY induced an influx of divalent cations ($Mg^{2+}$ in this case) as a primary event. There have been a number of suggestions in the literature that LKY may induce a $Ca^{2+}$ influx into macrophages, but direct measurements by Block *et al.*[9] using $^{45}Ca$ showed no enhanced uptake by test LKY over control LKY, although A23187 at $10^{-6}$ mol/l induced a 2.5-fold increase in intracellular $^{45}Ca$ over 30 min. However, it has been claimed that LKY does induce an enhanced $Ca^{2+}$ uptake[5,11] and thus this question still remains open and must be of central importance in determining the molecular mechanism of MIF action.

It was noted by Pick *et al.*[5] that the observed polymerization of macrophage tubulin may be mediated by either high or low intracellular $Ca^{2+}$ levels together with changes in the cyclic-GMP/cyclic-AMP ratio. We have shown that dibutryl cyclic AMP ($5\times10^{-4}$ mol/l) in the presence of theophylline ($10^{-3}$ mol/l) significantly inhibited LKY induced macrophage aggregation[8]. Many studies have been carried out on the effects of exogenous cyclic AMP and drugs raising its intracellular concentration on macrophage migration and inhibition of MIF activity. Although dibutryl cyclic AMP will inhibit macrophage migration at very high levels ($10^{-3}$ mol/l) there is no evidence that this plays a role as the second messenger of MIF activity. At lower levels, only at $10^{-4}$ mol/l will dibutryl cyclic AMP inhibit MIF activity, below this there is no effect and above this spontaneous migration is depressed[9]. The levels we have used ($5\times10^{4}$ mol/l) are high, but we have not measured the intracellular levels of cyclic AMP induced by this. Block *et al.* has shown an approximately fourfold increase in intracellular cyclic AMP levels over 20 h after addition of $10^{-4}$ mol/l dibutryl cyclic AMP and no change at $10^{-5}$ mol/l and lower, although they did not also add theophylline. It will await further work to determine the significance of this inhibition of aggregation by $5\times10^{-4}$ mol/l dibutryl cyclic AMP.

Compared with the work done on cyclic AMP, attention is only now turning to the possible role of cyclic GMP in MIF action. The idea that cyclic GMP may be involved came from speculation over the mechanism of tubulin polymerization induced by MIF[4,5] and by analogy with the role of cyclic GMP in modulating surface phenomena which are dependent on microtubule function in polymorphs[12]. Very recently it has been shown that leukocyte inhibiting factor (LIF) causes cyclic GMP levels in leukocytes[13]. Exogenous cyclic GMP was reported to have no effect on macrophage migration[14] at $10^{-3}$ to $10^{-7}$ mol/l. We have found a reproducible but only marginal inhibition of macrophage migration by dibutryl cyclic GMP at $10^{-3}$ mol/l ($25.4\pm3.9\%$, $p<0.01$). In the absence of further specificity controls this must be of doubtful significance, although it is of interest that macrophage aggregation can also be induced by dibutryl cyclic GMP[15], but only at $10^{-3}$ mol/l. Preliminary work on the direct measurements of cyclic AMP and cyclic GMP levels of aggregated macrophages at 30 min shows no test-control difference in cyclic AMP and only a marginal increase in cyclic GMP levels[15]. Thus it remains to be seen whether $Ca^{2+}$, $Mg^{2+}$ and/or cyclic GMP are involved in the reported increases in the polymerization of tubulin induced by MIF. At this early stage it is difficult to make any precise statements as to the mechanism of macrophage aggregation induced by LKY, although preliminary work suggests that there are similarities between this and the mechanisms of action of MIF. If this turns out to be the case then the quantitative measurement of LKY induced macrophage aggregation should prove a valuable method for the study of the early (<30 min) events in the perturbation of macrophage metabolism by LKY.

## References


1 Lolekha, S., Dray, S. and Gotoff, S. P. (1970). Macrophage aggregation *in vitro*: a correlate with delayed hypersensitivity. *J. Immunol.*, **104**, 296

2 Rouveix, B., Badenoch-Jones, P. and Turk, J. L. (1979). A sensitive technique for measuring specific macrophage aggregation: a comparison with macrophage migration inhibition, for the detection of lymphokine activity. *Immunology*, **36**, 589

3 Badenoch-Jones, P., Rouveix, B. and Turk, J. L. (1980). Studies on lymphokine-induced macrophage aggregation. Specificity and quantitative aspects. *Int. Arch. Allergy Appl. Immunol.* (In press)

4 Pick, E. and Abrahamer, H. (1973). Blocking of macrophage migration inhibitory action by microtubular disruptive drugs. *Int. Arch. Allergy Appl. Immunol.*, **44**, 215

5 Pick, E., Honig, S. and Griffel, B. (1979). The mechanism of action of soluble lymphocyte mediators. VI. Effect of MIF on macrophage microtubules. *Int. Arch. Allergy Appl. Immunol.*, **62**, 188

6 McCarthy, P. L., Shaw, J. E. and Remold, H. G. (1979). The role of microtubules in the response of macrophages to MIF. *Cell Immunol.*, **46**, 409

7 Snyder, J. A. and McIntosh, J. R. (1976). Biochemistry and physiology of microtubules. *Ann. Rev. Biochem.*, **45**, 699

8 Badenoch-Jones, P., Rouveix, B. and Turk, J. L. (1979). Studies on the mechanism of macrophage aggregation induced by lymphokines. *Immunology*, **37**, 361

9 Block, L. H., Aloni, B., Blemesderfer, D., Kashgarian, M. and Bitensky, M. W. (1978). Macrophage migration inhibition factor: interactions with calcium, magnesium and cyclic AMP. *J. Immunol.*, **121**, 1416

10 Hand, L. W., King, N. L., Johnson, J. D. and Lowe, D. A. (1977). Requirement for magnesium influx in activation of alveolar macrophages mediated by ionophore A23187. *Nature (London)*, **265**, 543

11 Greindeder, D. K. and David, J. R. (1977). The role of calciums in the action of MIF induced by neuraminidase-galactose oxidase. *Fed. Proc., Fed. Am. Soc. Exp. Biol.*, **36**, 1218

12 Oliver, J. M., Zuvier, R. B. and Berlin, R. D. (1975). Concanavalin A Cap formation on polymorphonuclear leukocytes of normal and beige mice. *Nature (London)*, **263**, 471

13 Bendtzen, K. and Klysner, R. (1979). Increased polymorphonuclear leukocyte c GMP levels induced by the human lymphokine, leukocyte migration inhibitory factor (LIF). *Immunopharmacology*, **1**, 323

14 Pick, E. and Manheimer, S. (1974). The mechanism of action of soluble lymphocyte mediators. II. Modification of macrophage migration and MIF action by drugs, enzymes and cationic environment. *Cell Immunol.*, **11**, 30

15 Rouveix, B., Badenoch-Jones, P., Larne, S. and Turk, J. L. (1980). Lymphokine-induced macrophage aggregation: the role of cyclic nucleotides. (In preparation)

# 38

# Inhibitory effect of benoxaprofen and BW 755C on rabbit PMN leukocyte lipoxygenase (Abstract)

J. R. WALKER AND W. DAWSON (UK)

Arachidonic acid is metabolized by rabbit peritoneal PMNs via both prostaglandin cyclo-oxygenase and fatty acid lipoxygenase pathways to yield a multiplicity of biologically active products. These activities have been well characterized for the prostaglandins and thromboxanes and recent attention has been directed to the activities of the many hydroxy substituted arachidonic acid metabolites including leukocyte chemotactic and chemokinetic stimulation and possible mediation of leukoctye aggregation[1,2].

The relationship of inhibition of either of these enzymes to the activity of clinically active anti-inflammatory drugs is of considerable interest and recent reports suggest that dual inhibition provides a novel spectrum of biological activity[3,4].

Quantitation of 5,12-diHETE and 5-HETE produced by rabbit peritoneal PMNs on exposure to calcium ionophore has been established[4]. Benoxaprofen, an anti-inflammatory drug with low prostaglandin cyclo-oxygenase inhibitory activity has been shown to inhibit rabbit PMN lipoxygenase product formation in a dose related fashion with an $IC_{50}$ of about $6 \times 10^{-5}$mol/l. BW 755C, previously reported to inhibit a horse platelet lipoxygenase, has now been shown to inhibit the rabbit PMN enzyme with an $IC_{50}$ of about $10^{-4}$mol/l. Indomethacin was much less active in this system with little effect at$10^{-5}$ mol/l. Relative to their $IC_{50}$s against prostaglandin cyclo-oxygenase (benoxaprofen $> 5 \times 10^{-5}$mol/l; BW 755C $5 \times 10^{-6}$mol/l; Indomethacin $5 \times 10^{-7}$ mol/l) it is clear that benoxaprofen and BW 755 are very different in their spectrum of activity. All three are potent in classical animal models of inflammation; benoxaprofen and indomethacin have both been used clinically and are effective in the treatment of inflammatory conditions in man and it is reasonable to suppose that they achieve these effects by different mechanisms of action.

## References

1 Goetzl, E. J. and Sun, F. F. (1979). *J. Exp. Med.* **150,** 406
2 Ford-Hutchinson, A. W., Bray, M. A. and Smith, M. J. H. (1979). *J. Pharm. Pharmacol.,* **31**, 868
3 Higgs, G. Flower, R. J. and Vane, J. R. (1979). *Biochem. Pharmacol.*, **28,** 1959
4 Walker, J. R. and Dawson, W. (1979). *J. Pharm. Pharmacol.*, **31,** 778

# 39

# Mechanism of inhibition of prostaglandin biosynthesis by anti-inflammatory steroids

M. DI ROSA, P. PERSICO, R. CARNUCCIO AND A. PINTO (ITALY)

Anti-inflammatory steroids inhibit prostaglandin (PG) biosynthesis in a variety of tissues and cultured cells. This inhibition is secondary to a suppression of phospholipase $A_2$, the enzyme which releases arachidonic acid from membrane phospholipids[1,2]. Recent reports show that the inhibition of PG biosynthesis and the anti-inflammatory effect of glucocorticosteroids depend on receptor occupancy and require RNA and protein synthesis[3–7].

We present evidence that glucocortisoids induce in rat leucocytes the release of a soluble 'second messenger', possibly a protein or non-dialisable polypeptide which mediates the anti-phospholipase effect of the steroids.

## METHOD

Male Wistar rats (weighing 150–200 g) were killed by exposure to ether and bled. The peritoneal cavity was washed with 20 ml of heparinized Krebs solution. The cell rich fluid was removed and centrifuged (50 g). The cells pooled from 10–15 animals were washed twice by re-suspending in Krebs solution enriched with bovine serum albumin (100 $\mu$g/ml). The final suspension contained 10 million of cells per ml (80% mononuclears and 20% polymorphonuclears).

The final cell suspension was divided into two samples. Hydrocortisone sodium phosphate (0.01–10 $\mu$g/ml) was added to one sample. No drug was present in the other sample. Incubation was carried out for 90 min at 37 °C in a metabolic shaker. Alternatively prednisolone (0.01–1 $\mu$g/ml) or dexamethasone (0.001–0.1 μg/ml), both as sodium phosphate salts, were also used.

After incubation the cells were removed by centrifugation and the supernatants were separately dialysed overnight at 4 °C against a large volume of Krebs solution replaced three times (supernatant/Krebs final ratio 1:300). PG in the supernatants were occasionally determined before and after the dialysis. In some experiments a small amount of labelled hydrocortisone ([1,2,6,7 (*n*) $^3$H]hydrocortisone, 90 mCi/mmol, C.E.A., France) was added to supernatants and the radioactivity measured before and after the dialysis.

A second pool of freshly collected peritoneal cells (test leukocytes) was suspended in Krebs albumin. A series of 3 ml samples was prepared by mixing 1 ml of cell suspension with 2 ml of dialysed supernatant from control or steroid-treated leukocytes and incubated for 120 min as above with killed bacteria (*Bordetella pertussis*) in a ratio of 1000 bacteria per cell[8].

After incubation the cells were removed by centrifugation. The supernatant was acidified to pH 3.0 with 0.1 N HCl, extracted twice with equal volume of ethyl acetate and evaporated. The residue was dissolved in 1 ml of Krebs solution and PG bioassayed using rat stomach strips suspended in Krebs solution containing a mixture of antagonists to prevent the action of other mediators[9]. The recovery of this procedure, evaluated with synthetic $PGE_2$ (Upjohn), was about 80%. In some experiments cycloheximide (1 μg/ml) or arachidonic acid (1 μg/ml) were also added to the incubation medium of either generator or test leukocytes.

## RESULTS

The amount of PG released into the medium by rat peritoneal leukocytes is in the range 2–4 ng per $10^6$ cells at 90 min. After dialysis supernatants of incubated cells do not contain detectable amounts of PG. Dialysis is also able to remove hydrocortisone from the supernatant for the initial radioactivity of labelled hydrocortisone after dialysis is reduced by 99%.

Test leukocytes, which are incubated with killed bacteria, release substantial amounts of PG (10–12 ng per $10^6$ cells at 120 min) since phagocytozing process stimulates PG production. The effect of dialysed supernatants from either control or hydrocortisone treated generator leukocytes on PG production by test leukocytes is summarized in Figure 39.1.

The PG release by test leukocytes is not affected by the dialysed supernatant from generator leukocytes incubated in Krebs albumin while it is greatly reduced by the dialysed supernatant from generator leukocytes incubated with 10 μg/ml hydrocortisone.

Cycloheximide (1 μg/ml) abolishes the ability of hydrocortisone to induce the formation of the inhibitor in generator leukocytes although this antibiotic does not modify the effect of the pre-formed inhibitor. The steroid induced inhibitor is not effective in presence of arachidonic acid (1 μg/ml).

| Cells | Drugs (μg/ml) | | | | | |
|---|---|---|---|---|---|---|
| Generator leucocytes | - | HCT (10) | HCT(10) +CXM(1) | CXM (1) | HCT (10) | HCT (10) |
| Test leucocytes | - | - | - | - | CXM (1) | AA (1) |

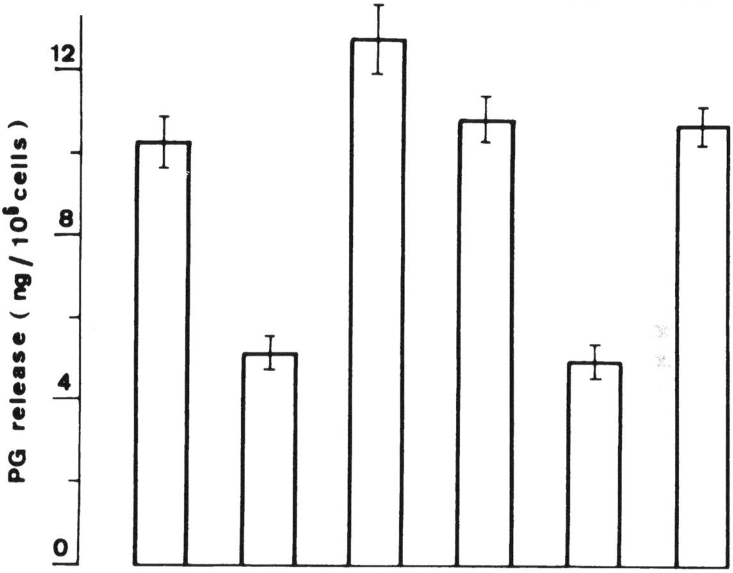


**Figure 39.1** Effect of dialysed supernatant from rat leukocytes incubated with hydrocortisone (generator leukocytes) on the PG release by rat leukocytes phagocytozing killed bacteria (test leukocytes). HCT: hydrocortisone; CXM: cycloheximide; AA: arachidonic acid. Results are expressed in terms of $PGE_2$ equivalents. Bars represent the mean value ± SE of 4–6 experiments

The effect of various concentrations of hydrocortisone on the release of the steroid induced inhibitor from generator leukocytes is shown in Figure 39.2. A concentration related response is observed in the range 0.01–10 μg/ml hydrocortisone. The release of the inhibitor is also induced by equipotent concentrations of prednisolone and dexamethasone (data not shown).

## DISCUSSION

Anti-inflammatory steroids inhibit PG biosynthesis by preventing the release and/or the activation of phospholipase $A_2$, the enzyme which releases fatty acids from phospholipids and therefore supplies the substrates for cyclo-

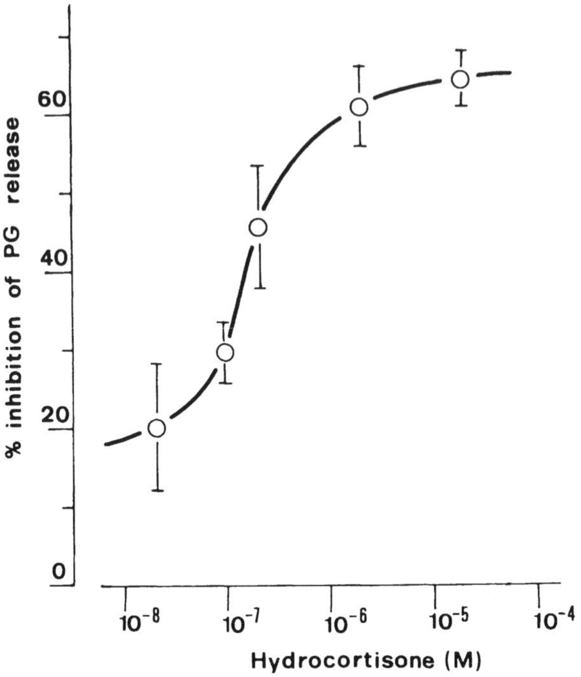


**Figure 39.2** Relationship between hydrocortisone concentration in the medium of generator leukocytes and the inhibition exhibited by the steroid induced inhibitor on the PG production by test leukocytes. Results are expressed in terms of $PGE_2$ equivalents. Each point represents the mean value ± SE of 4–6 experiments

oxygenase[1]. Recent findings have shown that the inhibition of phospholipase $A_2$ by anti-inflammatory steroids works through the same mechanism exhibited by steroid hormones on their target cells, i.e. stimulation of transcription and consequent induction of specific proteins[3–6].

Rat peritoneal leukocytes incubated with anti-inflammatory steroids (hydrocortisone, prednisolone, dexamethasone) release a non-dialysable inhibitor which mediates the anti-phospholipase effect of anti-inflammatory steroids. Arachidonic acid is in fact able to revert the inhibition of PG biosynthesis exhibited by the hydrocortisone induced inhibitor in rat leukocytes. The steroid induced inhibitor of phospholipase $A_2$ may be a protein or a polypeptide since its formation is prevented by cycloheximide. The release of the inhibitor from rat peritoneal leukocytes is induced by hydrocortisone concentrations ($10^{-6}$–$10^{-7}$ mol/l) which are known to produce physiological effects through specific steroid receptors.

The discovery of a steroid-induced inhibitor of PG biosynthesis in leukocytes, because of the key role played in inflammation by both PG and leukocytes, may contribute to clarify the control mechanisms of inflammatory response. A steroid induced phospholipase $A_2$ inhibitor has been recently reported to occur in guinea pig lungs[5]. It will be of great interest to further explore and compare the properties of these steroid induced inhibitors, generated, respectively, by guinea pig lungs and rat leukocytes.

## References


1 Flower, R. J. and Blackwell, G. J. (1976). The importance of phospholipase $A_2$ in prostaglandin biosynthesis. *Biochem. Pharmacol.*, **25,** 285

2 Gryglewski, R. J. (1976). Steroid hormones, anti-inflammatory steroids and prostaglandin. *Pharm. Res. Commun.*, **8,** 337

3 Danon, A. and Assouline, G. (1978). Inhibition of prostaglandin biosynthesis by corticosteroids requires RNA and protein synthesis. *Nature (London),* **273,** 552

4 Di Rosa, A. and Persico, P. (1979). Mechanism of inhibition of prostaglandin biosynthesis by hydrocortisone in rat leukocytes. *Br. J. Pharmacol.*, **66,** 161

5 Flower, R. J. and Blackwell, G. J. (1979). Anti-inflammatory steroids induce biosynthesis of a phospholipase $A_2$ inhibitor which prevents prostaglandin generation. *Nature (London)*, **278,** 456

6 Russo-Marie, F., Paing, M. and Duval, D. (1979). Involvement of glucocorticoid receptors in steroid-induced inhibition of prostaglandin secretion. *J. Biol. Chem.*, **254,** 8498

7 Tsurufuji, S., Sugio, K. and Takemasa, F. (1979). The role of glucocorticoid receptor and gene expression in the anti-inflammatory action of dexamethasone. *Nature (London)*, **280,** 408

8 Higgs, G. S., McCall, E. and Youlten, L. J. F. (1975). A chemotactic role for prostaglandins released from polymorphonuclear leukocytes during phagocytosis. *Br. J. Pharmacol.*, **53,** 539

9 Gilmore, N., Vane, J. R. and Wyllie, J. H. (1968). Prostaglandin release by the spleen. *Nature (London)*, **218,** 1135

# 40

# Selective control of formation of 1 and 2 series prostaglandins: a new concept in the regulation of inflammation and immunity

D. F. HORROBIN, M. S. MANKU, M. OKA
AND S. C. CUNNANE (CANADA)

## INTRODUCTION

The roles of prostaglandins (PGs) and thromboxanes (TXs) in inflammation are uncertain. There can be no doubt that these agents are formed in increased amounts in a wide variety of inflammatory conditions and that inhibition of that formation by steroids and by non-steroidal anti-inflammatory drugs (NSAID) is well correlated with relief of symptoms in both acute and chronic inflammatory conditions in humans and with suppression of some of the features of acute inflammation in animal models. On the other hand, there is equally no doubt that glucocorticoids and NSAID do not favourably influence the long-term course of most chronic inflammatory states in humans[1]. Furthermore there is a good deal of evidence that PGs can play anti-inflammatory roles[2–5].

Similar confusion exists in relation to the immune response, where PGs have been reported both to suppress and to enhance both cell-mediated and humoral immunity in human and animal cells *in vitro* and in a variety of *in vivo* animal models[6–11].

In contrast to the steroids and the NSAID there are other drugs, such as penicillamine, colchicine, levamisole, anti-malarials, zinc and gold salts, which do not, at clinically relevant concentrations, inhibit PG synthesis in a manner analogous to that of either the steroids or the NSAID. Penicillamine[12,13] and colchicine[14,15] have actions consistent with stimulation of PG synthesis. These drugs are almost all difficult to use: responses are erratic, side effects are common and some patients are made worse. On the other hand, when they do work they may have the greatly desired effect of actually changing for the better the long-term course of the disease. The most convincing and consistent results have occurred with colchicine, traditionally used in gout, but more recently employed with striking success in the management of familial Mediterranean fever (FMF)[16,17] and necrotizing vasculitis[18].

Most of the discussion about the roles of the different PGs in inflammation has centred on the question of whether the Es or the Fs are important. Little attention has been paid to the possibility that the important differences may be those between the series of PGs, the 1s formed from dihomogammalinolenic acid (DGLA), the 2s formed from arachidonic acid (AA), and the 3s formed from eicosapentenoic acid. However, the possible importance of different series is shown by the fact that in human platelets DGLA and its products have an overall anti-aggregatory effect while AA and its metabolites have an overall pro-aggregatory effect. A number of observations led us to suspect that at physiological concentrations *in vivo* $PGE_1$ might be a particularly effective inhibitor of chronic inflammation and regulator of the immune response. $PGE_1$ is a potent activator of adenyl cyclase and in contrast to $PGE_2$ it inhibits platelet aggregation[19]. $PGE_1$ is effective in controlling the chronic disease of the NZB/W mouse[9], and in inhibiting immunologically-mediated vasculitis[20]. Moreover it can inhibit the mobilization of arachidonic acid, possibly via cyclic AMP[21,22], and can regulate the movements of intracellular calcium[23,24] which are important in control of phospholipases and of lysosomes. These effects led us to wonder whether various chronic inflammatory states and disorders of immunity might relate to *reduced* formation of 1 series PGs coupled with a consequential *excess* formation of 2 series PGs, Most experimental studies could have missed such a possibility because many assays do not distinguish between PGs of the 1 and 2 series. We therefore investigated the selective effects of various agents on 1 and 2 series PG formation. Several compounds which modify the long term courses of inflammatory diseases selectively enhance the production of 1 series PGs.

## METHOD

There are two major rate-limiting steps in the formation of PG endoperoxides. The first is the mobilization of the PG precursors stored in the form of phospholipids to give free DGLA or AA. The second is the conversion of the free DGLA or AA to their respective endoperoxides. We have used two different techniques, one to study the mobilization of the precursors and one to investigate their onward conversion.

### Mobilization of AA and DGLA

In the isolated, perfused, mesenteric vascular bed of the rat[23,25], addition of

AA or DGLA in increasing concentrations to the perfusing fluid produces changes in vascular reactivity characteristic for each acid. These changes are blocked by adding NSAID to the fluid, are accompanied by increased output of PG-like material as assessed by rat stomach bioassay and can be imitated by $PGE_1$ in the case of DGLA and by $PGE_2$ in the case of AA[23]. We therefore assume that the reactivity changes are caused by conversion of the precursors to PGs. Glucocorticoids and lithium do not block formation of PGs from the acids or the biological activities of the acids.

The effects of AA and DGLA are quite different. The preparation is routinely tested by injecting a fixed dose of either noradrenaline or potassium into the perfusate: these injections cause vasoconstriction and a rise in pressure which can be accurately measured. Noradrenaline mainly acts by releasing intracellular or membrane-bound calcium to the contractile mechanism while potassium causes calcium entry from the extracellular fluid[23,25]. Increasing concentrations of AA cause progressively larger and larger responses to the same doses of noradrenaline and potassium. DGLA has no effect on potassium responses and a biphasic effect on noradrenaline responses, potentiating them at low concentrations and inhibiting them at high ones. $PGE_2$ imitates the effect of AA, and $PGE_1$ imitates the effect of DGLA (Figure 40.1). At $10^{-11}$ mol/l $PGE_1$ has a maximal effect in enhancing intracellular calcium release. At higher concentrations this effect is progressively reduced and then reversed.

With this preparation it is therefore possible to identify agents which release AA or DGLA and which modify the conversion of these precursors to PGs. Agents which act at the mobilization stage have their effects blocked by both steroids and NSAID. Agents which act at the cyclo-oxygenase stage still exert their effects when the preparation is perfused with a fixed amount of AA or DGLA to provide precursor material, and with a high steroid concentration to block mobilization of endogenous precursor.

### Conversion of AA and DGLA to their respective products

To study this stage we have used human platelets incubated with either [$^{14}$C]AA or [$^{14}$C]DGLA. Incubation and separation techniques are similar to those widely used by others and have been described in detail[26,27]

## AGENTS MODIFYING RELEASE OF DGLA AND AA

Using the above methods we have been able to demonstrate that the following agents selectively release DGLA as shown by the production of a PG-like material whose outflow is blocked by NSAID or by steroids and which has no effect on potassium responses but a biphasic effect on noradrenaline responses.

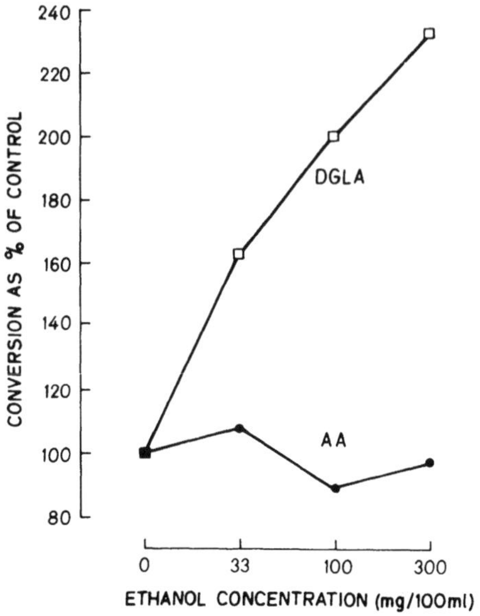


**Figure 40.1** The effects of increasing concentrations of ethanol on the conversion of labelled DGLA to the sum of $PGE_1$, $TXB_1$ and $PGF_{1}\alpha$, and on the conversion of AA to the sum of the corresponding 2 series PGs. Ethanol had no convincing effect on AA metabolism but caused a progressive increase in the conversion of DGLA to its products. Vitamin C had similar effects over the 10 to 100 μg/ml range[26,27]

(1) Prolactin[28] over the concentration range 25–800 ng/ml.
(2) Zinc[23] over the concentration range 0.01–10 μg/ml.
(3) Penicillamine[13,29] over the concentration range 1–100 μ/ml.
(4) Levamisole[29] over the concentration range 1–100 μg/ml.
(5) Phenformin[29] over the concentration range 0.1–15 μg/ml.

The effects of these agents seemed to be substantially greater during the winter months. In the case of zinc we have explored this seasonal variation in detail[30]. The variation is abolished by pinealectomy. Pinealectomized winter animals or intact summer animals can be made to behave like intact winter animals by treatmentof the animal *in vivo* or the preparation *in vitro* with melatonin. Melatonin alone enhances responses to noradrenaline without affecting those to potassium and when present in a fixed concentration it substantially potentiates the effectiveness of zinc. Low levels of colchicine seem to have effects similar to those of melatonin.

In contrast, the following agents have actions consistent with selective mobilization of AA. They have equipotent effects on noradrenaline and potassium responses with no evidence of a diphasic response at high concentrations. Their effects are blocked by NSAID and steroids and are accompanied by outflow of bioassayable PG-like material.

(1) Angiotensin II over[31] the concentration range $10^{-13} - 10^{-7}$ mol/l.
(2) Vasopressin[32] over the concentration range $10^{-13} - 10^{-7}$ mol/1.
(3) Myo-Inositol[33] over the concentration range $10^{-8} - 10^{-3}$ mol/1.

The effects of all the DGLA and AA releasing agents, with the sole exception of zinc, can be blocked by glucocorticoids. The effects of all the DGLA releasing agents, including zinc, can be readily blocked by lithium at concentrations in the 0.2–2 mol/1 range which are relevant to the use of lithium in psychiatry[23]. In contrast, lithium only weakly inhibits the effects of AA releasing agents[32]. We conclude that the AA and DGLA releasing systems are about equally steroid sensitive but that lithium has a selective action on DGLA. The zinc effect is insensitive to steroids but blocked by lithium. Beta-endorphin is able to block the effect of prolactin on the release of $PGE_1$ like material but we did not have sufficient material to dissect its mechanism of action further[34].

These results therefore challenge the conventional view that agents mobilizing one PG precursor will also mobilize another and strongly indicate that it is possible to enhance selectively the formation of either the 1 or the 2 series PGs. Evidence for selective mechanisms of AA mobilization has recently come from other directions. There seems to be a transfer of AA in phosphatidyl-inositol to a diglyceride, with a cleavage of the latter by a diglyceride lipase[35,36]. It is of interest that myo-inositol, which might be expected to modify inositol-containing phospholipids, led to selective mobilization of AA[33].

## CONVERSIONS OF AA OR DGLA TO PG AND TXS

Using human platelets we have found that a variety of agents are able to modify selectively the conversion of DGLA and of AA to their respective PGs. Ethanol and vitamin C (Figure 40.2) are both able to enhance substantially the formation of 1 series PGs at concentrations which have no effect on 2 series PG formation[26,27]. Results with a variety of other compounds are shown in Table 40.1. Each result represents the mean of three experiments. The important points to note are as follows:

(1) Colchicine at $10^{-5}$ mol/1 enhanced formation of 2 series PGs, a finding similar to that previously made by others[14,15]. However, $10^{-5}$ mol/l is 2–3 orders of magnitude higher than the maximal plasma concentrations achieved during human therapeutic use. At $10^{-7}$ mol/1, colchicine enhanced the formation of 1 series PGs, slightly inhibited the formation of $PGE_2$ and substantially inhibited production of $TXB_2$. Since $TXB_2$ is chemotactic[37] this effect could explain the inhibition of chemotaxis which is a major part of colchicine's action[38].

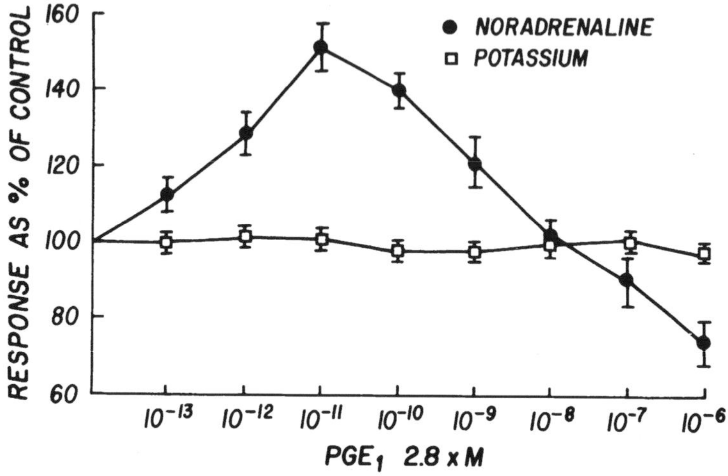


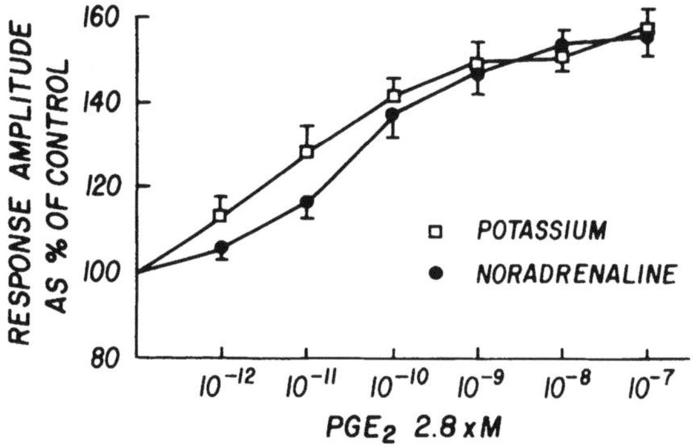


**Figure 40.2** The effects of $PGE_1$ and $PGE_2$ on vascular responses to a fixed dose of either noradrenaline or potassium in the perfused mesenteric vascular bed of the rat. $PGE_1$ had a biphasic effect on noradrenaline responses but no action on potassium ones. $PGE_2$ affected responses to both pressor agents equally and there was no evidence of a biphasic dose response curve

(2) Opiates. The biologically active (−)-isomer of levorphanol had a biphasic effect on formation of 1 series PGs, enhancing it at low concentrations and inhibiting it at high concentrations. It had no effect on AA metabolism. The opiate antagonist, naloxone, blocked both effects. The (+)-isomer which is without opiate activity had no effects. Levorphanol can activate different types of opiate receptor and it is possible that one type of opiate receptor enhances and another inhibits 1 series PG formation while having no effect on 2 series PG formation from their respective precursors. In the mesenteric preparation beta-endorphin blocked produc-

tion of $PGE_1$-like material in response to prolactin but had no effect on production of $PGE_2$-like material in response to vasopressin.

**Table 40.1** Effects of various agents on the conversions of DGLA to $PGE_1$ and $TXB_1$ and of AA to $PGE_2$ and $TXB_2$ in human platelets. Platelets were incubated with the labelled precursors and the products separated and counted as described in detail elsewhere[26,27]. Results are expressed as percentages of the control counts obtained when vehicle was added without the drug. Each figure is the mean of three determinations. NC means 'no change'

| *Precursor* | DGLA | DGLA | AA | AA |
|---|---|---|---|---|
| *Product* | $PGE_1$ | $TXB_1$ | $PGE_2$ | $TXB_2$ |
| (+)-levorphanol, 18 ng or 18 μg/ml | NC | NC | NC | NC |
| (−)-levorphanol, 18 ng/ml plus 10 μg/ml naloxone | NC | NC | NC | NC |
| (−)-levorphanol, 18 ng/ml | 123% | 120% | NC | NC |
| (−)-levorphanol, 18 μg/ml plus 10 μg/ml naloxone | NC | NC | NC | NC |
| (−)-levorphanol, 18 μg/ml | 72% | 76% | NC | NC |
| colchicine, $10^{-7}$ mol/l | 158% | 143% | 95% | 78% |
| colchicine, $10^{-5}$ mol/l | NC | NC | 138% | 146% |
| chloroquine, 2 μg/ml | 127% | 124% | NC | NC |

(3) Chloroquine enhanced formation of 1 series PGs but had no effect on formation of 2 series PGs.

(4) $PGE_2$ had no effect on conversion of AA, but enhanced the conversion of DGLA to $PGE_1$

These results leave no doubt that it is possible to regulate selectively the conversions of PG precursors to their products, just as it is also possible to mobilize those precursors selectuvely.

## FEEDBACK REGULATION OF PG SYNTHESIS

The effects of $PGE_2$ in stimulating $PGE_1$ formation and of $PGE_1$ in inhibiting AA mobilization suggest the possibility of an important feedback relationship between the 1 and the 2 series PGs. There is a good deal of evidence that $TXA_2$ exerts a feedback inhibitory control over the 2 series pathway by inhibiting the mobilization of AA, the conversion of AA to endoperoxides and possibly the conversion of endoperoxides to $TXA_2$[29,39]. The results reported here suggest that a receptor to which colchicine can bind may be important in modulating this $TXA_2$ effect.

When assessed by bioassay in the mesenteric vascular bed, colchicine has effects at low concentrations[40] which are consistent with increased biological activity of $TXA_2$. However, when directly tested in human platelets, colchicine directly inhibited $TXA_2$ formation. These different results may simply represent different tissue and/or species responses. A more interesting possibility is that colchicine is able to enhance some, but not all, of the biological actions of $TXA_2$. Thus, suppose a certain level of $TXA_2$ is required to exert feedback control over the arachidonate pathway. If colchicine were able to potentiate this effect, the feedback would occur at a lower level of $TXA_2$ and $TXA_2$ production would fall to that lower level, leading to a reduction in those biological actions of $TXA_2$ and $TXB_2$ (possibly including chemotaxis) not influenced by colchicine. Such a mechanism could explain the apparently opposite effects of colchicine in the mesentery and in the platelets.

There is clinical evidence that this proposed mechanism may exist. Colchicine and melatonin have similar actions in the mesentery and there is independent evidence that they can bind to the same sites[41]. This raises the possibility that low concentrations of colchicine may be able to activate receptors normally activated by melatonin: high concentrations of colchicine may have the opposite effect and block melatonin effects[42]. Patients with psoriasis have a substantial defect in control of AA mobilization and large amounts of free AA are found in the skin[44]. Patients with psoriasis have exceptionally low circulating melatonin levels and no normal nocturnal rise[43]. If melatonin is necessary for the $TXA_2$ control of AA mobilization, these two mechanisms could be reconciled. Colchicine has been used in the treatment of psoriasis. It causes hair loss as a side effect but this side effect disappears in September when endogenous melatonin production tends to rise[45]. Melatonin and colchicine also seem able substantially to enhance the effect of zinc on formation of 1 series PGs and in platelets colchicine increased 1 series PG production.

Putting these observations together leads to the hypothesis of regulation of PG synthesis shown in Figure 40.3. This is a self-regulating system which will

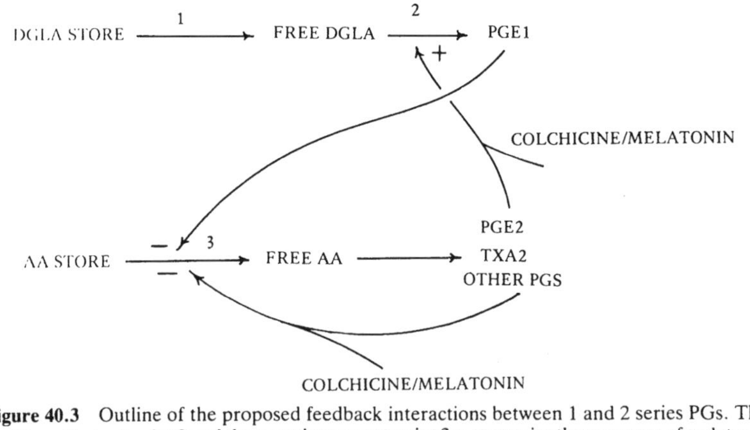


**Figure 40.3** Outline of the proposed feedback interactions between 1 and 2 series PGs. The positive effects at point 2 and the negative ones at point 3 may require the presence of melatonin or a ligand which can bind to melatonin receptors such as colchicine in low concentrations. Zinc, levamisole and penicillamine seem to act at point 1 by increasing the formation of free DGLA. It is stressed that this concept is at present expressed only in very general terms. Other PG products of each pathway are very likely to play roles in it and these roles may differ from tissue to tissue and species to species

ensure that production of the 1 and 2 series compounds remains in balance. This should not be regarded as more than a preliminary sighting shot at understanding regulation of PG formation and no doubt many other factors will be found to interact with the system. However, it does provide a framework for testing hypotheses and does lead to some interesting predictions. The way the system might work is shown in the following examples:

(1) A primary fall in $PGE_1$ formation will lead to increased AA mobilization, and hence enhanced production of $TXA_2$ and $PGE_2$ which will raise $PGE_1$ levels back to normal.

(2) A primary rise in $PGE_1$ synthesis will shut off AA mobilization, reduce formation of $PGE_2$ and $TXA_2$ and hence reduce formation of $PGE_1$.

(3) A primary rise in 2 series PG formation will enhance $PGE_1$.

(3) A primary rise in 2 series PG formation will enhance $PGE_1$ synthesis which will shut of AA mobilization and lower 2 series PG levels to normal.

(4) A primary fall in 2 series PG production will remove $PGE_2$ and $TXA_2$ stimulation of $PGE_1$ synthesis, enhance mobilization of AA and raise 2 series PG levels to normal.

Thus, provided that dietary supplies of DGLA and AA are adequate, provided that all the co-factors for the reactions are present, and provided the feedback loops remain intact, PG synthesis should be self-regulating with production of the 1 and 2 series held in balance. A number of factors could throw the system into disorder. Some examples are as follows:

(1) Inadequate provision of essential fatty acids in the diet or inadequate conversion of linoleic aid to gamma-linolenic acid because of inhibition of delta-6-desaturase by saturated fats and trans-fatty acids, by ageing, by insulin lack or by other factors[46]. Body stores of DGLA are much greater than those of AA. A partial inadequacy of essential fatty acid intake will therefore seriously deplete DGLA stores at a time when AA stores have hardly been affected. In consequence, $PGE_1$ levels will fall, control of AA mobilization will be lost and production of 2 series PGs will increase. Normally this would lead to a compensating rise in $PGE_1$ with a switch-off of AA mobilization but because of DGLA depletion this control will not operate. As a consequence there will be sustained elevation of 2 series PG production coupled with a deficiency in the 1 series. That this is a real rather than simply a theoretical possiblity is indicated by situation of children with cystic fibrosis[46,47]. Whether because of pancreatic failure or a metabolic error, these children are naturally partially deficient in essential fatty acids with low blood levels of linoleate. Yet, paradoxically, they have raised circulating levels of 2 series PGs[47]. Feeding linoleate, far

from exaggerating the PG abnormality as might be instinctively expected, actually brings the PG levels down to normal. This actually observed series of events is a directly predictable consequence of our proposed feedback loop. This might explain the reported effects of essential fatty acids in rheumatoid arthritis[48] and the fact that transformed cells which have lost their delta-6-desaturase[49] consistently show high rates of 2 series PG formation.

(2) Inadequate provision of the co-factors necessary for $PGE_1$ formation would lead to consequences similar to those described above. These required co-factors include pyridoxine, zinc and ascorbic acid, all of which may be consumed in marginally adequate amounts by those on a typical Western diet[46,50,51]. This might explain the reported effects of zinc in rheumatoid arthritis although no doubt many factors may be involved[52].

(3) Blockade of $TXA_2$ and/or $PGE_2$ receptors, and/or selective blockade of their formation beyond the endoperoxide level, would lead to loss of feedback control of arachidonate metabolism. Radiation has been reported to have one or other effects[52,53] possibly accounting for increased 2 series PG production after radiation.

(4) Blockade of the melatonin/colchicine receptors or loss of the melatonin or melatonin like ligands which seem important in inhibiting AA mobilization and enhancing $PGE_1$ formation could cause loss of regulatory control. This may be important in the excess AA mobilization in psoriasis (see previous section).

(5) Selective blockade of $PGE_1$ formation (e.g., by an opioid produced in response to stress) would lead to the consequences outlined in (1).

(6) Virus infection and radiation exposure have a number of features in common and it is possible that viruses could act by blocking $TXA_2/PGE_2$ formation or by blocking the feedback effects of these agents.

## PGs, THE IMMUNE SYSTEM AND FIBROUS TISSUE FORMATION

The effects of PGs on immunity are exceedingly complex. PGEs have been studied more extensively than PGFs which seem to be relatively inactive. $PGE_1$ and $PGE_2$ have many similar effects, which is partly to be expected from their structures and partly from the stimulation of $PGE_1$ formation by $PGE_2$. It is usually argued that the PGE effects are mediated by cyclic AMP but it is highly improbable that this is the whole story. As will become apparent we believe that the calcium effects are very important.

Detailed analysis of the effects of $PGE_1$ on humoral immunity suggests that very low levels enhance antibody formation while higher levels inhibit it[6–11]. It has recently been convincingly argued that the differences between helper and suppressor interactions between T lymphocytes and B lymphocytes are simply a matter of cell concentration[54]. Low cell concentrations enhance and high cell concentrations inhibit antibody formation and the apparent effects of cell separation may be simply due to the inevitable concentration changes produced by separation techniques. Since PG levels in a culture are likely to be a function of cell density it is very possible that PGs could be involved in this effect. Simply shaking a culture may convert helper into suppressor function[55], an observation consistent with the PG hypothesis since mechanical stimulation increases PG formation.

Similar observations have been made with respect to the effects of PGs on fibrous tissue and glycosaminoglycan formation. Moderate PG depletion by essential fatty acid deficient diets or moderate doses of NSAID may lead to increased fibrous tissue and glycosaminoglycan production[2,3,5,56]. Severe PG depletion, on the other hand, may lead to defective fibrous tissue and glycosaminoglycan formation[2,3,5,56]. Similar dual responses have been noted during vitamin C deficiency states, one of the effects of which will be to reduce $PGE_1$ levels[50]. Moderate ascorbic acid depletion increases fibrous tissue formation and enhances humoral immune responses with the development of auto-immune disease[50,57]. Severe vitamin C depletion produces immune failure and loss of normal fibrous tissue production. It seems possible that $PGE_1$ is particularly important in collagen formation since zinc and vitamin C, two factors critical for collagen production, act at successive points on the $PGE_1$ pathway.

$PGE_1$ seems particularly important for T lymphocyte function. The evidence has been reviewed in detail[46]. It includes the observations that the thymus is the only tissue which has been consistently found to contain high $PGE_1$ levels, that zinc and vitamin C which are necessary for T lymphocyte function are both necessary for $PGE_1$ formation, that $PGE_1$ and thymic hormone have a number of similar actions both *in vitro* and *in vivo*, and that $PGE_1$ can in part control the auto-immune disease in the NZB/W mouse which is associated with defective T lymphocytes[9].

Thus $PGE_1$ seems important in both the regulation of immunity and of fibrous tissue formation and its effects have repeatedly been shown to follow a 'bell-shaped' pattern, with low concentrations enhancing immune responses and net collagen production and high $PGE_1$ concentrations inhibiting these same parameters. It seems to us that the parallels with the effects of $PGE_1$ on intracellular calcium release are of particular interest (Figure 40.1). Calcium is an important regulator of many cell processes, through effects on membranes, effects on calcium-dependent regulator proteins, and effects on release of lysosomal enzymes and on mitochondrial function. The peak effect of $PGE_1$ in enhancing intracellular calcium release seems to occur in the region of $10^{-11}$ mol/l. Levels of $PGE_1$ in the vicinity of cells may well be in the

$10^{-10}$ – $10^{-8}$ mol/l range, to the right of this peak. Suppose that the $PGE_1$ effects on calcium, on lysosomes, on T cell helper functions and on fibrous tissue formation all reach a peak at around $10^{-11}$ mol/l. If normal $PGE_1$ levels are around $10^{-9}$ mol/l, then all these parameters will be less than maximally activated. Moderate reduction of $PGE_1$ levels such as might occur with dietary deficiencies, with opioid release in response to stress or with lithium, will move the situation leftwards up to the peak of the 'bell' with increased lysosomal activity, increased antibody and auto-antibody formation and increased fibrous tissue production. Severe reduction of $PGE_1$ levels will cause a leftwards move down from the peak with reduced evidence of inflammation and auto-immunity because of reduced mobilization of intracellular calcium. This may be the situation which occurs in schizophrenics who appear to have very seriously reduced rates of $PGE_1$ formation in platelets, coupled with evidence of resistance to inflammatory states such as rheumatoid arthritis[58].

## UNDERSTANDING DRUG EFFECTS

The work presented in this paper suggests new approaches to the understanding of diseases of inflammation and immunity and may possibly introduce a new logic into the therapeutic approaches to these diseases. The fundamental proposition is that most chronic disorders of inflammation and immunity are associated with reduced 1 series and increased 2 series PG production. Some of the problems are caused by the 2 series excess and some by the lack of 1 series compounds, notably $PGE_1$. Which particular disease syndrome affects a particular individual will depend on the genetic background and environmental exposures of that individual. This concept leads to the following comments on actions of drugs.

### NSAID

These will inhibit formation of both 1 and 2 series PGs. They will alleviate problems due to 2 series excess. They will worsen problems caused by $PGE_1$ deficiency or have no effect if 1 series PG levels are already low. They will prevent the development of normal feedback controls. Since they do not usually inhibit the lipoxygenases, NSAID may exaggerate problems caused by excess production of leukotrienes from mobilized AA.

### Steroids

These will also block both 1 and 2 series PG formation. they may be more potent than the NSAID since they inhibit AA mobilization and so block leukotriene as well as PG formation. Otherwise the problems are similar to those with the NSAID. The failure of the NSAID and steroids to modify the courses of chronic inflammatory states for the better may relate to their failure to increase $PGE_1$ production.

**Zinc and levamisole**

These agents seem able to enhance $PGE_1$ production by increasing AA mobilization. It should be noted that if the bell-shaped curve is important, they will be initially effective only in those whose endogenous $PGE_1$ levels are on the peak of to the *right* of it. The theory predicts that those whose $PGE_1$ levels are so low that they are down the left hand side of the bell will initially be made *worse* as they move up to the peak. Improvement may then follow if they can be pushed over on to the right hand side.

**Penicillamine**

This seems to activate $PGE_1$ synthesis by mobilizing DGLA but it is a zinc chelator and in the long-term *in vivo* may actually *decrease* $PGE_1$ production by mobilizing and excreting zinc. If this is the case then penicillamine may work in at least some patients by pulling them down the left side of the bell. This may explain why successful anti-inflammatory responses are often accompanied by signs of zinc deficiency and why zinc supplementation may nullify the effects of penicillamine[59].

**Anti-malarials**

These may enhance $PGE_1$ formation by increasing conversion of DGLA to $PGE_1$ and they may also have PG antagonist actions[60].

## LOGICAL APPROACHES TO THERAPY

If these proposals are correct, then steroids and NSAID should never be used in long-term therapy except as a last resort. They will prevent normal formation of $PGE_1$ and will block the development of normal feedback relationships. An ideal sequence of events in therapy might be as follows:

(1) Establish a state of optimum nutrition. Since normal feedback relationships cannot be established according to this concept in the absence of normal $PGE_1$ formation, adequate provision of the nutritional requirements for $PGE_1$ synthesis is a *sine qua non* for any therapy. Recent dietary studies of urbanized populations suggest that nutrients whose intake is particularly likely to be marginal include essential fatty acids, pyridoxine, vitamin C and zinc. These have been reviewed and promising preliminary results have been obtained by treating patients with Sjogren's syndrome with evening primrose oil (the richest natural source of essential fatty acids) and with vitamin C[46,57]. Attention to nutritional status may thus have therapeutic effects by itself. It is also likely to make patients more sensitive to agents which enhance $PGE_1$ production, thus enabling control to be achieved at lower and less toxic dose levels.

(2) Drugs effective in long term control of inflammation and auto-immunity.

Colchicine, which seems to sensitize the feedback mechanism, may well be the most under-utilized drug in this field. The relatively high doses used in acute gout have made people unduly aware of its potential toxicity. The much lower doses used in the prevention of inflammatory episodes in gout, FMF[16,17] and necrotizing vasculitis[18], seem to be effectively without toxicity even in children and pregnant women. There is some evidence that colchicine may also help in situations where there is excess fibrous tissue formation[61,62]. Histidine seems to be required for its action[40], and this may contribute to its ineffectiveness in rheumatoid arthritis in which histidine levels are low[63]. Penicillamine, zinc and levamisole may enhance $PGE_1$ formation at a point different from that of colchicine and so there are logical reasons for adding them to a colchicine regime, perhaps in lower doses than they are normally used. Antimalarials may perhaps be similarly employed.

(3) Since $TXA_2$ seems important in the feedback process, defective formation of $TXA_2$ would lead to loss of feedback control. Amantadine has actions consistent with enhancement of $TXA_2$ formation *in vitro*[29] and may enhance $TXA_2$ formation *in vivo*[64]. The possible importance of this is indicated by recent observations on the treatment of $NZB_1W$ mice with essental fatty acids and amantadine. $PGE_2$ in these mice controls many features of this disease but does not lower titres of anti-DNA antibodies. Essential fatty acids alone also failed to lower antibody titre, but the combination of essential fatty acids (evening primrose oil) and amantadine together was successful in correcting this abnormality[64].

(4) Only if control cannot be achieved by mechanisms which will maintain rather than break the feedback loops should NSAID and steroids be employed in the long term.

**Acknowledgments**

The experimental work on which this work is based was financially supported by the Muscular Dystrophy Association of Canada, by Dr David Roy, by Mrs Sydney Duder and by the Fisher Family Foundation.

## References

1 Lewis, G. P. (1978). Inflammation, with emphasis on its mediation. *Ann. R. Coll. Surg. Eng:* **60,** 192

2 Bonta, I. L. and Parnham, M. J. (1978). Time-dependent pro- and anti-inflammatory effects of prostagland in $E_1$ on experimental granulomata in rats. *Br. J. Pharmacol.*, **62,** 417P

3 Kulonen, E. and Potila, M. (1975). Effect of the administration of antirheumatic drugs on experimental granuloma in the rat. *Biochem. Pharmacol.*, **24,** 417P

4 James, G. W. L. and Church, M. K. (1978). Hyperalgesia after treatment of mice with prostaglandins and arachidonic acid and its antagonism by anti-inflammatory compounds. *Arzneim. Forsch.*, **28,** 804

5 Bonta, I. L., Bult, H., Parnham, M. J. and Vincent, J. E. (1978). Inflammatory models in rats depleted of endogenous precursors of prostaglandins. *Agents Actions*, **8,** 98

6 Goldyne, M. E. (1977). Prostaglandins and the modulation of immunological responses. *Int. J. Dermatol.*, **16**, 701

7 Ishizuka, M., Taeuchi, T. and Umezawa, H. (1974). Promotion of antibody formation by prostaglandin. *Experientia*, **30**, 1207

8 Plescia, O. J., Smith, A. H. and Grinwick, K. (1975). Subversion of immune system by tumor cells and role of prostaglandins. *Proc. Natl. Acad. Sci. (USA)*, **72**, 1848

9 Krakauer, K., Torrey, S. B. and Zurier, R. B. (1978). Prostaglandin $E_1$ treatment of NZB/W mice. III. *Clin. Immunol. Immunopathol.*, **11**, 256

10 Webb, E. R. and Osheroff, P. L. (1976). Antigen stimulation of prostaglandin synthesis and control of immune responses. *Proc. Natl. Acad. Sci. (USA)*, **73**, 1300

11 Quagliata, F, Lawrence, V. J. W. and Phillips-Quagliata, J. M. (1973). Prostaglandin $E_1$ as a regulator of lymphocyte function. *Cell. Immunol.*, **6**, 457

12 Famaey, J. P., Fontaine, J. and Reuse, J. (1976). The effects of D-penicillamine on ileal smooth muscle and their possible relationships with prostaglandins. In Munthe, E. (ed.) *Penicillamine: Research in Rheumatoid Disease*, pp. 50–57. (Rahway: Merck Sharp & Dohme).

13 Cunnane, S. C., Zinner, H. Horrobin, D. F. *et al.* (1979). Copper inhibits pressor responses to noradrenaline but not potassium. Interactions with prostaglandins $E_1$, $E_2$ and $I_2$ and penicillamine. *Can. J. Physiol. Pharmacol.*, **57**, 35

14 Robinson, D. R., Smith, H., McGuire, M. B. and Levine, L. (1975). Prostaglandin synthesis by rheumatoid synovia and its stimulation by colchicine. *Prostaglandins*, **10**, 67

15 Floman, Y. (1978). Prostaglandin E production by cultured inflamed rat synovium: stimulation by colchicine and inhibition by chloroquine. *Prostaglandins Med.*, **1**, 39

16 Goldfinger, S. E. (1972). Colchicine for familial Mediterranean fever. *New Eng. J. Med.*, **287**, 1302

17 Lehman, T. J. A., Peters, R. S., Hanson, V. and Schwabe, A. D. (1978). Long term colchicine therapy of familial Mediterranean fever. *J. Pediatr.*, **93**, 876

18 Hazen, P. G., and Michel, B. (1979: Management of necrotizing vasculitis with colchicine. *Arch. Dermatol.*, **115**, 1303

19 Kloeze, J. (1969). Relationship between chemical structure and platelet aggregation activity of prostaglandins. *Biochim. Biophys. Acta*, **187**, 285

20 Kunkel, S. L., Thrall, R. S., Kunkel, R. G. *et al.* (1976). Suppression of immune complex vasculitis in rats by prostaglandin. *J. Clin. Invest.*, **64**, 1525

21 Feinstein, M. B., Becker, E. L. and Fraser, C. (1977). Thrombin, collagen and A23187 stimulated platelet arachidonate metabolism: differential inhibition by $PGE_1$, local anesthetics and a serine-protease inhibitor. *Prostaglandins*, **14**, 1075

22 Minkes, M., Stanford, N., Chi, M. M. Y. *et al.* (1977). Cyclic adenosine monophosphate inhibits the availability of arachidonate to prostaglandin synthetase in human platelet suspensions. *J. Clin. Invest.*, **59**, 449

23 Manku, M. S., Horrobin, D. F., Karmazyn, M. and Cunnane, S. C. (1979) Prolactin and zinc effects on rat vascular reactivity: possible relationship to dihomogammalinolenic acid and to prostagland in synthesis. *Endocrinology*, **104**, 774

24 Kirtland, S. J. and Baum, H. (1972). Prostaglandin $E_1$ may act as a calcium ionophore. *Nature (London) New Biol.*, **236**, 47

25 Manku, M. S. and Horrobin, D. F. (1976). Indomethacin inhibits responses to all vasoconstrictors in the rat mesenteric vascular bed: restoration of responses by prostaglandin $E_2$. *Prostaglandins*, **12**, 369

26 Manku, M. S., Oka, M. and Horrobin, D. F. (1979). Differential regulation of the formation of prostaglandins and related substances from arachidonic acid and from dihomogammalinolenic acid. 1. Effects of ethanol. *Prostaglandins Med.*, **3**, 119

27 Manku, M.S., Oka, M. and Horrobin, D. F. (1979). Differential regulation of the formation of prostaglandins and related substances from arachidonic acid and from dihomogammalinolenic acid. 11. Effects of vitamin C. *Prostaglandins Med.*, **3**, 129

28 Horrobin, D. F. (1979). Cellular basis of prolactin action: involvement of cyclic nucleotides, polyamines, prostaglandins, steroids, thyroid hormones, Na/K ATPases and calcium: relevance to breast cancer and the menstrual cycle. *Med. Hypotheses*, **5**, 599

29 Horrobin, D. F. (1978). *Prostaglandins: Physiology, Pharmacology and Clinical Significance.* (Edinburgh: Churchill Livingstone)

30 Cunnane, S. C., Horrobin, D. F., Manku, M. S. *et al.* (1980). The vascular response to zinc

varies seasonally: effects of pinealectomy and melatonin. *Chronobiologia,* (In press)
31 Kondo, K., Manku, M. A., Horrobin, D. F. *et al.* (1977). Potentiation of the pressor effects of noradrenaline and potassium ions in rat mesenteric arteries by physiological levels of angiotensin II: effects of prostaglandin E2 and cortisol. *Clin. Sci. Mol. Med.,* **53,** 233
32 Karmazyn, M., Manku, M. S. and Horrobin, D. F. (1978). Changes of vascular reactivity induced by low vasopressin concentrations: interactions with cortisol and lithium and possible involvement of prostaglandins. *Endocrinology,* **102,** 1230
33 Karmazyn, M., Horrobin, D. F., Manku, M. S. *et al.* (1977). Myo-Inositol in physiological concentrations stimulates production of prostaglandin-like material. *Prostaglandins,* **14,** 967
34 Manku, M. S., Horrobin, D. F., Seidah, N. and Chretien, M. (1977). Beta-endorphin inhibits the effects of prolactin on synthesis of $PGE_1$-like material. Presented at the International Conference on Central Nervous System Effects of Hypothalamic Hormones and Other Peptides, Montreal, May 2.
35 Bell, R. L , Kennerly, D. A., Stanford, N. and Majerus, P. W. (1979). Diglyceride lipase: a pathway for arachidonate release from human platelets. *Proc. Natl. Acad. Sci. (USA),* **76,** 3238
36 Rittenhouse-Simmons, S. (1979). Production of diglycerides from phosphatidyl inositol in activated human platelets. *J. Clin. Invest.,* **63,** 580
37 Boot, J. R., Dawson, W. and Kitchen, E. A. (1976). The chemotactic activity of thromboxane $B_2$: a possible role in inflammation. *J. Physiol.,* **257,** 47P
38 Malawista, S. E. (1975). The action of colchicine in acute gouty arthritis. *Arthritis Rheum.,* **18,** 835
39 Horrobin, D. F., Manku, M. S., Karmali, R. A. *et al.* (1978). Thromboxane A2: a key regulator of prostaglandin biosynthesis and of interactions between prostaglandins, calcium and cyclic nucleotides. *Med. Hypotheses,* **4,** 178
40 Horrobin, D. F., Oka, M. and Manku, M. S. (1978). Thromboxane $A_2$ as a regulator of prostaglandin synthesis. Relevance to interactions between colchicine and histidine in the control of inflammation. *Eur. J. Rheum.,* **2,** 181
41 Fitzgerald, T. J. and Veal, A. (1976). Melatonin antagonizes colchicine-induced mitotic arrest. *Experientia,* **32,** 372
42 Malawista, S. E. (1971). The melanocyte model. Colchicine-like effects of other anit-mitotic agents. *J. Cell Biol.,* **49,** 848
43 Birau, N. and Schloot, W. (1979). Pathological nyctohemeral rhythm of melatonin secretion in psoriasis, Klinefelter's syndrome and spina bifida. *IRCS J. Med. Sci.,* **7,** 400
44 Hammarstrom, S., Hamberg, M., Duell, E. A. *et al.* (1975). Increased concentrations of non-esterified arachidonic acid, 12L-hydroxy-5,8,10,14-eicosatrienoic acid, prostaglandin $E_2$ and prostaglandin $F_2$ alpha in epidermis of psoriasis. *Proc. Natl. Acad. Sci. (USA),* **72,** 5130
45 Malkinson, F. E. and Lynfield, Y. L. (1959). Colchicine alopecia. *J. Invest. Dermatol.,* **33,** 371
46 Horrobin, D. F., Manku, M. S., Oka, M. *et al.* (1979). The nutritional regulation of T lymphocyte function. *Med. Hypotheses,* **5,** 969
47 Chase, H. P. and Dupont, J. (1978). Abnormal levels of prostaglandins and fatty acids in blood of children with cystic fibrosis. *Lancet,* **2,** 36
48 McCormick, J. N., Neill, W. A. and Sim, A. K. (1977). Immunosuppressive effect of linoleic acid. *Lancet,* **2,** 508
49 Dunbar, L. M. and Bailey, J. M. (1975). Enzyme deletions and essential fatty acid metabolism in cultured cells. *J. Biol. Chem.,* **250,** 1152
50 Horrobin, D. F., Oka, M. and Manku, M. S. (1979). The regulation of prostaglandin $E_1$ formation: a candidate for one of the fundamental mechanisms involved in the actions of vitamin C. *Med. Hypotheses,* **5,** 849
51 Horrobin, D. F. and Cunnane, S. C. (1980). Interactions between zinc, essential fatty acids and prostaglandins: relevance to acrodermatitis enteropathica, total parenteral nutrition, the glucagonoma syndrome, diabetes, anorexia nervosa and sickle cell anaemia. *Med. Hypotheses,* **6,** 277
52 Johnson, M., Jessup, R. and Ramwell, P. (1973). Ultraviolet light modification of the prostaglandin receptor. *Prostaglandins,* **4.** 593
53 Manku, M. S., Horrobin, D. F., Oka, M. *et al.* (1978). Ultra-violet radiation and 8-

methoxypsoralen have actions similar to those of known inhibitors of thromboxane $A_2$ synthesis in rat mesenteric blood vessels. *Prostaglandins Med.*, **1**, 86

54 Farrant, J. and Knight, S. C. (1979). Help and suppression by lymphoid cells as a function of cellular concentration. *Proc. Natl. Acad. Sci. (USA)*, **76**, 3507

55 Eardley, D. D., Staskawicz, M. O. and Gershon, R. K. (1976). Suppressor cells: dependence on assay conditions for functional activity. *J. Exp. Med.*, **143**, 1211

56 Dekel, S., Falconer, J. and Francis, M. J. O. (1980): The effect of anti-inflammatory drugs on glycosaminoglycan sulphation in pig cartilage. *Prostaglandins Med.*, **4**, 133

57 Horrobin, D. F. and Campbell, A. (1980). Sjogren's syndrome and the sicca syndrome: the role of prostaglandin $E_1$ deficiency. Treatment with essential fatty acids and vitamin C. *Med. Hypotheses*, **6**, 225

58 Horrobin, D. F. (1979). Schizophrenia: reconciliation of the dopamine, prostaglandin and opioid concepts and the role of the pineal. *Lancet*, **1**, 529

59 Mery, C., Delrieu, F., Ghozlan, R. *et al.* (1976). A controlled trial of D-penicillamine in rheumatoid arthritis – dose effect and the role of zinc. *Scand. J. Rheumatol.*, **5**, 241

60 Manku, M. S. and Horrobin, D. F. (1976). Chloroquine, quinine, procaine, quinidine, tricyclic antidepressants and methyl xanthines are prostglandin agonists and antagonists. *Lancet*, **2**, 1115

61 Alarcon-Segovia, D., Ibanez, G. and Kershenobich, D. (1974). Treatment of scleroderma by modification of collagen metabolism. A double blind trial with colchicine versus placebo. *J. Rheumatol*, **1**, 97

62 Trnavska, Z., Mikulikova, D. and Trnavsky, K. (1977). The effects of colchicine and its derivatives on collagen biosynthesis *in vitro*. *Agents Actions*, **7**, 563

63 Gerber, D. A. (1975). Low free serum histidine concentration in rheumatoid arthritis. A measure of disease activity. *J. Clon. Invest.*, **55**, 1164

64 Karmali, R. A., Hanrahan, R., Volkman, A. and Smith, N. (1980). Regulation of autoimmunity and development of antibodies to DNA in NZB/W mice (Submitted for publication)

# 41

# Human haptoglobin: an endogenous inhibitor of prostaglandin synthase

S. A. SAEED, P. A. DENNING-KENDALL,
W. J. McDONALD-GIBSON AND H. O. J. COLLIER (UK)

## INTRODUCTION

Human blood plasma haptoglobin (Hp) is a well-characterized glycoprotein present in the $\alpha_2$-globulin fraction of most mammalian plasma or serum. The most characteristic property of Hp is to bind haemoglobin (Hb) stoichiometrically and irreversibly. Several good reviews[9,17] have appeared on the chemistry and physiology of Hp. but its exact physiological function still remains uncertain. It is well known that Hp levels in the serum vary greatly in different conditions. It is usually elevated in inflammatory conditions and acute infections, but depressed in severe chronic liver disease and certain haemolytic conditions[7]. For the past few years we have been studying the inhibition of prostaglandin (PG) biosynthesis by human blood plasma or serum[7,14]. These studies demonstrated that Hp potently inhibits PG synthesis. This finding suggested that the biological function of Hp may be associated with the inhibition of PG synthesis *in vivo*. We have therefore evaluated the effects of purified Hp on several test systems used to study PG synthase inhibitors.

## METHODS

### Assay of bull seminal vesicle PG synthase activity

Two methods were used for the assay of PG synthase activity of bull seminal vesicle homogenate (BSV). The first was measurement of oxygen uptake during cyclo-oxygenation of arachidonic acid and the second was bioassay of $PGE_2$ on hamster fundic strip. The standard assay mixture used for both assays contained 50 mmol/l sodium phosphate buffer pH 7.4, 6 mg/ml BSV homogenate protein, 61 $\mu$mol/l sodium arachidonate as substrate, an appropriate amount of test substance and 1.3 mmol/l reduced glutathione (GSH) as co-factor.

*Preparation of enzyme*

Bovine seminal vesicles from non-castrated adult bulls, supplied either fresh or frozen from a local abattoir, were freed of fat and connective tissue at room temperature before the homogenate was prepared at 4 °C. The vesicles were cut into small pieces and put through a meat mincer. The coarsely ground mixture thus obtained was homogenized in a Kenwood food blender with three volumes of 50 mmol/l phosphate buffer pH 7.4. The resulting homogenate was clarified first by straining through cheesecloth and then by centrifugation at 600 g for 15 min. The supernatant was removed, saturated with oxygen-free nitrogen and stored in aliquots at −20 °C for up to 6 months. This preparation containing 24 mg/ml protein was used as a source of BSV PG synthase.

*Preparation of substrate*

Arachidonic acid (Grade I) was supplied by Sigma. A 10 mg ampoule (99% pure) was taken up in 1.0 ml of 96% ethanol and diluted to 10.0 ml with 0.2% w/v aqueous sodium carbonate. This solution was stored at −20 °C and diluted when required in 50 mmol/l phosphate buffer.

*Measurement of oxygen uptake by BSV homogenate (cyclo-oxygenase activity)*

The uptake of oxygen into arachidonic acid by BSV homogenate was determined by difference from measurements at 37 °C of oxygen saturation of the incubates with a Yellow Springs Instrument Co. Model 53 oxygen monitor and a Toshima electron flat-bed recorder. The instrument and recorder were calibrated with air saturated distilled water at 37 °C. A standard incubation volume of 4 ml was used and the reaction initiated by the addition of 1 ml of BSV homogenate at 37 °C after a 3 min pre-incubation of all other components, allowing them also to reach 37 °C. The addition of enzyme was followed immediately by insertion of the oxygen electrode, and the change in oxygen saturation of the incubate recorded for 15 min. The proportion of total oxygen uptake that could be attributed to cyclo-oxygenase activity in this test system was determined with indomethacin. The maximal inhibition of oxygen uptake by indomethacin (28 $\mu$mol/l was 51.9 ± 1.3% whereas inhibition of $PGE_2$ was complete. Since indomethacin is a known cyclo-oxygenase inhibitor it was assumed that this proportion of the oxygen consumption was directed towards the production of prostaglandins (cyclo-oxygenase). To calculate inhibition of cyclo-oxygenase activity, test samples were incubated both with and without indomethacin at 28 μmol/l. The negative control was an incubate containing substrate, co-factor, buffer but no enzyme.

*Bioassay of $PGE_2$ on hamster fundic strip*

PG activity was measured as described previously[2], using a standard assay mixture of 2 ml. The negative control was an incubate containing boiled (10 min) BSV homogenate. The reaction was started by addition of 61 μmol/l sodium arachidonate and the mixture was incubated aerobically with gentle shaking for 15 min at 37 °C. PGs were extracted in acidified ethyl acetate and assayed on hamster stomach strip, as described elsewhere[2,20]. Total PG activity was expressed in terms of a reference standard $PGE_2$.

**Measurement of haptoglobin**

Hp concentration in plasma, serum or purified Hp preparations was determined according to the peroxidase method of Connell and Smithies[3] and expressed as haemoglobin-binding capacity (HbBC). Briefly, this method depends on the peroxidase activity of haemoglobin–haptoglobin complexes. Hydrogen peroxide is the oxidizing substrate, and guaiacol the hydrogen donor. The reaction conditions are chosen so that the peroxidase activity of free haemoglobin (Hb) is essentially zero. The formation of teraguaiacol during the reaction was followed spectrophotometrically at 470 nm. In the present work the assay was calibrated with human plasma Cohn fraction $IV_4$ as a source of Hp and lyophilized human methaemoglobin (Sigma). It should be noted that the peroxidase activity of the complexes is independent of Hp phenotype[10].

**Tone of rat gastric fundus strip**

Since the intrinsic tone of the isolated rat gastric fundus strip is due to intramural generation of prostaglandins[6], this preparation can be used as an index of PG synthesis[2]. A strip of rat gastric fundus was suspended from a Harvard isotonic transducer (H386) under a tension of 1 g in a 4 ml organ bath at 37 °C, in Krebs solution bubbled with 5% $CO_2$ in oxygen and the response was recorded. After setting up, the preparation was washed repeatedly with Krebs solution for about 1 h, and, when the tone was constant, small volumes (0.005–0.2 ml) of sodium arachidonate, dissolved in ethanol, 10% in 0.2% $Na_2CO_3$ in water, were added in increasing concentration every 5 min until the tone was maximal (usual dose range, 4 to 657 μmol/l arachidonate). The concentration of arachidonate required to increase tone to 25% of maximum (SC25) under control conditions was determined graphically. To measure the effects of Hp the above procedure was repeated in the presence of test substance after 20 min pre-incubation with the test substance before addition of arachidonate, and the SC25 values were determined as before.

**Arachidonate or bradykinin induced bronchoconstriction in the guinea pig**

Male albino guinea pigs weighing 400–600 g each (Dunkin–Hartley strain) were anaesthetized by administration of sodium pentobarbitone, 60 mg/kg intraperitoneally. The trachea was cannulated for artificial ventilation by a Starling pump (5–8 ml) at 72 strokes/min via a Fleisch pneumatochograph. The difference in pressure across this device was measured with a Grass differential pressure transducer. This gives a flow signal which was fed into a Hewlett-Packard 8816A analogue computer. Transpulmonary pressure (TPP) was measured with another differential pressure transducer via side arms to the thoracic cavity and the tracheal cannula. The signals for low and TPP were applied to the analogue computer so that there was approximately 180° phase difference. The computer derived the dynamic compliance and resistance from the ingoing signals. Test substances were administered intravenously via the external jugular vein. Sodium arachidonate doses of 0.1–0.5 mg/kg or bradykinin as triacetate from Sigma at 1–5 $\mu$g/kg were given via the cannulated left external jugular vein and 'washed in' with 0.5 ml of 0.85% w/v sodium chloride solution (saline) containing 10 units/ml of heparin. These doses were given at 30 min intervals to produce a large but submaximal bronchoconstriction. After 2 or 3 similar responses to the same dose of challenge substance had been obtained, the test substance in saline (0.1–1 ml) was injected intravenously, and 45 s after another dose of challenge substance is given.

**Measurement of platelet aggregation**

Human blood obtained from healthy donors who had not taken any non-steroidal anti-inflammatory drugs for 1 week was immediately mixed with 10 units/ml of heparin and centrifuged at 200 g for 15 min. The platelet-rich plasma thus obtained was centrifuged at 600 *g* for 15 min and the resulting platelet pellet washed with saline. The pellet of washed platelets was then suspended in 0.5 volumes of 0.1 mol/l Tris–HCl buffer, pH 7.4. Platelet aggregation was monitored with a Born aggregometer. Haptoglobin or Cohn $IV_4$ was added to 0.5 ml of platelet suspension at 37 °C, the volume was made up to 0.7 ml with saline and the mixture pre-incubated at 37 °C for 5 min, prior to the addition of sodium arachidonate (aggregating agent). The percentage inhibition due to test substance compared with control (arachidonate alone) was calculated at 1, 2, 3 and 4 min after addition of arachidonate.

## RESULTS

**Purification of haptoglobin**

The procedure was based on extraction with 60 mmol/l Tris–HCl buffer, pH 7.3 ammonium sulphate precipitation followed by ion-exchange chromatography on DE-52 cellulose. The results of the purification steps are summarized in Table 41.1. All steps were peformed at 0–4 °C and centrifugation at 600 *g* for 30 min unless otherwise specified.

**Table 41.1** Purification of haptoglobin from human plasma Cohn $IV_4$

| | *Total protein* (mg) | *Recovery of protein* (%) | *Hp content* (% w/w) | *Recovery of Hp* (%) | $IO_{50}$* (μg/ml) |
|---|---|---|---|---|---|
| Cohn $IV_4$ | 2947 | 100.0 | 15.1 ± 0.2 | 100.0 | 475 ± 30 |
| Step 1: extraction with 60 m mol/l Tris-HCl buffer, pH 7.3 | 2510 | 85.1 | 18.7 ± 0.4 | 100.0 | 372 ± 46 |
| Step 2: ammonium sulphate precipitation | 370 | 12.5 | 47.6 ± 3.8 | 43.7 | 240 ± 25 |
| Step 3: ion exchange chromatography on DEAE cellulose (fractions 39–49) | 133 | 4.5 | 75.8 ± 0.9 | 23.9 | 140 ± 8.0 |

*The amount of material required to inhibit $PGE_2$ biosynthesis, by 50%, as measured by bioassay.
For other details, see Methods.

Step 1: *Extraction with Tris–HCl buffer*
3.74 g of human plasma Cohn fraction $IV_4$ containing 2.95 g protein) prepared from normal pooled plasma was extracted with 60 mmol/l Tris–HCl buffer, pH 7.3, and centrifuged to remove any insoluble matter. The supernatant was subsequently extensively against deionized water and lyophilized. The powder obtained was stored at −20 °C until used.

Step 2: *Ammonium sulphate precipitation*
To distilled water containing 10 mg/ml of human plasma Cohn $IV_4$ powder from step 1, solid pulverized ammonium sulphate was added in small portions with stirring each time, to 50% saturation, which precipitated most of the haptoglobin (Hp). After standing for 2 h at 4 °C the suspension was centrifuged for 60 min. The clear yellow supernatant was discarded and the precipitate dissolved in a small volume of distilled water, dialysed for 24 h against frequent changes of distilled water and lyophilized.

Step 3: *Ion-exchange chromatography on DE-52 cellulose*
The lyophilized powder from step 2 containing 370 mg protein was taken up in 15 ml of 0.01 mol/l sodium acetate buffer pH 5.0 and centrifuged to remove

any insoluble matter. The clear supernatant was layered onto a 2.7 × 70 cm DE−52 cellulose column equilibrated with 0.01 mol/l acetate buffer. The elution was carried out a flow rate of 60 ml/h with a linear gradient of 0.01–0.5 mol/l acetate buffer over 48 h. The fraction collector was operated on a time basis and set to collect 15 ml fractions. Protein concentration of the eluate fractions was followed by measuring absorption at 280 nm. Fractions containing protein were then assayed for inhibition of PG synthase and Hp content.

## Result of fractionation

The results of fractionation by this method are shown in Figure 41.1 and summarized in Table 41.1. In Figure 41.1 elution profile indicates the resolution obtainable. It is evident that the major protein peak coincides with the peaks of haptoglobin and its inhibition of $PGE_2$ biosynthesis. The fractions 39–49 (Figure 41.1), which contained most of the Hp were pooled, concentrated with carbowax 20 M and dialysed against 2 l of water which was changed every 15 h for 2 days. Fractions 50–59 (Figure 41.1) were also treated in the same way. The dialysed solutions were then lyophilized and finally stored at

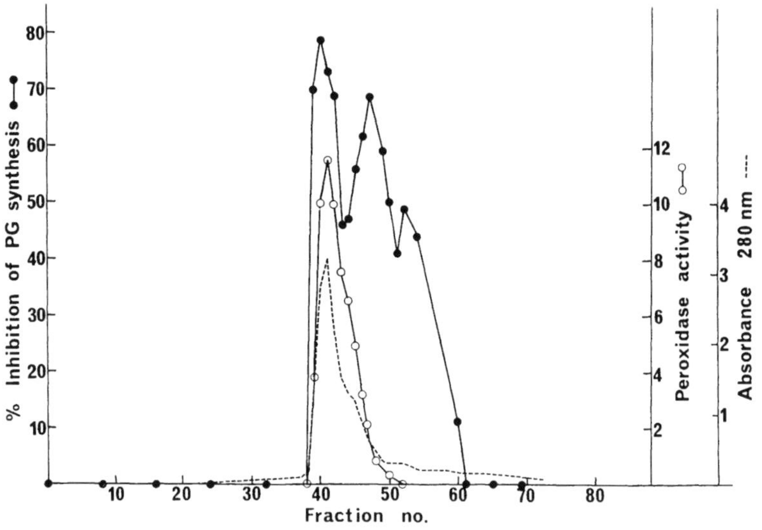


**Figure 41.1** Separation of haptoglobin on DEAE cellulose. 370 mg protein from step 2 was taken up in 15 ml of 0.01 mol/l sodium acetate buffer pH 5.0 and applied to a 2.7 × 70 cm column of DE-52 cellulose and eluted with a linear concentration gradient of 0.01–0.5 mol/l acetate buffer. Elution of protein from the column was followed by measuring absorbance at 280 nm. Inhibitory activity against $PGE_2$ biosynthesis was followed by testing aliquots of the fractions. Haptoglobin concentration was measured according to the peroxidase method of Connell and Smithies[3]

−20 °C until used for various biochemical studies. The material (fractions 39–49, Figure 41.1) prepared by this method achieved purification both of haptoglobin and its inhibitory potency of PG synthase.

Table 41.1 shows that the Hp content and its inhibitory activity on PG synthase increased at each stage of the purification procedure, the final product regularly containing 76% Hp and having over three times the inhibitory activity against PG synthase of the starting material. In Figure 41.1 it will be seen that fractions 50–60 also inhibited PG synthase. After dialysis, however, this inhibitory activity was lost. We attribute this dialysable activity to contamination by sodium acetate used as the elution buffer. The major contaminants in the 76% pure Hp preparation obtained above were: albumin 5%; glycoproteins 10%; transferrin, haemopexin and ceruloplasmin <5%. These contaminating proteins at the above concentration had no effect on PG synthase.

**Inhibition of bull seminal vesicle PG synthase by Hp**

Figures 41.2 a, b and c illustrate the concentration/response relationships for inhibition of cyclo-oxygenase activity and $PGE_2$ biosynthesis by human plasma, Cohn fraction $IV_4$ and purified Hp, respectively. It is evident that Hp was less potent against $PGE_2$ biosynthesis than against cyclo-oxygenase, but

**Table 41.2** Inhibition of increased airway resistance and decreased lung compliance induced by sodium arachidonate or bradykinin

| *Treatment* | *Dose* (mg/kg i.v.) | *Challenge Substance* | *Mean % inhibition + se of response to challenge* | |
|---|---|---|---|---|
| | | | *Resistance* | *compliance* |
| Haptoglobin (76% pure) | 5 | arachidonate sodium | 31.8 ± 4.7 | 24.4 ± 5.3 |
| | 20 | | 44.3 ± 6.7 | 34.3 ± 7.4 |
| | 50 | | 67.7 ± 0.3 | 49.0 ± 3.2 |
| | 100 | | 67.0 ± 8.0 | 64.0 ± 0 |
| Haptoglobin (76% pure) | 5 | bradykinin | 34.7 ± 1.7 | 19.5 ± 5.5 |
| | 20 | | 48.3 ± 4.4 | 33.4 ± 11.8 |
| | 50 | | 67.0 ± 0 | 73.2 ± 19.8 |
| | 100 | | 94.0 ± 6.0 | 86.5 ± 13.5 |
| Acetyl salicylate | 2 | arachidonate sodium | 85.5 ± 3.5 | 71.5 ± 6.5 |
| | 2 | bradykinin | 82.0 ± 9.6 | 80.7 ± 9.9 |
| Indomethacin | 0.03 | arachidonate sodium | 47.0 ± 15.8 | 58.7 ± 15.7 |
| | 0.1 | | 90.5 ± 9.5 | 85.5 ± 14.5 |
| | 0.01 | bradykinin | 35.5 ± 9.9 | 25.3 ± 8.2 |
| | 0.03 | | 58.0 ± 14.0 | 53.0 ± 3.0 |
| | 0.1 | | 83.5 ± 11.5 | 86.0 ± 6.0 |

For other details, see Methods.

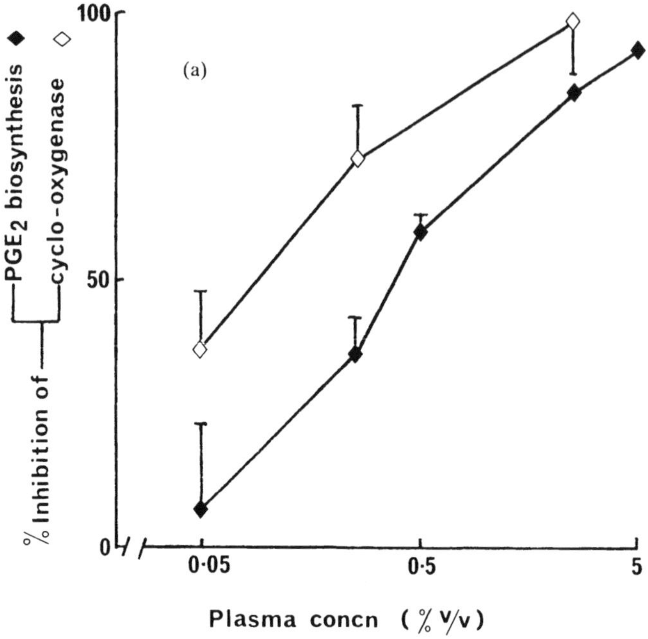
(a)
% Inhibition of
◆ PGE2 biosynthesis
◇ cyclo-oxygenase
100
50
0
0·05
0·5
5
Plasma concn (% v/v)

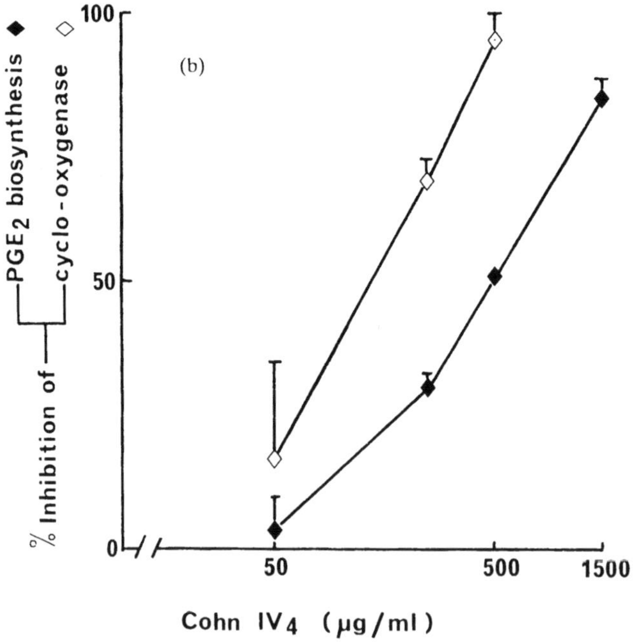
(b)
% Inhibition of
◆ PGE2 biosynthesis
◇ cyclo-oxygenase
100
50
0
50
500
1500
Cohn IV4 (µg/ml)

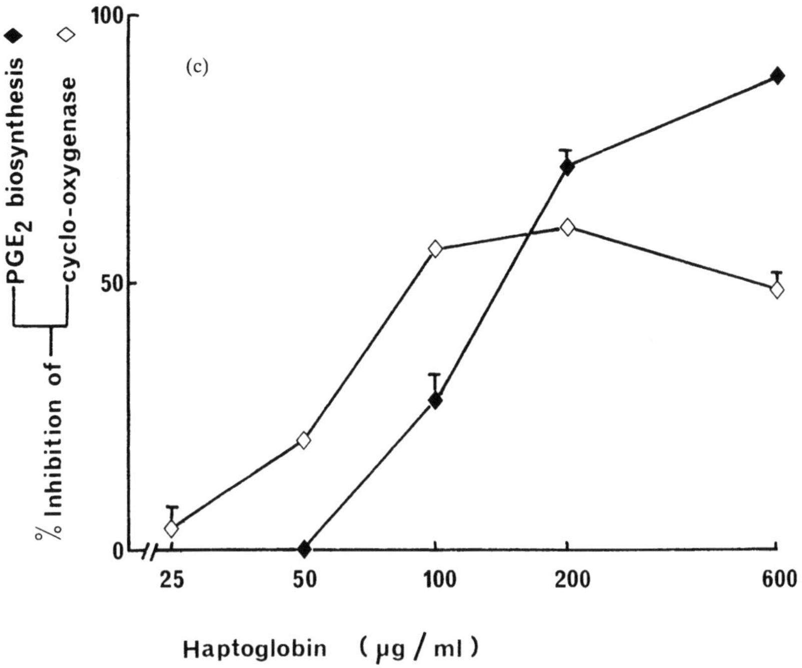


**Figure 41.2** Inhibition of $PGE_2$ biosynthesis (closed symbols) and of cyclo-oxygenase activity (open symbols) by BSV homogenate (see Methods). (a) Human plasma; (b) plasma Cohn $IV_4$; (c) haptoglobin (76% pure). Points represent the mean of at least three observations and vertical bars represent the standard error of the mean. Where no bar is shown, the error falls within the symbol

its inhibitory effect on cyclo-oxygenase was incomplete. With Cohn $IV_4$, however, virtually complete inhibition of cyclo-oxygenase was achieved.

In other experiments the time course of inhibition of $PGE_2$ by Hp was compared with that of Cohn fraction $IV_4$, using two concentrations of each inhibitor (Figure 41.3). Both Hp and Cohn fraction $IV_4$ exerted maximal effects between 10 and 15 min after the start of incubation. This compares favourably with the time course of acetyl salicylate, reported previously[14].

**Reversal by haemoglobin of inhibition of $PGE_2$ biosynthesis**

Figure 41.4 shows that human Hb, at 50 or 500 μg/ml, stimulates $PGE_2$ biosynthesis by BSV homogenate and almost completely reverses the inhibitory effect of Hp. It is evident that Hb (50 μg/ml) a concentration that completely bound Hp (100 μg/ml), abolished its inhibitory effect on $PGE_2$ biosynthesis. Neither noradrenaline nor reduced glutathione which, as cofactors of PG synthase, stimulate $PGE_2$ biosynthesis[12], antagonized the inhibitory activity of Hp (results not shown).

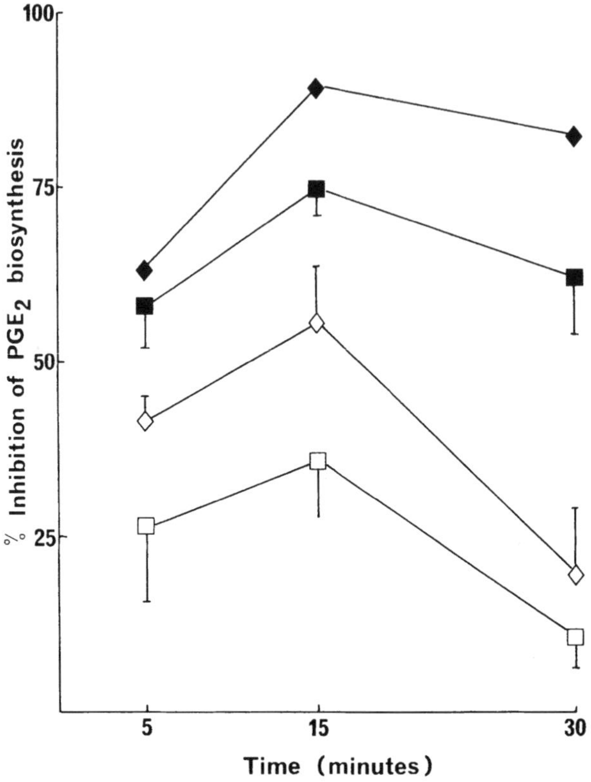


**Figure 41.3** Time course of the inhibition of $PGE_2$ biosynthesis by human plasma Cohn $IV_4$ and 76% pure haptoglobin. Two concentrations of each inhibitor: Cohn $IV_4$ 400 μg/ml ◇, and 1000 μg/ml ◆; haptoglobin 100 μg/ml □, and 200 μg/ml ■. Each point represents the mean of at least three observations

**Inhibition of tone of rat fundus strip**

Both acetyl salicylate and Hp inhibited sodium arachidonate (4–657 mol/l) induced increases in tone of the isolated rat gastric fundus strip in a dose-related manner, but on a weight for weight basis acetyl salicylate was more active than haptoglobin (Figure 41.5).

**Inhibition of bronchoconstriction**

Purified Hp when given intravenously (i.v.) to anaesthetized guinea pigs, in doses of 5, 20, 50 or 100 mg/kg, inhibited the increase of airway resistance and the decrease of lung compliance induced by i.v. injection of either 0.1–0.5 mg/kg of arachidonate or 1–5 μg/kg of bradykinin (Table 41.2). At doses effective in inhibiting bronchoconstriction induced by arachidonate or bradykinin, Hp did not inhibit bronchoconstriction induced by submaximal doses

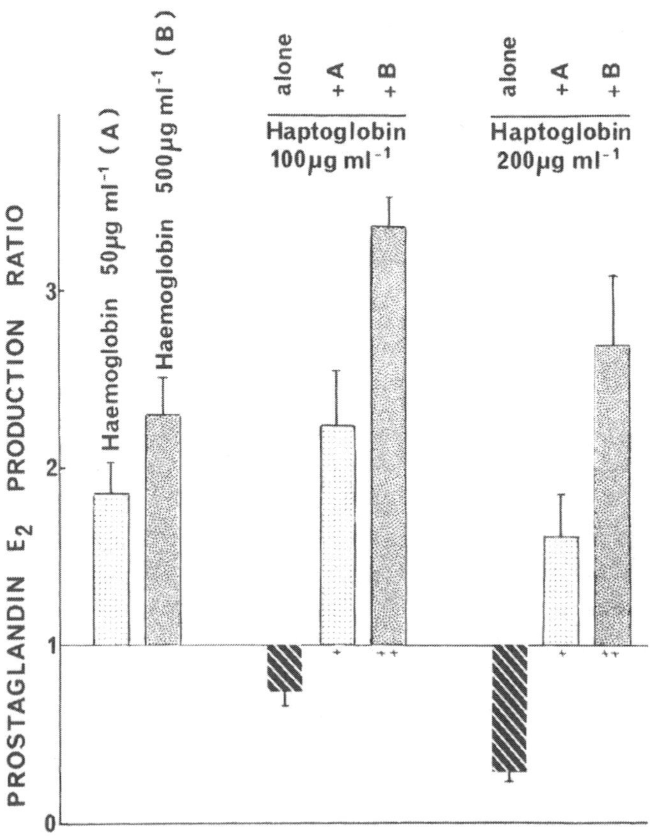


**Figure 41.4** Reversal by haemoglobin of the inhibition of $PGE_2$ biosynthesis by human haptoglobin (76% pure). (A) Human haemoglobin 50 μg/ml and (B) Human haemoglobin, 500 μg/ml. Results are expressed in terms of the prostaglandin $E_2$ biosynthesis ratio which was taken as 1 in the controls with no haemoglobin or haptoglobin. $^*p < 0.005$; $^{**}p < 0.0005$ for difference from the corresponding sample containing haptoglobin only

of $PGF_{2\alpha}$. Like Hp, indomethacin and acetyl salicylate, two well-known inhibitors of PG synthase, also inhibited the arachidonate or bradykinin-induced bronchoconstriction in the guinea pig (Table 41.2).

**Inhibition of arachidonate-induced platelet aggregation**

Aggregation induced by sodium arachidonate is known to be inhibited by acetyl salicylate, an inhibitor of cyclo-oxygenase[11]. It was found that Cohn fraction $IV_4$ and Hp which inhibited cyclo-oxygenase (Figures 41.2b, c), also inhibited arachidonate induced platelet aggregation in the absence of plasma (Table 41.3). Of the two protein fractions, however, Cohn fraction $IV_4$ was more potent in inhibiting aggregation.

**Effect of glucocorticoids on plasma Hp levels and PG synthase inhibitor activity**

We have previously demonstrated[14] that glucocorticoids increase the levels of inhibitor of PG synthase in plasma. To determine whether these changes in inhibitory activity are associated with parallel changes in Hp levels, we studied in rats the effects of intraperitoneal injections of dexamethasone sodium phosphate (24 mg/kg) and hydrocortisone sodium succinate (360 mg/kg) on plasma Hp levels and inhibitory activity. Groups of 4 or 5 rats were each given the drug or saline intraperitoneally in an injection volume of not more than 200 $\mu$l. After treatment, rats were bled individually (at 4, 24, 48 and 72 h intervals) into plastic tubes containing 500 $\mu$l of 1% (w/v) EDTA as an anti-coagulant. Plasma was separated by centrifugation at 600 *g* for 15 min and tested for inhibitory activity and Hp concentration by methods described already.

The results obtained show that administration of dexamethasone or hydrocortisone in rats causes an increase in plasma inhibitory activity as compared with saline-treated control rats. This increase in inhibitory activity and the corresponding increases in Hp concentrations are shown in Figure 41.6. It is evident that both glucocorticoids raised inhibitory activity and Hp concentrations to a similar extent and with comparable time courses.

## DISCUSSION

The $\alpha_2$-glycoprotein, Hp is present in normal plasma at a concentration[17] of approximately 1 mg/ml. Since Hp binds selectively and firmly to Hb both *in vivo* and *in vitro*, it has been proposed that the function of Hp is concerned with the prevention of loss of iron through the kidney[7]. This, however, is not its only property. Hp possesses significant inhibitory activity against cathepsin B[16] and also inhibits the haemagglutinating ability of influenza virus for chicken erythrocytes[5]. Recently we have shown that human plasma or serum powerfully inhibits PG biosynthesis[14]. The results of these and subsequent studies cited in this report suggest yet another function for haptoglobin, i.e. as an inhibitor of PG synthase.

By employing a variety of test systems commonly used to study PG synthase inhibitors, we found Hp to be capable of inhibiting the cyclo-oxygenation of arachidonic acid leading to PG formation mediated by bull seminal vesicle PG synthase (Figure 41.2c). The inhibitory effect of Hp on $PGE_2$ biosynthesis was completely reversed by Hb (Figure 41.4), a known stimulant of PG synthase. Like acetyl salicylate, Hp also inhibited the arachidonic acid-induced tone increases in the rat gastric fundic strip (Figure 41.5) and arachidonic acid and bradykinin induced bronchoconstriction in the guinea pig (Table 41.2).

Finally, plasma fraction Cohn $IV_4$ and Hp also inhibited the arachidonic acid induced aggregation of washed human blood platelets (Table 41.3). This

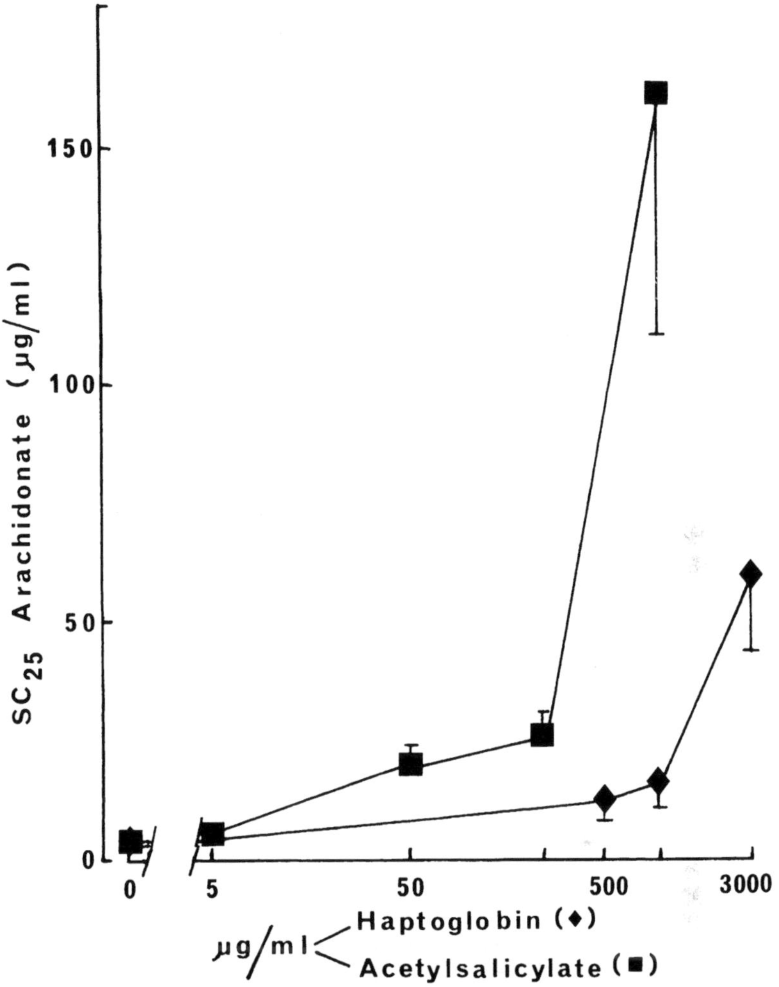


**Figure 41.5** Inhibition by acetyl salicylate (■) and 76% pure haptoglobin (◆) of increase in tone of rat gastric fundus strip induced by sodium arachidonate (4–657 µmol/l). The SC25 is the concentration of arachidonate required to increase tone to 25% of the maximal increase obtained in the preparation used. For other details see the text

result does not agree with the findings of Whittle[19], who, however, used platelet-rich plasma (PRP) for his aggregation studies. It is probable that the presence of plasma would protect platelets against aggregation by arachidonic acid. This explanation gains support from the work of Ts'ao and Holly[18], showing that plasma prevents arachidonic acid induced platelet lysis.

Further evidence that the PG synthase inhibitory activity of Hp was a prop-

**Table 41.3** Effect of human plasma Cohn fraction $IV_4$ and Hp on platelet aggregation induced by arachidonate

| *Plasma fraction* | *Concentration* (mg/ml protein) | *Percentage inhibition of aggregation; measured at various times (min) after addition of arachidonate* | | | |
|---|---|---|---|---|---|
| | | 1 | 2 | 3 | 4 |
| Cohn $IV_4$ | 1.13 | 60.0 ± 4.7 | 53.3 ± 5.6 | 51.4 ± 4.3 | 52.4 ± 2.8 |
| Cohn $IV_4$ | 2.81 | 90.8 ± 2.2 | 87.2 ± 4.9 | 84.8 ± 4.7 | 84.7 ± 3.8 |
| Hp (76% pure) | 3.6 | 34.0 ± 5.5 | 29.1 ± 10.0 | 32.2 ± 12.8 | 36.6 ± 12.3 |
| Hp (76% pure) | 7.2 | 54.8 ± 8.8 | 56.9 ± 10.5 | 56.7 ± 11.8 | 59.5 ± 10.9 |

Washed human platelets were incubated for 5 min with test proteins before the addition of sodium arachidonate (28 μg/ml). Platelet aggregation was measured as described in the Methods section. The percentage inhibition due to test protein compared with control (arachidonate alone) was calculated at 1, 2, 3 and 4 min after the addition of arachidonate. Results are mean values ± SE of three determinations.

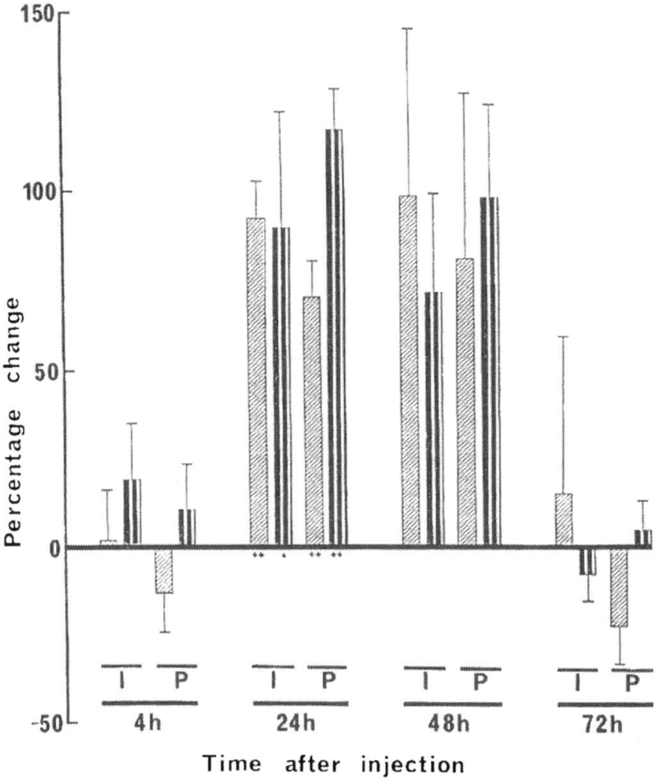


**Figure 41.6** Time course of the effect of hydrocortisone and dexamethasone on rat blood plasma PG synthase inhibitory activity (I) and peroxidase activity (P), as a measure of haptoglobin concentration. Hydrocortisone sodium succinate 360 mg/kg (cross-hatched columns) and dexamethasone sodium phosphate 24 mg/kg (striped columns). Results are expressed as percentage changes in PG synthase inhibitory activity as estimated by bioassay of $PGE_2$, and peroxidase activity, compared with saline injected controls. $^*p = 0.05$; $^{**}p = <0.0025$

erty of Hp and not a consequence of contamination by other proteins was provided by the finding that the 76% pure Hp preparation used in this study, when depleted of Hp by affinity chromatography on Hb–Sepharose, failed to inhibit $PGE_2$ biosynthesis. That Cohn $IV_4$ was more effective than haptoglobin inhibiting cyclo-oxygenase (Figures 41.2b and c) indicates, however, the possible presence of another inhibitor in Cohn $IV_4$.

Other workers have also provided evidence that Hp inhibits PG synthase. Shim[15] for example, reported that human Hp inhibits PG biosynthesis in the presence of reduced glutathione, but in the absence of tryptophan *in vitro*, Deby *et al.*[4] found a direct correlation between Hp levels and response to arachidonate induced hypotension in rabbits. Previously, we have reported[13] that foetal calf serum, which does not contain Hp, was completely devoid of PG synthase inhibitory activity. This and other evidence with glucocorticoids, which increase Hp levels and plasma PG synthase inhibitory activity to similar extents and with comparable time courses, provide further support that Hp inhibits PG synthase.

In summary, this unique property of Hp indicates that the function of Hp may be concerned with the endogenous control of PG production. The circumstances in which Hp may act in this way in the body remains to be determined; but it probably forms a part of a haemostatic control system that could help to curtail the progress of certain aggregatory or inflammatory reactions. We believe that further work in this area will provide useful information about natural regulatory mechanisms in diseases associated with imbalanced PG production and also lead to the development of suitable methods for detecting types of anti-inflammatory activity more relevant to human disease.

**Acknowledgments**

We thank Miss Julia B. Omer for technical help and Dr R. G. McDonald-Gibson of Brunel University for allowing the use of Born aggregometer.

**References**

1 Collier, H. O. J., Denning-Kendall, P. A., McDonald-Gibson, W. J. and Saeed, S. A. (1980). In Remuzzi, G., Mecca, G. and de Gactano, G (eds) *Hemostasis, Prostaglandins and Renal Diseases*, pp 257–267. New York: Raven Press
2 Collier, H. O. J., McDonald-Gibson, W. J. and Saeed, S. A. (1976). *Br. J. Pharmacol.*, **58,** 193
3 Connell G. E. and Smithies, O. (1958). *Biochem. J.*, **72.** 115
4 Deby, C., Caneghem Van, P. and Bacq, Z. M. (1978). *Biochem. Pharmacol.*, **27,** 613
5 Dobryszycka, W. and Lisowska, E. (1966). *Biochem. Biophys. Acta*, **121,** 42
6 Eckenfels, A. and Vane, J. R. (1972). *Br. J. Pharmacol.* **45,** 451
7 Higginbotham, T. W. (1975). *J. Tenn. Med. Assoc.*, **68,** 116
8 Laurell, C. B. and Nyman, M. (1957). *Blood*, **12,** 493
9 Lee, T. H. and Shim, B. S. (1973). *Postgrad. Med. Digest. (Seoul)*, **1,** 2, 72, 114 and 141
10 Nyman, M. (1959). *Scand. J. Clin. Lab. Invest*, **11** (Suppl.), 39
11 Roth, G. J. and Majerus, P. W. (1975). *J. Clin. Invest*, **56,** 624
12 Saeed, S. A. and Cuthbert, J. (1977). *Prostaglandins*, **13,** 565
13 Saeed, S. A., Kendall, P. A., McDonald-Gibson, W. J. and Collier, H. O. J. (1978). *Biochem. Soc. Trans.*, **6,** 1166
14 Saeed, S. A., McDonald-Gibson, W. J., Cuthbert, J., Copas, J. L., Schneider, C., Gardiner, P. J., Butt, N. M. and Collier, H. O. J. (1977). *Nature (London)*, **270,** 32
15 Shim, B. S. (1978). *Korean J. Biochem.*, **10,** 23
16 Snellman, O. and Sylven, B. (1967). *Nature (London)*, **216,** 1033
17 Sutton, H. E. (1970). The Haptoglobins. In Steinberg, A. G. and Bearn, A. G. (eds) *Progr. Med. Geet.*, **7,** pp. 163–216. New York: Grune & Stratton
18 Ts'ao, C. and Holly, C. M. (1979). *Prostaglandins*, **17,** 775
19 Whittle, B. J. R. (1978). *J. Pharm. Pharmacol.*, **30,** 467
20 Ubatuba, F. B. (1973). *Br. J. Pharmacol.*, **49,** 662

# 42

# Release of thromboxane $B_2$ and $PGE_2$ by rabbit polymorphonuclear leukoctyes (Abstract)

E. M. DAVIDSON, M. J. H. SMITH AND
A. W. FORD-HUTCHINSON (UK)

Rabbit polymorphonuclear leukocytes (PMNs) elicited by intraperitoneal injections of glycogen were prepared and suspended in Eagle's MEM (Davidson *et al.* (1978). *Br.J.Pharmacol.* **63,** 407P). PMNs were incubated in the presence and absence of serum opsonized zymosan (1 mg/ml) and/or $10^{-5}$ mol/l calcium ionophore (A23187) for 2 h at 37°C. Cells were removed by centrifugationa and aliquots of the supernatant removed for enzyme assays and radio-immunoassay of $PGE_2$. The remaining supernatant was acidified and extracted with diethyl ether. The ether extracts were either used for bioassay of PGE-like activity (rat fundic strip) or derivatized to form the methyl ester, methoxime, tertiary butyldimethylsilyl ethers of the prostaglandins and $TXB_2$ and the levels were measured by quantitative gas chromatography mass spectrometry (GC–MS).

| *Stimuli* | *$TXB_2$* | *ng/$10^7$ cells* *$PGE_2$* | *PGE-like activity* | *% total ß-glucuronidase* |
|---|---|---|---|---|
| Control | 1.8 | 0.1 | 0.5 | 5 |
| Zymosan | 3.6 | 0.3 | 1.5 | 26 |
| Ionophore | 5.6 | 1.2 | – | 53 |
| Zymosan + ionophore | 4.7 | 0.4 | – | 40 |

The only prostanoid consistently detected by GC–MS was $TXB_2$ although traces of $PGF_{2\alpha}$ were detected in some samples. $PGE_2$ concentrations in the samples were below the detection limit of this assay and were determined by radio-immunoassay and bioassay. Stimulation of the PMNs with either zymosan and/or ionophore resulted in increased $TXB_2$, $PGE_2$ and β-glucuronidase release with no loss of viability as measured by the release of lactate dehydrogenase or trypan blue exclusion.

# 43

# Prostaglandin and thromboxane production by rat macrophages (Abstract)

M. V. DOIG AND A. W. FORD-HUTCHINSON (UK)

Rat macrophages collected by peritoneal lavage were plated out at a concentration of $2 \times 10^7$ cells per 25 $cm^2$ in Medium 199 containing 5% fetal calf serum, 25 m mol/l HEPES pH 7.4 and antibiotics. The cells were aged for 24 h prior to use producing a pure macrophage population (>95%) as shown by the presence of Fc receptor sites, the ability to phagocytose sheep red blood cells and the presence of non-specific esterase staining granules. The cells were cultured for a further 48 h in fresh medium in the presence or absence of serum opsonized zymosan. Following removal of cells by centrifugation media were acidified and extracted with diethyl ether. The prostaglandins and thromboxane $B_2$ in the sample were then derivatized to form their methyl ester, methoxime, tertiary butyldimethylsilyl ethers and the levels of the prostaglandins and thromboxane $B_2$ were measured by quantitative gas chromatography/mass spectrometry.

Media from rat macrophages cultured for 48 h in the presence of serum opsonized zymosan contained 150–500 ng of 6-keto $PGF_{1\alpha}$, up to 80 ng of $PGE_2$, 20–80 ng $TXB_2$ and up to 40 ng of $PGF_{2\alpha}$ per $2 \times 10^7$ cells seeded. There was no evidence for the presence of $PGE_1$ or $PGD_2$ and no significant difference was found in prostaglandin and thromboxane production by the cells in the presence or absence of zymosan. Time course studies have been carried out following incubation of the macrophages for 3, 6, 9, 24 and 48 h. There was a time dependent release of $PGE_2$ and PG 6-keto $F_{1\alpha}$, maximum levels being reached after 24 h. The levels of thromboxane $B_2$ remained constant after 3 h and those of $PGF_{2\alpha}$ reached a maximum after 9 h. These results demonstrate that rat macrophages produce considerable amounts of 6-keto $PGF_{1\alpha}$ which implies that these cells synthesize $PGI_2$. This is of potential interest in relationship to inflammation as $PGI_2$ modulates cyclic AMP levels within luekocytes and has also been shown to be a modulator of vascular permeability responses, a potent hyperalgesic agent and a potent inhibitor of lymphocyte transformation.

# 44

# Specificity of glucocorticoid inhibition of synovial prostaglandin synthesis

R. M. McMILLAN, CONSTANCE E. BRINCKERHOFF AND EDWARD D. HARRIS, JR. (USA)

## INTRODUCTION

Inhibition of prostaglandin (PG) synthesis contributes to the anti-inflammatory activity of a number of anti-rheumatic compounds. Inhibition of PG synthesis by non-steroidal anti-inflammatory drugs (e.g. aspirin, indomethacin) has been observed in experiments with cell-free preparations of PG synthase as well as in intact tissues and cells[1-3]. These agents appear to act primarily by blocking the enzyme cylo-oxygenase which catalyses the initial step in synthesis of PGs from their fatty acid precursor, arachidonic acid[4].

In contrast, glucocorticoids have no effect on PG synthesis in cell-free systems but, in many intact cells and tissues, they inhibit PG production[5-7], possibly by blocking a phosopholipase which releases arachidonate from phospholipids[8]. Recent studies have revealed that anti-inflammatory steroids induce production of an inhibitor of PG formation[9,10] by a mechanism that involves RNA and protein synthesis[9,11].

Corticosteroids exert a number of effects on lipid synthesis and metabolism[12,13], and we believed it was important to determine whether inhibition of PG synthesis by glucocorticoids was a selective effect or a reflection of non-specific changes in lipid turnover. We elected to investigate this question by studying the effect of a glucocorticoid, dexamethasone, on PG synthesis and fatty acid release in monolayer cultures of synovial fibroblasts. We report here that dexamethasone selectively inhibits arachidonate release and metabolism in this system but does not inhibit release of other fatty acids.

## METHODS

### Cell culture

Rabbit synovial cells were prepared from explants or by enzyme dissociation and cultured in 60 mm dishes in Dulbecco's Modified Eagles medium (DMEM) containing 20% foetal calf serum (FCS). Fibroblast-like cells growing to confluence were trypsinized and cultured for up to six passages in DMEM containing 10% FCS with penicillin and streptomycin.

### Metabolism of radiolabelled arachidonate

Synovial fibroblasts (approximately $2 \times 10^5$/35 mm dish) were incubated with 1 μCi [$^3$H]arachidonic acid or 0.5 μCi [$^{14}$C]arachidonic acid for 20 h at 37 °C in DMEM–10%FCS. Under these conditions the cells incorporated 50–80% of the radioactivity. The cell monolayers were washed three times with serum-free culture medium and then incubated with phorbol myristate acetate (PMA) or bradykinin in DMEM containing 0.2% lactalbumin hydrolysate (LH). After 20 h culture media were acidified and lipids were extracted with ethyl acetate. Organic extracts were dried under nitrogen, reconstituted in ether:methanol (9:1) and applied to silica gel plates (Eastman). Lipids were separated by thin-layer chromatography (TLC) using benzene:dioxane:acetic acid (60:30:3) and visualized with iodine vapour. Areas of the TLC plate corresponding to authentic standards were removed for quantitation of radioactivity.

### Measurement of fatty acid release

Synovial fibroblasts (approximately $10^6$/60 mm dish) were incubated with 1 μCi [$^3$H]arachidonate, [$^{14}$C]oleate, [$^{14}$C]linoleate or [$^{14}$C]palmitate for 24 h in DMEM–10%FCS. After incorporation of fatty acids, cells washed twice and incubated with PMA or bradykinin for a further 20 h. Replicate subsamples of culture media were removed to determine release of radioactive lipids (fatty acids + metabolites).

## RESULTS AND DISCUSSION

Monolayer cultures of synovial fibroblasts may be induced to release high levels of PGs by exposure to inflammatory agents[5,14] such as bradykinin or PMA. Table 44.1 shows results of TLC analysis of [$^3$H]arachidonic acid metabolism induced by these agents. PMA caused approximately a 4-fold increase in release of radioactive lipids (arachidonate + metabolites). This increased radioactivity was localized primarily in the area corresponding to authentic $PGE_2$ which increased approximately 15-fold and accounted for over 60% of the radioactivity released from PMA-stimulaed synovial cells. Bradykinin stimulated total radioactivity release by 1.5-fold; [$^3$H]PGE$_2$, which was stimulated nearly 3-fold by bradykinin, again accounted for most of the increased radioactivity.Addition of PMA or bradykinin to cells pre-labelled with [$^{14}$C]arachidonate yielded comparable data to those obtained with [$^3$H]arachidonate.

**Table 44.1** Stimulation of [$^3$H]arachidonate metabolism in rabbit synovial fibroblasts

| *Treatment* | *PGF$_{2\alpha}$* | *PGE$_2$* | *TxB$_2$* | *PGD$_2$* | *ARA* | *Total* |
|---|---|---|---|---|---|---|
| Control | 87<br>± 7 | 274<br>± 32 | 100<br>± 6 | 80<br>± 3 | 556<br>±62 | 1466 |
| PMA | 229<br>±30 | 3527<br>±545 | 291<br>±61 | 152<br>±15 | 790<br>±68 | 5790 |
| Bradykinin | 169<br>+51 | 725<br>+76 | 94<br>+12 | 75<br>± 7 | 578<br>±29 | 2129 |

Synovial fibroblasts were pre-labelled with [$^3$H]arachidonate and then incubated with PMA ($10^{-8}$mol/l) or bradykinin ($10^{-7}$mol/l) for 20 h in DMEM–0.2% LH. Lipids were extracted and separated by TLC. Radioactivity in areas corresponding to authentic standards was determined. Results are expressed as c.p.m. (mean values ± SD; $n$=3); $TxB_2$=thromboxane B$_2$; $ARA$=arachidonic acid

The data shown in Table 44.1 indicate that bradykinin induced less marked stimulation of arachidonate metabolism in synovial cells than did PMA. In addition bradykinin exerted a more selective action (Figure 44.1). Bradykinin produced a 1.5-fold stimulation of radioactivity release from cells pre-labelled with [$^3$H]arachidonate but not from cells labelled with other fatty acids. PMA stimulated release of all four fatty acids tested (Figure 44.1). In four separate experiments, with three different synovial fibroblast lines, the mean values (±SD) for PMA-induced stimulation of arachidonate, linoleate, oleate and palmitate release were, respectively, 2.25±0.24, 1.85±0.50, 1.40±0.21 and 1.35 ± 0.10.

Treatment of synovial cells with PMA usually resulted in contracted cells and it is conceivable that fatty acid release might result from turnover of membrane phospholipids associated with this morphological change. If this were the case, then increased incorporation of lipid precursors might also occur. However, we have found no evidence for an effect of PMA on uptake of radio-labelled arachidonate, oleate, linoleate or palmitate[18]. Thus enhanced fatty acid release induced by PMA is likely to be a consequence of non-specific lipase activation rather than a generalized increase in phosopholipid turnover.

The non-selective release of fatty acids induced by PMA provided a useful model for investigating the specificity of glucocorticoid inhibition of PG synthesis. In three experiments with rabbit synovial cells pre-labelled with

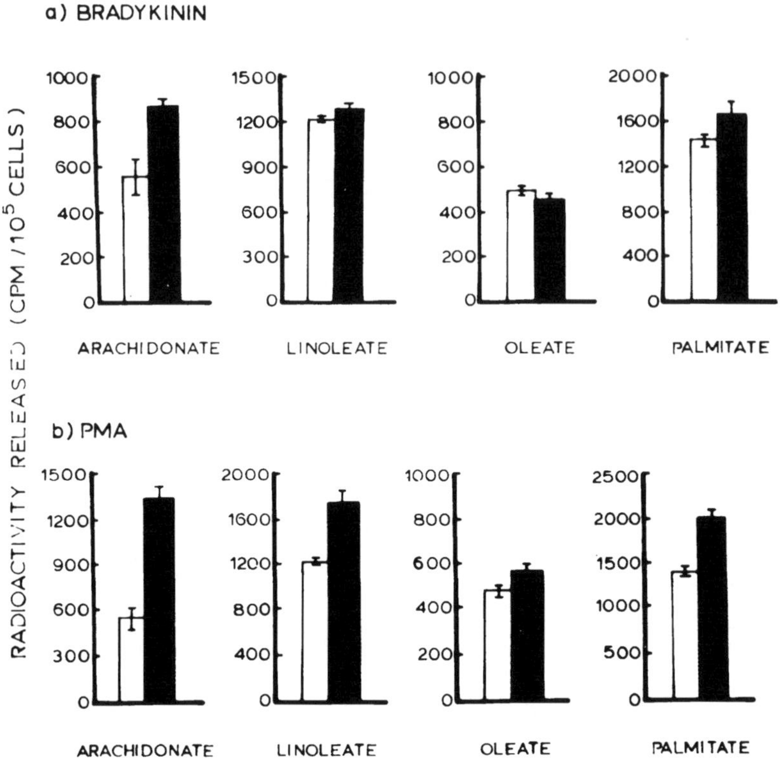


**Figure 44.1** Fatty acid release from synovial fibroblasts induced by bradykinin and PMA. Synovial fibroblasts were pre-labelled with radioactive arachidonate, linoleate, oleate or palmitate and then incubated with PMA ($10^{-8}$ mol/l) or bradykinin ($10^{-6}$ mol/l) for 20 h in DMEM–0.2% LH. Bars represent mean values ± SD ($n = 3$)

[$^3$H]arachidonate PMA induced a 2–4-fold increase in total radioactivity released and this was abolished by a 2 h pretreatment with $10^{-7}$ mol/l dexamethasone. Table 44.2 illustrates the effect of dexamethasone on [$^3$H] arachidonate metabolism. In this experiment, [$^3$H]PGE$_2$ release induced by PMA was inhibited by 82% and [$^3$H]arachidonic acid levels were reduced by 42%. In four other experiments, using rabbit or human synovial cells, dexamethasone always produced a more marked effect on [$^3$H]PGE$_2$ levels than on [$^3$H] arachidonate. This suggests that, in this system, dexamethasone interferes with PG synthesis partly by phospholipase inhibition and partly by an additional mechanism that may involve inhibition of cyclo-oxygenase, an effect previously reported in studies of rheumatoid synovial tissue[10].

To determine whether glucocorticoid inhibition of arachidonate release and metabolism was selective, we investigated the effect of dexamethasone

**Table 44.2** Effect of dexamethasone on [$^{3}$H]arachidonate release and metabolism in rabbit synovial fibroblasts

| | *Control* | *PMA* | *PMA* +DEX ($10^{-7}$mol/l) |
|---|---|---|---|
| [$^{3}$H]PGE$_2$ | 166 ± 80 | 1541 ± 179 | 284 ± 51 (18%) |
| [$^{3}$H]ARA | 191 ± 13 | 210 ± 33 | 123 ± 33 (58%) |

Synovial fibroblasts, pre-labelled with [$^{3}$H]arachidonate, were pre-incubated with dexamethasone (DEX) for 2 h in DMEM–0.2% LH before addition of PMA ($10^{-8}$mol/l) for an additional 20 h. Lipids were extracted and separated by TLC. Radioactivity in areas corresponding to PGE$_2$ and arachidonic acid is expressed as c.p.m. (mean values ± SD; $n$=3). Figures in parenthesis show PMA + DEX data as percentages of results obtained with PMA alone

on release of radiolabelled fatty acids (Figure 44.2). PMA-induced release of radioactivity from [$^{3}$H]arachidonate cells was inhibited by pretreatment with the steroid. Release of other fatty acids was not inhibited; indeed dexamethasone potentiated release of radioactivity from synovial cells labelled with [$^{14}$C]oleate. The mechanism of this enhancement is unclear but one possibility is that increased oleate release in some way compensates for the decreased levels of arachidonate release during glucocorticoid treatment.

Our data demonstrate that PG formation in synovial fibroblasts can be a sequel to either selective release of arachidonate (e.g., with bradykinin) or non-specific release of fatty acids (with PMA). Similar data have been reported in two other systems. Needleman and co-workers found that ischaemia stimulated release of both arachidonate and oleate from cardiac and renal tissues[15,16].

More recently, Hong and Deykin reported that ionophore $A_{23187}$ caused non-selective release of fatty acids from transformed mouse fibroblasts[17]. In these systems bradykinin also released only arachidonate and both groups proposed the existence of cellular lipases with different fatty acid specificities. In these previous studies it was not possible to determine whether non-selective stimuli activate several phospholipases or a single phosopholipase with a broad spectrum of action. The data presented here indicate the existence of numerous cellular lipases which have different fatty acid specificities and which may be independently activated or inhibited by pharmacologic agents.

Our demonstration of an arachidonate-selective inhibition by dexamethasone suggests that anti-inflammatory steroids exert a highly specific effect on PG generation. This action is not accompanied by non-specific depression of phosopholipid metabolism such as would accompany membrane stabilization. The precise mechanisms of corticosteroid inhibition of arachidonate

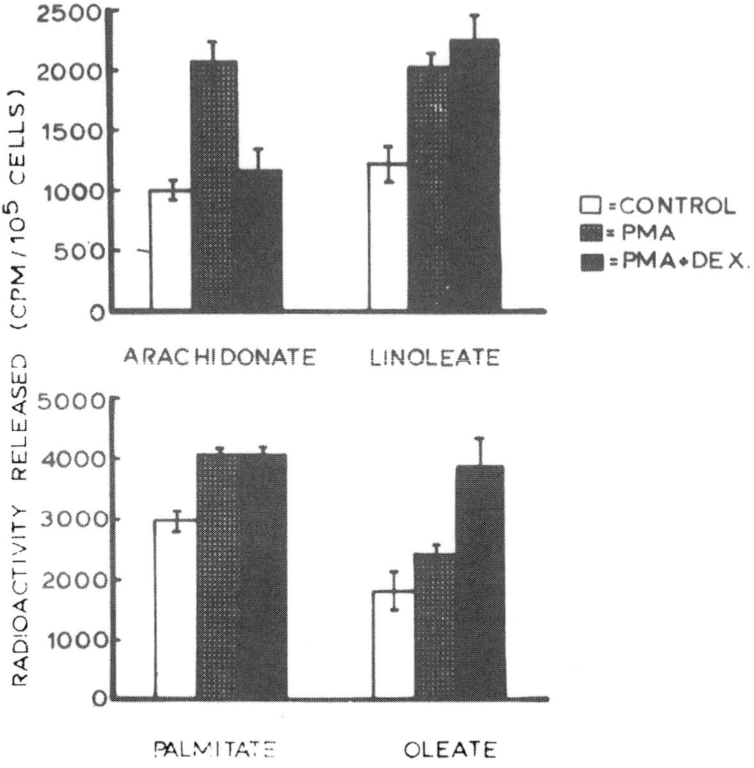


**Figure 44.2** Effect of dexamethasone on fatty acid release. Synovial fibroblasts were prelabelled with radioactive arachidonate, linoleate, oleate or palmitate. Cells were then incubated with dexamethasone ($10^{-7}$ mol/l) for 2 h in DMEM–0.2% LH before addition of PMA ($10^{-8}$ mol/l) for a further 20 h

release and metabolism remains to be clearly established, and, in this system, may involve both cyclo-oxygenase and phospholipase inhibition. In view of the specificity of the effects reported here, we believe that synovial fibroblasts may provide a model system for characterizing the sequence of events leading from glucocorticoid receptor binding to possible changes in protein synthesis and blockade of PG release.

**Acknowledgments**

We are grateful to Dr. Allan Munck, Dr. John V. Fahey and Ms. Carol A. Vater for their constructive criticisms during this project; to Ms. Jeanie Hahn for preparing the figures and to Ms. Robin Scribner for typing the manuscript. This work was supported by USPHS Grants 5RO1 AM14780–09 and 5 P60 AM 20641–03; by Biomedical Research Support Grant RR–05392 from the NIH Biomedical Research Support Branch; by grants from the National and

New Hampshire Chapters of the Arthritis Foundation and by the KROC Foundation, Santa Ynez, California. R.M. McMillan is an Arthritis Foundation Postdoctoral Fellow.

## References


1 Vane, J. R. (1971). Inhibition of prostaglandin synthesis as a mechanism of action for aspirin-like drugs. *Nature (London), New Biol.*, **231**, 232

2 Ferreira, S. H., Moncada, S., and Vane, J. R. (1971). Indomethacin and aspirin abolish prostaglandin release from the spleen. *Nature (London), New Biol.*, **231**, 237

3 Smith, J. B. and Willis, A. L. (1971). Aspirin selectively inhibits prostaglandin production in human platelets. *Nature (London), New Biol.*, **231**, 235

4 Roth, G. J., Stanford, N., and Majerus, P. W. (1975). Acetylation of prostaglandin synthase by aspirin. *Proc. Natl. Acad.Sci. (USA)*. **72**, 3073

5 Newcombe, D. S. Fahey, J. V. and Ishikawa, Y. (1977). Hydrocortisone inhibition of the bradykinin activation of human synovial fibroblasts. *Prostaglandins*, **13**, 235

6 Tashjian, A. H., Jr., Voelkel, E. F., McDonough, J., and Levine, L. (1975). Hydrocortisone inhibits prostaglandin production by mouse fibrosarcoma cells. *Nature (London)*, **258**, 739

7 Kantrowitz, F., Robinson, D. R., McGuire, M. B., and Levine, L. (1975). Corticosteroids inhibit prostaglandin production by rheumatoid synovia. *Nature (London)*, **258**, 737

8 Blackwell, G. J., Flower, R. J. Nijkamp, R. P., and Vane, J. R. (1978). Phospholipase $A_2$ activity of guinea-pig isolated perfused lungs: stimulation and inhibition by anti-inflammatory steroids. *Br. J. Pharmacol*, **62**, 79

9 Flower, R. J., and Blackwell, G. J. (1979). Anti-inflammatory steroids induce biosynthesis of a phosopholipase $A_2$ inhibitor which prevents prostaglandin generation. *Nature (London)*, **278**, 456

10 Robinson, D. R., Bastian, D. and Servello, L. (1979). Mechanism of corticosteroid inhibition of prostaglandin synthesis by rheumatoid synovial tissue. *Arthritis Rheum*, **22**, 650

11 Danon, A., and Assouline, G. (1978). Inhibition of prostaglandin biosynthesis by corticosteroids requires RNAand protein synthesis. *Nature (London)*, **273**, 552

12 Foley, J. E., Jeffries, M., and Munck, A. (1980). Glucocorticoid effects on incorporation of lipid and protein precursors into rat thymus cell fractions. *J. Steroid Biochem.* (In press)

13 Jenrenaud, B. and Renold, A. E. (1960). Studies on rat adipose tissue *in vitro*. VII. Effects of adrenal cortical hormones. *J. Biol. Chem.*, **235**, 2217

14 McMillan, R. M., Fahey, J. V., Brinckerhoff, C. E., and Harris, E. D., Jr. (1980). Secretion of inflammatory mediators from synovial fibroblasts: dissociation of collagenase and prostaglandin release. Samuelsson, B. Ramwell, P. W. and Paoletti, R. (eds.) In *Advances in Prostaglandin and Thromboxane Research*. Vol 8, p1701. (New York: Raven Press)

15 Hseuh, W., Isakson, P. C. and Needleman, P.(1977). Hormone selective lipase activation in the isolated rabbit heart. *Prostaglandins*, **13**, 1073

16 Needleman, P. (1978). Characterization of the reaction sequence involved in phospholipid labeling and deacylation and prostaglandin synthesis and actions. *J. Allergy Clin. Immunol.*, **62**, 96

17 Hong, S. L. and Deykin, D. (1979). Specificity of phospholipases in methylcholantrhene-transformed mouse fibroblasts activated by bradykinin, thrombin, serum and ionophore $A_{23187}$. *J. Biol. Chem.*, **254**, 11463

18 McMillan, R. M.and Harris. E. D., Jr. (unpublished data)

# 45

# Collagenase release from synovial fibroblasts: relationship to fatty acid release and prostaglandin synthesis

R. M. McMILLAN, CONSTANCE E. BRINCKERHOFF AND EDWARD D. HARRIS, Jr. (USA)

## INTRODUCTION

Rheumatoid synovium has proliferative and destructive characteristics *in vivo*. These capabilities are also evident in tissue culture studies in which cultured explants of rheumatoid synovium have been shown to invade normal tendon[1] and release substances which stimulate bone resorption[2]. There are numerous biochemical differences between normal and inflamed synovia but it is likely that the destructive capacity of rheumatoid tissues is related in part to formation of high levels of prostaglandins (PGs) and collagenase[3,4]. $PGE_2$, released from cultured rheumatoid synovium, stimulates bone resorption[2] and collagenase is believed to be the major enzyme responsible for cartilage degradation associated with rheumatoid arthritis[5,6].

Numerous cell and tissue culture studies have revealed a close relationship between PGs and collagenase secretion. Concomitant release of PGs and collagenase occurs in a number of cell types, including adherent cells derived from rheumatoid synovium, and, in some systems, collagenase release has been shown to be mediated by PGs[8].

Previous studies[9–11] in our laboratory have demonstrated that fibroblasts from normal synovium release very little collagenase but produce high levels of the enzyme following treatment with a variety of diverse agents, including phorbol myristic acetate (PMA), polyethylene glycol (PEG) and cytochalasin B. PMA treated rabbit synovial fibroblast cultures appear to be a reasonable model for stimulated mesenchymal cells found as part of the synovial lesion in rheumatoid arthritis.

In the present study we report that these collagenase inducers also stimulate PG synthesis, apparently via non-specific activation of phospholipases. PGs do not mediate collagenase release in this system but the possibility that non-prostanoic lipid metabolites may have a role in collagenase induction is discussed.

## METHODS

Synovium from the knee joints of 3–4 week old New Zealand white rabbits were cultured as explants or dissociated enzymatically. Fibroblast-like cells were grown to confluence in Dulbecco's Modified Eagles medium (DMEM) containing 20% foetal calf serum (FCS). At confluence, cells were trypsinized and cultured for up to 6 passages in DMEM–10% FCS.

For induction of collagenase with PMA or cytochalasin B, cultures were washed three times with Hanks Balanced Salt Solution (HBSS) and medium was replaced with DMEM containing 0.2% lactalbumin hydrolysate (LH). Cells were then incubated with PMA or cytochalasin B and medium was removed after 48 h for measurement of collagenase and $PGE_2$. In experiments to induce multi-nucleate giant cell formation, actively growing cells were treated with PEG–6000 (50%; w/v) for 1 min at 25 °C. Cells were washed three times in DMEM, cultured for 24 h in DMEM–20% FCS and subsequently incubated in DMEM–0.2% LH.

Collagenase is normally released from rabbit synovial fibroblasts in latent form. Latent collagenase in culture media was activated with 10 $\mu$g/ml TPCK trypsin for 30 min at room temperature followed by 40 $\mu$g/ml soybean trypsin inhibitor. Collagenase was assayed by measuring lysis of radio-labelled collagen fibrils at 37 °C[12]. One unit of collagenase activity represented enzyme sufficient to degrade 1 $\mu$g fibrillar collagen/h. Collagenase activity was expressed with respect to intracellular TCA-precipitable protein as determined by the method of Lowry *et al.*[13]

Release of $PGE_2$ was measured by radio-immunoassay using a modification of the technique of Dray *et al.*[14]. Rabbit anti-$PGE_2$ antiserum (Institut Pasteur, Paris, France), $[^3H]PGE_2$ (New England Nuclear, Boston, USA), samples and standards were prepared in 0.1 mol/l phosphate buffer, pH 7.4, containing 0.9% NaCl, 0.1% sodium azide and 0.2% bovine gammaglobulins. Incubation procedures and measurement of bound radioactivity were carried out as previously described[9]

Fatty acid release was measured from cells that had incorporated $[^3H]$arachidonate, $[^{14}C]$oleate, $[^{14}C]$linoleate or $[^{14}C]$palmitate. Following fatty acid incorporation, cells were washed twice with HBSS and incubated with stimuli for 24 h in DMEM–0.2% LH. Samples of culture media were removed for determination of total radioactivity released (fatty acids and metabolites).

## RESULTS

Cultures prepared from explants or enzyme dissociation of normal rabbit synovium yield monolayers of fibroblast-like cells that produce low or undetectable amounts of collagenase and low levels of $PGE_2$. Treatment of these cells with PMA, PEG or cytochalasin B stimulated release of collagenase and $PGE_2$. PEG and PMA increased collagenase release 40-fold and stimulated $PGE_2$ synthesis 30–50-fold over control values. Cytochalasin B produced a similar enhancement of collagenase release but increased $PGE_2$ release by only 3-fold (Table 45.1).

**Table 45.1** Induction of collagenase and prostaglandin $E_2$ release from rabbit synovial fibroblasts

| | *Collagenase* (units/mg *cell protein*) | $PGE_2$ (ng/mg *cell protein*) |
|---|---|---|
| Control | 7.2 ± 4.8 | 17.5 ± 4.2 |
| PMA | 325 ± 25 | 469 ± 59 |
| Control | 0 | 1.1 ± 0.1 |
| PEG | 101 + 26 | 544 ± 110 |
| Control | 0 | 4.1 ± 0.2 |
| CB | 237 ± 24 | 12.1 ± 2.4 |

Synovial fibroblasts were treated with PMA ($10^{-8}$mol/l), PEG (30%) or cytochalasin B (1.5 μg/ml) as described in Methods. Results represent cumulative collagenase and $PGE_2$ levels after 48 h treatment with PMA or cytochalasin B or after 48 h incubation with PEG-induced giant cells. Mean values ± SD 1($n$ = 3)

Using PMA-stimulated synovial fibroblasts we observed temporal differences in $PGE_2$ and collagenase release (Table 45.2). High levels of collagenase and $PGE_2$ release were induced by treating cells with PMA for 3 days; PMA was then removed and incubations were continued for a further 6 days. After removal of PMA, collagenase release was maintained for 2 days and then declined, although release was still evident 6 days after PMA was removed. In contrast, 2 days after PMA removal $PGE_2$ release was less than 5% of levels detected during induction.

Figure 45.1 shows the time course of induction of $PGE_2$ and collagenase release. PMA caused no significant release of $PGE_2$ within 12 h. This lag was

**Table 45.2** Collagenase and $PGE_2$ release from rabbit synovial fibroblasts treated with PMA

| *Days in Culture* | Collagenase (units/mg *cell protein*) | $PGE_2$ (ng/mg *cell protein*) |
|---|---|---|
| 0–3 | 891 ± 32 | 1032 ± 106 |
| 3–5 | 755 ± 48 | 49.6 ± 7.2 |
| 5–7 | 174 ± 53 | 10.4 ± 0.8 |
| 7–9 | 32 ± 29 | 8.4 ± 1.0 |

Synovial fibroblasts were incubated with PMA ($10^{-8}$ mol/l) for 3 days in DMEM–0.2% LH to induce collagenase and $PGE_2$ release. PMA was then removed and cells were maintained for a further 6 days in DMEM–0.2% LH. Collagenase and $PGE_2$ levels were measured after induction and at 2 day intervals after PMA removal. Results are mean values ± SD ($n = 3$)

followed by a burst of $PGE_2$ release which was maximal by 24 h. Collagenase release was characterized by a 24 h lag followed by continued enzyme secretion.

In order to determine whether PGs played a role in enzyme induction we investigated the effect on collagenase release of agents that inhibit $PGE_2$ formation (Figure 45.2). Treatment of synovial fibroblasts with aspirin or indomethacin virtually abolished $PGE_2$ formation but did not affect collagenase release. Other data (not shown) also indicated that collagenase release in this system was not mediated by PGs: addition of $PGE_2$ ($10^{-6}$ mol/l) to cultures of synovial fibroblasts did not induce collagenase, and bradykinin ($10^{-6}$ mol/l), which stimulated arachidonic acid metabolism, primarily to $PGE_2$ did not cause collagenase secretion.

Marked differences were noted between the responses of synovial cells to bradykinin and to collagenase inducers—

(1) Treatment of synovial fibroblasts with cytochalasin B, PMA or PEG resulted in pronounced morphologic changes – cytochalasin B produced rounded cells with mutiple processes, PMA caused the cells to adopt a contracted appearance and PEG induced fusion of synovial fibroblasts to form multinucleate giant cells. Addition of bradykinin to cultures of synovial fibroblasts caused no detectable change in the morphology of the cells.

(2) $PGE_2$ release induced by bradykinin results from activation of a specific phospholipase that releases arachidonic acid but not other fatty acids[15]. In contrast, treatment of synovial fibroblasts with PMA or cytochalasin B stimulated release of other fatty acids in addition to arachidonate;

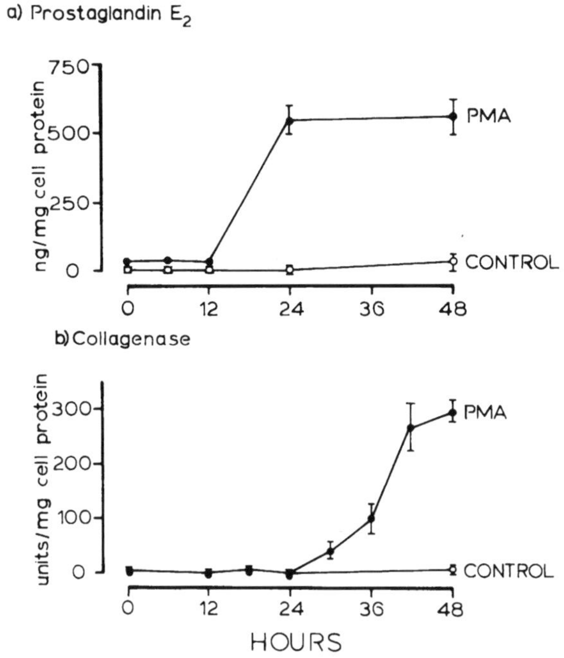


**Figure 45.1** Induction of collagenase and $PGE_2$ release by PMA. Synovial fibroblasts were incubated with PMA ($10^{-8}$mol/l) for various times in DMEM–0.2% LH. Points represent cumulative levels of collagenase and $PGE_2$ (mean values ± SD, $n = 3$)

indeed, cytochalasin B produced a more marked effect on palmitate and linoleate release than on arachidonate (Figure 45.3). It is worth noting that in cells pre-labelled with [$^3$H]arachidonate, PMA stimulated greater release of radioactivity than did cytochalasin B. This is consistent with their relative potencies as inducers of $PGE_2$ synthesis as shown in Table 45.1.

## DISCUSSION

The levels of $PGE_2$ and collagenase release observed in this study with stimulated synovial fibroblasts are comparable to the high values spontaneously produced by rheumatoid synovial cells[7,16,17]. Our results showing dissociation of PGs and collagenase with non-steroidal anti-inflammatory drugs are also similar to data obtained with rheumatoid cells. Using cells derived from rheumatoid synovium, Dayer *et al.* demonstrated that collagenase release was usually maintained in the presence of indomethacin[16,17]. In contrast, the levels of collagenase and $PGE_2$ released by stimulated macrophages are up to

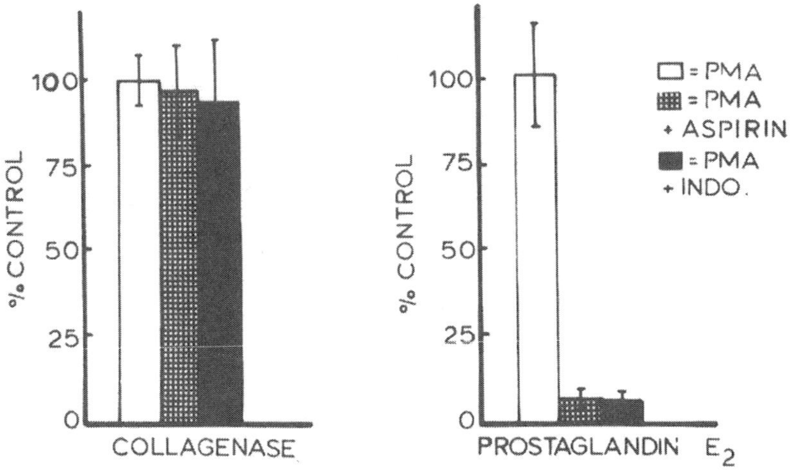


**Figure 45.2** Effect of inhibitors of PG synthesis on collagenase release. Synovial fibroblasts were incubated with aspirin ($10^{-5}$mol/l) or indomethacin ($10^{-7}$mol/l) for 2 h in DMEM–0.2% LH before addition of PMA for a further 2 days. Collagenase and $PGE_2$ release is expressed as per cent control values induced by PMA in the absence of PG synthesis inhibitors. Bars represent mean values ± SD ($n$ = 3)

100 times less, on a cellular basis, than those shown here, and in macrophages indomethacin abolishes collagenase release[8]. These data suggest that fibroblasts or fibroblast-like cells are likely to be more important than macrophages as a source of collagenase and PGs in inflamed synovia.

Collagenase release from rabbit synovial fibroblasts may be stimulated by a number of diverse agents, and, in order to determine the mechanisms involved in enzyme induction, it is important to establish similarities in the responses produced by the various stimuli. Two common properties of all collagenase inducers so far tested in this system are their ability to produce marked changes in the morphology of synovial cells and to stimulate arachidonate release and metabolism to $PGE_2$. Some of the drug-induced morphologic changes in rabbit synovial cells are similar to the 'dendritic' or 'stellate' cells found in rheumatoid synovial cell cultures[18,19]. These cells have been shown by immunofluorescent studies to have abundant collagenase in cell processes and on collagen substrate adjacent to the cells[20,21].

We demonstrate here that arachidonate release in response to two inducers of collagenase (PMA and cytochalasin B) is accompanied by release of other fatty acids, indicating that they cause non-selective stimulation of cellular lipases. Studies are in progress to determine whether PEG, and other collagenase inducers produce a similar pattern of fatty acid release.

The morphologic changes are early events that usually precede $PGE_2$ and collagenase release[10,22]. We believe that membrane perturbation produced by collagenase inducers gives rise to broad, non-specific activation of phos-

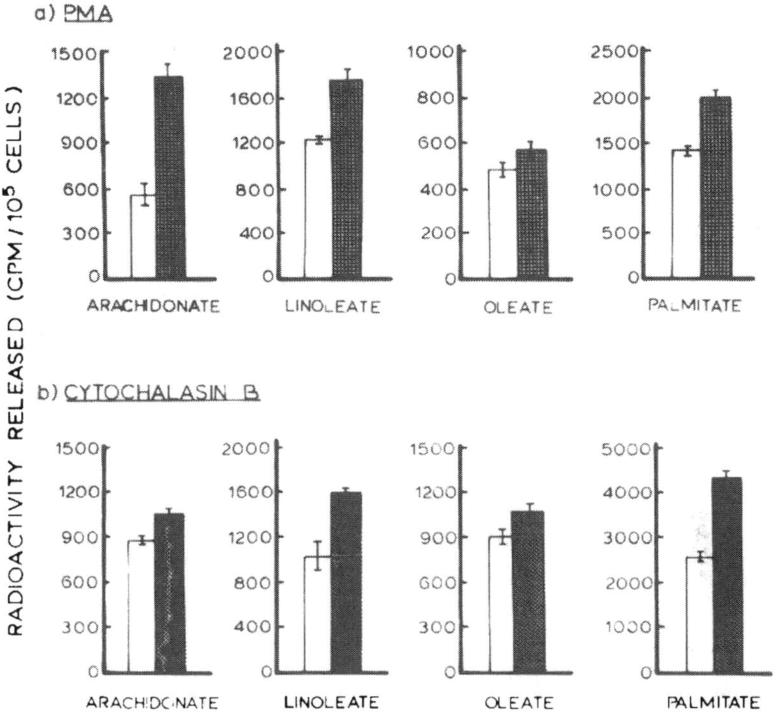


**Figure 45.3** Fatty acid release induced by PMA and cytochalasin B. Rabbit synovial fibroblasts were pre-labelled with radioactive arachidonate linoleate, oleate or palmitate and then incubated with PMA ($10^{-8}$mol/l) or cytochalasin B (1.5 μg/ml) for 20 h in DMEM–0.2% LH. Bars represent mean values ± SD ($n$ = 3)

pholipid metabolism of which $PGE_2$ release is one result. We do not yet know whether there is a causal relationship between lipase activation and collagenase release in this system. However, preliminary experiments from our laboratory indicate that treatment of synovial fibroblasts with lysolecithin results in collagenase induction[23]. This raises the intriguing possibility that release of collagenase from synovial cells is mediated not by PGs but by lysophospholipids or related products of phospholipase activation.

**Acknowledgments**

We are grateful to Dr John V. Fahey and Ms. Carol A. Vater for their advice and constructive criticisms and to Ms. Jeanie Hahn for preparing the figures. This work was supported by USPHS grants AM14780 and AM20641; by Biomedical Research Support Grant RR-05392 from the NIH Biomedical Research Support Branch; and by grants from the National and New Hampshire Chapters of the Arthritis Foundation and the Kroc Foundation, Santa Ynez, California. R. M. McMillan is an Arthritis Foundation Postdoctoral Fellow.

## References


1 Harris, E. D., Jr., DiBona, D. R. and Krane, S. M. (1970). A mechanism for cartilage destruction in rheumatoid arthritis. *Trans. Assoc. Am: Physicians*, **83**, 267

2 Robinson, D. R. Tashjian, A. H., Jr. and Levine, L. (1975). Prostaglandin-stimulated bone resorption by rheumatoid synovia. *J. Clin. Invest.*, **56**, 1181

3 Robinson, D. R. and McGuire, M. B. (1975). Prostaglandins in the rheumatic diseases. *Ann. N. Y. Acad Sci.*, **256**, 318

4 Evanson, J. M., Jeffrey, J. J. and Krane, S. M. (1967). Human collagenase: identification and characterisation of an enzyme from rheumatoid synovium in culture. *Science*, **158**, 499

5 Harris, E. D., Jr. and Krane, S. M. (1974). Collagenases. *N. Engl. J. Med.*, **291**, 557, 605, 652

6 Woolley, D. E. and Evanson, J. M. (1977). Collagenase and its natural inhibitors in relation to the rheumatoid joint. *Connective Tissue Res.*, **5**, 31

7 Dayer, J.–M., Krane, S. M., Russell, R. G. G. and Robinson, D. R. (1976). Production of collagenase and prostaglandins by isolated adherent rheumatoid synovial cells. *Proc. Natl. Acad. Sci. (USA)*, **73**, 945

8 Wahl, L. M., Olsen, C. E., Sandberg, A. L. and Mergenhagen, S. E. (1977). 'Prostaglandin regulation of macrophage collagenase production'. *Proc. Natl. Acad. Sci. (USA).*, **74**, 4955

9 Brinckerhoff, C. E., McMillan, R. M., Fahey, J. V. and Harris, E. D., Jr. (1979). Collagenase production by synovial fibroblasts treated with phorbol myristic acetate. *Arthritis Rheum.*, **22**, 1109

10 Brinckerhoff, C. E. and Harris, E. D. Jr. (1978). Collagenase production by cultures containing multinucleate giant cells derived from synovial fibroblasts. *Arthritis Rheum.*, **21**, 745

11 Harris, E. D. Jr., Reynolds, J. J. and Werb, Z. (1975). Cytochalasin B increases collagenase production by cells in vitro. *Nature (London)*. **257**, 243

12 Harris, E. D. Jr., DiBona, D. R. and Krane, S. M. (1969). Collagenase in human synovial fluid. *J. Clin. Invest.*, **48**, 2104

13 Lowry, O. H., Rosebrough, N. J., Farr, A. L. and Randall, R. J. (1951). Protein measurement with the folin reagent. *J. Biol. Chem.*, **193**, 265

14 Dray, F., Charbonnel, B. and MacLouf, J. (1975). Radioimmunoassay for prostaglandins F, E1 and E2 in human plasma. *Eur. J. Clin. Invest.*, **5**, 311

15 McMillan, R. M., Brinckerhoff, C. E. and Harris, E. D., Jr. (1980). Specificity of glucocorticoid inhibition of synovial prostaglandin synthesis. (This volume ch. 44)

16 Dayer, J.-M., Robinson, D. R. and Krane, S. M. (1977). Prostaglandin production by rheumatoid synovial cells. Stimulation by a factor from human mononuclear cells. *J. Exp. Med.*, **145**, 1399

17 Dayer, J.-M. and Krane, S. M. (1978). Interaction of immunocompetent cells and chronic inflammation as exemplified by rheumatoid arthritis. *Clin. Rheum. Dis.*, **4**, 517

18 Dayer, J.-M., Goldring, S. R. and Krane, S. M. (1978). Connective tissue resorption and rheumatoid arthritis: synovial cell culture as a model. Horton, Tarplay and Davis (eds) *Proceedings, Mechanisms of Localized Bone Loss*. Special supplement to *Calcified Tissue Abstracts*, p. 305.

19 Werb, Z., Mainardi, C. L., Vater, C. A. and Harris, E. D., Jr. (1977). 'Endogenous activation of latent collagenase by rheumatoid synovial cells. Evidence for a role of plasminogen activator. *N. Engl. J. Med.*, **296**, 1017

20 Woolley, D. E., Harris, E. D., Jr. Mainardi, C. L. and Brinckerhoff, C. E. (1978). Collagenase immunolocalization in cultures of rheumatoid synovial cells. *Science*, **200**, 773

21 Woolley, D. E., Brinckerhoff, C. E., Mainnardi, C. L., Vater, C. A., Evanson, J. M. and Harris, E. D., Jr. (1979). Collagenase production by rheumatoid synovial cells: morphological and immunohistochemical studies of the dendritic cell, *Ann. Rheum. Dis.* **38**, 262

22 McMillan, R. M., Fahey, J. V., Brinckerhoff, C. E. and Harris, E. D., Jr. (1980). Secretion of inflammatory mediators from synovial fibroblasts: dissociation of collagenase and prostaglandin release. In Samuelsson, B., Ramwell, P. W. and Paoletti, R. (eds.) *Advances in Prostaglandin and Thromboxane Research*. Vol. 8, p. 1701. (New York: Raven Press)

23 McMillan, R. M., Brinckerhoff, C. E. and Harris, E. D. (unpublished data)

# 46

# Observations on the influence of anti-oxidant compounds on prostaglandin biosynthesis (Abstract)

M. V. TORRIELLI, J. S. FRANZONE, T. NATALE
R. CIRILLO AND L. SENA (ITALY)

A number of anti-oxidant agents and/or free radical scavengers exert an anti-inflammatory activity that is displayed in various models of acute and chronic experimental inflammation in diverse fashion [1]. Three of the most active compounds for preventing acute inflammatory reactions appear to be propyl gallate (PG), 2-mercaptopropionylglycine (2MPG) and *N,N'*-diphenyl-*p*-phenylendiamine (DPPD). These chemicals significantly depress hind paw oedema induced acutely in the rat by injection of carrageenin, bradykinin, serotonin or dextran. In addition, PG and 2MPG are able to restrict, respectively, the phlogistic process following the injection of 4-hydroxy-2, 3-*trans*-penten-1-al and malealdehyde, while some non-steroidal anti-inflammatory agents are ineffective. The aldehydes mentioned above are thought to be among the final products of lipid peroxidation. An interpretation of the mechanisms of action of the above chemicals derives from data showing that lipid peroxidation plays a role in inflammation. Furthermore, such compounds could act by inhibiting the production of endoperoxides during the biosynthesis of prostaglandins. Recently, the pivotal role of $PGE_2$ in inflammation has been stressed[2].

Data here reported refer to a series of experiments carried out to evaluate the influence of PG, 2MPG and DPPD on $PGE_2$ formation from arachidonic acid compared to the effects of some non-steroidal anti-inflammatory agents.

Our results indicate propyl gallate, 2-mercaptopropionylglycine and *N,N'*-diphenyl-*p*-phenylendiamine inhibit, to different extents, $PGE_2$ production The most effective compound appears to be PG, which was more active than flufenamic acid and acetyl salicylic acid. A minor inhibitory activity was displayed by 2MPG and DPPD. These data suggest that tested compounds can interfere with the inflammatory reaction also by influencing prostaglandin biosynthesis.

## References

1 Dianzani, M. U., Torrielli, M. V., Paradisi, L. and Franzone, J. S. (1978). *Eur. J. Rheum. Inflamm.,* **1,** 187

2 Kuehl, F. A., Humes, J. L., and Egan, R. (1977). In Willoughby, D. A., Giroud, J. P. and Velo, G. P. (eds.) *Perspectives in Inflammation* p. 331 (Lancaster: MTP Press)

# 47

# Preliminary data on the influence of thyroid function on prostaglandin biosynthesis (Abstract)

J. S. FRANZONE, T. NATALE, L. SENA
AND M. V. TORRIELLI (ITALY)

The thyroid may influence, to different degrees, the development of acute inflammatory reactions, as produced by carrageenin injection, and interferes with the chronic inflammatory process, like the cotton pellet induced granuloma in the rat[1]. In addition, treatment with non-steroidal anti-inflammatory agents resulted in a significantly modified response to the pharmacological effect of these drugs of hyper- and hypothyroid rats as compared to euthyroid rats.

In an attempt to understand better the mechanism by which thyroid hormones can interfere with the inflammatory reactions, we studied prostaglandin synthesis in thyroparathyroidectomized and in tri-iodo-L-thyronine treated rats.

The hyperthyroid state significantly increases the biosynthesis of $PGE_2$ from arachidonic acid while hypothyroidism did not exert any influence as evaluated *in vitro* by rat stomach strip preparations[2]. In addition, in hypothyroid rats indomethacin, oxametacine and phenylbutazone were less effective in inhibiting $PGE_2$ formation while the hyperthyroid state slightly increased the inhibitory action of indomethacin.

## References

1 Sena, L., Franzone, J. S., Paradisi, L. and Torrielli, M. V. (1978). *Eur. J. Rheum. Inflamm.*, **1**, 278
2 Flower, R., Cryglewski, R., Hervaezynska-Cedro, K. and Vane, J. R. (1972). *Nature (London), New Biol.*, **238**, 104

# Discussion

**Professor G. P. Lewis (Chairman)** invited Dr Ford-Hutchinson to open the discussion with a brief account of lipoxygenase.

**Dr A. W. Ford-Hutchinson (UK)** said that they had adopted the view that because of the wide variety of lipoxygenase products so far discovered it was unwise to measure a particular product. They had therefore set up two bioassays; a PMN aggregation test which was an assay of chemotactic factors, and a chemokinesis assay using an agarose micro-droplet system. The generating system was rat PMNs treated with calcium ionophore and dilutions of up to 1 in 1000 of supernatants from these polymorph cells produced significant chemokinesis or aggregation of separate PMN populations. The time course of release of these activities was very rapid and drugs known to inhibit lipoxygenase pathways inhibited such activities whereas non-steroidal anti-inflammatories had no effect. HPLC showed that more than 95% of the activity was in a single peak with a characteristic triplet structure in the UV spectrum and mass spectrometry identified it as leukotriene B or 5, 12-dihydroxyeicosatetraenoic acid. Dose response studies showed it to be active down to 5 pg/ml with an $ED_{50}$ between 150–200 pg/ml which was 100–1000 times more active than 5-HETE, the most potent chemokinetic agent known previously. The chemokinetic activity for human PMNs was stimulated random movement. So far they had not examined directed movement. The PMN aggregation test used a standard aggregometer with nephelometry and showed a transient aggregation response after 45 s which had diminished to zero after 5 min. On being asked about assay data for the product, he said they had a complete mass spectrum for leukotriene B. The HPLC retention time was identical to that reported by Samuelsson. The UV spectrum showed three absorbent peaks, indicating a conjugated triene structure. Other assay data also defined it as identical to that material reported by Samuelsson as leukotriene B.

**Dr G. Higgs (UK)** considered the general scheme of arachidonic acid peroxidation. If endoperoxides were to be formed, then it was necessary to have peroxidation in the 11-position before there could be formation of G2, H2 and the conventional cyclo-oxygenase products. If cyclization did not occur, then the 11-peroxy acid would be available for hyper-peroxidation and the formation of a stable 11-HETE. There was now some evidence that the enzyme involved in the formation of these products was significantly different from that involved in reactions of other parts of the molecule. Siegel and co-workers had shown that 11-HETE was being produced by a microsomal enzyme which was previously thought to be exclusively cyclo-oxygenase and they would also present evidence that indomethacin prevented the formation of 11-HETE at the same concentrations as it prevented the formation of the cyclo-oxygenase product HHT. The chemokinetic and chemotactic activity to which Dr Ford-Hutchinson had referred resided in compounds like 12-HETE and 5-HETE. The interesting possibility also existed of slow reacting substance and eosinophil chemotactic factor being derived from the same pathway with the incorporation of either glutathione or another peptide or perhaps a single amino acid with the 5, 6-epoxide of arachidonic acid. There appeared to be very good evidence that lipoxygenase II products were very potent modulators of leukocyte function but in terms of drug development the trend in anti-inflammatories should probably be in the area of total inhibition of lipid peroxidation rather than selective cyclo-oxygenase inhibition, as was the case with indomethacin.

**Dr M. I. Siegel (USA)** said that for the synthesis of 15-HPETE or 11-HPETE, the initial rate-limiting step was the making labile of the hydrogen atom at position 13. The same was true of the cyclo-oxygenase reaction and so it was not surprising that one might find similar drug inhibition patterns. On adding an activated oxygen molecule at position 11 one arrived at the 11-derivative which Samuelsson had originally proposed as the putative intermediate or transition state on the way to prostaglandin endoperoxide. If that 11-peroxide were accessible to water or the enzyme had the capability of releasing it, the result was 11-HETE: On the other hand, if the enzyme added the activated oxygen to the 15-position after labilization of the hydrogen at the 13-position, one arrived at 15-HETE. In effect, this amounted to having a similar active site for all three species; prostaglandins, 11- and 15-HETE. He believed that the 15- derivatives were also produced via lipoxygenase I because he had found that in rat neutrophils, production of 11-HETE, 15-HETE and any of the cyclo-oxygenase products were all irreversibly inhibited by the same agents, aspirin and indomethacin. There was no evidence in neutrophils of any production of 12-HETE. 5-HETE did not occur in the basal state although it did occur after ionophore and some other treatments.

**Dr Higgs** pointed out that to have initial peroxidation in the 11-position one must have abstraction of hydrogen in the 15-position. In those conditions, peroxidation was facilitated at the 15-position as well as the 11-position. It was therefore very likely that the common trigger for 11-and 15-HETE production and endoperoxide production was abstraction of hydrogen at position 13. He thought it very feasible that the lipoxygenase I type of reaction existed and that aspirin-like drugs would inhibit it as well as inhibiting cyclo-oxygenase. In relation to the relevance of these findings to the cellular components of inflammation, it was necessary to consider these possible activities of 11-HETE and 15-HETE in terms of cell migration and he invited Mr Palmer to describe the relative potencies of lipoxygenase I and II products in this regard.

**Mr R. M. J. Palmer (UK)** had examined the activity of a number of monohydroxy products using a chemokinetic assay developed at King's College, London. The 5-hydroxy acid was the most potent, potency then declining progressively through the 8, 9, 11 and 12-derivatives and being absent in the 15-products. Thus it appeared that lipoxygenase I products were comparatively inactive in the human system. This structural specificity did not exist in rabbits or rats for reasons which were not clear. In the rabbit, the 15-acid was among the more potent. The possibility existed that it might be metabolized further to act as a substrate for lipoxygenase I. These species differences did call into question the relevance of monohydroxy acid as cell recruiting agents in inflammation.

**Dr Ford-Hutchinson** said that further metabolites, going beyond the dihydroxy and possibly the trihydroxy fatty acids, might eventually turn out to be far more important than the monohydroxy acids themselves. Using the same assay system they had found a $10^4$ times greater difference in potency between the 5, 12-dihydroxy and the 5-hydroxy acid. It was not entirely clear how the 5, 12-product was formed, though he believed that lipoxygenase would not enter into its production.

**Dr I-F. Skidmore (UK)** asked how important biologically were such lipid molecules. In particular, how important were they in acute inflammation with neutrophil infiltration or in inflammation where one might expect release of lipids, for example in radiation damage? Undoubtedly their activity had been demonstrated but it was now time to assess whether such activity were biologically relevant.

**Dr Ford-Hutchinson** speculated that they would not be particularly important in chronic inflammation. They would probably be more important in regard to violent stimuli such as sudden formation of antigen–antibody complexes during anaphylactic reactions. Such products were much more chemotactic towards eosinophils and their key action might be in bringing eosinophils towards such sites in anaphylaxis.

**Dr Higgs** did not completely agree. Many types of chronic inflammatory disease involved relapse and remission and during the relapse one might find so-called acute signs recurring, such as cell infiltration and cell migration into the inflamed area. He therefore saw a continuing role for the generation of these chemotactic factors by PMNs or by inflamed tissue, or indeed by the chronic inflammatory cells such as macrophages. Although understanding of their importance in inflammation was still far from complete, their effect at very low concentrations on leukocyte function had certainly been demonstrated.

**Dr R. J. Walker (UK)** said that his own work wholly substantiated previous findings. The rabbit PMN presumably had considerable lipoxygenase II activity but very little 11- or 12-HETE was formed. In the incubation conditions initially used the 5- and 5, 12-HETE made up 40% of the products. Benoxaprofen, in concentrations found in plasma, was capable of producing a dose related inhibition of both 5- and 5, 12-HETE and BW755 also inhibited the formation of these compounds.

**Dr Siegel** said that lipoxygenase metabolites might well serve roles other than acting as intermediates on the pathway to hydroxy fatty acids. Within the inflammatory reaction, it appeared that such hydroperoxides might also be involved in the release of histamine and several groups had shown their potency in causing tracheal or lung constriction. Thus it was necessary to consider the transient hydroperoxides themselves, as well as the hydroxy fatty acid end product.

**Dr R. Vinegar (USA)** said that despite many attempts using prostaglandins $E_1$, $E_2$, prostacyclin and 5- or 11-HETE, he had found none of them chemotactic, nor even truly inflammatory. For him they were merely oedemagens when injected subcutaneously.

**Professor Lewis** asked how specific were the enzyme inhibitors such as aspirin and BW755 in their effects on this relatively new pathway. The literature now reported lipoxygenase inhibitors where it previously reported cyclo-oxygenase inhibitors, presumably because of the close relation of these pathways. He wondered whether there would have to be a reassessment of the specificity of these drugs.

**Dr Higgs** said that indirect evidence suggested that aspirin, indomethacin and other non-steroidal anti-inflammatories might well have non-specific effects at high concentrations. At very low doses, indomethacin specifically inhibited the production of cyclo-oxygenase products but on increasing the dose it exerted an effect on cell migration, first a potentiation then a reduction. This might well be due to effects on lipoxygenase. He hoped that BW755 would give anti-inflammatory activity more akin to the steroids in that it would prevent arachidonic acid oxygenation by all pathways whereas steroids were perhaps working by preventing the release of arachidonic acid in the first place. It was hoped that a compound like BW755 might produce a steroid type of anti-inflammatory effect without the unwanted side effects of sodium retention and effects on protein synthesis. The drug inhibited both lipoxygenase I and II pathways and cyclo-oxygenase.

On being asked what evidence there was that steroids acted primarily by inhibiting arachidonic acid release, he said that in the early 1970s they had been tried against cyclo-oxygenase and lipoxygenase, both without effect. Increasing evidence now suggested that release of arachidonic acid was being effected, perhaps through stimulation of protein synthesis, resulting in a factor which inhibited phospholipase.

# DISCUSSION

**Dr M. Glatt (Switzerland)**, noting that benoxaprofen had been used in rather high dosage, wondered whether it was necessary, in order to obtain an effect, to increase the level so as to obtain the same inhibition of cyclo-oxygenase as had been obtained with indomethacin. In other words, the possibility might exist that this particular pathway was not important.

**Dr Walker (UK)** said that cyclo-oxygenase inhibition occurred at much greater concentrations than those required to inhibit lipoxygenase, the latter being achieved at therapeutic levels.

**Professor Lewis** again asked for clarification of the steps taken to identify the products of lipoxygenase activity.

**Dr J. A. Salmon (UK)** said that in the initial stages characterization was by HPLC, GlC and mass spectrometry. Thereafter they developed a screen which involved labelled arachidonate and thin-layer chromatography and after establishing the Rf of particular hydroxy acids that information could then be used in the screen. Because of their difference in UV absorption characteristics, hydroxy acids and leukotriene B could also be assayed after HPLC using this technique.

**Dr Ford-Hutchinson** recommended the use of a bioassay involving PNM aggregation which allowed handling of 150 samples a day much more readily than a chemical assay. While it was true that other substances would give the same result, he nonetheless thought the method was valuable for routine screening use where interfering compounds were unlikely to be present.

**Dr D. N. Hall (UK)** said that benoxaprofen appeared preferentially to inhibit the mononuclear rather than the polymorphonuclear leukocytes. He wondered what significance this had with regard to lipoxygenase activity.

**Dr S. C. R. Meacock (UK)** was unable to answer the question since work had principally been done on the PMN. It would be necessary to examine the mononuclear cell to establish whether its pathways were identical before the question could be answered.

**Dr Dunn (France)** said that it seemed well established that the products of the cyclo-oxygenase pathway were associated with gastric function and that inhibition of this pathway by non-steroidal anti-inflammatory agents might be one of the explanations for their ulcerogenic properties. He wondered whether there was any evidence that the products of the lipoxygenase pathway had any influence on gastric function. If not, it might be advisable to search for anti-inflammatory agents which worked preferentially on this latter pathway since they might be less ulcerogenic, although still anti-inflammatory.

**Dr Higgs** said that BW755 had no significant ulcerogenicity at doses 5–10 times the anti-inflammatory $ED_{90}$. It was not clear whether it influenced the lipoxygenase pathway but there did seem to be selective inhibition of inflammatory cyclo-oxygenase without any effect on prostacyclin production in the gastric mucosa. They hoped selectively to inhibit the generation of prostaglandins in inflammation without impairing the intestinal or gastric mucosal cyclo-oxygenase. Any drug which could achieve such an effect would be very welcome.

**Dr P. A. Bacon (Co-chairman)** asked whether benoxaprofen given with a standard non-steroidal agent such as indomethacin would show any additional clinical benefit.

**Dr Meacock** said it was important to realize that although benoxaprofen was a lipoxygenase inhibitor it had other effects too. So far they could not describe its total mechanism and thus were unable to answer the question.

**Dr Higgs** agreed. The information which was so far missing involved the actual measurement of drug effects on the generation of lipoxygenase products *in vivo*. They were attempting to do so but the assay problems were considerable. Biological activities, apart from leukocyte function, were fairly low and difficult to measure and so far they had had to rely on analytical techniques which were tedious and required a great deal of material. Preliminary evidence suggested that some of the monohydroxy acids were produced in the carrageenin induced inflammation in rats but this finding, and the effects of drugs on it, required further clarification.

**Miss E. M. Davidson (UK),** on being invited by the Chairman to comment on thromboxane production in PMNs, said that in rabbit PMNs arachidonic acid metabolism by the cyclo-oxygenase pathway did not seem to produce any prostaglandins. Even with the stimulus of ionophore and zymosan, thromboxane was found only in low nanagram levels.

**Dr P. Badenoch-Jones (UK)** was asked to comment on his work on lymphokine induced macrophage aggregation. They believed that by measuring macrophage aggregation they were measuring the same material as caused macrophage migration inhibition, the difference being that one could measure unlimited numbers of samples for macrophage aggregation. The aggregating activity occurred within 30 min whereas the migration inhibition took 6–16 h to become apparent. Preliminary experiments showed that colchicine would inhibit both migration inhibition and aggregation and there was some similarity in the effects of calcium ionophore which caused both an aggregation and an inhibition of macrophage migration. Reports in the literature suggested that calcium influx might be involved, together with an altered ratio of cyclic AMP to GMP in the mechanism of action of migration inhibition factor (MIF).

**Professor Lewis** said that macrophages did not aggregate *in vivo*, and so he questioned the relationship between a test measuring aggregation and true *in vivo* macrophage behaviour.

**Dr Badenoch-Jones** said that two aspects were relevant. It had been found in the early 1960s that when a sufficiently sensitized animal which had previously been injected with oil to cause an increase in the number of peritoneal macrophages received specific antigen intraperitoneally, one observed after 1–5 h an aggregation of macrophages to each other and also to the lining of the peritoneal cavity. Secondly, it was necessary to consider the relevance of MIF activity to the pathogenesis of chronic inflammation *in vivo*. Although perhaps naive, it was possible that increased adhesiveness of macrophages would cause them to stick together and hence to migrate out of the granuloma more freely than they migrated in.

**Mr M. A. Bray (UK)** had started to examine the behaviour of monocytes which appeared to show parallel behaviour to PMNs. They aggregated in the presence of ionophore but he did not know what relevance this had to lymphokines.

**Dr Dunn** had also observed the macrophage disappearance reaction referred to by DrBadenoch-Jones. The important point, however, was that this aggregation phenomenon could be completely abolished by anti-coagulants. He thought this to be quite different from the other results being discussed which involved such entities as cyclic nucleotides.

**Dr Badenoch-Jones** agreed that the macrophage disappearance reaction displayed a number of special features. Aggregation *in vitro* was observed after 1 h which was probably too early for active synthesis of lymphokines. Nonetheless, lymphokine (whose presence was shown by a potent MIF activity) would aggregate macrophages, a reaction which could be almost completely abolished by colchicine at $10^{-5}$ mol/l.

**Dr D. F. Horrobin (Canada)** and his group had been interested in the possibility of major differences between the series 1 and series 2 prostaglandins. There were three reasons why he believed that the series 1 prostaglandins might have favourable effects in chronic inflammation. First, Karim and others had found that, in all species, the 1 series prostaglandins were present at higher concentrations in the thymus than the 2 series, suggesting that they might have a special importance in the immune system. Secondly, the work of Dr Zurier in Connecticut showed very effective control of inflammation by $PGE_1$. $PGE_1$ was an effective inhibitor of the inflammatory response in the adjuvant arthritis model in rats, in mice, and in passively transferred vasculitis. Thirdly, $PGE_1$ could activate cyclic AMP, inhibit arachidonic acid mobilization and inhibit lysosomal activity, which also suggested that it might be a potent anti-inflammatory factor. His own group had used two test systems. One had compared the mobilization of di-homo-γ-linolenic acid, the precursor of the 1 series, with mobilization of arachidonic acid using rat vascular tissue. The other system had examined the conversion by human platelets of both acids to their respective prostaglandins. Surprisingly, they had found that a number of agents affected these systems differently. Zinc and levamisole appeared to influence the mobilization in the vascular system of di-homo-γ-linolenic but not arachidonic acid, while colchicine was able to enhance the formation of 1 series prostaglandins from the former without changing the formation of the 2 series from the latter. This was true at levels of colchicine used in gout or familial Mediterranean fever ($10^{-8}$–$10^{-7}$mol/l). at higher concentrations ($10^{-6}$–$10^{-5}$ mol/l) which were never used in clinical situations, the reverse effect occurred, with colchicine enhancing the formation of the 2 rather than the 1 series prostaglandins. Thus, a number of agents with long-term effects on the control of inflammatory processes were able selectively to increase the production of 1 series prostaglandins. Since both steroids and non-steroidal anti-inflammatory agents blocked the production of both the 1 and 2 series this might be why they were not effective in the chronic situation. Their group would argue that what were required were agents which would enhance series 1 production but inhibit that of series 2.

**Dr Bray** said that he knew of no recent evidence for the generation of 1 series prostaglandins by any cell type known to be involved in the inflammatory reaction. In addition, Dr Zurier had used large amounts of material injected into arthritic rabbits and rats.

**Dr Horrobin** said that although many believed that there was no circulating $PGE_1$ in man, Dr Lagarde in France had demonstrated its presence using a specific immunossay and had shown that human platelets actually produced more $PGE_1$ and $PGE_2$. Workers in Nashville had also demonstrated circulating $PGE_1$ at concentrations which were biologically active *in vitro*. The problem had been that most of the assays were non-specific, measuring the 1 and 2 series together. They had recently shown that $PGE_2$ greatly enhanced the conversion of di-homo-γ-linolenic acid to $PGE_1$ although having no effect on the conversion of arachidonic acid to $PGE_2$. Thus, $PGE_2$ would enhance the production of $PGE_1$ which raised very interesting questions about feedback relations between the two series.

**Miss M. V. Doig (UK)** said that with quantitive mass spectrometry of rat peritoneal macrophages they had not been able to find any evidence for prostaglandin $E_1$ or $E_2$ production.

**Professor T. C. Dray (France),** despite the use of a very specific immunoassay, had not been able to show the presence of $PGE_1$ in human blood. His level of sensitivity was 2 pg/ml. In Dr Lagarde's case, the prostaglandin might have come from platelets but he doubted if it were true circulating $PGE_1$.

**Dr M. K. Jasani (UK)** said that at a site of inflammation, parenchymal as well as inflammatory cells were present, and so far no one had ruled out the possibility that in inflamed tissue these parenchymal cells might be producing $PGE_1$.

**Dr S. A. Saeed (UK),** being asked to describe his work on an endogenous inhibitor of the prostaglandin system, said that they proceeded from the fact that human blood plasma or serum powerfully inhibited prostaglandin synthesis. They discovered that this activity was mainly associated with the albumin and haptoglobin factions of plasma. They suggested that haptoglobin inhibition, itself antagonized by haemoglobin, could be part of the natural system controlling prostaglandin synthesis. Haptoglobin acted mainly on cyclo-oxygenation of arachidonic acid, the reaction leading to endoperoxides.

**Dr Bacon** pointed out that haptoglobin was an acute phase reactant and there had been some discussion about the desirability of controlling acute phase reactants to help rheumatoid patients.

**Dr Saeed** agreed. It had been known for many years that haptoglobin increased in a variety of inflammatory situations. It was presumably part of the defence mechanism. The normal level of haptoglobin in the plasma was 1 mg/ml and he had found that 100 μg/ml of a haptoglobin preparation 76% pure inhibited bovine PG synthetase. He had obtained a good dose-response curve between 100 and 200 μg, levels below those in the serum. However, albumin in the plasma also contributed to PG synthesis inhibition and the two proteins together might give additive effects.

**Dr Billingham** took up the issue of acute phase reactants. The physician's role must not be to lower the level of such reactants artificially but rather to treat chronic disease in such a way that they were reduced as a secondary consequence. In rheumatoid arthritis haptoglobin could show a 10-fold increase, so if it had a role in damping down for the acute manifestations of inflammation, it was not doing so very effectively.

**Professor Lewis** then directed discussion to the mode of action of anti-inflammatory steroids. Some years previously, when it was first found that they prevented release of prostaglandins, work had been done on membrane permeability to steroids but they had not been able to detect any reaction between steroids and lipoproteins which might lead to an alteration in lipoprotein associated enzymes.

**Professor Di Rosa (Italy)** said that it was certainly known that corticosteroids inhibited prostaglandin biosynthesis in intact cells. There was increasing evidence that such inhibition required DNA-dependent RNA synthesis and protein synthesis. They had shown that rat peritoneal macrophages treated with hydrocortisone released into the medium the factor responsible for the anti-phospholipase effect. Dr Flower had found that in the effluent retrieved from lung perfused with dexamethasone there was a factor similarly inhibiting phospholipase. The release of this factor in his own system could be prevented by cyclohexamide or actinomycin D. The factor did not show effective inhibition in the presence of arachidonic acid. He believed that it was a protein or large polypeptide and the concentration range of hydrocortisone inducing its formation was $10^{-6}$ to $10^{-7}$ mol/l. Chromatographic and other assays performed with Dr Flower did not rule out the possibility that the lung inhibitor and the macrophage inhibitor might be very similar. So far they had not tested its effects on purified preparations in phospholipids.

**Dr Skidmore** warned against the increasingly common assumption that the anti-inflammatory effects of steroids were necessarily associated with their ability to inhibit arachidonic acid release from phospholipids. If this were the primary mechanism of action of steroids then replacement of arachidonic acid should reverse the anti-inflammatory effects in the same way that it had been shown that the anti-inflammatory effect of indomethacin could be reversed by administration of prostaglandins. He had used two systems to test this notion. First was the carrageenin oedema and secondly the influx of PMNs into a CM cellulose pouch in the rat. They had tried to reverse the anti-inflammatory effects by administration of exogenous arachidonic acid but in neither of these situations was a reversal effected. However, reversal of the carrageenin oedema could be achieved with prostaglandins. This suggested to him that the anti-inflammatory effect of steroids in simple acute models of inflammation was largely independent of reduction in arachidonic acid release.

**Dr Higgs** said that the interpretation of those experiments depended entirely on the premise that exogenously administered arachidonic acid was metabolized in the same way as endogenous acid. He believed there were indications that that was not so.

**Dr R. McMillan (USA)** was invited to describe his own work on the action of steroids. He said that they had been trying to make normal synovial cells biochemically resemble those cell types which could be taken from a rheumatoid joint, especially in regard to collagenase release. They had found that phorbol myristate acid

(PMA), cytochalasin B and polyethylene glycol would induce collagenase production when added to normal synovial cells. The change was accompanied by formation of prostaglandins giving two similarities between the modified cells and the rheumatoid synovial cells described by others. In addition, non-steroidal anti-inflammatory agents did not alter the collagenase pathway but did block prostaglandin production, again similar to effects seen in rheumatoid cells. However, some dissociation in effect was seen in that bradykinin, for example, would induce prostaglandin production but not collagenase in synovial cells. Bradykinin had been found to exert a specific effect, releasing arachidonic acid which was metabolized to prostaglandin $E_2$. In contrast, the collagenase inducers PMA and cytochalasin B induced wide changes in phospholipid metabolism leading to the release not only of arachidonic acid but also of oleate, linoleate and palmitate. The collagenase inducers all made dramatic changes to the morphology of the cell whereas bradykinin did not change its morphology. Their hypothesis was that prostaglandin production associated with collagenase inducers was a reflection of these dramatic changes in phospholipid metabolism which were probably related to changes in cell morphology. Thus it seemed that prostaglandin production stimulated by collagenase inducers in synovial cells was due to non-specific changes in phospholipid metabolism. This might explain why indomethacin was not active in inhibiting collagenase formation because it acted on only one part of the pathway. In addition, they had used PMA stimulated synovial cells and monitored release of different fatty acids to establish how specific was the dexamethasone inhibition of prostaglandin production. Dexamethasone inhibited arachidonic acid release and metabolism but did not affect the release of oleate, linoleate or palmitate. Dexamethasone actually potentiated the release of oleate by PMA so that its inhibition of prostaglandin production in this system was highly specific. It was not simply the result of stabilizing the membrane, which would inhibit all the fatty acid release.

**Professor Lewis** had found using fat cell ghosts that steroids produced an inhibition of phospholipase activity but there was also an increase in the activity of neutral lipase, so the amount of arachidonic acid released from neutral triglycerides was actually increased at the same time that the release of arachidonic acid from phospholipids was reduced. He wondered if Dr McMillan believed in the existence of a specific lipase to release arachidonic acid.

**Dr McMillan** said that his findings would support that hypothesis. The lipase for arachidonic acid was probably different from that for other fatty acids since dexamethasone could inhibit it selectively.

On being asked how he knew that the collagenase and prostaglandins were produced by the same type of cell, he agreed that he had not been dealing with a single cell type, although the cells were far more homogeneous than those found in rheumatoid arthritis.

**Dr I. J. Zeitlin (UK)** was invited to discuss his work on histamine. Initially they had devised an adjuvant arthritis model which permitted the study of permeability changes during various phases of development. In order to examine the relative importance of different mediators at different stages of arthritis they tested indomethacin, to block cyclo-oxygenase, and cimetidine to block histamine. To their surprise, since histamine was not thought to be very important in rat inflammation, they found that cimetidine produced a marked inhibition of adjuvant arthritis in rats. In order to test the specificity of the effect they examined the influence of intraperitoneal cimetidine on $H_1$ and $H_2$ agonists injected into the paw. On measuring paw volume, they found cimetidine was specific for the $H_2$ receptor, and that the $H_2$ agonist was much more effective in producing rat paw oedema than either histamine or the $H_1$ agonist.

On being asked whether this was an effect on the proposed histamine receptors of inflamed cells he said that if that were so one would expect cimetidine to potentiate the inflammatory response. It seemed more likely to be associated with vascular changes and so they developed a rabbit model which permitted changes in permeability and vascular tone to be examined simultaneously in relation to the synovium. In this model, the permeability changes seemed to be independent of blood flow changes produced by histamine and secondary to them. Histamine or antagonists were infused into the synovium and the appearance of labelled albumin in the perfusate or the accumulation of labelled erythrocytes in the synovial vasculature was measured. The concentrations of histamine were such that the permeability changes examined were not related to changes in overall systemic blood pressure. It seemed to him clear that the role of histamine and some other mediators in rheumatoid arthritis should be re-examined.

**Dr J. F. Franzoni (Italy)** was invited to describe his work on the anti-inflammatory activity of some anti-oxidant compounds. He said that the finding that certain anti-oxidants were able to prevent or depress acute or chronic inflammation suggested that they might interfere with prostaglandin biosynthesis. The 3 anti-oxidants with the most marked action in preventing inflammatory reactions did influence $PGE_2$ synthesis from arachidonic acid but their effects were not great. Compared with some non-steroidal anti-inflammatory agents only propyl gallate exerted a significant interference with prostaglandin biosynthesis, an effect which appeared more significant than those of flufenamic or acetyl salicylic acid.

# Section V
# Experimental Models of Inflammation and Chemotaxis

CHAIRMAN: L. E. Glynn
CO-CHAIRMAN: J. P. Giroud

# 48

# Effect of pharmacological agents on macrophage accumulation

N. ACKERMAN, A. TOMOLONIS, L. MIRAM, J. KHEIFETS, S. MARTINEZ AND A. CARTER (USA)

## INTRODUCTION

Rheumatoid arthritis is characterized by an influx of both polymorphonuclear (PMN) and mononuclear leukocytes into various inflammatory sites[1,2]. These infiltrating cells are, in part, responsible for a number of pathological events resulting ultimately in protease release and connective tissue catabolism. Over the past 10 years a number of *in vivo* models of leukocyte infiltration have been described[3-5]. Most have been aimed at PMN accumulation and the effects of pharmacological agents on this process. In the current studies, a model of macrophage accumulation was developed; in addition, the effects of steroidal and non-steroidal anti-inflammatories and anti-rheumatic agents were determined.

## MATERIALS AND METHODS

The procedure used to induce a pleural inflammatory reaction is outlined in Figure 48.1. In some experiments, peripheral blood samples were removed from the abdominal aorta and leukocyte number and type determined. A 0.5% carboxymethylcellulose vehicle was used in all pharmacological studies.

### Sources

The following reagents were used during these studies: carrageenin (Viscarin), dextran (MW=255000), vitamin E, acridine orange and α-naphthyl butyrate (Sigma); tricalcium phosphate (Baker); thioglycollate

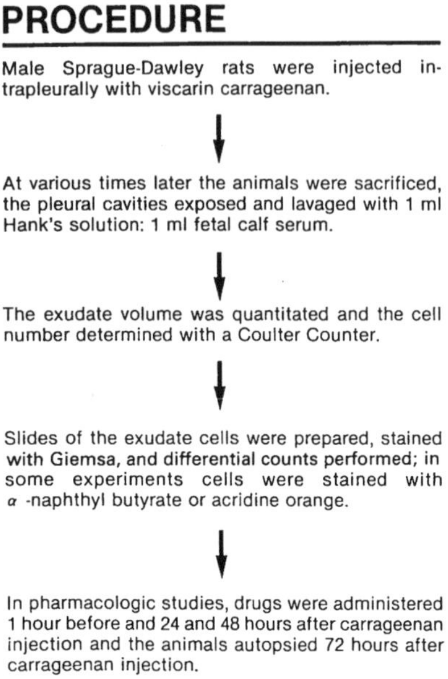


**Figure 48.1** Procedure for inducing a pleural macrophage response in rats

and complete Freund's adjuvant (Difco); dexamethasone, indomethacin and gold sodium thiomalate (Merck Sharpe and Dohme); naproxen (Syntex); levamisole (Pittman Moore); hydroxychloroquine (Winthrop); d-penicillamine (Calbiochem); dl-penicillamine (Aldrich).

## RESULTS

### Development of the pleural inflammatory reaction

In preliminary studies a number of agents were tested as inducers of a mononuclear cell infiltrate 48 and 72 h after introduction into the rat pleural space. Of the agents tested, 0.15 ml of a 1.0% carrageenin solution induced the largest number of mononuclear cells (Table 48.1). Over 90% of the mononuclear cells were macrophages as determined by morphological or histochemical criteria[6,7]. Thioglycollate and vitamin E, which induce large numbers of macrophages in the mouse peritoneal cavity[8] and rat paw[9], respectively, were much less effective than the carrageenin. Based on these and other results described elsewhere[10], a 72 h carrageenin-induced pleurisy was established as a macrophage accumulation model.

### Characteristics of the carrageenin reaction

The pleural cavity of the non-injected rat contained 8.9 ± 1.1 × (mean

**Table 48.1** Effects of selected agents on inducing cell infiltrate 48 h post-injection*

| *Potential stimulus* | *Concentration* (%) | *Volume injected* (ml) | *Number of animals* | *Number of Mononuclear cells*† ($\times 10^6$) |
|---|---|---|---|---|
| Saline | — | 0.5 | 10 | 8.0 ± 0.5 |
| Carrageenin | 1.0 | 0.15 | 10 | 102.2 ± 9.2 |
| Dextran | 10.0 | 1.0 | 10 | 15.0 ± 0.9 |
| Tricalcium phosphate | 1.0 | 1.0 | 8 | 43.4 ± 6.9 |
| Thioglycollate | 3.0 | 0.5 | 6 | 26.5 ± 0.9 |
| Complete Freund's adjuvant | 0.2 | 0.5 | 6 | 36.4 ± 6.6 |
| Vitamin E | 2.0 | 0.5 | 6 | 16.4 ± 0.8 |

*Groups of 6–10 rats were injected intrapleurally with various potential inflammatory stimuli. 48 h later the animals were sacrificed, the pleural cavities opened and lavaged, and the number of leukocytes determined. Slides were prepared and stained with Giemsa. The percentage of mononuclear cells was determined and the total number of intrapleural mononuclear cells calculated.

†Values indicate mean ± SE

± SE, $n = 6$) of which 71% were macrophages, 12% were lymphocytes and 14% were eosinophils. 6 h following injection of 0.3 ml carrageenin, the total pleural cell number was elevated to $284 \pm 34 \times 10^6$ cells (Figure 48.2). Almost 85% of these cells were PMNs, 2% were lymphocytes and 14% were macrophages. Macrophages were identified on the basis of morphological, histochemical and fluorescent characteristics. The total number of macrophages at this time was approximately $40 \times 10^6$. 24 h after the injection of carrageenin, $367.1 \pm 24.6 \times 10^6$ cells were present in the pleural cavity; 66% were PMNs and 33% were macrophages. The number of PMNs declined rapidly thereafter until they constituted only 8% of the total exudate cells at 72 h post-carrageenin injection. Macrophages constituted over 80% of the total exudate count at this time.

**Pharmacologic effects on 3 day pleural inflammation steroids**

Animals treated with dexamethasone, 0.005 (mg/kg)/day p.o., administered 1 h before and 24 and 48 h post-carrageenin, had 54 ± 9% fewer pleural macrophages than did vehicle treated animals ($p < 0.01$; Table 48.2). Total peripheral leukocyte and monocyte counts were unaffected. Animals treated with dexamethasone, 0.05 (mg/kg)/day p.o., showed a comparable response. The results indicate that dexamethasone was acting as an inhibitor of cell migration, or an inhibitor of the generation of one or more chemotactic factors. Willoughby and co-workers have demonstrated that, in rats, steroids

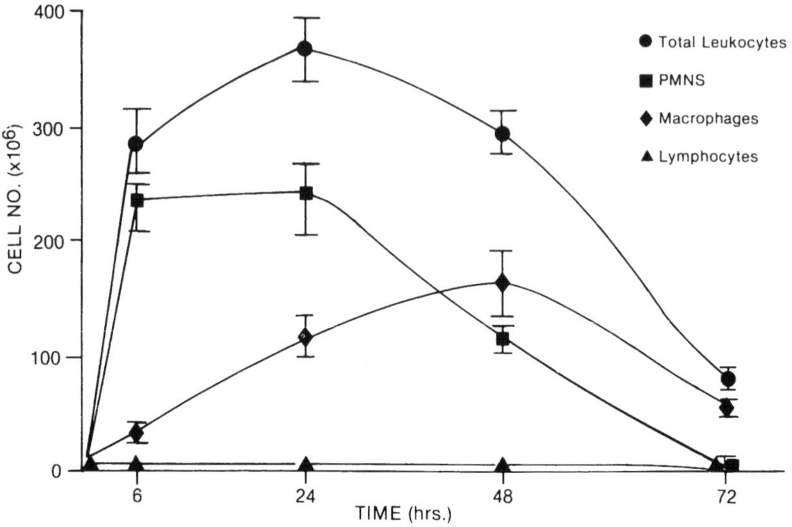


**Figure 48.2** Peripheral blood samples were removed from groups of 5–6 rats and quantitated; 0.3 ml viscarin carrageenin was injected intrapleurally. Various times later peripheral blood samples were removed and the animals autopsied. The pleural cavity was exposed and lavaged with Hank's solution plus fetal calf serum (1:1) and the peripheral blood and pleural exudate samples quantitated. Each value indicates mean ± SE of the cell type indicated within the pleural cavity

markedly reduced both the generation of chemotactic factors selective for monocytes, and the monocyte response to chemotactic factors obtained from non-drug treated animals[5]

**Non-steroidal anti-inflammatory agents**

Animals treated with indomethacin, 0.5 and 5.0 (mg/kg)/day p.o., had $82.7 \pm 7.6 \times 10^6$ and $102.7 \pm 8.4 \times 10^6$ pleural macrophages versus $47.7 \pm 6.3 \times 10^6$ in the vehicle controls ($p < 0.01$, Table 48.2). Animals treated with naproxen, 1 and 10 (mg/kg)/day, also had an elevated number of intrapleural macrophages (Table 48.2). This class of drugs have been shown to reduce the PMN accumulation in the carrageenin injected rat pleural cavity[11–13] One possible explanation for the enhanced macrophage response may be related to the activity of these drugs in blocking the cyclo-oxygenase pathway of prostaglandin biosynthesis. This could lead to an elevated production of certain lipoxygenase pathway products such as 12-L-hydroxy-5,8,10,14-eicosatetraenoic acid (HETE) which have been shown selectivity chemotactic for human eosinophils[14] Perhaps HETE or similar products (e.g. SRS-A) may be selectively chemotactic for rat monocytes.

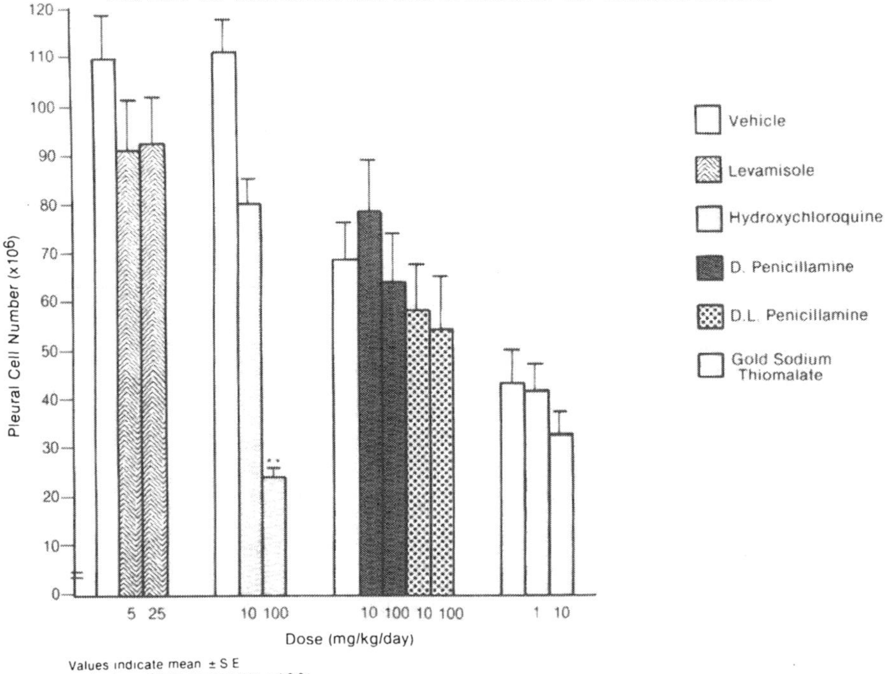


**Figure 48.3** Groups of 6–10 rats were injected intrapleurally with 0.3 ml carrageenin, and 3 days later autopsied and the number of pleural exudate cells quantitated. Drugs were administered orally (levamisole, hydroxychloroquine, D- and DL-penicillamine) or s.c. (gold sodium thiomalate) one hour before and 24 and 48 h after carrageenin injection. Values indicate mean ± SE.* indicates $p < 0.05$, ** indicates $p < 0.01$

**Anti-rheumatic agents**

Levamisole, 5 and 25 (mg/kg)/day p.o., D-and-DL-penicillamine, 10 and 100 (mg/kg)/day p.o., and gold sodium thiomalate, 1 and 10 (mg/kg)/day s.c., had no statistically significant effect on pleural cell accumulation (Figure 48.3). Hydroxychloroquine, 10 and 100 (mg/kg)/day p.o., caused a dose dependent decrease in pleural cell accumulation (Figure 48.3). At the higher dose, the cellular infiltrate was reduced over 80%; no changes in the peripheral blood picture were observed. The antimalarials, of which hydroxychloroquine is an example, are thought to become localized intracellularly within lysosomes. Perhaps they are reducing the synthesis and/or activities of one or more proteases required for the activation of complement and thereby inhibit the generation of chemotactic factors[15].

## CONCLUSIONS

A model of macrophage accumulation using a carrageenin induced pleurisy is

**Table 48.2** Effects of dexamethasone and selected non-steroidal anti-inflammatories on macrophage accumulation in a 3-day pleural reaction*

| *Drug* | *Dose* [(mg/kg)/day] | *n* | *Route* | *Percent reduction in the number of pleural macrophages*† |
|---|---|---|---|---|
| Dexamethasone | 0.005 | 7 | p.o. | 54 ± 9‡ |
| | 0.050 | 8 | p.o. | 57 ± 5§ |
| Indomethacin | 0.5 | 8 | p.o. | −73 ± 7§ |
| | 5.0 | 8 | p.o. | −115 ± 9§ |
| Naproxen | 1.0 | 7 | p.o. | −65 ± 3‡ |
| | 10.0 | 7 | p.o. | −99 ± 4§ |

*Animals were injected intrapleurally with 0.15 ml carrageenin and sacrificed 3 days later. The pleural cavities were lavaged and the total number of cells determined. Differential counts were performed on Giemsa-stained preparations, and the total number of pleural macrophages calculated. Total pleural cell number in vehicle treated animals was $60.2 \pm 6.0 \times 10^6$ (mean ± SE, $n = 21$); 87.6% of these cells were macrophages.

†A indicates a stimulation in pleural cell number.

‡$p < 0.05$ as determined with Student's $t$-test.

§$p < 0.01$ as determined with Student's $t$-test.

described. A number of pharmacological agents, such as dexamethasone and hydroxychloroquine, reduced the number of macrophages present at an inflammatory site. It is hoped that agents demonstrating this activity will reduce the size of the pannus in rheumatoid arthritis and be of significant therapeutic benefit.

## References


1 Hadler, N. M., Spitznagel, J. K., Quinet, R. J. (1979). Lysosomal enzymes in inflammatory synovial effusion. *J. Immunol.*, **123,** 572

2 Kobayashi, I., Ziff, M. (1975). Electron microscopic studies of the cartilage-pannus junction in rheumatoid arthritis. *Arthritis Rheum.*, **18,** 475

3 Borel, J. F., Feurer, C. (1978). *In vivo* effects of anti-inflammatory and other drugs on granulocyte emigration in the rabbit skin. *J. Pathol.*, **124,** 85

4 Parente, L., Kohm, M. S., Willoughby, D. A., Kitchen, A. (1979). Studies on cell motility in inflammation. I. The chemotactic activity of experimental, immunological and non-inflammatory exudates. *Agents Actions*, **9,** 190

5 Parente, L., Koh, M. S., Willoughby, D. A., Kitchen, A. (1979). Studies on cell motility in inflammation. II. The *in vivo* effect of anti-inflammatory and anti-rheumatic drugs on chemotaxis *in vitro*. *Agents Actions*, **9,** 196

6 Koski, I. R., Poplack, D. G., Blaese, R. M. (1976). A monospecific esterase stain for the identification of monocytes and macrophages. In Bloom, B. R. and David, J. R. (eds.) In Vitro *Methods in Cell Mediated and Tumor Immunity*, pp. 359–363 (New York: Academic Press)

7 Allison, A. C. (1976). Fluorescence microscopy of lymphocytes and mononuclear phagocytes and the use of silica to eliminate the latter. In Bloom, B. R. and David J. R. (eds.) In Vitro *Methods in Cell Mediated and Tumor Immunity*, pp. 395–404 (New York: Academic

Press)
8 Web, Z. and Gordon, S. (1975). Elastase reaction by stimulated macrophages. *J. Exp. Med.*, **142,** 361
9 Berkenkopf, J. W. and Lutsky, B. N. (1979). Vitamin E-induced chronic inflammation in rats. *Agents Actions*, **9,** 350
10 Ackerman, N., Tomolonis, A., Miram, L., Kheifets, J., Martinez, S. and Carter, A. (1981). Three day pleural inflammation: A new model to detect drug effects on macrophage accumulation. *J. Pharm. Exp. Ther.* (In press)
11 Ammendola, G., Di Rosa, M. and Sorrentino, L. (1975). Leucocyte migration and lysosomal enzyme release in rat carageenan pleurisy. *Agents Action*, **5,** 250
12 Koh, M. S., Parente, L. and Willoughby, D. A. (1979). Immunological and non-immunological pleural inflammation: The effects of anti-inflammatory and anti-rheumatic drugs. *Eur. J. Rheum. Inflamm.* **1,** 286
13 Ackerman, N. (Personal observations)
14 Goetzl, E. J., Woods, J. M. and Gorman, R. R. (1977). Stimulation of human eosinophil and neutrophil polymorphonuclear leukocyte chemotaxic and random migration by 12-L.hydroxy-5,8,10,14-eicosatetraenoic acid. *J. Clin. Invest.*, **59,** 179
15 Thomas, C. A., Yost, F. J. Jr., Snyderman, R., Hatcher, V. and Lazarus, G. S. (1977). Cellular serine proteinase induces chemotaxis by complement activation. *Nature (London)*, **269,** 521

49

# The histology of cotton pellet and polyvinyl sponge induced granulomas in rats (Abstract)

E. A. BOYLE, AND F. R. MANGAN (UK)

Sections have been taken from granulomas induced by the subcutaneous implantation of sterile cotton-wool pellets and polyvinyl sponges and these have been stained with the haematoxylin/eosin and Weigert/Van Gieson procedures. The granulomas have been removed at 9, 15 and 21 days after implantation and show a different pattern of formation in the two models. In the pellet a dense granuloma forms in and around the peripheral zone, completely encapsulating the cotton wool and barely penetrating into the centre. In the sponge, on the other hand, granuloma tissue has gradually penetrated the entire area. In the sponge random bundles of collagen fibres can be seen contrasting with the more organized fibrous sheath surrounding the pellet. Giant cells appeared in much greater frequency in the pellet, which had the characteristics of a typical foreign body granuloma, in contrast to that of the sponge, which was more characteristic of an irritant fibrosis.

# 50

# A biochemical and morphological study of the cotton pellet granuloma in the rat: effects of dexamethasone and indomethacin (Abstract)

P. J. BAILEY, ANITA STURM AND B. LOPEZ-RAMOS (USA)

The subcutaneous implantation of a cotton pellet into the rat results in the formation of a granuloma at the site of the implant. The early events comprise an accumulation of fluid and proteinaceous material together with an infiltration of neutrophils. The granuloma formed by day 7 is characterized by the formation of a vascularized fibrous capsule containing fibroblasts, giant cells and infiltrating mononuclear cells. Granuloma development was quantitated by dry weight measurements and its cellular content measured by assaying activity of *N*-acetyl-B-D-glucosaminidase (NAG) and total nucleic acid content. Nucleic acid determinations and histological examination show that cell infiltration into the granuloma takes place at a virtually constant rate over a 7 day period. In contrast the NAG activity does not change significantly until after day 5 when a large increase in the amount of enzyme extractable from the granuloma is seen. Systemic treatment of the animal with dexamethasone or indomethacin results in an inhibition of granuloma weight gain, NAG activity and nucleic acid levels. Drug treatment on days 0–3 results in suppression of granuloma formation whereas treatment on days 4–7 is without affect. This suggests that the two drugs are acting during the early phases of granuloma development. Histological examination shows clear differences between the action of dexamethasone and indomethacin. Dexamethasone profoundly inhibits the early infiltration of granulocytes and the later vascularization, infiltration of mononuclear cells and formation of the capsule. With indomethacin treatment, however, the early infiltration of granulocytes takes place, vascularization and encapsulation occurs but the later influx of mononuclear cells and the formation of giant cells is markedly reduced.

# 51

# Neutrophil interactions with particulate materials: an *in vitro* model for inflammatory arthritides

R. TURNER, G. COUNTS, J. JOHNSON,
E. WEST AND W. TREADWAY (USA)

## INTRODUCTION

Previous studies by our group[1] and others[2] have established *in vitro* systems for examining the interactions between neutrophils and immunoglobulin G aggregates or monosodium urate crystals which may be important in the inflammatory processses occurring in rheumatoid arthritis and gout. The present studies utilize a previously described[3] neutrophil monolayer system to quantitate the uptake of these particulate materials along with their subsequent effects on cellular adherence and enzyme release.

## MATERIALS AND METHODS

Neutrophils were obtained from normal subjects with their informed, written consent. All studies were carried out according to the Declaration of Helsinki.

**Insoluble IgG Aggregate preparation**

Insoluble IgG aggregates were prepared as previously described.[1] A solution of 20 mg/ml IgG (human gammaglobulins, fraction II, US Biochemical Corporation, Cleveland, Ohio) was prepared by suspending the IgG in 0.85% NaCl at 25 °C. This solution was centrifuged at 10 000 × *g* for 20 min to remove all remaining insoluble material. For studies requiring radiolabelled IgG, approximately 20 $\mu$Ci of 1.3 mol/l $^{51}CrCl_3$ (New England Nuclear, Boston, Massachusetts, specific activity approximately 375 Ci/g Cr) were added to each millilitre of solution ($1 \times 10^6$ (ct/min)/ml). The labelled or unlabelled IgG solutions were heat aggregated in a 63 °C water bath for 45 min, allowed to cool to room temperature and centrifuged at $10\,000 \times g$. The supernatant was discarded and the insoluble IgG precipitate was washed twice with 0.85% NaCl. The IgG solutions were brought to a concentration of 2.4 mg/ml in Dulbeccho's phosphate buffered saline (PBS). The protein content was measured by the Lowry technique[4].

**Monosodium urate crystal preparation**

The urate crystals were prepared by the method described by Seegmiller *et al.*[5]. This entailed dissolving 8 g of uric acid (Fisher Scientific Company) in 1600 ml of boiling water containing 49 ml of 1.0 N NaOH. The pH was adjusted to 7.2. The solution was cooled slowly to room temperature with stirring and stored overnight at 5 °C. The crystals were dried at room temperature and then dessicated. Examination under a polarizing microscope revealed a mean crystal length of 5–7 $\mu$m. The crystals were heated for 3 h at 180 °C before use to minimize possible pyrogen contamination.

**Monolayer studies**

Normal human neutrophils were obtained in 70–90% purity as previously described[1]. The cells were suspended to $5 \times 10^6$ polymorphonuclear leukocytes/ml in Dulbeccho's PBS containing 10% autologous serum. Monolayers were prepared by placing 2.5 ml of this cell suspension in 35 × 10 mm polyethylene petri dishes and incubating them for 45 min at 37 °C with periodic gentle agitation. The monolayers were washed twice in a PBS reservoir to remove non-adherent cells. A 1.5 ml volume of PBS 10% serum was gently layered over each monolayer prior to an additional 30 min 37 °C incubation. For the phagocytosis studies, 1.5 ml of either 2.4 mg/ml [$^{51}$Cr]IgG or 0.2 mg/ml urate crystals in PBS were layered over each dish. They were then incubated at 37 °C for 2, 15, 30, 45, 60 or 90 min and washed in PBS. Phagocytic activity was measured either by determining the number of adherent cells containing urate crystals, or, for the IgG studies, by scraping the surface of the monolayer into a counting tube and assaying the radioactivity in a gamma counter.

For the enzyme studies, the monolayers were not washed after the final incubation, but the fluid was gently aspirated from the cell layer so that aliquots could be taken for the determination of enzyme release. The remaining fluid was returned to the monolayer and the cells lysed by the addition of 0.1% Triton X-100. The total enzyme activity was determined by assaying aliquots of the cell lysate utilizing methods previously described[6].

Adherence was determined by microscopically counting the remaining cells after the final incubation and washing. One-way analysis of variance was performed on the data and the Tukey's multiple comparison test was employed in order to test the significance of all possible comparisons of experimental groups.

## RESULTS

Figure 51.1 shows the time curve of insoluble IgG aggregate phagocytosis. This curve is similar to the one reported[7] for neutrophils and IgG aggregates in tubes at the 'Future trends in inflammation III' meeting in 1977. As in the previous studies, there are wide standard errors with phagocytosis increasing with time and reaching statistical significance ($p < 0.05$) at 60 min and remaining significant at 90 min. Figure 51.2 shows the time curve of urate crystal phagocytosis. As shown in this figure, there is less variation at each time interval, with significantly greater ($p < 0.05$) phagocytosis above the 2 min value at each 15 min interval until the 45 min value, which does not differ significantly from the 60 or 90 min value. A similar time sequence has been reported by Shumacher[8] utilizing the electron microscope with apparent large increases to 30 min but with less thereafter. Significant IgG aggregate uptake had been previously demonstrated at 30 min with larger test groups[3], therefore adherence studies were performed in greater numbers at this time interval with the results shown in Figure 51.3. As is seen in this figure, control monolayers incubated in PBS alone maintained good adherence at 87 ± 4%. An insignificant decrease in adherence to 78 ± 5% was observed for monolayers incubated with PBS containing insoluble IgG aggregates. Urate crystals caused a marked decrease in adherence to 62 ± 5% which was statistically ($p < 0.05$) different from the PBS and insoluble IgG values. Figure 51.4 shows the time related increase in the release of the azurophilic granular enzyme β-glucuronidase, the azurophilic and specific granular enzyme lysozyme, and the cytoplasmic enzyme LDH on exposure of neutrophil monolayers to insoluble IgG aggregates. The points on the curve represent the average of two representative experiments. β-glucuronidase release and lysozyme release, as previously described by our group[6,9] and others[2] utilizing IgG aggregates and neutrophils in tubes, appears to be enhanced by the presence of aggregates in the system. The release of cytoplasmic enzyme LDH appears to be lessened by the presence of the aggregates in the system. Extensive release of lysozyme and LDH at 90 min has not been present in previous studies and may be a result of unexplained early cell death in one of these studies. Figure 51.5 shows the time curve of urate crystal induced enzyme release from neutrophil monolayers. As with IgG aggregates, these studies show the mean of two representative experiments and suggest that there is enhancement of the release of lysosomal enzymes by the crystals. LDH release does not appear to be significantly affected except at 45–90 min when cell death may account for

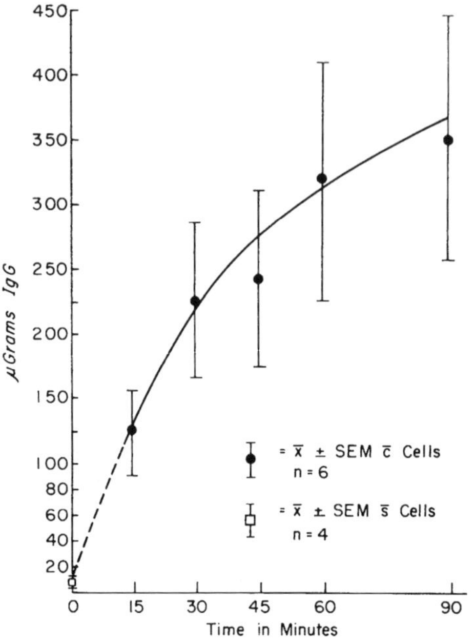


**Figure 51.1** Time curve of insoluble IgG phagocytosis

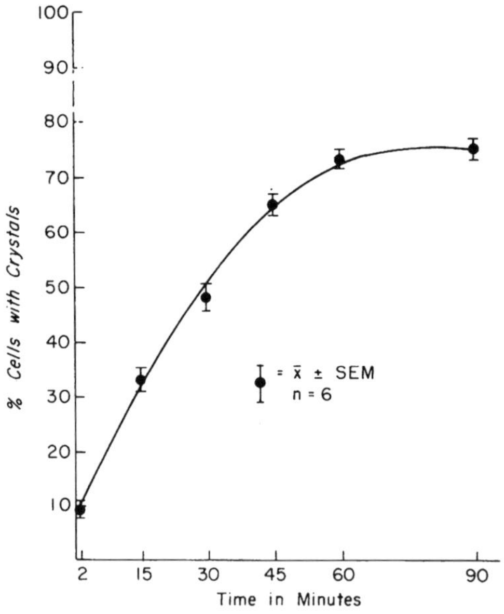


**Figure 51.2** Time curve of urate crystal phagocytosis

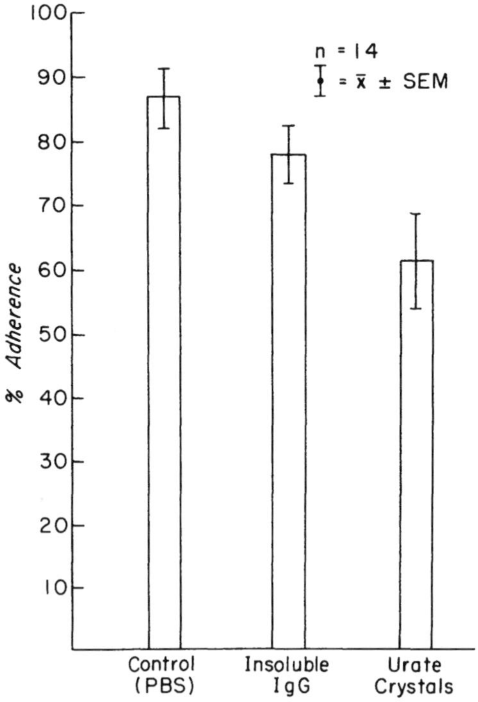


**Figure 51.3** Differing particle effects on cellular adherence

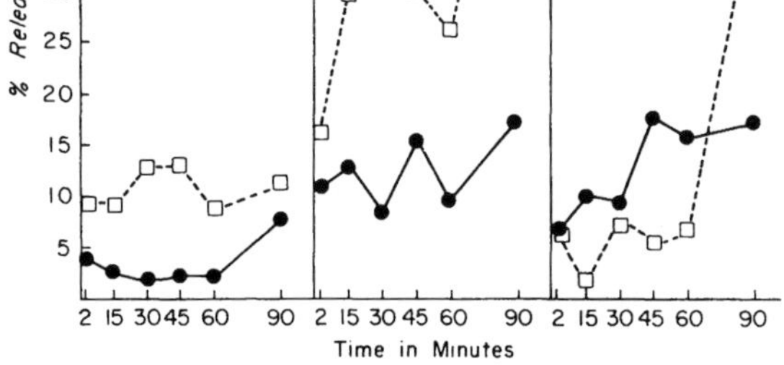


**Figure 51.4** Time curves of insoluble IgG induced enzyme release

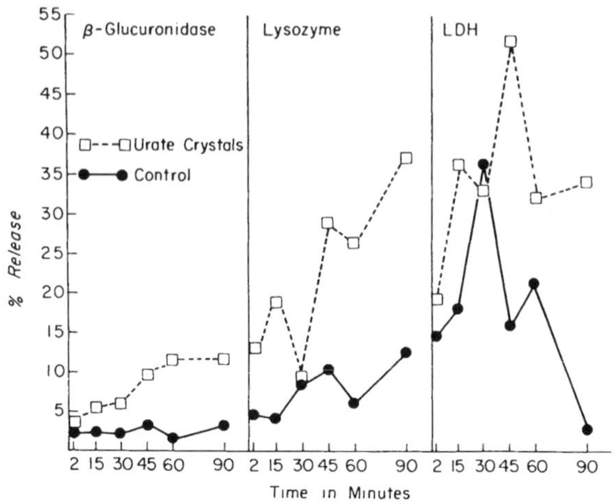


**Figure 51.5** Time curves of urate crystal induced enzyme release

the findings. Previous studies by others[2,10] have not shown selective release of the lysosomal enzymes with urate crystals and have not shown cell death at the time intervals utilized in our studies. It should be noted that these previous studies utilized neutrophils and urate crystals in tubes and not the monolayer system utilized here.

## CONCLUSIONS

The studies have (1) described a neutrophil monolayer system which may be utilized to delineate the sequential uptake of insoluble IgG aggregates and monosodium urate crystals, (2) documented the effect of this uptake on cellular adherence, and (3) demonstrated the uptake-induced release of azurophilic and specific granular enzymes which may be important in the inflammatory process occurring in the joints of patients with rheumatoid arthritis and/or gout.

### Acknowledgements
This work was supported in part by grants from the Easter Seal Research Foundation of the National Easter Seal Society for Crippled Children and Adults. The authors wish to thank the Medicine Satellite Center for excellent and timely help in the preparation of this manuscript.

### References
1 Turner, R., Collins, R., Browner, S., *et al.* (1976). Neutrophil and rheumatoid factor-immunoglobulin G insoluble complex interactions: phagocytosis and sequelae. *J. Rheumatol.*, **3**, 109

2 Weissmann, G., Zurier, R., Spieler, T. and Goldstein, I. (1971). Mechanisms of lysosomal enzyme release from leukocytes exposed to immune complexes and other particles. *J. Exp. Med.*, **134**, 149s

3 Turner, R., Counts, G., Mashburn, H., Treadway, W., and DeChatelet, L. (1980). Drug and rheumatoid factor effects on the uptake of immunoglubulin G aggregates by neutrophil monolayers. *Inflammation* (In press)

4 Lowry, O. H., Rosebrough, N. J., Farr, A. L. and Randall, R. (1951). Protein measurement with the Folin phenol reagent. *J. Biol. Chem.*, **193**, 265

5 Seegmiller, J. E., Howell, R. R. and Malawista, S. E. (1962). The inflammatory reaction to sodium urate. Its possible relationship to the genesis of gouty arthritis. *J. Am. Med. Assoc.*, **180**, 469

6 Turner, R., Martin, M., Schroff, J., Treadway, W. and DeChatelet, L. (1979). Neutrophil enzyme activities in rheumatoid inflammation. *Inflammation*, **3**, 219

7 Turner, R., Mashburn, H., Collins, R. *et al.* (1977). Rheumatoid factor immunoglobulin G complex precipitation and neutrophil stimulation: an *in vitro* model for rheumatoid inflammation. In Willoughby, D. A. (ed.) *Perspectives in Inflammation – Future Trends and Developments*, pp.39–46. (Lancaster: MTP Press)

8 Shumacher, H., Fishbein, P., Phelps, R. *et al.* (1975). Comparison of sodium urate and calcium pyrophosphate crystal phagocytosis by polymorphonuclear leukocytes. *Arthritis Rheum.*, **18**, 783s

9 Treadway, W., Collins, R. L., Turner, R. A. and DeChatelet, L. (1979). Polymorphonuclear leukocyte secretory and metabolic responses to immunoglobulin aggregates. *J. Rheumatol.*, **6**, 636

10 Kosen, F., Kinsburg, M. and Skosey, J. (1979). Polymorphonuclear leukocyte responses to monosodium urate crystals: modification by absorbed serum proteins. *J. Rheumatol.*, **6**, 519

# 52

# An *in vitro* mouse macrophage model for use in assessing the effects of anti-inflammatory drugs

D. D. WHITE, P. K. FOX AND P. LIVINGSTON (UK)

## INTRODUCTION

Mononuclear phagocytic cells are implicated in many chronic inflammatory diseases[1]. In rheumatoid arthritis these cells, stimulated by inflammatory products, engulf immune complexes accumulating in the diseased joint, accompanied by a selective secretion of lysosomal acid hydrolases[2]. These have the capacity to activate complement and kinin pathways as well as inducing the destruction of the proteoglycan matrix of the joint[3]. Inhibition of the release of these hydrolases by lysosomal membrane stabilizing drugs may be an important means of reducing joint destruction in chronic arthritis[3]. Many anti-inflammatory drugs, e.g. hydrocortisone, dexamethasone, phenylbutazone and flufenamic acid, have been reported to stabilize lysosomal membranes[4–6]. With some of these compounds a correlation has been demonstrated between lysosomal stabilization effects *in vitro* and their anti-inflammatory activities *in vivo* in animal models[4].

A model is described here in which macrophages are obtained from mouse peritoneal exudates after intraperitoneal injection of brain-heart infusion mixture. Opsonized zymosan particles are then used to stimulate phagocytic activity in these cells, the extent of which is measured in terms of the number of intracellular particles using a Coulter Counter. The specific zyosan induced release of lysosomal enzymes is monitored by measuring the extracellular activity of the marker enzyme β-*N*-acetylglucosaminidase (β-NAG) present at high activity in human rheumatoid synovial fluid[7].

Reduction in secretion of lysosomal enzymes from macrophages, dependent upon such processes as membrane stabilization, may be a beneficial property of any potential anti-arthritic drug.

## MATERIALS AND METHODS

### Materials

The following drugs were used in this study: auranofin (Smith, Kline & French Ltd.); myocrisin and ketoprofen (May & Baker Ltd.); dapsone (Aldrich Chemical Co. Ltd.), and hydrocortisone (Organon Laboratories Ltd.). All drugs were dissolved in Hanks' balanced salt solution without phenol red (HBSS) except auranofin (in ethanol, diluted with HBSS to a final ethanol concentration of 1%) and dapsone (in DMSO, diluted with HBSS to a final DMSO concentration of 0.05%). At these concentrations the solvents had no effect on enzyme activity or release.

### Macrophage preparation

Brain–heart infusion mixture (Difco, 1.0 ml.) was injected intraperitoneally into male CFLP mice (30–35 g) 3 days before harvesting cells by peritoneal lavage with 2.0 ml of ice-cold Waymouth's MB752/1 culture medium supplemented with 5% v/v heat inactivated foetal calf serum, 100 IU/ml penicillin and streptomycin (Flow), 2.5 μg/ml amphotericin β (Flow) and 30 units/ml heparin. The cell suspensions were pooled and 1.5 ml aliquots added to each well of a multiwell plate (Linbro, 6 wells, 3.5 cm diameter) before being incubated in an atmosphere of 5% $CO_2$ in air at 37 °C for 2 h. Non-adherent cells were removed by washing with warm HBSS and after replacement with 2.0 ml of warm culture medium, the incubation was continued for a further 22 h. Again non-adherent cells were removed by washing with warm HBSS and replaced with 2.0 ml of this salt solution.

### Zymosan induced phagocytosis

Zymosan (10 mg/ml) was boiled for 30 min, washed, mixed with 5% fresh mouse serum in saline and incubated at 37 °C for 30 min. The particles were washed twice in saline before being re-suspended in HBSS at a concentration of 1 mg/ml. After incubating the adherent macrophages in drug or HBSS for 0.5 h at 37 °C, opsonized zymosan particles ($2 \times 10^7$ particles) were added to each culture and re-incubated for 1 h. The extracellular medium was then removed for enzyme analysis. The cells were washed with warm HBSS (5 × 1 ml) to ensure complete removal of non-ingested zymosan before hypotonic lysis in 1.0 ml distilled water. Each culture plate was scraped with a polypropylene rod and the resulting lysate containing suspended zymosan was ultrasonically homogenized (100 W, 10 s, Labsonic 1510, Braun, Germany) to aid membrane dispersion and zymosan disaggregation.

### Zymosan particle counting

Aliquots (0.1 ml) from each lysate were diluted 1:50 with Isoton (Coulter

Electronics Ltd.) and transferred to a Coulter Counter, Model ZB, for measurement of zymosan particles. Duplicate determinations were performed using the following settings; orifice tube size, 50 µm; $T_L$, 8, $T_H$, 80; current, 0.354; amplitude, 2.

The contribution of the blank cell lysate (cell lysate containing no zymosan) was subtracted from each value and the number of ingested particles per microgram protein was calculated for each lysate. Percentage change was then expressed as a percent of control values.

### Measurement of enzyme activity

The activity of β-NAG selected as a marker of macrophage lysosomal enzyme activity was determined in the extracellular fluid from each culture using *p*-nitrophenyl-*N*-acetyl β-D-glucosaminide as substrate 8. β-Glucuronidase activity was measured, using phenolphthalein β-D-glucuronide as substrate 8. Activities were expressed as nmol substrate hydrolysed per hour per microgram protein and any drug induced change in activity calculated as a percent of control values.

The activity of the cytoplasmic enzyme lactate dehydrogenase was also measured[9] in the extracellular fluid and expressed as nmol of pyruvate reduced/h/µg protein and the extracellular activity calculated as a percentage of the total cell activity.

### Protein estimation

The protein content of each lysate was determined by the method of Miller[10] and expressed as microgram protein per lysate, after subtraction of the small quantity of protein bound to the zymosan during opsonization.

### Quantitation of adhering macrophage numbers

The number of adhering cells (macrophages) in the original cell suspension was measured by first adding an 0.1 ml aliquot of the cell suspension to each of 6 treated glass coverslips (1.5 cm diameter) in multiwell plates (Linbro, 24 wells, 1.6 cm diameter). After incubation and washing as described above, the adhering cells were fixed in acetic acid–alcohol solution (1:3) and stained in aceto-orcein (2% orcein in 50% acetic acid). The mean number of adhering cells per unit area was measured from 4 × 20 fields from each of 6 coverslips with the use of the Quantimet 720 image analyser[11] The results were expressed in terms of the number of adhering cells per millilitre of original cell suspension.

### Cell viability

The viability of adhering macrophages was assessed by microscopic examination of the cells 5 min after the addition of a drop of 0.5% trypan blue in saline.

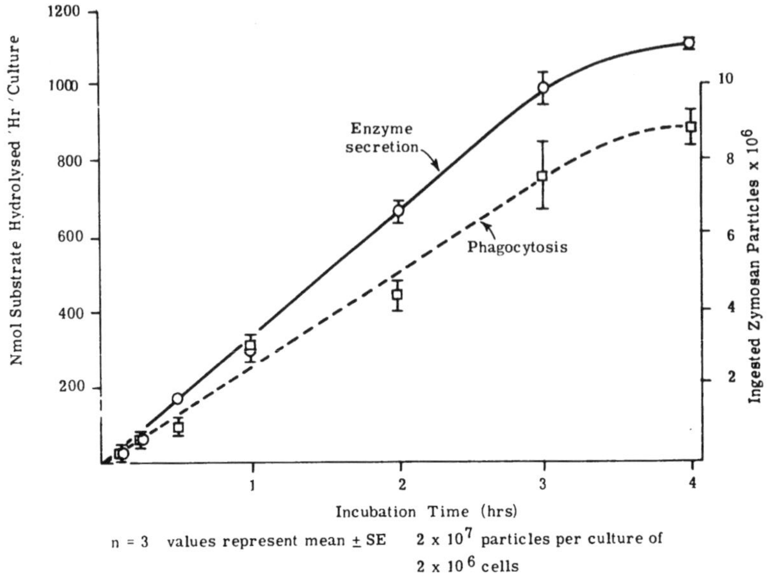


**Figure 52.1** Time course of β-*N*-acetylglucosaminidase secretion from one phagocytosis by mouse macrophages

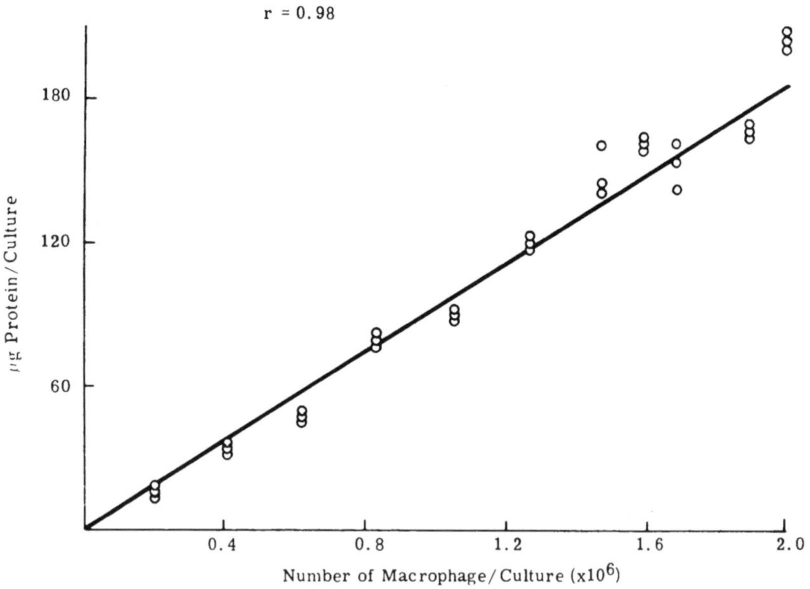


**Figure 52.2** Correlation of macrophage cell numbers with protein content ($r = 0.98$)

## RESULTS

### Preliminary experiments

*Correlation between phagocytosis, lysosomal enzyme release and time*

The number of ingested zymosan particles and the level of extracellular β-NAG activity were measured simultaneously in a number of cultures after incubation periods of up to 4 h. Both parameters were proportional to time (Figure 52.1) up to 3.5 h, a period in excess of the 1 h used in the methodology.

*Efficiency of removal of non-ingested zymosan*

Recognizing the difficulty of removing all extracellular zymosan particles from a cell culture, in a preliminary experiment *N*-ethylmaleimide (NEM) at 10 mol/l final concentration, an agent known to specifically inhibit the ingestion phase of phagocytosis in macrophages[12] was added to a number of cell cultures followed by 3 × 1 ml washings with HBSS. The number of zymosan particles in cultures in the presence and absence of NEM was measured (Table 52.1). In all other experiments this constant number of zymosan particles was subtracted from values determined in each lysate.

**Table 52.1** Effect of *N*-ethylmaleimide on zymosan uptake by mouse macrophages

| *Particle distribution* | *No of particles/culture* $\times 10^3$ | |
|---|---|---|
| | *control* | *+ NEM* |
| Extracellular medium | 2330 ± 291 | 7913 ± 49 |
| Non-adherent removed by washing | 3463 ± 137 | 2300 ± 152 |
| Cell lysate | 5653 ± 150 | 12 ± 61 |
| Total particles | 11446 | 10925 |
| Lysate content as % of total | 49% | 6% |

Mean ± SE, $n = 6$. Addition of $1 \times 10^7$ particles to each culture of $2 \times 10^6$ adhering cells.

*Correlation between macrophage numbers and their protein content*

To account for the variation in cell numbers between cultures, the protein concentration of each culture was measured. In this preliminary experiment the number of adhering macrophages and their protein concentration was determined in several cell cultures (Figure 52.2). A linear relationship was observed between the two parameters permitting lysate protein concentration to be used as a measure of cell numbers.

### Drug effects

The orally active anti-arthritic gold compound, auranofin, markedly inhibited lysosomal enzyme secretion of β-NAG and β-glucuronidase at $10^{-6}$ mol/l

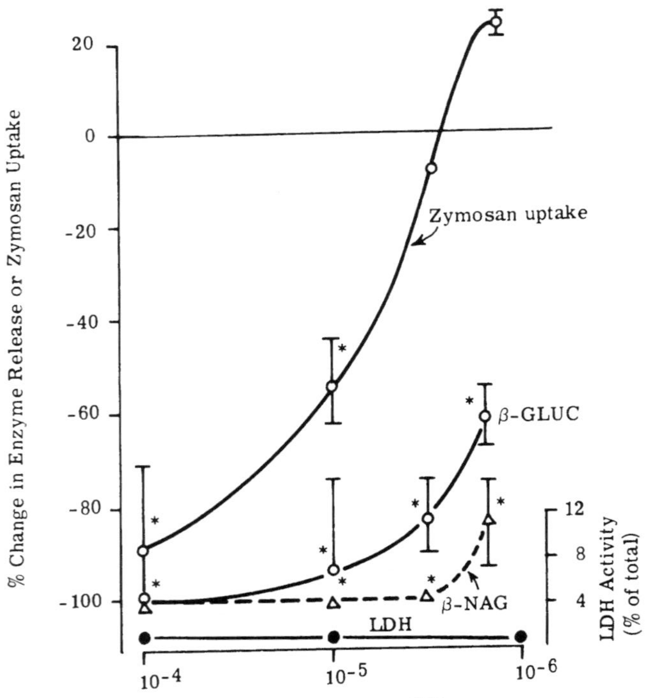


* = $p < 0.05$ Each point represents the mean ± SE of 5 cultures

**Figure 52.3** Auranofin

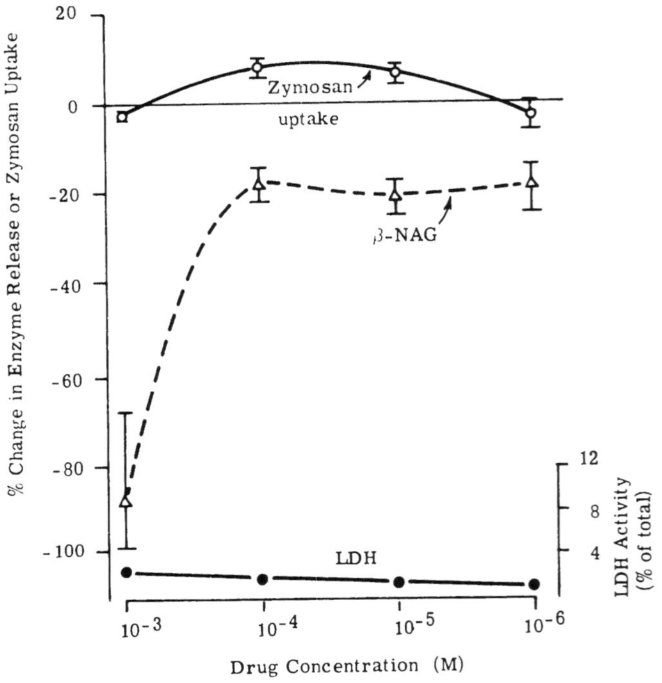


* = $p < 0.05$ Each point represents the mean ± SE of 5 cultures

**Figure 52.4** Myocrisin

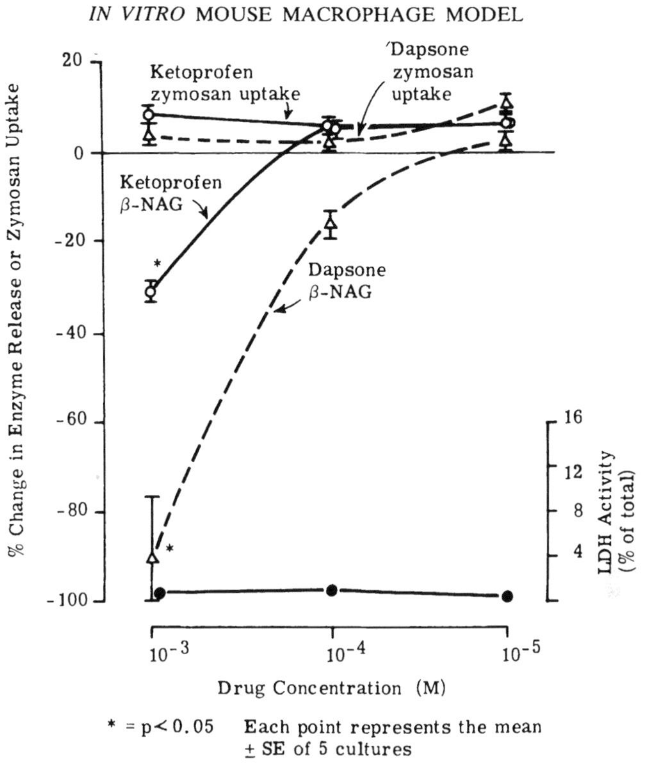


**Figure 52.5** Dapsone and ketoprofen

without affecting phagocytosis (Figure 52.3). At higher concentrations both processes were inhibited. The other anti-arthritic gold compound, myocrisin, reduced enzyme release to a lesser extent than auranofin, mainly at concentrations > $10^{-4}$ mol/l (Figure 52.4). This effect was also shared with the anti-inflammatory drugs dapsone and ketoprofen (Figure 52.5). The steroidal compound hydrocortisone (Figure 52.6) displayed a different profile by inhibiting both parameters. No compounds examined in this study reduced cellular integrity by raising extracellular lactate dehydrogenase activity.

## DISCUSSION

In this model, mouse peritoneal macrophages were stimulated to release lysosomal enzymes (represented by measuring β-*N*-acetyl glucosaminidase activity) by the phagocytosis of opsonized zymosan particles, and the effects

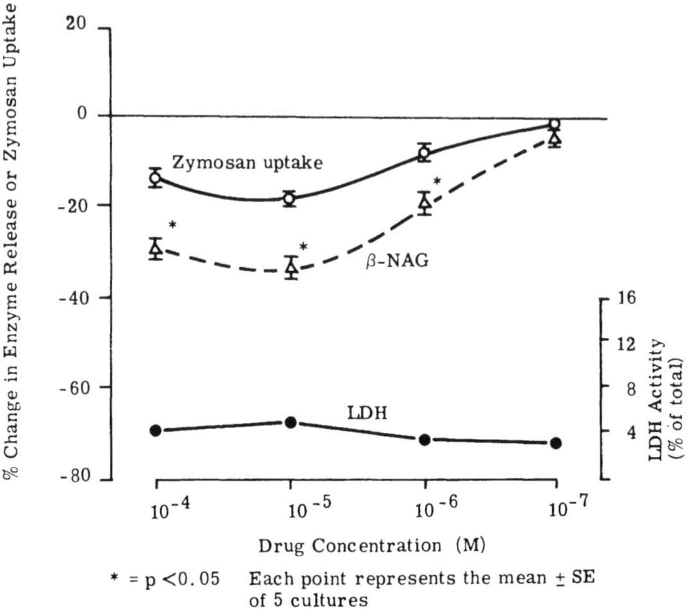


**Figure 52.6** Hydrocortisone

of drugs on these macrophage functions were studied. Zymosan particles were selected because they induce a higher level of lysosomal enzyme release than other stimuli such as bacteria or immune complexes[5] In addition, the extracellular activity of the cytoplasmic enzyme lactate dehydrogenase was monitored as an indicator of drug related cytotoxicity

In the preliminary experiments, both zymosan-stimulated phagocytosis and release of lysosomal enzyme activity were linear with time up to 3.5 h (Figure 52.1). This suggests that cellular lysosomal enzyme release occurs at the same time as, and not subsequent to, the process of phagocytosis. The level of residual zymosan particles present in the cultures, after phagocytosis had been inhibited by NEM and the cells washed with salt solution, was calculated to be 6% of the total particles in the cultures. In recent studies this figure has been reduced to 2% after more exhaustive washing of the cells. Subtraction of this figure from that obtained for the lysâte zymosan content gives a more realistic figure for intracellularly-incorporated zymosan. A third preliminary experiment showed that the lysate protein concentration was proportional to adhering cell numbers, providing that zymosan-bound opsinin protein was subtracted. It was therefore felt justified to express cell numbers in culture in terms of the protein concentration. Thus, in the drug studies, any tendency for them to reduce cellular adherence could be noted and corrected in the expression of the results.

All the anti-inflammatory drugs studied, with the exception of hydrocortisone, inhibited lysosomal enzyme release without affecting phagocytosis or cell viability at various concentrations tested, with auranofin proving the most active inhibitor. Hydrocortisone reduced both parameters. As no release of the cytoplasmic marker enzyme was observed with any of the drugs at the doses tested, it is assumed that reduction in secretion of lysosomal enzyme activity was a consequence of a direct non-cytotoxic (stabilizing) effect on lysosomal membranes.

Although phagocytosis and enzyme release may be related, the two processes can be independently inhibited by chemical agents. For example, cytochalasin B, by interfering with microfilment integrity, can inhibit phagocytosis without affecting enzyme release in neutrophils[13] while latex beads, ingested by macrophages, do not induce lysosomal enzyme secretion[14]

In rheumatoid arthritis, lysosomal enzyme activity released into an extracellular environment in the joints by infiltrating monocytes and tissue macrophages have the capacity, before being inactivated by serum inhibitors, to enhance the chronic inflammatory state and induce considerable destruction of the joint matrix. In addition, removal of immune complexes by phagocytic cells shown by others[2] may be considered to be a beneficial process in this disease condition. The premise may therefore be made that an ideal antiarthritic drug could be one which preferentially inhibits the extracellular release of lysosomal enzyme activity relative to phagocytosis. Such a premise is supported by the differential activity displayed by the drugs in this study. Furthermore, our results for the gold compounds may indicate that the greater potency of the orally active auranofin, as compared with myocrisin, reflects the former's superior effectiveness in animal studies[15] and in the treatment of rheumatoid arthritis[16, 17]

In conclusion, it is suggested that this model may be of value in detecting potential anti-arthritic drugs.

## References


1 Loeui, G. (1975). Inflammatory arthritis: immunology and inflammation at the cellular level. In Holt, P. J. L. (ed.) *Current Topics in Connective Tissue Diseases*, p. 48. (London: Churchill-Livingstone)

2 Davies, P. and Allison, A. C. (1976). The macrophage as a secretory cell in chronic inflammation. *Agents Actions*, **6**, 60

3 Weissman, G. (1971). Lysosomes and the mediation of tissue injury in arthritis. In Muller, W., Harwerth, H. G. and Fehr, K. (eds.) *Rheumatoid Arthritis*, p. 141. (London: Academic Press)

4 Tanaka, K. and Iizuka, Y. (1968). Suppression of enzyme release from isolated rat liver lysosomes by non-steroidal anti-inflammatory drugs. *Biochem. Pharmadol.*, **17**, 2023

5 Ringrose, P. S., Parr, M. A. and McLaren, M. (1975). Effects of anti-inflammatory and other compounds on the release of lysosomal enzymes from macrophages. *Biochem. Pharmacol.*, **24**, 607

6 Smith, R. J. (1977). Phagocytic release of lysosomal enzymes from guinea-pig neutrophils – regulation by corticosteroids, autonomic neurohormones and cyclic nucleotides. *Biochem. Pharmacol.*, **26**, 2001

7 Burkhardt, D., Stephens, R. S., Ghosh, P. and Taylor, T. K. F. (1978). Inhibition of synovial fluid lysosomal glycosidases by anti-arthritic gold preparations. *Agents Actions*, **8,** 251

8 Barrett, A. J. (1972). Lysosomal enzymes, In Dingle, J. T. (ed.) *Lysosomes, a Laboratory Handbook*. (Amsterdam: North-Holland Publishing)

9 Sigma Technical Bulletin No. 500. (1975). The quantitative colorimetric determination of lactate dehydrogenase. Sigma Chemical Co., St. Louis

10 Miller G. L. (1959). Protein determination for large numbers of samples. *Anal. Chem.*, **31,** 964

11 Picton, W., Devitt H. and Forgie M. A. (1976). Practical applications of the Quantimet 720, an image analysing computer in the field of investigative dermatology. *Br. J. Dermatol.*, **95,** 341

12 Walters, M. N.-I. and Papadimitriou, J. M. (1978). Phagocytosis; a review. *CRC Crit. Rev. Toxicol.*, **5,** 377

13 Smith, R. J. (1979). The guinea-pig neutrophil calcium-dependent lysosomal enzyme secretory process. Inhibition by non-steroidal anti-inflammatory agents. *Biochem. Pharmacol.*, **28,** 2739

14 Dean, R. T., Hylton, W. and Allison, A. S. (1979). Lysosomal enzyme secretion by macrophages during intracellular storage of particles. *Biochem. Biophys. Acta*, **584,** 57

15 Walz, D. T., Di Martino, M. J., Chakrin, L. W., Sutton, B. M. and Misher, A. (1976). Antiarthritic properties and unique pharmacologic profile of a potential chrysotherapeutic. Agent, S.K.&F. D-39162. *J. Pharmacol. Exp. Ther.*, **197,** 142

16 Finklestein, A. E., Walz, D. T., Batista, V., Mizraji, F., Roisman, F., and Misher, A. (1976). Auranofin. A new oral gold compound for treatment of rheumatoid arthritis. *Ann. Rheum. Dis.*, **35,** 251

17 Berglöf, F-E., Berglöf, K. and Walz, D. T. (1978). Auranofin; an oral chrysotherapeutic agent for the treatment of rheumatoid arthritis. *J. Rheumatol.*, **5,** 68

# 53

# Monosodium urate monohydrate stimulates release of lysosomal enzymes and prostaglandins from macrophages

R. M. McMILLAN, P. HASSELBACHER AND
EDWARD D. HARRIS, Jr (USA)

## INTRODUCTION

Ingestion of monosodium urate monohydrate (MSUM) crystals causes release of lysosomal and cytoplasmic enzymes from polymorphonuclear leukocytes[1,2]. These processes are well characterized and are believed to mediate many manifestations of acute gout[3]. In contrast, the mechanisms of tissue destruction in chronic gouty arthritis are poorly understood and there is little information about the interaction of MSUM with chronic inflammatory cells such as mononuclear phagocytes.

The secretory responses of mononuclear phagocytes have been extensively studied and numerous reports have indicated that lysosomal enzyme release from this cell type occurs in response to phagocytic stimuli[4–6]. We report here that phagocytosis of MSUM by macrophages induces selective secretion of lysosomal enzymes and stimulation of prostaglandin (PG) synthesis. These processes occur in the absence of serum but may be modified by serum proteins.

## METHODS

Mouse peritoneal macrophages were prepared as described elsewhere[7] and maintained overnight in Dulbecco's modified Eagle's medium (DMEM) containing 10% fetal calf serum (FCS). MSUM crystals were prepared as previously described[8] and zymosan suspensions were prepared according to the method of Weissmann *et al.*[4]. Stock suspensions of zymosan and MSUM (5 mg/ml) in phosphate buffered saline (PBS) were stored at 4 °C. For experiments with protein-coated crystals, MSUM was incubated with PBS, serum, IgG (15 mg/ml) or albumin (40 mg/ml) for 30 min at 37 °C, then washed 5 times and resuspended in PBS at a concentration of 5 mg/ml.

For stimulation of secretion, macrophages were usually washed twice with HBSS, then incubated with crystals in serum-free DMEM containing 0.2% lactalbumin hydrolysate (LH). Aliquot portions of conditioned medium were removed at various times for measurement of enzyme release and $PGE_2$ synthesis.

Lysosomal enzyme release was measured fluorimetrically using β-N-acetylglucosaminidase (NAG) as the marker enzyme[7]. One unit of NAG was defined as enzyme sufficient to degrade 1 nmol substrate/hour at 37 °C. As an index of cell lysis lactate dehydrogenase (LDH), a cytoplasmic enzyme, was assayed photometrically as previously described[9]. Intracellular enzyme analyses were performed after digesting the cells with 0.2% Triton X-100. Release of $PGE_2$ was measured by radio-immunoassay using a specific rabbit anti-$PGE_2$ antiserum (Institut Pasteur, Paris, France). Samples, antiserum and $[^3H]PGE_2$ (New England Nuclear, Boston, USA) were prepared in 0.1 mol/l phosphate buffer, pH 7.4, containing 0.9% NaCl 0.1% sodium azide and 0.2% bovine gammaglobulins. Assay incubations and determination of bound PGs were carried out as previously described[9].

## RESULTS

Incubation of peritoneal macrophages with MSUM or zymosan resulted in particle phagocytosis and release of lysosomal enzymes. Figure 53.1 shows a representative time course of NAG release induced by MSUM and zymosan. Stimulation of lysosomal enzyme release was observed within 90 min of exposure to either stimulus. NAG release was time dependent and essentially maximal by 9 h when MSUM and zymosan had induced 54% and 43% release, respectively (control value = 21%). A further increase in NAG release (~10%) was detected after 20 h, but a comparable increase was also seen in control cultures. Enzyme release in other experiments followed a similar time course although the absolute values of release varied considerably.

NAG release was not primarily a consequence of cell lysis. Figure 53.2 shows lysosomal and cytoplasmic enzyme release induced by 150 μg/ml MSUM or zymosan. After 3 h treatment with MSUM, release of NAG was around 35% compared to a control value of 11%. In contrast virtually no LDH release was observed at this time. By 26 h NAG release in response to

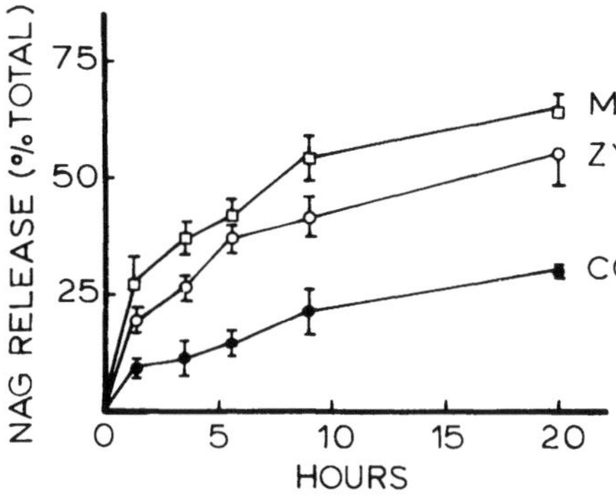


**Figure 53.1** Release of lysosomal enzymes from mouse peritoneal macrophages. Cells were incubated with MSUM (150 µg/ml) or zymosan (150 µg/ml) in DMEM–0.2% LH. Release is expressed as % of total NAG (cells + medium) in control cultures. Points represent mean values ± SD

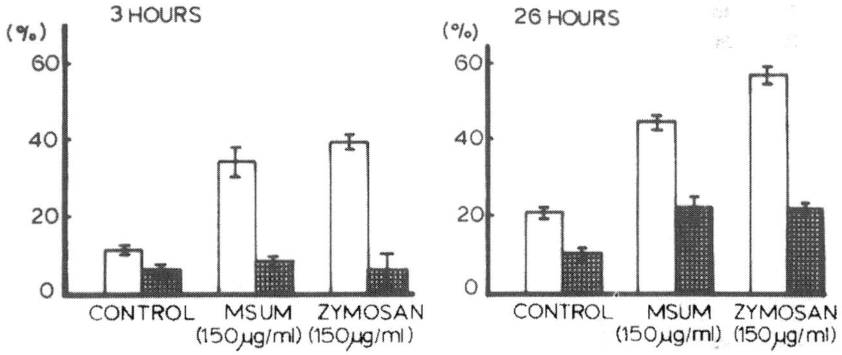


**Figure 53.2** Release of lysosomal and cytoplasmic enzymes from mouse peritoneal macrophages. Cells were incubated with MSUM or zymosan in DMEM–0.2% LH. Release of NAG (open bars) and LDH (shaded bars) are expressed as % of total enzyme (cells + medium) in control cultures. Bars represent mean values ± SD

MSUM was 45% (control value of 21%); this was accompanied by around 20% release of LDH (control value of 11%). Similar results were obtained with zymosan treated cells.

LDH release induced by 150 µg/ml MSUM was variable and was always less marked than release of NAG. In the experiment depicted in Table 53.1, this concentration of MSUM caused little release of LDH even after 24 h. Higher doses of MSUM caused little further increase in release of NAG but caused marked stimulation of LDH release. A 24 h treatment of macrophages with 500 µg/ml MSUM produced release of similar amounts of NAG and LDH (Table 53.1).

**Table 53.1** Release of lysosomal and cytoplasmic enzymes from mouse peritoneal macrophages induced by monosodium urate monohydrate

NAG

| | Enzyme release (%) | |
|---|---|---|
| | 4 h | 24 h |
| Control | 11.6 ± 2.1 | 23.6 ± 0.7 |
| MSUM (150 μg/ml) | 17.1 ± 0.7 | 35.2 ± 5.7 |
| MSUM (500 μg/ml) | 26.9 ± 9.5 | 37.0 ± 11.0 |

LDH

| | Enzyme release (%) | |
|---|---|---|
| | 4 h | 24 h |
| Control | NT | 10 ± 0.8 |
| MSUM (150 μg/ml) | NT | 12.8 ± 0.5 |
| MSUM (500 μg/ml) | NT | 38.9 ± 2.5 |

Cells were incubated with MSUM in DMEM – 0.2% LH. Release of NAG and LDH is expressed as % total enzyme (cells + media) in control cultures. Results are mean values ± SD. NT = not tested.

NAG release induced by MSUM was accompanied by synthesis and secretion of $PGE_2$. Table 53.2 shows NAG and $PGE_2$ release induced by 150 μg/ml zymosan or MSUM. Zymosan provoked slightly more NAG release than MSUM and stimulated 2-fold greater secretion of $PGE_2$. Higher doses of MSUM caused enhanced $PGE_2$ release (data not shown), but, as described above, this concentration also induced substantial LDH release.

The experiments described were carried out in serum-free media. However, it was possible that serum proteins might modulate enzyme release. In order to investigate this possibility, macrophages were washed in HBSS then incubated overnight in serum-free DMEM-0.2% LH. The next day the cells were washed in DMEM-0.2% LH and then incubated for 2 h in DMEM with 150 μg/ml MSUM crystals which had been pre-incubated with different protein preparations. This crystal concentration and incubation time ensured selective lysosomal enzyme release. NAG release induced by MSUM was enhanced by pretreating the crystals with IgG. Pretreatment of MSUM with serum, heat-inactivated serum or albumin did not enhance NAG release; in fact a slight decrease in enzyme release was observed (Table 53.3).

**Table 53.2** Release of NAG and $PGE_2$ from peritoneal macrophages

NAG

| | Enzyme release (units/$10^5$ cells) | |
|---|---|---|
| | 3 h | 26 h |
| Control | 4.0 ± 0.5 | 5.0 ± 0.9 |
| MSUM (150 μg/ml) | 14.0 ± 0.7 | 16-0 ± 1.4 |
| Zymosan (150 μg/ml) | 17.6 ± 0.8 | 20.6 ± 0.8 |

$PGE_2$

| | $PGE_2$ release (ng/$10^5$ cells) | |
|---|---|---|
| | 3 h | 26 h |
| Control | 0.78 ± 0.12 | 0.51 ± 0.25 |
| MSUM (150 μg/ml) | 1.49 ± 0.19 | 2.33 ± 0.11 |
| Zymosan (150 μg/ml) | 3.90 ± 0.21 | 4.95 ± 0.85 |

Cells were incubated with MSUM or zymosan in DMEM–0.2%LH. Results are mean values ± SD

**Table 53.3** Effect of serum proteins on NAG release induced by MSUM

| *Cell treatment* | *NAG release* (units/$10^5$ cells) |
|---|---|
| Control | 1.72 ± 0.56 |
| MSUM/PBS | 4.50 ± 0.36 |
| MSUM/serum | 4.16 ± 0.34 |
| MSUM/heat inactivated serum | 4.30 ± 0.20 |
| MSUM/IgG | 5.30 ± 0.12 |
| MSUM/albumin | 4.02 ± 0.44 |

MSUM crystals, pre-coated with proteins, were added to cells for 2 h in DMEM. Results are mean values ± SD

## DISCUSSION

Selective release of lysosomal enzymes from macrophages has been demonstrated using a variety of agents known to induce chronic inflammation including zymosan[4], immune complexes[6], carrageenins[10,11] and phorbol myristic acetate[12]. In the present study we demonstrate that crystals of MSUM, the cause of acute gouty arthritis, also stimulate lysosomal enzyme release from macrophages.

The characteristics of MSUM-induced lysosomal enzyme release were very similar to the response of another stimulus to phagocytosis, zymosan. Release induced by both agents was time dependent and was maximal about 9 h after addition of particles to cells. Initial release of lysosomal enzymes induced by MSUM (~3 h) was not accompanied by leakage of cytoplasmic constituents; thus release was not a direct consequence of cell lysis. However, prolonged exposure of macrophages to crystals resulted in some leakage of cytoplasmic enzymes. This was also observed with zymosan but not in studies with phorbol myristate acetate, a soluble inducer of lysosomal enzyme release[20]. We believe that this apparent cytotoxic effect is probably mediated by ingested crystals, perhaps via intracellular release of lysosomal enzymes. The concentration of MSUM used for these studies was critical. In most experiments, a concentration of 150 μg/ml was used and this gave qualitatively similar data to those obtained with zymosan. In contrast, higher concentrations of MSUM caused more pronounced toxicity. Prolonged incubation of cells with 500 μg/ml MSUM produced release of similar amounts of cytoplasmic and lysosomal enzymes.

Lysosomal enzyme release induced by MSUM was accompanied by synthesis and secretion of $PGE_2$. This was also observed with zymosan and has been demonstrated using other lysosomal enzyme inducers[13,14]. Stimulation of PG production by MSUM has also been reported by Newcombe and coworkers, who demonstrated that crystal phagocytosis was accompanied by release of [$^{14}$C]$PGE_2$ from macrophages that were pre-labelled with [14C] arachidonate[15,16]. Our data support their view that, since MSUM stimulates little PG release from polymorphonuclear leukocytes, synovial membrane macrophages may be a major source of the increased PG levels in gouty synovial fluid[15].

MSUM induced release of lysosomal enzymes occurred in the absence of serum and did not require activation of serum proteins (e.g. complement, immunoglobulins). However, pretreatment of crystals with IgG potentiated lysosomal enzyme release. This was not a non-specific protein effect since albumin-coated crystals did not evoke increased enzyme secretion. This suggests that enhanced lysosomal enzyme release by IgG-coated MSUM is mediated via a specific membrane interaction such as binding to cellular receptors for the Fc portion of IgG as has been suggested to occur with neutrophils[17] and platelets[18]. Treatment of crystals with fresh or heat-inactivated serum did not produce increased lysosomal enzyme release. This was surprising since MSUM selectively absorbs IgG from serum[19]. It appears that other serum protein(s) may cause a 'masking' effect that prevents the interaction of IgG-coated MSUM with macrophage Fc receptors.

There have been numerous reports from several laboratories that MSUM stimulates lysosomal enzyme release from polymorphonuclear leukocytes[1,2] and this is believed to be an important mechanism in acute gouty inflammation[3]. The data presented here indicate that MSUM-induced release of lysosomal enzymes from macrophages is much slower than the similar process in neutrophils, which is complete within 30–60 min[17]. Other differences were also noted.

(1) In the absence of serum, MSUM induces rapid release of lysosomal and cytoplasmic enzymes from neutrophils[17]. In macrophages, MSUM induced selective lysosomal enzyme release although prolonged incubations or high MSUM doses produced cytotoxicity.

(2) Prior incubation of MSUM with IgG or serum enhances lysosomal enzyme release from neutrophils and inhibits cytoplasmic leakage[17]. Our data suggest that the effects of IgG in macrophages are more complex and may be masked by other serum components. However, in future studies it will be important to investigate the effect of IgG on the delayed release of LDH from macrophages induced by MSUM.

The data presented here demonstrate that low concentrations of MSUM induce selective release of lysosomal enzymes from macrophages and that this is accompanied by stimulated PG synthesis. Phagocytosis of MSUM by macrophages, and subsequent release of inflammatory mediators, may have a patho-physiologic role in urate deposition disease. Since it is in chronic gout that the bulk of joint destruction occurs, the interactions of MSUM with mononuclear phagocytes and other chronic inflammatory cells are worthy of further studies.

**Acknowledgments**
We are grateful to Dr Constance E. Brinckerhoff and Ms. Carol A. Vater for their constructive criticism, and to Ms Jeanie Hahn for preparing the figures. This work was supported by USPHS grant AM14780; a Clinical Investigator Award 7-KO8-AM-00587 from the National Institutes of Health; a Multipurpose Arthritis Center Grant from the National Institutes of Health, and grants from the National and New Hampshire chapters of the Arthritis Foundation and from the Kroc Foundation, Santa Ynez, California. R. M. McMillan is an Arthritis Foundation postdoctoral fellow.

## References


1 Shirahama, T. and Cohen, A. S. (1974). Ultrastructural evidence for leakage of lysosomal contents after phagocytosis of monosodium urate crystals. *Am. J. Clin. Pathol.*, **76,** 501
2 Hoffstein, S. and Weissmann, G. (1975). Mechanisms of monosodium urate crystals with dog, fish and human leukocytes. *Arthritis Rheum*, **18,** 153
3 Weissmann, G. (1971). The molecular basis of acute gout. *Hosp. Pract.*, **6,** 43
4 Weissmann, G., Dukor, P. and Zurier, R. B. (1971). Effect of cyclic nucleotides on release of lysosomal enzymes from phagocytes. *Nature (London), New Biol.*, **231,** 131
5 Davies, P., Page, R. C. and Allison, A. C. (1974). Changes in cellular enzyme levels and extracellular release of lysosomal acid hydrolases in macrophages exposed to group A streptococcal cell wall substance. *J. Exp. Med.*, **139,** 162
6 Cardella, C. J., Davies, P. and Allison, A. C. (1974). Immune complexes induce selective release of lysosomal hydrolases from macrophages *in vitro. Nature (London)*, **261,** 48
7 McMillan, R. M., MacIntyre, D. E., Beesley, J. E. and Gordon, J. L. (1980). Regulation of macrophage lysosomal enzyme release: role of arachidonate metabolites, divalent cations and cyclic AMP. *J. Cell. Sci.* (In press)
8 Hasselbacher, P. (1979). C3 activation by monosodium urate monohydrate and other crystalline material. *Arthritis Rheum.*, **22,** 571
9 Brinckerhoff, C. E., McMillan, R. M. Fahye, J. V. and Harris, E. D., Jr. (1979). Collagenase production by synovial fibroblasts treated with phorbol myristate acetate. *Arthritis Rheum.*, **22,** 1109
10 Schorlemmer, H. U., Ferluga, J. and Allison, A. C. (1977). Interactions of macrophages and complement components in the pathogenesis of chronic inflammation. In Willoughby, D. A., Giroud, J. P., and Velo, G. P., (eds.) *Perspectives in Inflammation–Future Trends and Developments.*, p. 191. (Lancaster: MTP Press)
11 Gordon, J. L., MacIntyre, D. E. and McMillan, R. M. (1977). Stimulation of platelets and macrophages by carrageenin. *Br. J. Pharmacol.*, **61,** 140P.
12 Bonney, R. J., Wightman, P. D., Davies, P., Sadowski, S. J., Dahlgren, M. E., Kuehl, F. A., Jr., and Humes, J. L. (1978). Secretion of inflammatory mediators by macrophages as a function of their state of stimulation. *J. Cell Biol.*, **75,** 96a
13 Bonney, R. J., Wightman, P. D., Davies, P., Sadowski, S. J., Kuehl, F. A., Jr. and Humes, J. L. (1978). Regulation of prostaglandin synthesis and of the selective release of lysosomal hydrolases by mouse peritoneal macrophages. *Biochem. J.*, **176,** 433
14 Brune, K., Glatt, M., Kalin, H. and Peskar, B. A. (1978). Pharmacological control of prostaglandin and thromboxane release from macrophages. *Nature (London)*, **274,** 261
15 Fine, I., Wigley, F., Chang, J. and Newcombe, D. (1980). Crystal-induced synthesis of prostaglandin (PG) $E_2$ by macrophages. *Proceedings of the 4th International Prostaglandin Conference*
16 Fine, I., Sannes, P. and Newcombe, D. (1980). Human synovial fibroblasts and macrophages: urate phagocytosis and prostaglandin release. *Clin. Res.*, **28,** 146A
17 Kozin, F., Ginsburg, M. H. and Skosey, J. L. (1979). Polymorphonuclear leukocyte responses to monosodium urate crystals: modification by absorbed serum proteins. *J. Rheu-*
18 Ginsburg, M., Henson, P., Henson, J. and Kozin, F. (1979). Mechanisms of platelet response to monosodium urate crystals. *Am. J. Pathol.*, **94,** 549
19 Hasselbacher, P. (1979). Binding of IgG and complement protein by monosodium urate monohydrate and other crystals. *J. Lab. Clin. Med.*, **94,** 532
20 McMillan, R. M., Hasselbacher, P. and Harris, E. D., Jr. (unpublished data)

# 54

# Comparison between calcium pyrophosphate and monosodic urate induced inflammations of the palatal connective tissue

J. L. JOUVIN AND A. DANIEL (FRANCE)

Suspensions of calcium pyrophosphate (CPPD) and monosodic urate (MS) induce an inflammatory response when injected subcutaneously[1,2]. CPPD deposits in man induce arthritides called pseudogout. The arthritis of pseudogout may last from 1 to 4 weeks and is lower in intensity than the arthritis of gout induced by MSU crystal deposits[3]. The clinical differences between gout and pseudogout suggest that pathophysiological processes of these diseases may differ. It seems that CPPD and MSU crystals are not treated in the same way by the surrounding tissues and cells.

Therefore it was interesting to evaluate quantitatively by stereologic analysis, the modifications of palatal connective tissue during crystal induced inflammation and to compare the CPPD and MSU effects.

## MATERIAL AND METHOD

The experiment was performed on 39 young adult male guinea pigs weighing between 200 and 300 g and divided into several groups.

(1) Three healthy animals, in order to evaluate the physiological conditions.

(2) Six control animals sacrificed 6 h and 24 h (three animals per stage) after 500 μl Tyrode injections in order to evaluate the effects of injection trauma.

(3) 15 animals injected with a CPPD crystal saline suspension (500 μl) in the palatal mucosa and sacrificed 1, 3, 6, 12, and 24 h after the injections (three animals per stage).

(4) 15 animals injected with a MSU crystal saline suspension (500 μl) in the palatal mucosa and sacrificed under the same conditions as the CPPD injected groups.

CPPD and MSU crystals were synthesized following the technique described by Denko and Whitehouse[2] in 1976. The CPPD crystal preparation was made using sodium pyrophosphate and calcium nitrate and the MSU crystal preparation was made using uric acid and soda.

The particles obtained measured between 10 and 20 μm for the CPPD crystals (Figure 54.1) and between 20 and 40 μm for the MSU crystals (Figure 54.2). The ultrastructural aspect of the native crystals are shown in Figures 54.3 to 54.6. Then the crystals were ground to reduce their size to between 0.25 and 3 μm (Figures 54.7 and 54.8). The microcrystals were suspended in Tyrode and 500 μl of this suspension (20 mg/ml) were injected in the palatal mucosa between the two first molars following the technique described by Daniel and Fournier[4].

The animals were killed by decapitation and the palatal mucosa was immediately dissected and fixed in Carnoy's solution within 24 h at 4°C. The tissue was dehydrated in ethanol and embedded in paraffin. Serial 3 μm frontal sections of the intermolar palatal mucosa were stained using the Masson trichrome technique. The sections were analysed using a stereological technique described by Weibel *et al.*[5]. For each animal, ten sections were randomly selected and examined in random order to avoid bias. The standardized pattern of selected fields for morphometric analysis is illustrated in Figure 54.9. The aim of this analysis was to arrive at the volumetric densities of the different constituents of the connective tissue (collagen, oedema, vessels, fibroblasts, mononuclear cells, polymorphonuclear leukocytes, lymphocytes and plasmocytes).

All the specimens were prepared in the same conditions, and therefore comparison between the different groups was possible, especially the oedema and vessels volume fractions depending on the biopsy procedure, the fixation technique and the histological preparation.

The morphometric evaluation was performed at two levels.

(1) Level 1 (magnification 500 and a lattice comprising 100 light points): volume fractions occupied by collagen, oedema and vessels.

(2) Level 2 (magnification 760 and a lattice comprising 100 light points): volume fractions occupied by the different cells.

Estimations of volumetric densities of the various components were calcu-

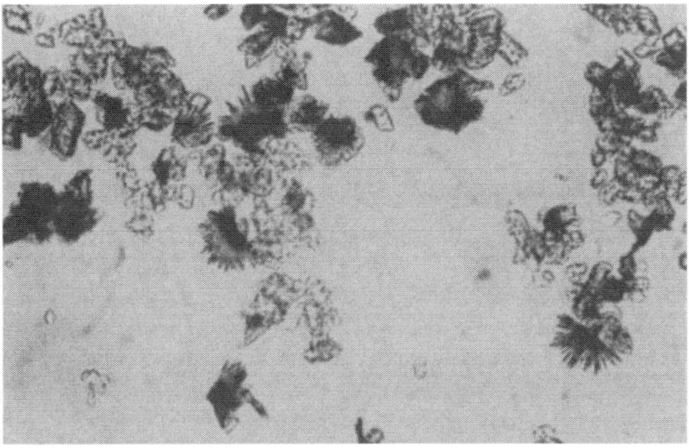

**Figure 54.1** Structural aspect of native CPPD crystals

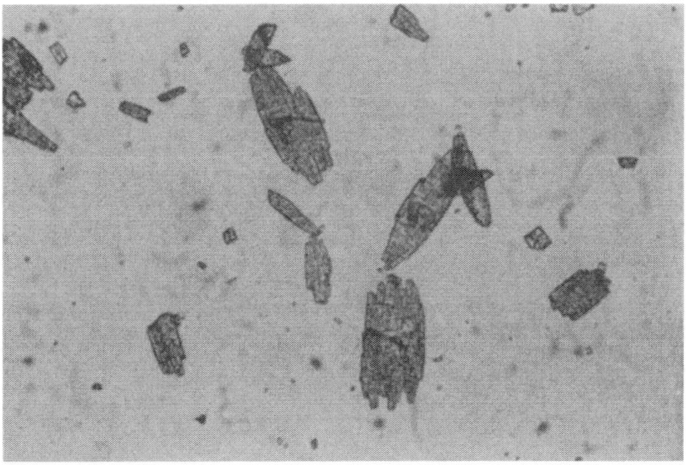

**Figure 54.2** Structural aspect of native MSU crystals

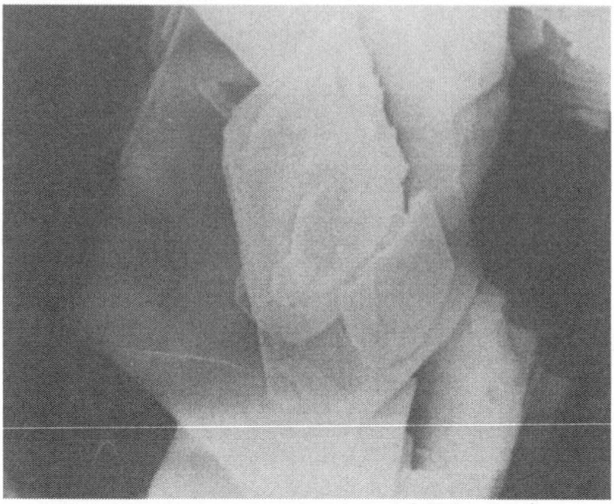

**Figure 54.3** Ultrastructural aspect of CPPD crystals

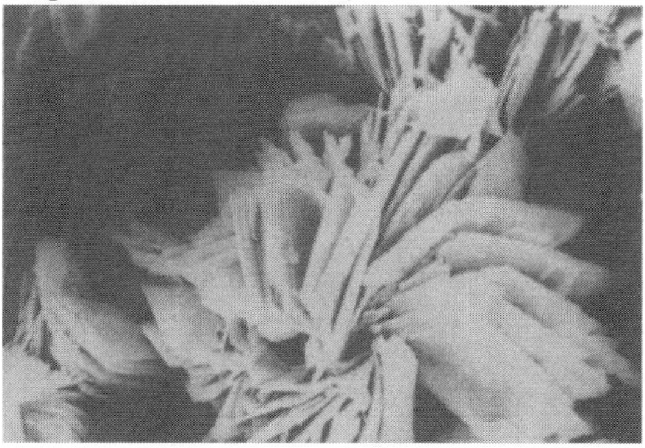

**Figure 54.4** Ultrastructural aspect of CPPD crystals

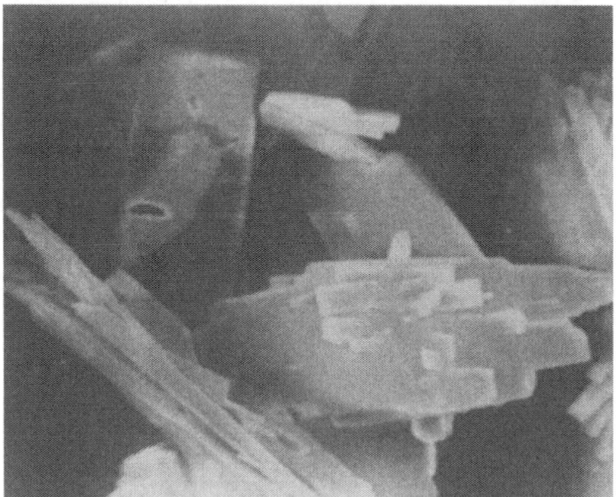

**Figure 54.5** Ultrastructural aspect of MSU crystals

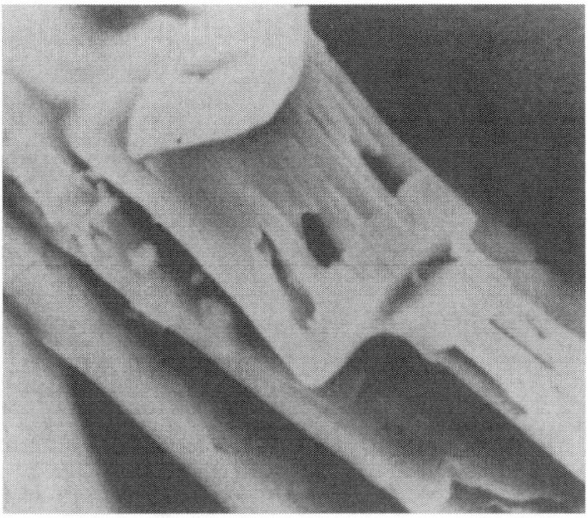

**Figure 54.6** Ultrastructural aspect of MSU crystals

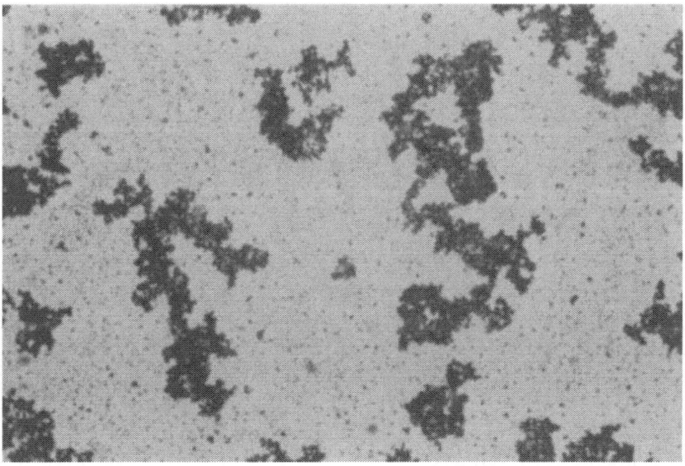

**Figure 54.7** Ground CPPD crystals

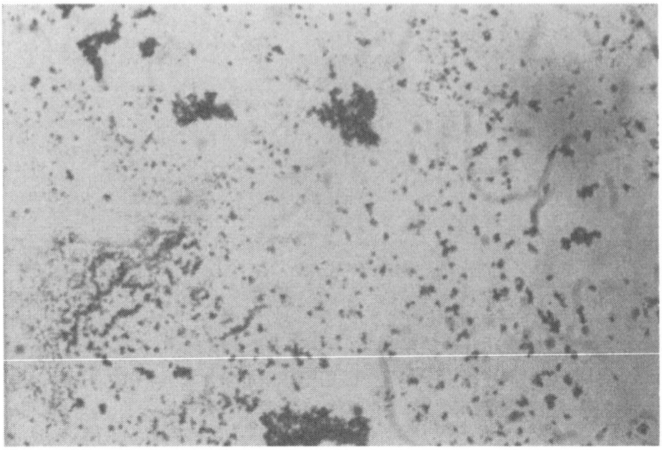

**Figure 54.8** Ground MSU crystals

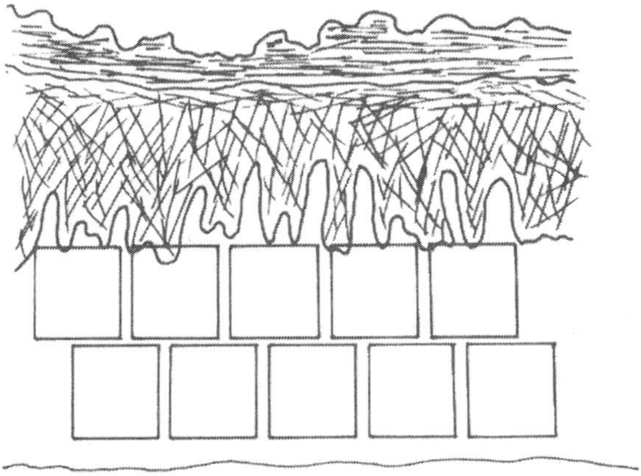

**Figure 54.9** Pattern of the fields for morphometric analysis

lated by applying respective stereological formulae which have been described by Weibel *et al.*[5]. Statistical analysis has been performed using Student's *t*-test and analysis of variance.

## RESULTS

### Histological observation

The morphology of all specimens representing healthy mucosa had a uniform pattern. The epithelium was orthokeratinized and marked rete pegs could be

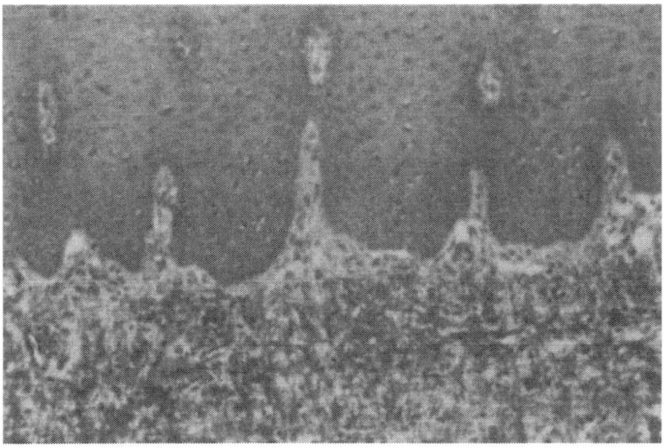

**Figure 54.10** Healthy mucosa

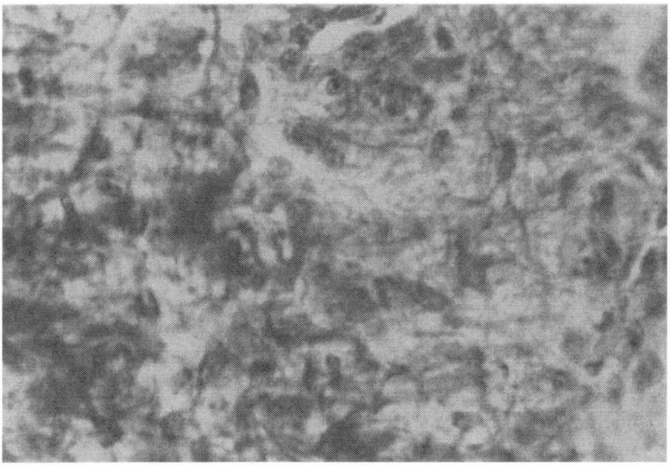

**Figure 54.11** Healthy mucosa

observed at the interface between epithelium and connective tissue (Figure 54.10). The entire connective tissue was filled with a dense network of collagen fibre bundles (Figure 54.11). Some vessels were noted but microscopic examination revealed the absence of inflammatory infiltrate.

**Developing inflammations**

One hour after the CPPD injection, many polymorphonuclear leukocytes were already detectable in the connective tissue. Dilated vessels were also noted. After the MSU injection, inflammatory cells, but mainly monocytes, could also be detected in connective tissue with dilated vessels.

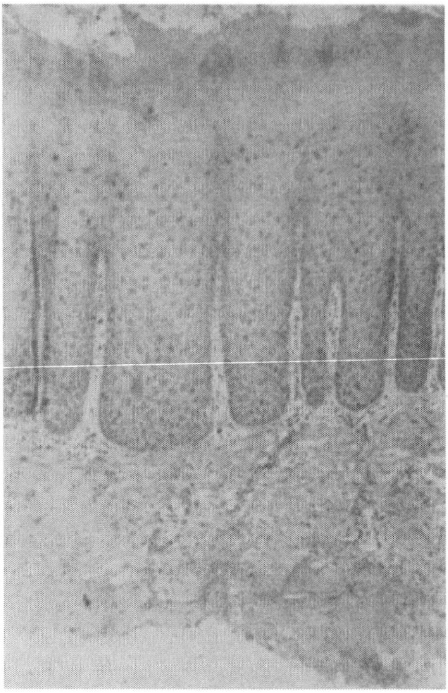

**Figure 54.12** Palatal mucosa 3 h after CPPD injection

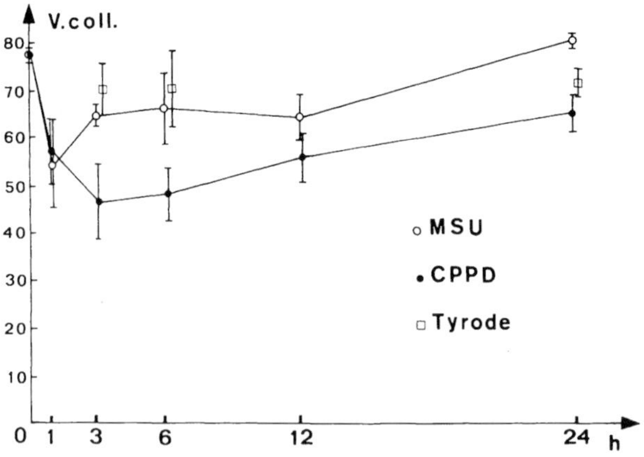


**Figure 54.13** Collagen volume fraction evolution

With CPPD induced inflammation, the maximal oedematous reaction is observed especially around the vessels, 3 h after the injection ·Figure 54.12). During the next stages (6 and 12 h), the oedema decreased and monocytes were mainly present. 24 h after the injection, inflammatory symptoms were always present, in particular the vessels were dilated and few oedema and monocytes were present.

The MSU induced inflammation presented a different pathway. 3 h after the injection, the inflammatory reaction seemed lower than 1 h after injection but at the 12 h stage a new step of inflammation development could be observed. Then, in the next few hours, the inflammatory process decreased. In conclusion, MSU induced inflammation can be regarded as a 2-step inflammatory process, the maximal intensity being observed 1 h after the crystal injection and a second spike occurring 12 h after the initial injection.

**Morphometric parameters**

The morphometric parameters characterizing healthy guinea pig palatal connective tissue are:

| | |
|---|---|
| Collagen | 78.8% |
| Oedema | 4.7% |
| Vessels | 2.6% |
| Fibroblasts | 12.7% |
| Monocytes | 4.1% |
| Polymorphonuclear leukocytes | 0.5% |
| Lymphocytes | 0% |
| Plasmocytes | 0% |

One hour after CPPD and MSU injections, the volumetric densities of collagen similarly decrease (Figure 54.13), but during the next stages the collagen volume fraction decrease is lower with the MSU. The volumetric densities of oedema (Figure 54.14) follow an opposite pattern. Again we find that the MSU induced inflammation is of a lower intensity.

Few differences are noted when we consider the vessels' volumetric densities (Figure 54.15). Nevertheless, the value obtained 24 h after the crystal injection is higher than the healthy mucosa value.

The fibroblast volume fractions' study (Figure 54.16) confirms the lower intensity of the MSU reaction, especially 6 h after the injection, but we can already observe with this curve the two stages of inflammation induced by MSU. This phenomenon is confirmed by the monocytes' volumetric fraction curves (Figure 54.17).

When we consider the polymorphonuclear leukocytes' volumetric densities (Figure 54.18), another difference appears between the two crystal induced inflammations. With the MSU, during the first stages (1 and 3 h) monocytes are more numerous than polymorphonuclear leukocytes.

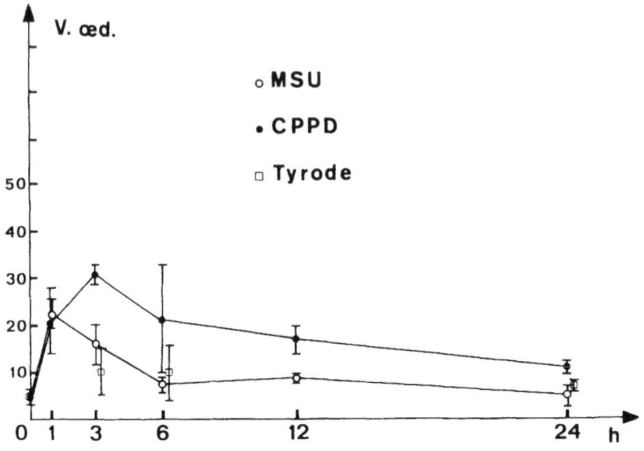


**Figure 54.14** Oedema volume fraction evolution

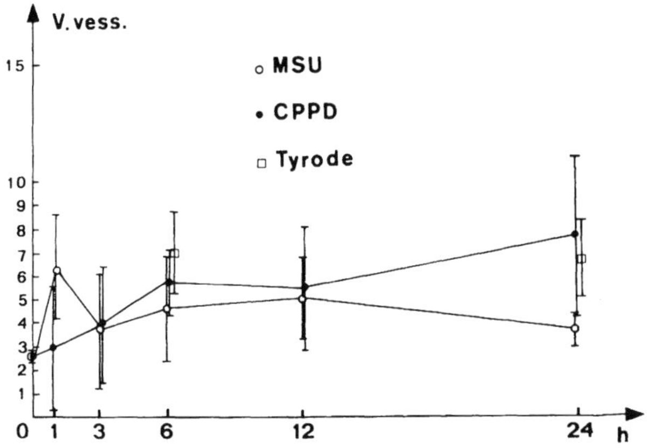


**Figure 54.15** Vessels' volume fraction evolution

However, these cells are mainly observed during the first stages after the CPPD injection.

Few remarks can be made about the lymphocytes (Figure 54.19) and the plasmocytes (Figure 54.20), as these cells are rarely observed with the present experimental model.

## DISCUSSION

The present investigation demonstrates that it is possible to induce inflammation of the palatal mucosa of guinea pigs by CPPD and MSU crystal suspension injections (the comparison between crystal injected mucosae and Tyrode

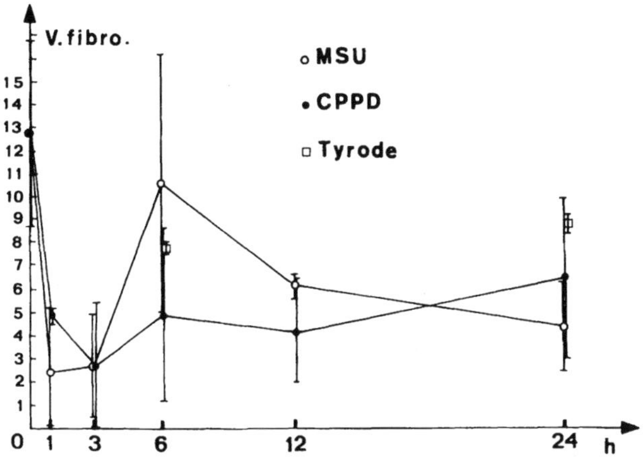


**Figure 54.16** Fibroblasts' volume fraction evolution

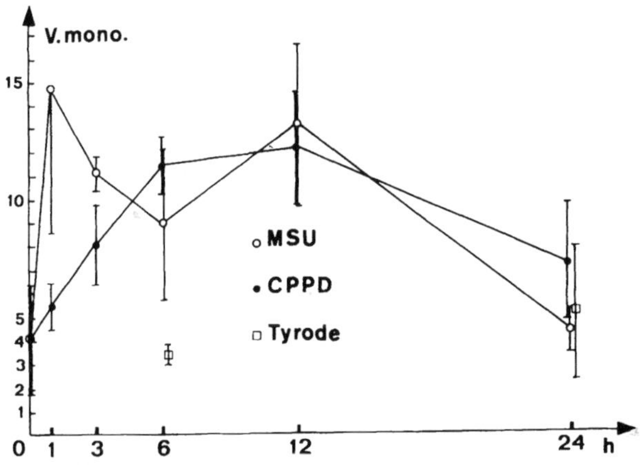


**Figure 54.17** Monocytes' volume fraction evolution

injected mucosae obviously shows the phenomenon), and that the differences between CPPD and MSU induced inflammations should be noted.

With CPPD induced inflammation, the maximum intensity is observed 3 h after the crystal injection, but the maximum intensity is as soon as 1 h after the injection for MSU crystals. These observations must be related to the clinical symptoms of pseudogout arthritides (induced by CPPD deposits in man) and gouty arthritis (induced by MSU deposits). The pseudogout lasts for a longer time than the gouty arthritis. This is in agreement with our findings on the CPPD induced inflammation of the palatal connective tissue which is present 24 h after injection when, with MSU crystals, there is a complete absence of

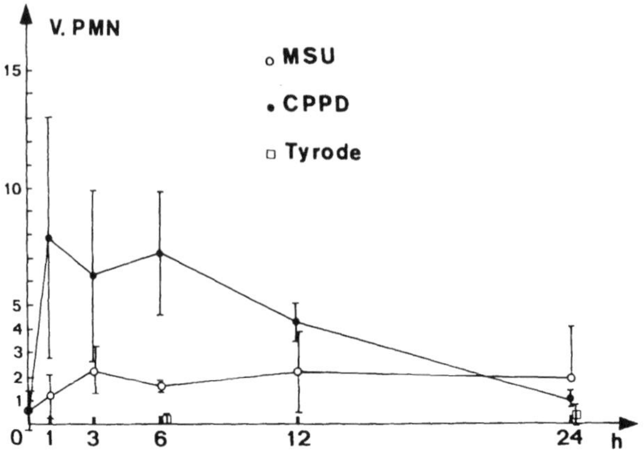


**Figure 54.18** Polymorphonuclear leukocytes' volume fraction evolution

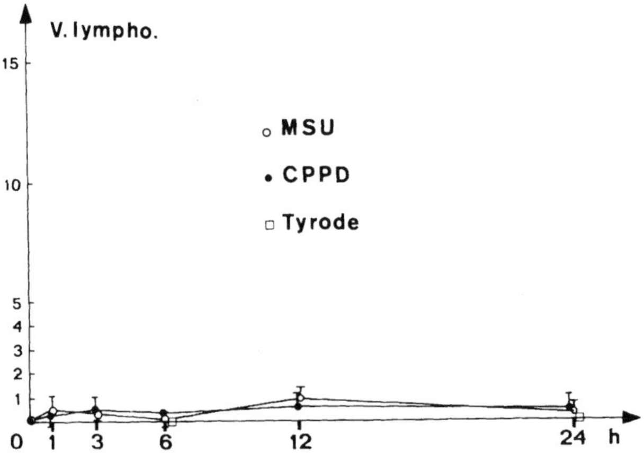


**Figure 54.19** Lymphocytes' volume fraction evolution

inflammatory signs at the same stage. On the other hand, the maximum intensity observed 1 h after the MSU crystal injection is in agreement with the clinical symptoms of the gouty arthritis, which occurs suddenly.

Ultrastructural studies have shown *in vitro* a rapid destruction of polymorphonuclear leukocytes after MSU crystal phagocytosis. The cells are probably killed by phagolysosome membrane lysis which leads to cell death[6,7]. The CPPD crystals present a lower membranolytic effect than MSU crystals without cellular death. All these features can explain the differences between inflammations induced by the two kinds of crystals[8].

The second spike observed during the MSU inflammation development,

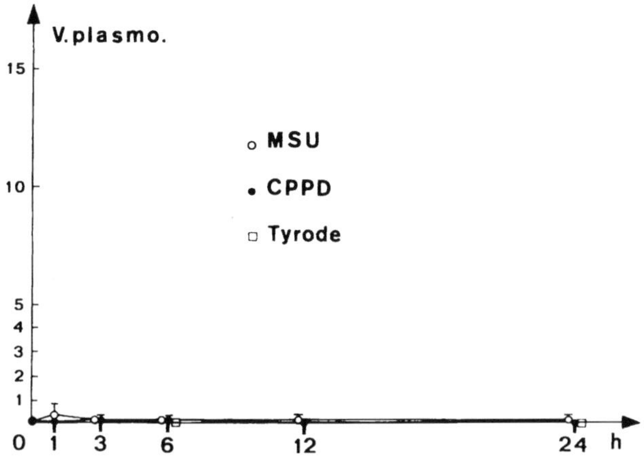


**Figure 54.20** Plasmocytes' volume fraction evolution

especially observed with the study of the phagocytic cells volume fractions (monocytes and polymorphonuclear leukocytes) could be caused by the chemotatic activity exerted by the PMN cellular rests after the initial lysis of these cells by ingested MSU crystals.

## References

1 MacCarty, D. J. and Kozini, F. (1976). An overview of cellular and molecular mechanism in crystal induced inflammation. *Arthritis Rheum.*, **18**, (Suppl.), **757**

2 Denko, C. W. and Whitehouse, M. W. (1976). Experimental inflammation induced by naturally occuring microcristalline calcium salts. *J. Rheumatol.*, **3**, 54

3 Cats, A. and Van de Putte, L. B. A. (1977). Athritis: a clinical model of inflammation. In Bonta, I. L., Thompson, J. and Brunek (eds.) *Inflammation: mechanisms and their impact on therapy. Agents Actions Suppl.*, **3**, (Basel: Birkhäuser Verlay)

4 Daniel A. and Fournier, B. (1978). Quantitative parameters of carrageenin induced inflammation of guinea-pig palatal mucosa. *J. Dent. Res.*, **57**, Special Issue A, 223

5 Weibel, E. R., Kistler, G. S. and Scherle, W. F. (1966). Practical stereological methods for morphometric cytology. *J. Cell Biol.*, **30**, 23

6 Weissmann, G. and Rita, G. (1972). Molecular basis of gouty inflammation: interaction of monosodium urate crystals with lysosomes and liposomes. *Nature (London) New Biol.*, **240**, 167

7 Schumacher, H. R., Fishbein, P., Phelps, D., Tse, R. and Krauser, R. (1975). Comparison of sodium urate and calcium pyrophosphate crystals phagocytosis by polymorphonuclear leukocytes. *Arthritis Rheum*, **18**, (Suppl.), 783

8 Mandel, N. S. (1976). The structural basis of crystal induced membranolysis. *Arthritis Rheum.*, **19**, (Suppl.), 439

# 55

# Intracellular killing of micro-organisms by phagocytic cells: the effect of extracellular stimuli (Abstract)

P. C. J. LEIJH, M. TH. VAN DEN BARSELAAR, TH. L. VAN ZWET AND R. VAN FURTH (NETHERLANDS)

The rate of intracellular killing of micro-organisms by monocytes and granulocytes can be measured independently from the rate of ingestion. This method allowed us to study the effect of extracellular factors (serum proteins and lectins) on intracellular killing. The intracellular killing of micro-organisms by human granulocytes and monocytes proved to be dependent on the presence of extracellular serum. In the absence of serum, killing of *S. aureus* by monocytes did not occur and was sub-optimal for granulocytes. In the presence of heat-inactivated serum the killing index lay between the values obtained in the absence of serum and in the presence of fresh serum. The killing in the presence of inactivated serum is very probably dependent on an interaction between the Fc part of IgG and the Fc receptor in the cell membrane, as indicated by the following findings: (1) IgG preparations were as active as inactivated serum: (2) p-Fc fragments of IgG stimulated intracellular killing, whereas (Fab')$_2$ fragments were inactive in this respect; (3) only IgG subclasses $IgG_1$ and $IgG_3$ were stimulatory, and the cells only carry receptors for these subclasses. Complement component C3b also stimulated the intracellular killing of *S. aureus* ingested by monocytes and granulocytes. In case of the monocytes, C3b is generated via the alternative pathway, whereas for the granulocytes factors of the classical as well as the alternative pathway are involved in this process. Incubation of phagocytes containing ingested *S. aureus* in the presence of various lectins also resulted in the stimulation of intracellular killing of ingested bacteria. However, this was only found for those lectins for which receptors were demonstrable on the cell surface. Together, these results indicate that the intracellular killing by phagocytes is regulated by an extracellular stimulus interacting with a membrane receptor.

# 56

# *In vivo* studies on the influence of antigen induced joint inflammation on patellar hyaline articular cartilage

W. B. VAN DEN BERG, M. W. M. KRUIJSEN AND L. B. A. VAN DE PUTTE (NETHERLANDS)

## INTRODUCTION

Loss of articular cartilage is a major complication of chronic joint inflammation, leading to joint dysfunction and deformity. Enzymatic degradation of proteoglycans[1] and collagen[2] is currently thought to play an important role in cartilage destruction. Recent data have also implicated altered chondrocyte function as a possible contributing factor, since cartilage slices from rabbits with antigen induced arthritis were shown to have a decreased rate of proteoglycan synthesis *in vitro*[3]. Whether this inhibition of the synthetic capacity of articular chondrocytes also occurs *in vivo* and contributes to loss of hyaline articular cartilage remains to be verified.

The aim of the present investigation was to study the influence of chronic experimental allergic arthritis on chondrocyte metabolism *in vivo*. Arthritis was induced with methylated bovine serum albumin (mBSA) in C57B mice as described by Brackertz[4], and incorporation of intravenously administered $^{35}S$ was seen on autoradiographs of whole joint sections as a measure of chondrocyte function. Since autoradiographs of serial sections of whole knee joints from normal mice showed a large variation in $^{35}S$ incorporation in all joint cartilage structures, with the exception of patellar cartilage, the labelling of patellar chondrocytes was chosen to compare the incorporation of $^{35}S$

in inflamed versus saline injected control joints.

## MATERIALS AND METHODS

### Animals and induction of arthritis

Male C57B mice 6–8 weeks of age were immunized with 100 μg methylated bovine serum albumin (mBSA, Sigma Chemical Company, St. Louis, Missouri, USA) emulsified in 0.1 ml Freund's complete adjuvant (FCA) containing mycobacterial strain H37RA (Difco Laboratories, Detroit, Michigan, USA), by divided injections into the footpads of the two forelegs and the flank skin. After 7 days 0.1 ml of mBSA in FCA was injected into two different dermal sites of the flank. On both occasions $2 \times 10^9$ *Bordatella pertussis* organisms (RIV, Bilthoven, the Netherlands) were administered i.p. as an additional adjuvant. On day 21 arthritis was induced by intra-articular injection of 100 μg mBSA in 10 μl physiological saline (sterlized by Millipore filtration) into the right knee joint. Contralateral knee joints were injected with physiologic saline only.

### Histology and grading of arthritis

At various time intervals (indicated in the results section) after induction of arthritis, mice were killed by ether anaesthesia. Both knee joints were removed *in toto* and fixed in 4% phosphate-buffered formalin. After decalcification of the joints in formic acid the tissues were processed and embedded in paraffin wax. Total joint sections (6 μm) were prepared and stained with Haematoxylin and Eosin. Arthritis was noted semi-quantitatively in a standardized frontal section of the knee joint which included both menisci, cruciate ligaments and the patella.

The extent of cellular infiltration of the synovial tissue was graded on a scale of 0 to 3 according to the proportion of tissue densely infiltrated with cells. Cellular exudate within the joint space was graded on a similar scale of 0 to 3. In addition, sections were stained with Alcian Blue in order to detect proteoglycan depletion in articular cartilage.

### Autoradiography

Each mouse was injected intravenously in the tail vein with 50 μCi $Na_2{}^{35}SO_4$ in 0.2 ml physiological saline, 6 h before sacrifice. Animals were killed by ether anaesthesia and blood samples were taken to verify proper i.v. administration of radioactivity. Total knee sections were prepared as described above. Comparable sections of the arthritic joint and the contralateral saline-injected control joint of one animal were mounted on the same slide in similar position, dipped in K 5 emulsion (Ilford) and exposed for 1–3 weeks. After this period the slides were placed in developer for 10 min and stained with Haematoxylin and Eosin. The $^{35}S$ labelling of the patellar chondrocytes was noted semi-quantitatively. The extent of incorporation in the arthritic knee was expressed relative to the incorporation in the saline-injected control joint on the same slide and graded on the following scale:

- 0 similar incorporation
- 1 minor decreased
- 2 definite decreased
- 3 severe decreased

## RESULTS

Histological data on arthritic and non-arthritic knees are shown in Figure 56.1. The initial phase (1–7 days) of inflammation was characterized by cell-rich exudate in the joint space, infiltration of neutrophils and mononuclear cells in synovial tissue and synovial lining cell hyperplasia. Later on, local fibroblast proliferation predominated and progressive joint destruction was seen. Histology of the patella showed no gross abnormalities during the first 4 days of arthritis. Thereafter, chondrocyte death, especially in the central part of the patellar hyaline articular cartilage, was observed in several arthritic specimens, unrelated to the nearby presence of pannus. Alcian Blue staining showed clear cut proteoglycan depletion starting at day 4 after arthritis induction.

Results of autoradiographs are also shown in Figure 56.1. Up to day 14 after arthritis induction most of the patellar hyaline cartilage of inflamed joints showed decreased $^{35}S$ content as compared to saline-injected control joints. At day 28 labelling of patellar hyaline articular cartilage areas showing histologically intact chondrocytes returned to normal values.

## DISCUSSION

The loss of joint function associated with chronic arthritis, e.g. rheumatoid arthritis, is at least in part due to erosion of the articular cartilage surface. This lesion is thought to be predominantly enzymatically mediated via protease activity generated from cells infiltrating synovial membrane, synoviocytes, cells in synovial exudates, or enzymes from the cartilage itself[5].

The present study strongly suggests that a decreased proteoglycan content of cartilage during joint inflammation may also result from an inhibition of proteoglycan biosynthesis. In mice with antigen induced arthritis the labelling of patellar cartilage after i.v. administration of $^{35}S$ was markedly decreased. This could not merely be due to enzymatic breakdown of newly formed (labelled) proteoglycan, because Alcian Blue staining showed only minor proteoglycan depletion on the first days of arthritis induction, when $^{35}S$

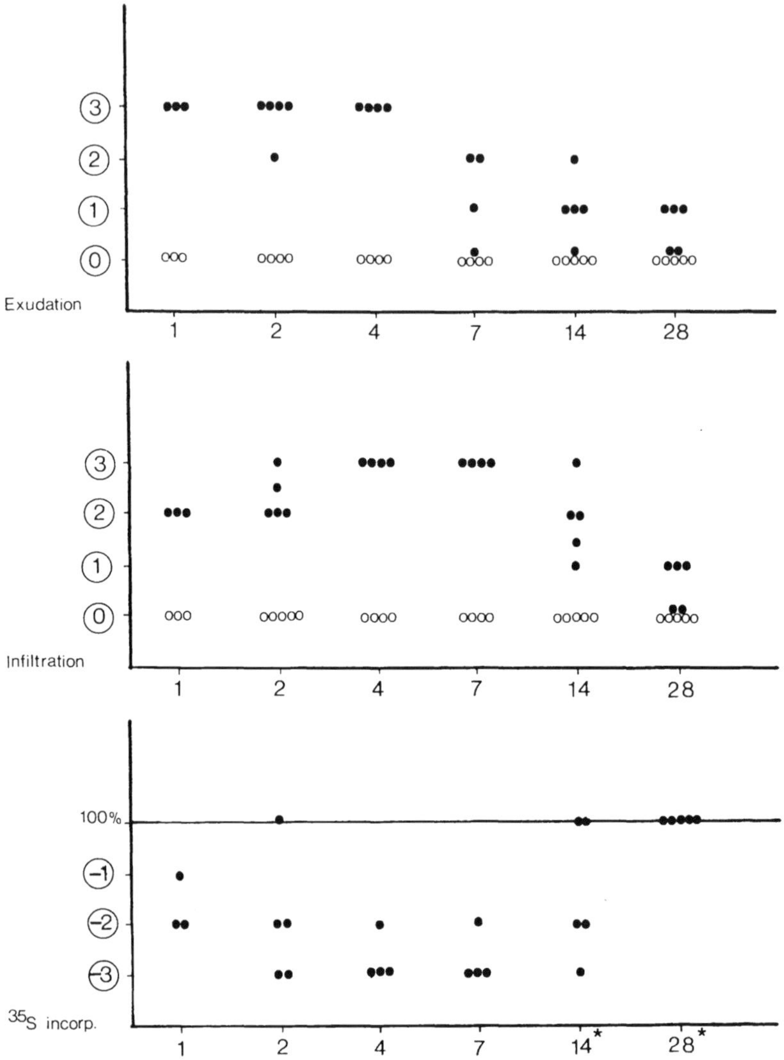


**Figure 56.1** Histological data on arthritic and non-arthritic knees
○ control joint
● inflamed joint
* labelling in areas showing intact chondrocytes

labelling had already clearly decreased. Clear cut proteoglycan depletion only occurred as early as 4 days after arthritis induction. Furthermore, chondrocyte death became apparent, especially in the central part of the patella, at the 7th day of the arthritis, which is compatible with a decreased function of these cells in earlier stages of the inflammation.

The inhibition of proteoglycan synthesis may be either reversible or irreversible, dependent on the survival of chondrocytes during the active phase of joint inflammation. At later stages of the arthritis normal labelling of patellar cartilage was found in areas with histologically intact chondrocytes.

The mechanism of the inhibition of proteoglycan synthesis during antigen induced arthritis in unknown. Possible mediators of this effect include hyaluronic acid, oligosaccharides derived from it, lymphokines, prostaglandins and humoral factors released from synovium[3,6], which were all shown to inhibit *in vitro* proteoglycan synthesis by articular chondrocytes. In addition, toxic effects on chondrocytes cannot be excluded. Using electron microscopic techniques Ohno[7] showed early chondrocyte damage in antigen induced arthritis in rabbits. In the present investigation histological chondrocyte death could be clearly observed at the 7th day after arthritis induction. A direct toxic action of mBSA is improbable since injection of mBSA in non-immunized animals does not cause chondrocyte death. Local production of lymphokines with cytotoxic properties (lymphotoxin) is one possible explanation, which is currently under investigation.

Analysis of autoradiographs of patellar cartilage from arthritic specimens showed striking regional differences. The most marked inhibition of $^{35}S$ incorporation and chondrocyte death was often found in the central part of the patella. Sometimes central chondrocytes of normal patellae also showed decreased incorporation of $^{35}S$. This probably indicates that the central chondrocytes are less metabolically active and that the influence of inflammation was most pronounced at these sites.

Of notice is the occurrence of chondrocyte death without nearby presence of pannus, whereas metabolically active chondrocytes are found in cartilage beneath pannus tissue. This indicates that next to enzymatic degradation the turning-off of chondrocyte function also contributes to cartilage destruction, an effect that seems to be unrelated to pannus formation.

## References


1 Lowther D. A. and Gillard G. C. (1976). Carrageenin-induced arthritis. The effect of intraarticular carrageenin on the chemical composition of articular cartilage. *Arthritis Rheum.* **19,** 769

2 Woolley D. E., Crossley M. J. and Evanson J. M. (1977). Collagenase at sites of cartilage erosion in the rheumatoid joint. *Arthritis Rheum.*, **20,** 1231

3 Lowther D. A., Sandy J. D., Santer V. B. and Brown H. L. G. (1978). Antigen induced arthritis. Decreased proteoglycan content and inhibition of proteoglycan synthesis in articular cartilage. *Arthritis Rheum.*, **21,** 675

4 Brackertz D., Mitchell G. F. and Mackay I. R. (1977). Antigen-induced arthritis in mice. I induction of arthritis in various strains of mice. *Arthritis Rheum.*, **20,** 841

5 Dingle J. T. (1979). Heberden oration 1978. Recent studies on the control of joint damage. *Ann. Rheum. Dis.*, **38,** 201

6 Jubb R. W. (1979). The effect of synovium on proteoglycan synthesis by human articular cartilage. Abstract, Heberden oration

7 Ohno O., Tateishi H. and Cooke T. D. (1978). Pathogenesis of chronic inflammation in experimental ferritin-induced arthritis. *Arthritis Rheum.*, **21**, 81

# 57

# A stereological analysis of collagen phagocytosis in a model of chronic inflammation in rats (Abstract)

D. A. DEPORTER (CANADA)

It is well established that the phagocytosis and intracellular degradation of collagen by fibroblasts is an important mechanism in the normal remodelling and turnover of a variety of soft connective tissues (Cate, T. and Deporter, D. A. (1975). *Anat. Rec.*, **182,** 1). Furthermore, using electron microscope stereology, we have recently demonstrated that there is a positive correlation between the collagen phagocytic activity of a tissue and its rate of mature collagen turnover (Svoboda, Shiga and Deporter. (1980). *Anat. Rec.* In press).

Significant resorption of soft connective tissue collagen occurs during chronic inflammation. Both macrophages and fibroblasts have been observed to phagocytose collagen during experimental chronic inflammation (Pérez-Tamayo, (1970). *Lab. Invest.*, **22,** 142; Soames and Davies, J. (1977). *Periodont. Res.*, **12,** 378; Deporter and Brown (1980). *J. Periodont. Res.* In press). The present study was undertaken to compare the collagen phagocytic activity in inflamed versus control periodontal tissues of rats. By eliciting a localized periodontal inflammation on one side of the mouth, it was possible to use each animal as its own control.

Tissues were analysed using EM stereology. The results indicate a dramatic increase in collagen phagocytic activity in inflamed periodontal tissues, and suggest that the phagocytic mechanism may be of central importance in the resorption of soft tissue collagen that occurs during chronic inflammatory disorders.

# 58

# Modification of chemotaxis and peptide binding during pathophysiological state of polymorphonuclear leukocytes

M. ROCH-ARVEILLER, J. P. ABITA,
D. BRADSHAW AND J. P. GIROUD (FRANCE)

## INTRODUCTION

Local recruitment of polymorphonuclear leukocytes (PMNs) to inflammatory sites is essential to the host in its defence against injury. The activation of directed migration of cells (chemotaxis) along a chemical gradient is determined by a variety of attractants such as serum factors[1], particularly a fragment of the fifth component of complement[2], bacterial metabolites[3], cell derived materials from sensitized lymphocytes[4], or PMNs and denatured proteins[5]. Recently Schiffman *et al.*[6] have shown that small synthetic *N*-formylmethionyl peptides, which may be related to natural bacterial leukoattractants, induce leukocyte chemotaxis. Williams *et al.*[7] with human PMNs and Aswanikumar *et al.*[8], with rabbit PMNs have demonstrated that membrane receptors appear to mediate chemotaxis induced by both natural bacterial peptides and formylated synthetic peptides.

In the present report we have compared, with two different methods of assessment, the chemotactic response of 'normal' and inflammatory rat PMNs, and we have studied the interaction of the chemotactic agent f-Met-Leu-Phe with specific cellular receptors.

## MATERIALS AND METHODS

f-Met-Leu-Phe was purchased from UCB, Bruxelles, Belgium, f-Met-Leu-[$^3$H]Phe was obtained by catalytic dehalogenation of *N*-formyl-Met-Leu-Phe(C1)-OH (Bachem, Switzerland) and was shown to be 100% pure by thin-layer chromotagraphy. Its specific activity was 24 Ci/mmol and it was biologically indistinguishable from unlabelled f-Met-Leu-Phe.

### Cell collection

Cells were collected from the rat pleural cavity 4 h after the injection of either 1 ml of isologous serum (for 'normal' cells) or 1 ml of 1% calcium pyrophosphate (CaPP) in saline (for inflammatory cells). The cells were then washed three times with medium NCTC 135 containing fetal calf serum (30% v/v) and then resuspended in this medium. They were then incubated at 37 °C for 15 min and their chemotactic responsiveness assessed as described below.

### Chemotaxis assessment

Two methods were performed in parallel:

*Method 1*

Chemotaxis was first assessed by the method described initially by Bessis[9] and modified by Giroud *et al.*[10], whereby the movement of PMN towards a laser-lysed erythrocyte is followed under the phase-contrast microscope. To quantify the response a chemotactic ratio was calculated which represented the ratio between the number of cells on the target red cell 10 ms after lysis and the number in the fields initially, multiplied by 100. The difference between this ratio, obtained for control cells, was subtracted from that obtained for treated cells to give a quantitative and qualitative indication of the effect of treatment. This 'ratio difference' which is positive for a stimulation of chemotaxis and negative for an inhibition was used for statistical analysis between individual experiments using a paired *t*-test. The speed of the cells was determined from a measurement of the distance travelled by individual cells over a 3 min period.

*Method 2*

Chemotaxis was also assessed by using $^{51}$Cr-labelled granulocytes, as described by Gallin *et al.*[11], in a modified Boyden chamber with two cellulose nitrate filters (Millipore Corp., France) of pore size 5 μm and 3 μm on top of each other. The $^{51}$Cr-labelled neutrophils, at a concentration of $2–3\times10^6$/ml in solution A were placed in the upper compartment of the chemotactic chamber. The chemotactic peptide was diluted from a stock solution at $2\times10^{-3}$ mol/l in DMSO, in solution A (Hanks' solution, buffered at pH 7.2 with 50 mmol/l HEPES, containing 2% bovine serum albumin) and used in the lower compartment at a concentration of $10^{-8}$ mol/l. The chambers were incubated for 3 h at 37 °C in 100% humidity and 5% $CO_2$. At the end of the incubation period the lower filters were removed, rinsed, and counted in a gamma counter (Kontron Electronics CG 4000). Results are expressed as ct/min in lower filter/total ct/min put in the upper chamber.

**f-Met-Leu-[$^3$H]Phe binding assay**

All binding studies were performed in solution A at 22 °C in plastic microcentrifuge tubes (Beckman) at a final volume of 200 μl. Neutrophils were incubated with increasing concentrations of f-Met-Leu-[$^3$H]Phe for 30 min. The incubation was started by addition of cells and terminated by dilution with 1 ml of ice-cold Hanks' solution, followed by centrifugation (10s at 12000 rev/min). The supernatant was discarded by aspiration and the cell pellet was then washed rapidly with 1 ml of ice-cold Hanks' solution and separated again by 10s centrifugation. The cell pellets were then dissolved in aqueous sodium dodecyl sulphate (205 μl; 0.1%) and transferred to counting vials containing 10 ml of Instagel. Radioactivity was measured in a liquid scintillation spectrophotometer (Kontron Electronic SL 3000). Non-specific binding was defined as the amount of binding not inhibited by 50 mmol/l unlabelled f-Met-Leu-Phe and was usually equal to 10–15% of the total counts bound. Specific binding was defined as the total amount of f-Met-Leu-[$^3$H]Phe bound minus the non-specific binding.

## RESULTS

Table 58.1 presents the results obtained with both techniques performed in parallel. In the necrotaxis experiments we have measured the chemotactic ratio defined as the percentage of cells on the target red cell, 10 min after lysis, related to the number of cells in the fields initially, multiplied by 100.

We observed that the chemotactic ratio of normal cells is higher than that of inflammatory cells. This 'ratio difference' indicates an inhibition of the chemotactic responsiveness of the inflammatory cells. The statistical analysis of the results for all the experiments ($n$=150) is highly significant ($p$<0.001).

We observed identical results with the Boyden chamber technique. The number of inflammatory cells migrating towards the chemotactic peptide is twice less than the number of normal cells.

The specific binding of f-Met-Leu-[$^3$H]Phe to normal and inflammatory PMN was a time dependent process reaching a maximum binding level after 30 min at 22 °C. It was found to be concentration dependent and saturable (Figure 58.1). Scatchard analysis of the binding curve gave a straight line (Figure 58.2) indicating that the peptide binds to a single population of sites.

The dissociation constants $K_D$ derived from the Scatchard plots are $4.8\times10^{-8}$ mol/l and $7\times10^{-8}$ mol/l for normal and inflammatory PMN, respectively. The number of binding sites per PMN was calculated to be about 140 000 and 184 000 for normal and inflammatory cells, respectively. These values

**Table 58.1** Comparison of chemotactic responsiveness of 'normal' cells and inflammatory cells measured by necrotaxis and by radioassay in Boyden chambers

| *Necrotaxis* | |
|---|---|
| *Cells* | *% of cells on the target at t + 10 min* |
| Normal | 62 ± 11 |
| Inflammatory | 44 ± 7 |
| *Boyden chamber* | |
| Normal | 4.6 ± 1 |
| Inflammatory | 2.15 ± 0.15 |

can be compared with that found for rabbit[8] peritoneal PMN (120 000) and human[12] peripheral blood PMN (40 000).

## DISCUSSION

It has been demonstrated[13] that calcium pyrophosphate crystals may induce an acute inflammatory reaction in the rat pleural cavity. In this report we have compared the chemotactic behaviour of 'inflammatory cells' harvested in the rat pleural cavity 4 h after administration of calcium pyrophosphate to the chemotactic responsiveness of 'normal' cells harvested in the same cavity 4 h after administration of isologous serum. These cells may be called normal because they are not morphologically modified by contact with isologous serum even after separation of the PMN by fractionation on Ficoll-Hypaque gradient.

We have demonstrated that inflammatory cells show a diminished chemotactic responsiveness in the necrotaxis assay as well as in the Boyden chamber assay when the synthetic peptide f-Met-Leu-Phe is used as chemoattractant.

Using radio-labelled f-Met-Leu-Phe we have been able to exhibit the presence of specific receptor sites on rat PMN. Our binding experiments have shown that inflammatory cells have a slightly higher number of total binding sites for f-Met-Leu-[$^3$H]Phe than 'normal' cells. These results indicate that the diminished chemotactic responsiveness of inflammatory cells compared to normal cells cannot be due to a loss of binding sites for the chemoattractant.

These data are reminiscent of the 'chemotactic deactivation' obtained when PMN are pre-incubated with high concentrations of a chemoattractant[14]. Using human peripheral blood PMN, Abita and Morgat[12] have demonstrated that the decreased chemotactic responsiveness seen when these cells are incubated with high concentrations of f-Met-Leu-Phe and then washed is not correlated with a loss of binding sites for this radiolabelled peptide.

Recently, Fehr and Dahinden[15] have described an analogous phenome-

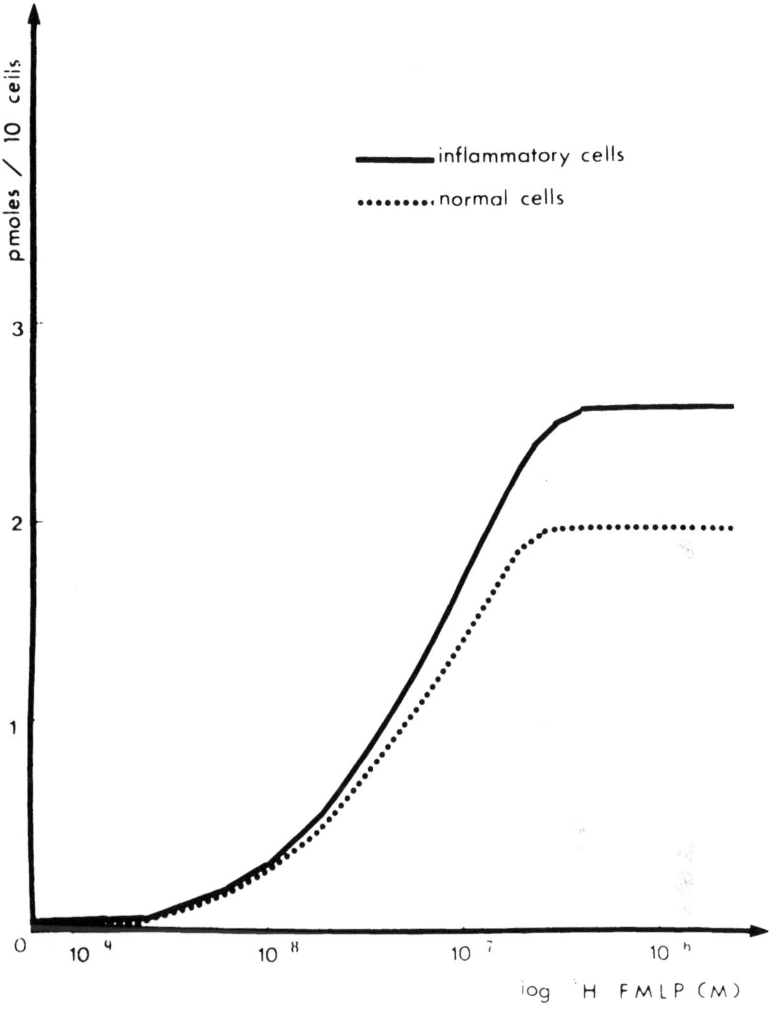


**Figure 58.1** Binding of f-Met-Leu-[³H]Phe to rat PMN as a function of increasing concentrations of f-Met-Leu-[³H]Phe

non with human neutrophils. They also found that these deactivated cells do not respond chemotactically to a gradient of complement-derived factors. Since these chemoattractants (essentially $C_{5a}$ and $C_{3a}$ according to Fernandez *et al.*[16]) are totally unrelated to f-Met-Leu-Phe and have different specific receptors on the neutrophils[2], it is highly improbable that a loss of binding sites for f-Met-Leu-Phe would impair neutrophil chemotaxis towards the complement derived factors. The explanation for chemotactic deactivation

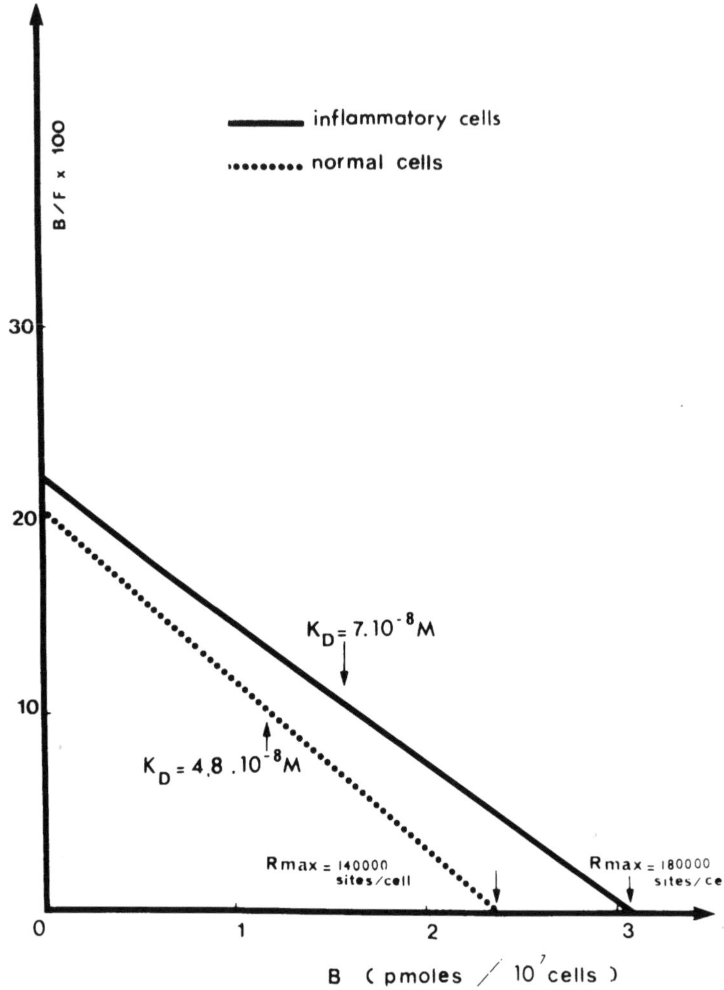


**Figure 58.2** Scatchard's analysis of the binding of f-Met-Leu-[$^3$H]Phe on rat PMN

claimed by Fehr and Dahinden[15] was that high concentrations of f-Met-Leu Phe render the cells hyperadhesive leading to profoundly diminished directed and random migration. On the other hand, Lentneck *et al.*[17] had shown that adherence to nylon fibre columns of granulocytes from patients with acute inflammatory diseases was twice the normal rate.

In preliminary experiments we have also shown that our inflammatory cells present an increased adherence on plastic compared to 'normal' ones.

In conclusion the data presented here show by direct binding experiments with f-Met-Leu[$^{3}$H]Phe that the decreased chemotactic responsiveness of rat inflammatory PMN is not due to a loss of binding sites for this peptide. One of the most probable explanations for this observation might be a consequence of increased cell adhesiveness.

**Acknowledgments**

This work was supported by grant from INSERM ATP No. 69.78.101 and by grant INSERM CRL No. 78.4.046.33 from one of us (J.P.A.)

**References**

1 Keller, H. U. and Sorkin, E. (1966). Studies on chemotaxis. IV The influence of serum factors on granulocyte locomotion. *Immunology*, **10,** 409
2 Chenoweth, D. E. and Hugli, T. E. (1978). Demonstration of specific $C_{5a}$ receptor on intact human polymorphonuclear leukocytes. *Proc. Natl. Acad. Sci.* (USA), **75,** 3943
3 Keller, H. U. and Sorkin, E. (1967). Studies on chemotaxis. V On the chemotactic effect of bacteria. *Int. Arch. Allergy Appl. Immunol.*, **31,** 505
4 Ward, P. A., Remold, H. G. and David, J. R. (1970). The production by antigen-stimulated lymphocytes of a leukotactic factor distinct from migration inhibitory factor. *Cell Immunol.*, **1,** 162
5 Wilkinson, P. C. and McKay, I. C. (1972). The molecular requirements for chemotactic attraction of leukocytes by proteins. Studies of proteins with synthetic side group. *Eur. J. Immunol.*, **2,** 570
6 Schiffmann, E., Corcoran, B. A. and Wahl, S. M. (1975). *N*-formylmethionyl peptides as chemoattractants for leukocytes. *Proc. Natl. Acad. Sci. (USA)*, **72,** 1059
7 Williams, L. T., Snyderman, R., Pike, M. C. and Lefkowitz, R. J. (1977). Specific receptor sites for chemotactic peptides on human polymorphonuclear leukocytes. *Proc. Natl. Acad. Sci. (USA)*, **74,** 1204
8 Aswanikumar, S., Corcoran, B., Schiffmann, E., Day, A. R., Freer, R. J., Showell, H. J. and Becker E. L. (1977). Demonstration of a receptor on rabbit neutrophils for chemotactic peptides. *Biochem. Biophys. Res. Commun.*, **74,** 810
9 Bessis, M. (1974). Necrotaxis, chemotaxis towards an injured cell. *Antibiot. Chemother. (Basel)* **19,** 369
10 Giroud, J. P., Roch-Arveiller, M. and Muntaner, O. (1978). Prélèvement répété des polynucléaires dans la cavité pleurale du rat. Application à l'étude du chimiotactisme. *Nelle Rev. Fse. Hématol.*, **20,** 535
11 Gallin, J. P., Clark, R. A. and Kimball, H. R. (1973).Granulocyte chemotaxis an improved in vitro assay employing $^{51}$Cr labelled granulocytes. *J. Immunol.*, **110,** 233
12 Abita, J. P. and Morgat, J. L. (1980). On the mechanism of human polymorphonuclear leukocytes deactivation of chemotaxis by the synthetic peptide formyl-methionyl-leucyl-phenylalanine. *FEBS Lett.*, **111,** 14
13 Willoughby, D. A., Dunn, C. J., Yamamoto, S., Capasso, F., Deporter, D. A. and Giroud, J. P. (1975). Calcium pyrophosphate-induced pleurisy in rats: a new model of acute inflammation. *Agents Actions*, **1,** 35
14 Ward, P. A. and Becker, E. L. (1968). The deactivation of rabbit neutrophils by chemotactic factor and the nature of the activariable esterase. *J. Exp. Med.*, **127,**
15 Fehr, J. and Dahinden, C. (1979). Modulating influence of chemotactic factor-induced cell adhesiveness on granulocyte function. *J. Clin. Invest.*, **64,** 8
16 Fernandez, H. N. Henson, P. M., Otani, A. and Hugli, T. E. (1978). Chemotactic response to human $C_{3a}$ and $C_{5a}$anaphylatoxins. *J. Immunol.*, **120,** 109
17 Lentnek, A. L., Schreiber, A. D. and McGregor, R. R. (1976). The induction of augmented granulocyte adherence by inflammation. *J. Clin. Invest.*, **57,** 1098

# 59

# Diverging effects of chemotactic serum peptides and synthetic f-Met-Leu-Phe on neutrophil locomotion and adhesion (Abstract)

H. U. KELLER (SWITZERLAND), J. H. WISSLER AND B. DAMERAU (WEST GERMANY)

The chemotactic serum peptides CAT 1.6.1. and $C5a_{desArg}$ induced marked directional locomotion over a wide concentration range. They had, however, no significant effects on random locomotion and adhesion of human neutrophils. In contrast, f-Met-Leu-Phe produced marked negative chemokinetic effects and its capacity to induce directional locomotion was more limited with respect to magnitude and concentration range. Migration inhibition as induced by f-Met-Leu-Phe was related to its dose-dependent effects on spreading and cell adhesion. The results suggested that chemotactic serum peptides are more suitable than f-Met-Leu-Phe to study reactions which are specifically related to chemotaxis, at least under the test conditions used.

# 60

# Correlation between aggregative and chemotaxis inducing activities of five chemotactic peptides (Abstract)

B. DAMERAU, E. GRÜNEFELD, AND W. VOGT (WEST GERMANY)

---

Aggregation of leukocytes by chemotactic agents is possibly the *in vitro* equivalent of leukocyte adherence *in vivo*, the first step of leukoycte migration to inflammatory sites. We therefore compared the aggregative and the chemotaxis inducing activity of five chemotactic peptides, namely the complement-derived peptide C3a and C5a and the synthetic *N*-formyl-methionyl peptides f-Met-Leu-Phe-OH, f-Met-Leu-Leu-OH and f-Met-Leu-OH, using identical cell preparations in both assays. Peripheral human leukocytes were prepared by sedimentation of blood in a dextran-containing medium, suspended in Gey's solution with 0.5% human serum albumin to a final concentration of $10^7$ cells/ml in the aggregation assay (nephelometric determination in an aggregometer) or to a concentration of $10^6$ cells/ml in the Boyden chamber experiments (filters of 3 μm pore size; leading front method).

All the peptides studied induced chemotaxis *and* aggregation of leukocytes; dose-response relations for each peptide were very similar in both activities. This strongly indicates that chemotactic agents produce both chemotaxis and aggregation by similar mechanisms, the latter effect being most probably the *in vitro* equivalent of leukocyte adherence *in vivo*. This view is further supported by the similar inhibition profiles in chemotaxis and aggregation by the SH-reagents *p*-chloromercuribenzoate (which only slightly inhibited both processes at a concentration of $3\times10^{-5}$mol/l and *N*-ethylmaleimide (which caused total inhibition at the same concentration).

The protease inhibitors tosyl-lysyl-chloromethylketone (blocking trypsin-like activity) and tosyl-phenylalanyl-chloromethly-ketone (blocking chymotrypsin-like enzymes) also reduced the aggregating and chemotactic activities of C5a and f-Met-Leu-Phe-OH in similar dose-response relations.

# 61

# On the mechanism of human polymorphonuclear leukocyte deactivation of chemotaxis by the synthetic peptide formyl-methiony-leucyl-phenylalanine

J. P. ABITA (FRANCE)

## INTRODUCTION

Polymorphonuclear leukocytes respond chemotactically *in vitro* to a variety of compounds including denatured proteins[1] factors derived from complement[2], bacterial products[3] and synthetic peptides, the most potent being the peptide formyl-methionyl-leucyl-phenylalanine (f-Met-Leu-Phe)[4,5]. In addition f-Met-Leu-Phe induces granule enzyme secretion and superoxide production when added with cytochalasin B to rabbit neutrophils in suspension[4,6] and aggregates these cells[7]. There is evidence that all these functions result from the interaction of the peptide with a common membrane receptor[4,6–8] which has been demonstrated, by direct binding studies, to exist on the cell surface of rabbit[9] and human neutrophils[10].

Using rabbit peritoneal neutrophils, Ward and Becker reported that if the cells were incubated with high concentrations of a chemoattractant derived from complement and were then washed, the cells showed a diminished chemotactic responsiveness towards the same stimulus[11]. This phenomenon had been termed 'chemotactic deactivation'[11] and although it has been noted with other chemotactic factors, including f-Met-Leu-Phe[12], it has not yet received a satisfactory explanation. However, Showell *et al.*[13] have demonstrated that the deactivation of neutrophils is not restricted to chemotaxis. If rabbit peritoneal neutrophils are incubated with f-Met-Leu-Phe and are then washed before being rechallenged with the same peptide and cytochalasin B, the cells show a decreased secretory responsiveness. These authors have suggested that this deactivation might be related to a loss of binding sites for the peptide.

Since in many other systems [for a review see reference 14] deactivation (or desensitization or refractoriness) has been shown to be effectively related to a loss of binding sites on the cells for the effector, we have decided to see if this was true also for chemotactic deactivation.

In the present study we show, using human peripheral blood neutrophils, that there is a time and dose-dependent decrease in the chemotactic responsiveness of these cells towards f-Met-Leu-Phe when they are pre-incubated with the same peptide and then washed. However, these changes in chemotactic responsiveness are neither accompanied by a loss of binding sites for this peptide nor by a difference in the affinity for its receptor.

## MATERIALS AND METHODS

F-Met-Leu-Phe was purchased from UCB, Bruxelles, Belgium. f-Met-Leu-[$^3$H]Phe was prepared by catalytic dehalogenation of the peptide f-Met-Leu-Phe-(I)-OH (Bachem, Switzerland) and was shown to be 100% pure by thin-layer chromatography and amino acid analysis. Its specific activity was 24 Ci/mmol and it was biologically indistinguishable from unlabelled f-Met-Leu-Phe.

Polymorphonuclear neutrophils were obtained from heparinized peripheral blood of human volunteers using the method described by Williams *et al.*[10] and were at least 98% pure.

Neutrophils were washed twice and resuspended in solution A (Hanks' balanced salt solution buffered with 50 mmol/l HEPES at pH 7.2 containing 2% bovine serum albumin) at a concentration of $15 \times 10^6$ cells/ml and incubated, at 37 °C, in solution A alone or in solution A containing different concentrations of the chemotactic peptide. At the end of the incubation period, the cells were collected by centrifugation (350 *g* for 10 min) and resuspended in 40 ml of solution A. After 10 min at 37 °C the sedimentation and resuspension were repeated. After an additional 10 min at 37 °C, the cells were again centrifuged for 10 min at 350 *g* and resuspended in solution A. Final cell concentrations at the end of the washings were $10–12 \times 10^6$ cells/ml. Aliquots of this suspension of washed cells were used to study f-Met-Leu-[$^3$H]Phe binding on chemotaxis towards fresh f-Met-Leu-Phe.

Chemotaxis was measured by using $^{51}$Cr labelled neutrophils as described by Gallin *et al.*[15], in a modified Boyden chamber (Celloplex, Basel, Switzerland) with two cellulose nitrate filters of pore size 3 μm and 5 μm on top of each other. The $^{51}$Cr labelled neutrophils at a concentration of $4 \times 10^6$ cells/ml were placed in the upper compartment of the chemotactic chamber. The chemotactic peptide was diluted, from a stock solution at $10^{-3}$ mol/l in dimethylsulphoxide, in solution A and used in the lower compartment of the chamber at a final concentration of $10^{-8}$ mol/l. The chambers were incubated for 3 h at 37 °C in 100% humidity and 5% $CO_2$. At the end of the incubation the lower filters were removed, rinsed and counted in a gamma counter (Kontron Electronics CG 4000). Results are expressed as ct/min in lower filter/total ct/min put in the upper compartment of the chamber.

All binding studies were performed in solution A at 22 °C in plastic microcentrifuge tubes (Beckman) in a final volume of 0.2 ml. Neutrophils were incubated with increasing concentrations of f-Met-Leu-[$^3$H]Phe for 30 min. The incubation was started by addition of cells and terminated by dilution with 1 ml of ice-cold Hanks' solution followed by centrifugation (10s at 12 000 rev/min). The supernatant was discarded by aspiration and the cell pellets were then washed rapidly with 1 ml of ice-cold Hanks' solution and separated again by 10s centrifugation. The cell pellets were then dissolved in aqueous sodium dodecyl sulphate (250 $\mu$l, 0.1%) and transferred to counting vials containing 10 ml of Instagel. Radioactivity was measured in a liquid scintillation spectrophotometer (Kontron Electronics SL 3000). Non-specific binding was defined as the amount of binding not inhibited by 50 $\mu$mol/l unlabelled f-Met-Leu-Phe and was usually equal to 10–15% of the total counts bound. Specific binding was defined as the total amount of f-Met-Leu-[$^3$H] Phe bound minus the non-specific binding.

## RESULTS

Table 61.1 presents the results of experiments in which various suspensions of neutrophils were incubated at 37 °C with f-Met-Leu-Phe or in solution A alone. After washing, the cells were tested for chemotaxis towards the same fresh peptide. There is a time and dose-dependent inhibition of chemotaxis when the cells are preincubated with f-Met-Leu-Phe at concentrations of $10^{-8}$ mol/l and higher.

After pre-incubation and washing, we also determined the peptide receptor concentration per cell by incubating the washed cells at 22 °C for 30 min (a time which we have shown to be necessary to reach equilibrium) with increasing concentrations of f-Met-Leu-[$^3$H]Phe (Figure 61.1). It can be seen that f-Met-Leu-[$^3$H]Phe binding to cells that had been pre-incubated with $10^{-8}$ mol/l f-Met-Leu-Phe for 1 h, or with $10^{-6}$ mol/l peptide for 30 min, was identical to that of cells that had not been exposed to the peptide (Figure 1A). Analysis of the Scatchard's plots (Figure 1B) indicates that there is neither decrease in the effective concentration of receptors, nor alteration in affinity. With either set of cells, the equilibrium dissocation constant, $K_d$, was $2.2 \times 10^{-8}$ mol/l. At saturation, the $1.8 \times 10^6$ cells present in the incubation mixture are capable of binding 118 fmoles of f-Met-Leu-[$^3$H]Phe. This value corresponds to about 40 000 sites per cell.

**Table 61.1** Effect of pre-incubation of neutrophils with f-Met-Ieu-Phe on locomotion towards the same peptide

| *Cells migrating towards* | *Time of pre-incubation* (min) | *No peptide* | *Cells pre-incubated with f-Met-Leu-Phe* | | | | |
|---|---|---|---|---|---|---|---|
| | | | $10^{-10}$ mol/l | $10^{-8}$ mol/l | $10^{-7}$ mol/l | $10^{-6}$ mol/l | $10^{-5}$ mol/l |
| | | | % of cells migrating in the lower filter | | | | |
| No peptide<br>f-Met-Leu-Phe $10^{-8}$ mol/l | 0 | 1.45<br>8.66 | – | – | – | – | – |
| No peptide<br>f-Met-Leu-Phe $10^{-8}$ mol/l | 5 | 1.51<br>7.60 | 1.61<br>7.83 | 1.63<br>8.27 | 1.58<br>5.78 | 1.55<br>4.34 | 1.53<br>2.12 |
| No peptide<br>f-Met-Leu-Phe $10^{-8}$ mol/l | 15 | 1.63<br>8.33 | 1.58<br>7.44 | 1.51<br>7.72 | 1.43<br>3.29 | 1.33<br>1.66 | 1.61<br>1.91 |
| No peptide<br>f-Met-Leu-Phe $10^{-8}$ mol/l | 30 | 1.93<br>8.79 | 1.55<br>7.32 | 1.93<br>5.86 | 1.46<br>2.9 | 1.55<br>1.71 | 1.74<br>1.93 |
| No peptide<br>f-Met-Leu-Phe $10^{-8}$ mol/l | 60 | 1.52<br>7.43 | 1.71<br>7.60 | 1.34<br>2.15 | 1.55<br>2.01 | 1.37<br>1.43 | 1.58<br>1.65 |

Each figure is the mean of four different determinations done in duplicate

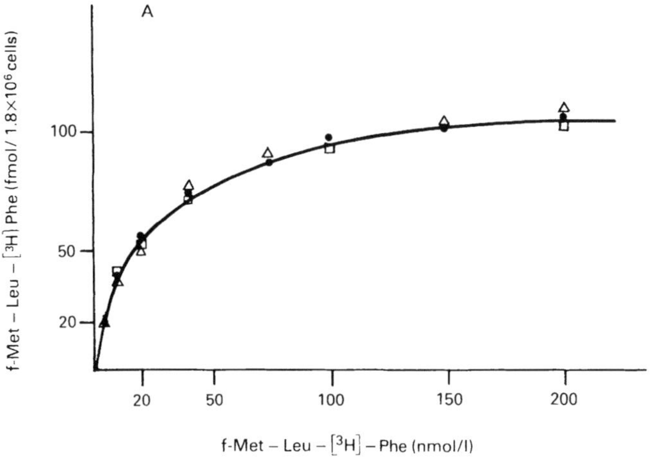


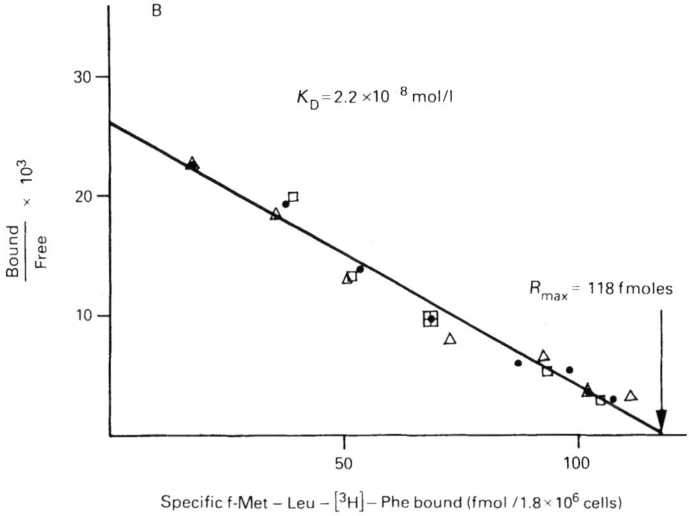


**Figure 61.1(A)** Binding of f-Met-Leu-[$^3$H]Phe to neutrophils as a function of concentration of f-Met-Leu-[$^3$H]Phe. f-Met-Leu [$^3$H]Phe at the indicated concentrations was incubated with human neutrophils for 30 min at 22 °C and specific binding was measured. (●——●) indicates cells which had been incubated for 1 h at 37 °C in solution A alone; (□——□) indicates cells which had been incubated for 1 h at 37 °C in the presence of f-Met-Leu-Phe $10^{-8}$ mol/l and then washed. (△——△) indicates cells which had been incubated for 30 min at 37 °C in the presence of f-Met-Leu-Phe $10^{-6}$ mol/l and then washed. Each value shown represents the mean of three determinations done in duplicate.
(B) The data are plotted according to Scatchard's analysis

In a further set of experiments we tested the ability of our washing procedure to reverse the binding of f-Met-Leu-[$^3$H]Phe. 15 × $10^6$ cells were incubated, in duplicate, with f-Met-Leu-[$^3$H] Phe 4 × $10^{-8}$ mol/l in 1 ml of solution A. After 1 h at 37 °C, two 100 μl aliquots were removed, washed with ice-cold Hanks' solution and their radioactivity determined. The 800 μl left were diluted with 40 ml of solution A at 37 °C and washed twice as described in methods. At the end of the washing procedure, the cell pellet was resuspended in 1 ml of solution A at 22 °C. Two 100 μl aliquots were immediately removed, washed with ice-cold Hanks' solution and their radioactivity measured. The remaining cells were separated in three 190 μl fractions on which the total and non-specific binding of fresh f-Met-Leu-[$^3$H]Phe, 4 × $10^{-8}$ mol/l were measured as described in methods. Cells pre-incubated in solution A alone were treated under the same conditions. The results of these experiments are presented in Table 61.2. It can be seen that cells pre-incubated either in solution A alone or in the presence of f-Met-Leu-[$^3$H]Phe can bind the same amount of fresh radio-labelled peptide corroborating the results of Figure 61.1. It can be seen also that cells pre-incubated with f-Met-Leu-[$^3$H]Phe and then washed thoroughly at 37 °C keep an amount of radioactivity slightly higher than the non-specific binding. This result and our data (not shown) on the kinetics of binding of f-Met-Leu-[$^3$H]Phe on human neutrophils suggest that a certain amount of peptide is interiorized after its association with the cells.

## DISCUSSION

We have demonstrated that human peripheral blood neutrophils pre-incubated with the synthetic chemotactic peptide f-Met-Leu-Phe and then washed, lose, in a time and dose-dependent fashion, their ability to respond chemotactically to the same peptide. This deactivation of chemotaxis is already manifest after 5 min of pre-incubation of cells with peptide concentrations higher than $10^{-8}$ mol/l.

Using radio labelled f-Met-Leu-Phe we have shown that our washing procedure is able to displace all the peptide that was originally bound to the cells during the pre-incubation period. Thus neutrophils which had been pre-incubated with f-Met-Leu-Phe at concentrations up to $10^{-5}$ mol/l and then washed have the same total binding capacity for f-Met-Leu-[$^3$H]Phe than do cells pre-incubated in buffer alone.

Our results are in accord with those published recently by Fehr and Dahinden[16] (while this manuscript was in preparation) who also found that human neutrophils pre-incubated with high concentrations of f-Met-Leu-Phe are chemotactically deactivated. They also found that these deactivated cells do not respond chemotactically to a gradient of complement-derived factors. Since these chemoattractants (essentially C5a and C3a[17]) are totally unrelated to f-Met-Leu-Phe and have different specific receptors on the neutrophils[18] it

**Table 61.2** Reversal of f-Met-Leu-[$^3$H]Phe binding by the washing procedure

| *Cell treatments* | *ct/min/2 × 10$^6$ cells* |
|---|---|
| Cells pre-incubated with f-Met.Leu-[$^3$H]Phe 4 × 10$^{-8}$ mol/l at 37 °C for 1 h, washed at 0 °C and counted | 1834 |
| Cells pre-incubated with f-Met-Leu-[$^3$H]Phe 4 × 10$^{-8}$ mol/l at 37 °C for 1 h, washed twice at 37 °C and counted | 590 |
| Cells pre-incubated with f-Met-Leu-[$^3$H]Phe 4 × 10$^{-8}$ mol/l at 37 °C for 1 h, washed twice at 37 °C and rechallenged with fresh f-Met-Leu-[$^3$H]Phe 4 × 10$^{-8}$ mol/l for 30 min at 22 °C | 1920 |
| Cells pre-incubated and washed at 37 °C as above and rechallenged with fresh f-Met-Leu[$^3$H]Phe 4 × 10$^{-8}$ mol/l and f-Met-Leu-Phe 5 × 10$^{-5}$ mol/l for 30 min at 22 °C | 680 |
| Cells pre-incubated in solution A alone for 1 h at 37 °C, washed twice at 37 °C and challenged with f-Met-Leu-[$^3$H]Phe 4 × 10$^{-8}$ mol/l for 30 min at 22 °C | 1433 |
| Cells pre-incubated in solution A alone for 1 h at 37 °C, washed twice at 37 °C and challenged with f-Met-Leu-[$^3$H]Phe 4 × 10$^{-8}$ mol/l and f-Met-Leu-Phe 5 × 10$^{-5}$ mol/l for 30 min at 22 °C | 199 |

Each value is the mean of two different determinations done in duplicate.
1433 ct/min/2 × 10$^6$ cells represent 80 fmoles of peptide bound on the cells.

is highly improbable that a loss of binding sites for f-Met-Leu-Phe would impair neutrophil chemotaxis towards the complement-derived factors. The explanation for chemotactic deactivation of human neutrophils claimed by Fehr and Dahinden[16] was that high concentrations of f-Met-Leu-Phe render the cells hyperadhesive leading to profoundly diminished directed and random migration.

Another explanation put forward by Spilberg *et al*[12], using human neutrophils and two chemoattractants totally unrelated to f-Met-Leu-Phe, was that deactivation is the functional manifestation of an unorganized chemotactic factor-sensitive microtubule assembly and not the blockade of available receptors. On the other hand, Wilkinson[19] has recently published results which seem to indicate that levamisole and the calcium ionophore A23187, if present during the preincubation of neutrophils with f-Met-Leu-Phe, could prevent the inhibition of chemotaxis. Since neither drug interferes with the binding of f-Met-Leu-[$^3$H] Phe (our data not shown) it is possible that cyclic nucleotides or calcium, or both, may be involved in the molecular mechanism of neutrophil deactivation.

In conclusion, the data presented in this study show, by direct binding experiments with f-Met-Leu-[$^3$H] Phe, that the chemotactic deactivation of human neutrophils, induced by pre-incubation of the cells with the peptide, is not due to a loss of binding sites for the chemoattractant. Whatever the molecular mechanism for this deactivation of chemotaxis, it certainly involves a step beyond the binding of the peptide to its membrane receptor. Work is in progress in our laboratory to investigate this problem.

**Acknowledgments**

The authors wish to thank Miss H. Tomachevsky for excellent technical assistance. Dr. P. Kaplan for carefully reading the manuscript and Prof. Y. Najean for fruitful discussions. This work was supported by grant C.R.L. 78–4, 046.33 from I.N.S.E.R.M.

## References

1 Wilkinson, P. C. (1974) In *Chemotaxis and inflammation*, p. 54. (Edinburgh: Churchill Livingston)
2 Snyderman, R., Phillips, J. and Mergenhagen, S. E. (1970). *Infect. Immun.* **1,** 521
3 Keller, H. V. and Sorkin, E. (1967). *Int. Arch. Allergy*, **31,** 505
4 Showell, H. J., Freer, R. J., Zigmond, S. H., Schiffman, E., Aswanikumar, S., Corcoran, B. A. and Becker, E. L. (1976). *J. Exp. Med.*, **143,** 1154
5 Spilberg, I., Mandell, B., Mehta, J., Sullivan, T. and Sinckowitz, L. (1978). *J. Lab. Clin. Med.*, **92,** 297
6 Becker, E. L., Sigman, M. and Oliver, J. M. (1979). *Am. J. Pathol*, **95,** 81
7 O'Flaherty, J. T., Showell, H. J., Kreutzer, D. L., Ward, P. A. and Becker, E. L. (1978). *J. Immunol.* **120,** 1326
8 Becker, E. L. (1976) *Am. J. Pathol.*, **85,** 385
9 Aswanikumar, S., Corcoran, B., Schiffmann, E., Day, A. R., Freer, R. J., Showell, H. J., Becker, E. L. and Pert, C. (1977). *Biochem. Biophys Res. Commun.*, **74,** 810
10 Williams, L. T., Snyderman, R., Pike, M. C. and Lefkowitz, R. J. (1977). Proc. Natl. Acad. Sci. (USA) **74,** 1204
11 Ward, P. A. and Becker, E. L. (1968). *J. Exp. Med.*, **127,** 693
12 Spilberg, I., Mandell, B. and Hoffstein, S. (1979). *J. Lab. Clin. Med.* **94,** 361
13 Showell, H. J., Williams, D., Becker, E. L., Naccache, P. H. and Sha'afi, R. (1979). *J. Reticuloendothelial Soc.*, **25,** 139
14 Kahn, R. C. (1976). *J. Biol. Chem.*, **70,** 261
15 Zigmond, S. H. and Sullivan, S. J. (1979). *J. Cell. Biol.* **82,** 515
16 Fehr, J. and Dahinden, C. (1979). *J. Clin. Invest.*, **64,** 8
17 Fernandez, H. N., Henson, P. M., Otani, A. and Hugli, T. E. (1978). *J. Immunol.*, **120,** 109
18 Chenoweth, D. E. and Hugli, T. E. (1978). *Proc. Natl. Acad. Sci (USA)* **75,** 3943
19 Wilkinson, P. C. (1979). *Immunology*, **36,** 579

62

# Dynamics of membranes in viable leukocytes associated with cellular recognition and biological memory in chemotaxis and promotion of locomotion in chemokinesis(Abstract)

J. H. WISSLER AND E. LOGEMANN (WEST GERMANY)

---

A basic feature of the inflammatory process is the oriented migration to and accumulation at the site of tissue injury of the different types of leukocytes. Transitions from random to directional locomotion of leukocytes comprise cellular direction finding (cellular recognition) with processing of chemical information (metastable, dissipative conformer phases), and positional information (dissipative physical structures of chemical information in form of concentration non-equilibria as gradients and boundaries) residing in the solution of the chemoattractant. Concerning basic biological terms governing cell migration, classical anaphylatoxin-associated serum-derived chemotactic solutes highly purified and crystallized according to Wissler 1971. *Experientia 27: 1447. (Eur. J. Immunol*, **2,** 73), are biologically specific and exclusively induce this transition in neutrophil granuloytes: neither cellular locomotion itself, nor aggregation and adhesion of cells is influenced. Stimulation by this chemoattractant obeys Weber–Fechner's law and expresses memory effects, i.e., repeated stimulation by same concentrations of the chemoattractant give little or no biological response (tachyphylaxis) in terms of direction finding (Keller, Wissler, Hess and Cottier, (1978). *Eur. J. Immunol.* **8,** 1). Hence, this recognition process in direction finding is different from stimulation of locomotion of leukocytes (chemokinesis); e.g., by positive chemokinetic solutes like porcine and human serum albumin which allows no direction finding and is not subject to cellular refractoriness (tachyphylaxis). The molecular events involved in the interaction of leukocyte membranes with dissipative anaphylatoxin conformer phases and serum albumin solutions were studied by total intensity and polarization of fluorescence on a quantum basis by pulse or continuous excitation of various probes (Wissler and Logemann (1978): *Z. Physil. Chemie.*, **360**, 1204) which exhibit selective affinity for proteins, hydrocarbon regions and for different transverse regions of phosphatidyl choline bilayers in cell membranes. As derived from Perrin plots, lipid-hydrocarbon surface membrane layers of viable normal porcine and canine peripheral neurophils kept in Gey's balanced salt solution (pH 7.10, 37 °C) have an average microviscosity $\pi$ of 0.15 Pa s and a low fusion activation energy (< 2 kcal/mol). In the biologically active dose range (1 nmol/l–1 μmol/l), porcine serum-derived chemoattractant does not noticeably interact with this lipid layer, but several mobile membrane protein entities, not preformed intact single receptors, are the primary and major target sites which are held together multivalently by single or clusters of anaphylatoxin molecules and which thus form one receptive unit (domain) at the membrane surface. The metastable association of the membrane proteins is the result of direct information transfer from dissipative (metastable) anaphylatoxin conformer phases in solution and extrusion of structured water molecules. Chemotactic solutes act directly and independently of albumin as positive chemokinetic solute. Neither is complex formation between albumin and anaphylatoxin conformers a necessary principle for the recognition process in chemotaxis. Major targets of albumin as chemokinetic solute are lipid-hydrocarbon layers at the cell surface which thus are shielded from exposure to water molecules. Chemoattractant induces hysteresis (memory) in fluorescence of protein probes.

# Discussion

**Dr N. R. Ackerman (USA)** described his work on a model of macrophage accumulation involving injection of carrageenin into the pleural cavity and monitoring the cellular response for 4 days. At 3 days they observed a cellular reaction of $10^8$ cells, of which 80–85% were macrophages as determined on the basis of morphology and staining characteristics. Using this test system they then examined a variety of anti-inflammatory and anti-rheumatic agents to see whether they would specifically affect accumulation of macrophages at an inflamed site. Dexamethasone at 5 (μg/kg)/day reduced the number of macrophages by 52%. At this dose there was no effect on the peripheral monocyte population, indicating that it was probably the result of chemotaxis. Surprisingly, non-steroidal anti-inflammatory agents in clinically effective doses (indomethacin 5 mg/kg or naproxen 10 mg/kg) gave a stimulation of macrophage numbers of 50–60%, which was exacerbated further at higher doses. The anti-rheumatic compound hydroxychloroquine gave some inhibition at 10 (mg/kg)/day and significant inhibition at 100 (mg/kg)/day. Levamisole, penicillamine and gold sodium thiomalate were inactive in this test system.

**Professor J. P. Giroud (Co-Chairman)** said that carrageenin had many different pharmacological properties but that different workers often used different preparations. He enquired about the specificity of Dr Ackerman's preparation.

**Dr Ackerman** said he had used a Sigma preparation, a combination of kappa and lambda forms. They chose it only after trying a number of other pro-inflammatory materials, none of which gave an infiltrate of comparable size or macrophage specificity.

In response to a question about the timing of drugs he said that they had been given at -1 h, 24 h and 48 h after carrageenin and autopsies were performed at 72 h. They had performed the work because there was very little in the literature on the effects of anti-rheumatic agents on accumulation of macrophages at an inflammatory site. Most studies were on PMN accumulation over much shorter time periods.

**Dr E. A. Boyle (UK)** was invited to discuss his work on pellet and sponge induced granuloma in rats. He said that the two models were set up in an attempt to examine collagen levels in animals following drug treatment. The porous polyvinyl sponge had proved much easier to use than the cotton wool pellet and much easier to remove at 9 days, when there was an appreciable amount of collagen already laid down in the granuloma. Although collagen levels were very similar in the two models, the pattern of granuloma formation appeared different. There was encapsulation around the cotton wool pellet but in the porous sponge the inflammatory cells and collagen had infiltrated into the middle. They had been able to show that d-penicillamine and beta-aminoproprionitrile both increased soluble collagen levels in the sponge.

As to differences in response to the two types of implant, they had found that DNA levels from day 2 onwards were far higher in the cotton pellet. He was not sure whether the early cellular responses were different in the two models because it was very difficult to remove cells from the cotton pellet and they had not performed any autoradiographic studies.

**Dr P. Bailey (USA)** had also used the cotton pellet granuloma assay as a measure of chronic inflammation in the rat but had concentrated on cellular events occurring within the pellet, using levels of the enzyme *N*-acetyl-β-D-glucosaminidase (NAG) which had a particularly high specific activity in mononuclear phagocytic cells. He had also measured total nucleic acids as an index of total cell infiltration. Measurement of enzyme levels showed clear inhibition of infiltration using pharmacological doses of indomethacin, a phenomenon difficult to demonstrate using only dry or wet weight measurements. They had also studied the time relationship of the interactions. Dosing with indomethacin during the first 3 days produced inhibition of granuloma development at day 7. However, dosing with dexamethasone or indomethacin between days 4 and 7 produced no inhibition. This underlined the important events taking place during the early phases of granuloma development. They were now able to give indomethacin doses on days 0 and 1 and obtain full inhibition of granuloma formation on day 7. The model also suggested differences in the mechanism of action of steroidal and non-steroidal agents. Treating with dexamethasone on day 7 produced a completely acellular granuloma with no development of a fibrous capsule. Treatment with indomethacin, however, athough it also inhibited the movement of inflammatory cells into the cotton, did not prevent the development of the fibrous capsule. So far they had not been successful in recovering cells from the granuloma to study them *in vitro* nor had they used other enzyme markers. They were not inferring that NAG was a mediator of inflammation but simply a marker of inflammatory cell infiltrate. The $ED_{50}$ for pre-dosing with dexamethasone was 35 μg/kg/day. The first dose was given subcutaneously 4 h after implantation of the pellet.

**Dr Boyle** said that he had used dexamethasone to reduce granuloma and although he could reduce collagen levels a great deal of granulomatous tissue still remained, even after giving 45 μg of the drug.

**Professor I. B. Lorenzen (Denmark)** questioned the value of using sponges and cotton pellets in which a capsule developed for the study of drug effects on the formation of granulation tissue. In his view, when the granuloma became encapsulated then it was effectively sealed off from the action of the drug. When investigating the effect of the drug in such a model one might actually simply be measuring the effect on capsule formation.

**Dr Bailey** said that this might be true, but it was still part of the inflammatory response.

**Dr R. Turner (USA)** was invited to describe his work on neutrophil interactions with particulate material. He said that he believed that neutrophil interactions with such particulate material as insoluble immune complexes in rheumatoid arthritis and monosodium urate crystals in gout were important aspects of the inflammatory process. From their original test tube system they had now developed a system of plastic petri dishes using neutrophil monolayers. They were exposed to particulate materials and he measured the effects on adherence of the cells to the petri dishes and release of lysosomal or cytoplasmic enzymes: Monosodium urate crystals at 30 min caused a decreased adherence of the cells but insoluble IgG aggregates did not appear to affect it. There appeared to be selective release of lysosomal enzymes caused by both crystals and aggregates and at 45 min there was a release of LDH cytoplasmic enzyme induced by monosodium urate crystals but not insoluble aggregates. So far they had not established the dose-response curve with the aggregates but they knew that 1.2 mg/ml was sufficient to produce significant release in the original tube assays. In the monolayers, the amount required was less than milligram quantities.

In response to a question about a cell-derived chemotactic factor he said that such a factor with a molecular weight of less than 10 000 susceptible to protease inhibitors did exist. It attracted neutrophils.

In answer to a question about whether he had examined abnormal cells he said that they had not yet done so with a monolayer system. In 1971 he had reported that rheumatoid neutrophils had a decreased phagocytic capacity as judged in the tube tests. That led to the present studies in an attempt to quantitate whether the uptake of complexes was responsible. They found that neutrophils exposed to immune complexes could not phagocytoze as well as those exposed to uric acid crystals, which led to the present *in vitro* studies.

**Dr D. White (UK)** was invited to describe his mouse *in vitro* macrophage model. Macrophages were elicited from the peritoneal cavity by brain-heart infusion. Three hours later the accumulated macrophages were cultured and treated with various types of drugs. The parameters examined were phagocytosis of opsonized zymosan and the ensuing release of lysosomal enzymes using the marker NAG. LDH release was measured as a test of cellular integrity. Auranofin, an orally active gold compound, dramatically inhibited lysosomal enzyme release at a concentration of $10^{-6}$ mol/l, at which concentration it did not affect phagocytosis. At higher concentrations, both processes were inhibited. The gold compound myocrisin would inhibit enzyme release at higher concentrations but had no effect on phagocytosis. Dapsone inhibited lysosomal release only at concentrations approaching $10^{-3}$ mol/l and a similar profile was observed with ketoprofen. In contrast, hydrocortisone inhibited both parameters. He agreed that this model had similar properties to some others but they hoped that by using opsonized zymosan the level of phagocytosis and therefore ingestion was increased, which might be more akin to the ingestion of immune complexes in rheumatoid arthritis. In answer to a specific question he said that the brain–heart infusion mixture had similar properties to the thioglycolates and other media used to elicit macrophages and its effects were very reproducible.

**Dr R. M. McMillan (USA)** had performed investigations which extended this theme. He said that there was very little information on the interaction of urate crystals with chronic inflammatory cells. In an attempt to understand the mechanisms involved in chronic gouty arthritis they had investigated the effect of adding monosodium urate crystals at a concentration of 150 μg/ml to monolayers of peritoneal macrophages. Within 1 h there was phagocytosis of all types of particles with measurable release of NAG. The effect of urate in inducing lysosomal release was not a direct effect upon the cell membrane. At 4 h the release was relatively selective, and after 24 h it had not greatly increased. Prolonged incubation of the cells with the crystals would however cause lysis as witnessed by the LDH release. Initial results were obtained in serum free media but treatment of the crystals with various serum proteins produced different effects. Coating the cells with serum did not potentiate lysosmal enzyme release, nor did treating the crystals with albumin. However, pre-treatment of the crystals with IgG did potentiate lysosomal enzyme release. These results suggested that one should examine the interaction of urate not only with mononuclear phagocytes, but also with other chronic inflammatory cells.

**Dr J. L. Jouvin (France)** was invited to describe his work on the effect of calcium pyrophosphate (CPPD) and monosodium urate (MSU) on gingival tissue. He said that they had induced an inflammatory response by subcutaneous injection of suspensions in the palatal mucosae of guinea pigs. The investigation was prompted by the belief that CPPD and MSU crystals were not handled in the same way by the surrounding tissues and cells. They therefore performed a quantitative evaluation by stereological methods of the modifications to palatal connective tissue during such crystal induced inflammation. In the early stages with MSU they found that monocytes were more numerous than PMNs. The reverse situation was seen after CPPD injection.

In answer to a question he said that the CPPD was triclinic calcium pyrophosphate. Particle size was 10–30 μm.

**Professor J. P. Giroud (France)** said that it was extremely important that workers on crystal deposition disease should make sure that they were all using the same substances and thus avoid the problem which had for some years plagued users of carrageenin.

**Dr A. Daniel (France)** said that one of the principle characteristics of palatal connective tissue was that it was fibrous and very similar to gingival tissue. It was because of its similarity to gingival tissue that they had used it.

**Dr C. J. Dunn (France)** found the use of triclinic calcium pyrophosphate surprising because in peudo-gout the predominant crystal form was the monoclinic dihydrate. In addition, crystals 10–30 μm were very difficult to phagocytoze.

**Dr Daniel** agreed. 10–30 μm referred to the native crystals. Before injection they were ground to particles 1–3 μm in diameter. With native crystals, no inflammatory reaction appeared.

**Dr P. C. J. Leijh (Netherlands)** was invited to describe his work on intracellular killing by monocytes. He had incubated monocytes in various media and studied the killing of previously phagocytozed bacteria. Optimal killing of *Staphylococcus aureus* was achieved only in the presence of fresh serum. The factors in the serum which appeared to be responsible were IgG which interacted with Fc receptors on the monocyte membrane and the complement component C3b. There appeared to exist a phenomenon with extracellular stimuli inducing intracellular killing of bacteria by interaction with receptors on the monocyte membrane.

In answer to a question about other bacteria, he said that streptococci were killed intracellularly without extracellular stimulation. He believed the same to occur in patients with chronic granulomatous disease where streptococci were killed as a result of their own hydrogen peroxide formation in the phagosomes. In answer to a further question, he said that they had gone to considerable lengths to distinguish bacteria on the surface of the cell from those which had been ingested and he had no doubt that they were dealing with true intracellular killing.

**Dr B. W. van den Berg (Netherlands)** was invited to review his work on antigen induced joint inflammation. He had studied incorporation of radioactive sulphates into patella chondrocytes in the mouse as a measure of *in vivo* chrondrocyte metabolism during joint inflammation. In this model there was depression of chondrocyte function during chronic inflamation, a depression which seemed to be unrelated to the formation of pannus. Inhibition and chrondrocyte death was found in the central part of the patella where no pannus tissue was present, while normally functioning chondrocytes were found under the pannus tissue at lateral sites. He had no data on the mediators responsible for this inhibition of chondrocyte function although lymphokines and prostaglandins might both be implicated.

In answer to questions he said that mice were immunized by the methylated form of bovine serum albumin with Freund's complete adjuvant. The disease generally lasted from 3–6 months and they were currently screening various strains of mice for susceptibility to arthritis. They had never found arthritis in the saline control joint but they were currently studying the effect of systemic injection with methylated bovine albumin.

**Dr D. A. Deporter (Canada)** was invited to review his finding on collagen phagocytosis. This had been demonstrated in a variety of tissues but it had been largely regarded as a curiosity rather than a significant mechanism. They had demonstrated a direct correlation between the quantity of collagen being phagocytozed in three different soft connective tissues and the rate of mature collagen degradation occurring in those tissues as determined biochemically. Moving on to the inflammatory situation of peridontal disease in the rat, they had been able to demonstrate a dramatic increase in phagocytosis of collagen in the inflamed as compared to the control sites. He wished to challenge the general concensus that the primary mechanism of collagen absorption during collagen inflammation was due to the secretion of enzymes by inflammatory cells such as macrophages.

**Dr McMillan** said that macrophages were a relatively poor source of collagenase. It was more appropriate in this context to consider synovial lining cells. In his view, collagen phagocytosis in rheumatoid arthritis was a curiosity, rather than the underlying mechanism of collagen degradation.

**Dr D. E. Woolley (UK)** believed that even in peridontal disease collagenase activity existed. Recent immunoreactive techniques had shown that collagenase existed extracellularly in those tissues which were resorbing. In his view, extracellular and intracellular mechanisms might both occur. The collagen fibres themselves were comparatively large and one would expect at least some breakdown before they were phagocytozed.

**Dr Deporter** agreed that it was possible to demonstrate extracellular enzyme but he felt nonetheless that the phagocytic mechanism was more important than had generally been assumed.

**Dr M. Roch-Arveiller (France)** was invited to describe her study of rat PMNs obtained from the pleural cavity 4 h after injection of 1 ml of serum, compared to those similarly obtained after injection of calcium pyrophosphate. Measurement of chemotaxis by two different methods suggested that the latter cells showed a significant decrease in their chemotactic response. Their results suggested that this decrease in chemotactic response was not related to the number of chemotactic peptide binding sites present.

**Dr G. O. Till (Germany)** said that these results related to two quite different cell populations. Those produced in response to calcium pyrophosphate had migrated into the pleural cavity and phagocytozed material deposited there. It was well known that cells which had phagocytozed did not respond well to chemotactic agents.

**Dr A. W. Ford-Hutchinson (UK)** had performed similar experiments comparing peripheral PMNs with peritoneal cells and he too had found decreased chemotaxis but enhanced aggregation of the inflammatory cells.

**Dr P. C. Wilkinson (UK)** said that there was a marked change in adhesiveness in cells when they moved into the peritoneum, which might account for differences in locomotion.

**Professor Keller (Switzerland)** agreed. He too had found that exudate cells moved slower than blood cells. He had the impression that there was little or no effect on chemotaxis but a considerable decrease in speed of locomotion. They had been studying the response of human neutrophils to 3 chemotactic factors; f-Met-Leu-Phe and two serum peptides, one called C5a desArg and the other CAC161. All factors produced increased accumulation on the lower side of the filter, but f-Met-Leu-Phe was significantly less active than the other two. The synthetic peptides produced a dose-dependent decrease in the rate of locomotion and a dose-dependent increase in the cell adhesion to glass. In contrast, the serum peptides neither decreased the rate of locomotion nor changed adhesion to the surface. Thus, there existed factors which had chemotactic effects without having effects on adhesion, whereas f-Met-Leu-Phe increased adhesion and decreased locomotion. The effect of locomotion was detectable at $10^{-8}$ mol/l and complete immobilization was produced at $10^{-5}$ mol/l.

**Dr Wilkinson** noted that Professor Keller had used protein-coated glass. He had found a dose-dependent change with f-Met-Leu-Phe in that at $10^{-9}$ mol/l the maximally active chemotactic concentration, there was a reduction in adhesion when compared to control but at $10^{-6}$ mol/l adhesiveness to protein-coated glass was higher than the control. In addition, he found a reduction of adhesion at 10 min followed by an increase at 60 min. Thus, the adhesiveness changed with time. Cell adhesiveness to substrata was an extremely complicated phenomenon which depended not only on the substratum but also on changes in the cell's physiology.

**Professor Keller** agreed that the environment influenced chemokinesis and adhesion and that one could not make absolute statements. Nonetheless, it had proved possible to dissociate the two phenomena.

**Dr Skidmore** asked what was the relationship between the movement of cells in the gradient of the chemotactic agent and adhesion of the cells to an artificial surface. He also wondered what was the relationship of either of these events to the adherence of a leukocyte in the blood to the endothelial wall.

**Dr Wilkinson** said he felt that these were three different phenomena. Measuring cell adhesion to an artificial substratum was quite different from measuring adherence of cells to the endothelium. It was important to start using physiological substrata like endothelium *in vitro*.

**Dr B. Dammerau (Germany)** was invited to describe his findings from a comparable analysis of five chemotactic peptides. He had compared the effects of two complement derived chemotactic peptides and three synthetic formyl methionyl peptides. He had found that the dose–response relations in both chemotaxis and in aggregation of isolated peripheral human leukocytes were almost identical for all five substances. From these results they concluded that there must be a strong correlation in the mechanism of both of these actions. In addition, they found that *p*-chloromercurobenzoate only slightly inhibited aggregation and had only a minor effect on random migration of leucocytes whereas *N*-ethylmaleimide induced a dose-dependent total inhibition of chemotaxis aggregation and random migration.

**Dr Ford-Hutchinson** said that these results demonstrated that aggregation was an adhesion phenomenon since it represented adhesion of PMNs to each other. A similar phenomenon occurred *in vivo* where intravenous injection of chemotactic substances produced margination of the neutrophils throughout the vasculature.

**Dr Wilkinson** did not entirely agree. The temporal sequence of the two events were similar but it was premature to suggest that neutrophil to neutrophil adhesion was related to adhesion of neutrophils to endothelial cells. Workers in Connecticut could not obtain a change in adhesion of neutrophils to the endothelium at times when they had aggregation of neutrophils to each other.

**Dr Skidmore** said that there was also evidence that when neutrophils stuck to the vascular endothelial surface as a result of an inflammatory reaction the change took place primarily in the vascular endothelium and not in the neutrophil.

**Dr J. P. Abita (France)** was invited to review his work on loss of chemotactic response in neutrophils. He said that neutrophils pre-incubated with a chemoattractant, then washed, lose their ability to respond chemotactically to it. This phenomenon was called chemotactic deactivation. He investigated whether this absence of a response could be correlated with the loss of binding sites for chemo-attractants. Neutrophils were pre-incubated at 37 °C with different concentrations of f-Met-Leu-Phe and after washing they were assayed for chemotaxis and for binding to tritiated f-Met-Leu-Phe. There was a time- and dose-dependent decrease in chemotactic responsiveness of the neutrophil but the decrease was not accompanied by a loss of binding sites for the peptide. The figure of 40 000 binding sites per cell remained constant. Thus chemotactic deactivation necessitated a step beyond the binding of a peptide to its membrane receptor on the neutrophil.

**Dr Wilkinson** said that they could not deactivate neutrophils with f-Met-Leu-Phe in bivalent cation depleted media. In their hands it seemed to be a calcium dependent phenomenon.

**Dr J. H. Wissler (Germany)** was invited to describe his work on leukocyte membranes. He said that they had studied the effect of serum proteins on the membranes of viable leukocytes by direct measurement of the intensity of polarization of fluorescence emitted by introduced markers. Human serum albumin interacted with the lipid layer of the leukocyte to protect it from exposure to the aqueous solution of the cellular environment. This was a feature of chemokinetic solutes. Chemotactic solutes, in contrast, did not interact with distinct pre-formed receptors but several mobile protein units were asociated by the anaphalatoxin molecule and thus a receptive unit was formed during the recognition process in chemotaxis.

In answer to a question, he said that the associated units were proteins although they had not as yet been isolated. The anaphalatoxin molecule interacted in a multivalent way with these proteins. He also believed that f-Met-Leu-Phe was a large enough molecule to make many multivalent interactions with proteins in the membrane. However, the interaction of f-Met-Leu-Phe seemed more complex than that with anaphalatoxin conformers. At the least, it seemed to interact in a somewhat different way with the membrane.

# Section VI
# Measurement of Human and Experimental Inflammation

CHAIRMAN: E. C. Huskisson
CO-CHAIRMAN: M. Lequesne

# 63

# Quantitative assessment of experimentally induced arthritis in guinea pigs using microfocal radiography

J. C. BUCKLAND-WRIGHT, C. H. CASHIN, N. S. DOHERTY AND B. L. JEFFRIES (UK)

## INTRODUCTION

The assessment of joint damage in experimentally induced inflammatory arthritis has always been difficult and has usually involved a combination of quantitative and qualitative methods, for example, (1) the measurement of joint diameter, (2) serial histological sections, and (3) radiography. The limitations of these methods are, first, joint diameter does not always reflect the damage in the joint; second, histology is time consuming and it is difficult to obtain an evaluation of joint damage in three dimensions; third, the resolution of the radiographs produced by clinical machines enables the alterations in arthritic joints to be described qualitatively and/or by simple mensural assessments such as scoring systems, cortical indices and densitometric analyses.

A non-destructive method is required for precise quantitative assessment of the anatomical changes in arthritis and this is provided by new developments in high definition magnification radiography. The new microfocal X-ray unit[1-3] produces high definition stereo-projection radiographs at magnifications between 1 to 100 and at a theoretical resolution equivalent to the X-ray source size of 5–10 μm. The three dimensional appearance of the structures in the joint is obtained by examining the stereo-pair radiographs under a stereoscope.

## APPLICATION 1: TIME COURSE STUDY

Microfocal radiography was used for the quantitative evaluation of the pathogenesis of a cell mediated immune arthritis in guinea pigs.

### Materials and methods

*Animals*

Thirty five male guinea pigs (Dunkin–Hartley strain) were used, of which five were controls.

*Immunisation and induction of arthritis*

Animals were immunized by the intra-articular injection of 2 mg heat killed *Mycobacterium tuberculosis* (Human strains, C, DT and PN, Central Veterinary Laboratories, Weybridge, Surrey) in a dose volume of 0.05 ml into the left knee. The *M. tuberculosis* was suspended in saline, homogenized and autoclaved before use. For the injection the guinea pigs were lightly anaesthetized with ether.

Arthritis was induced 21 days later by a challenge dose into the right knee of 0.2 mg *M. tuberculosis* in 0.05 ml of saline. Five guinea pigs were sacrificed, 3, 15, 28 and 43 days post challenge. The hind limbs were removed, skinned and fixed in 10% formal saline.

*Radiography*

Lateral and antero-posterior stereo-projection radiographs were taken of each right knee on Cronex NDT 55 (Dupont Photoproducts, UK) fine grained X-ray film at a primary magnification of X8. The X-ray unit was operated at 30 kV, 1 mA and at 18 s exposure. The stereo-pair radiographs were examined under a Sokkisha mirror stereoscope MS 27.

*Measurements*

The parameters measured are illustrated diagramatically in Figures 63.1 and 63.2. The measurements were divided into two groups:

Those related to cyst formation and erosive changes

(1) Width of intercondylar fossa (A in Figure 63.1).
(2) Total number of force bearing trabeculae in the epiphyses of the femur and tibia (the large diameter trabeculae intersecting lines B – C and D – E in Figure 63.1).

*Osteoporosis in the femoral shaft*

(1) Number of trabeculae in a cross-section of the femoral metaphysis (intersecting lines F – G in Figure 63.2).
(2) Cortical index (total femoral width (M– N) /total thickness of cortical bone (M – O) + (P – N), in Figure 63.2).

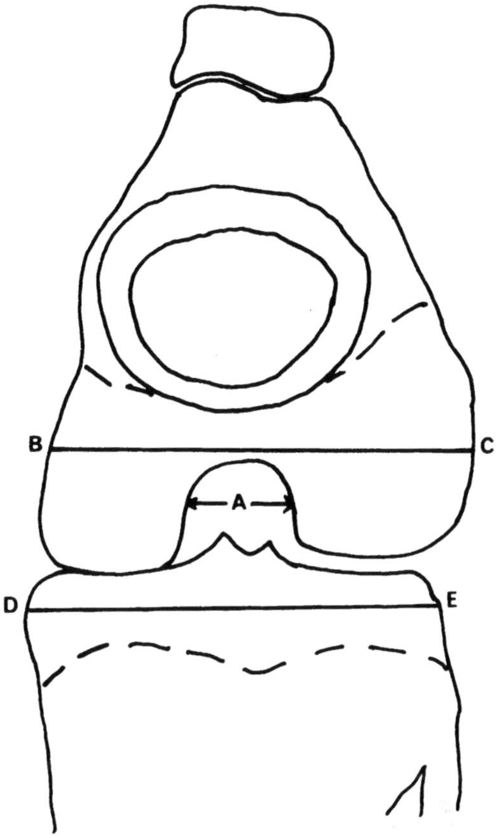


**Figure 63.1** Antero-posterior view of the guinea pig knee showing measurements used for assessing bone erosion. For explanation of figure refer to text.

## Results

*Radiographic observations*

The stereo-projection radiographs showed that the pathological changes in the experimentally induced arthritis paralleled those in human rheumatoid arthritis.

(1) The synovial membrane increased in size with the formation of numerous villi, these were particularly well developed in the popliteal region and suprapatella bursa (1 in Figure 63.3).

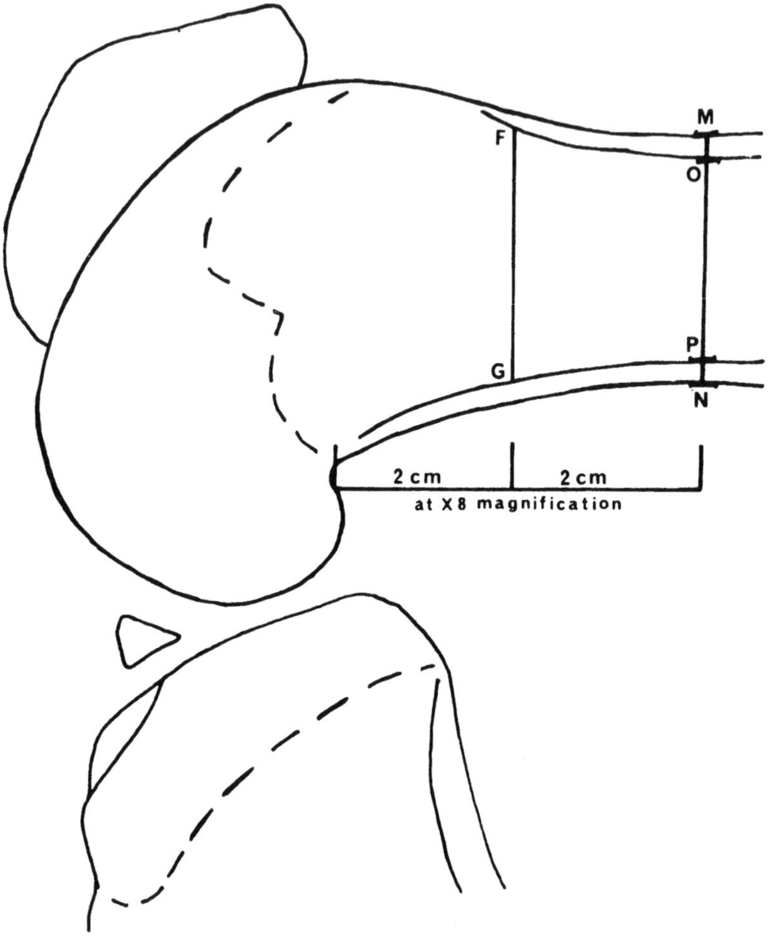


**Figure 63.2** Lateral view of the guinea pig knee showing the measurements used for assessing osteoporosis

(2) The formation of sub-periosteal erosions and cysts (2 in Figure 63.3).

(3) The formation of sub-chondral cysts in the femur and tibia (3 in Figure 63.3).

(4) The loss of bone from the epiphyseal plates in the femur and tibia (4 in Figure 63.3), this was frequently associated with the enlargement of cystic erosions.

(5) Displacement of gastrocnemius sesamoid bones (5 in Figure 63.3) due to

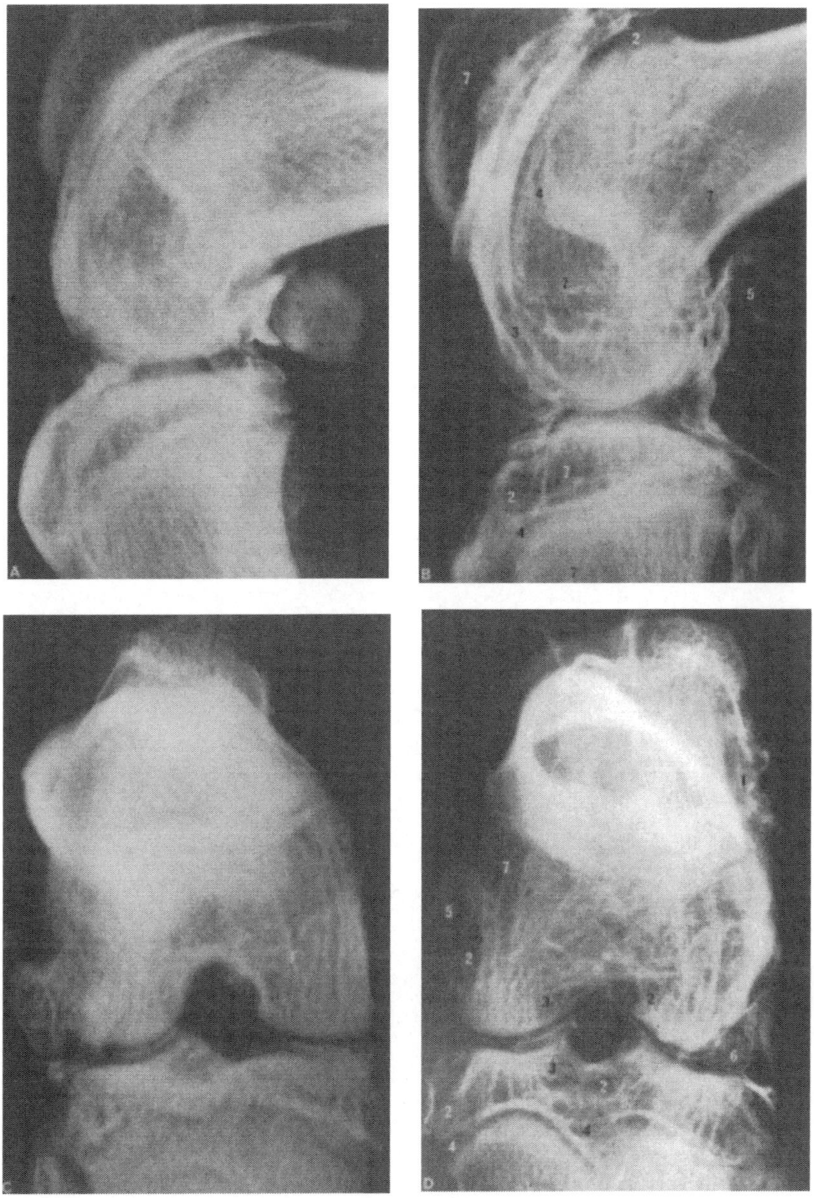

**Figure 63.3** (A) and (B) are lateral, (C) and (D) are antero-posterior microfocal radiographs of the guinea pig knee joint. (A) and (C) are normal, (B) and (D) illustrate the effects of the induced inflammatory arthritis 15 days post challenge. The joint capsule has been outlined by an intra-articular injection of contrast medium. (F) is a large force-bearing trabecula. For explanation of figure refer to text. Primary X-ray magnification × 8, reproduced × 4.5.

swelling within the joint capsule and laxity in the tendons of the gastrocnemius muscles.

(6) Displacement of the articular menisci and sub-luxation of the knee joint (6 in Figure 63.3) resulting from the inflammation of the periarticular ligaments leading to joint looseness.

(7) Osteoporosis (7 in Figure 63.3). The latter was seen as a reduction in the number of trabeculae recorded in the juxta-articular bones, including the patella, gastrocnemius sesamoid bones and in the calcified portions of the menisci.

*Measurements*

Figures 63.4 and 63.5 are graphs showing that the erosion of bone by the pannus in the juxta-articular region reached a maximum 28 days after the onset of the arthritis in the right knee. Figures 63.6 and 63.7 are graphs which illustrate that osteoporosis reached a maximum 15 days after the onset of the arthritis.

**Conclusion**

The time course study showed that the development of the lesions was gradual in the challenged knee over a period of about 28 days. As the extent of the osteoporosis reached a maximum 15 days post challenge and was measured at sites fairly remote from the joint, it suggests the release of a humoral osteoporotic factor by the inflamed tissues.

The X-ray technique measured changes in the bone which are of major importance in drug assessment, i.e. erosion and osteoporosis, which cannot be measured by conventional pharmaceutical techniques.

## APPLICATION 2: DRUG EVALUATION

**Materials and methods**

Seventy male guinea pigs (Dunkin–Hartley strain) were used in this study. Ten were kept as controls. Arthritis was induced in the remainder as described above in the time course study. The animals were divided into six groups, of which one was the arthritic control.

*Drug treatment*

Drug dosing commenced on the tenth day after sensitization and continued to the end of the experiment on the 49th day, i.e. 28 days post challenge.

The drugs administered were D-penicillamine (dista), 100mg/kg p.o.; dexamethasone (Sigma), 0.1 mg/kg i.p.; sodium aurothiomalate (May & Baker), 2 mg/kg i.m.; aspirin, 100 mg/kg p.o.; chloroquine diphosphate (Sigma), 30 mg/kg p.o.

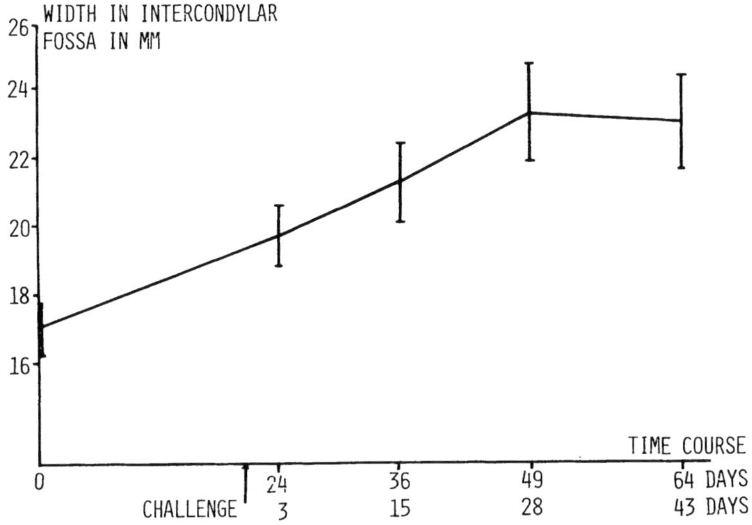


**Figure 63.4** Mean and standard deviation of the intercondylar fossa width, in the right knees during the time course study. The arrow indicates when the challenge dose was given

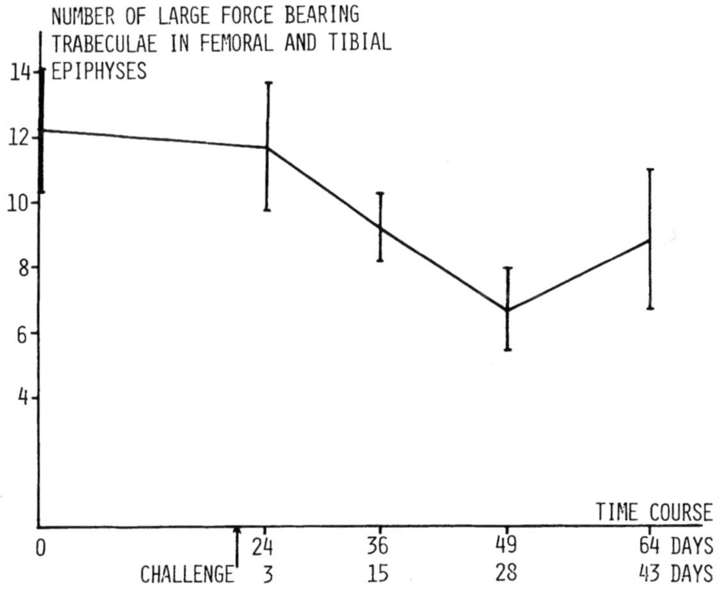


**Figure 63.5** Mean and standard deviation of the number of large force bearing trabeculae in the femoral and tibial epiphyses, in the right knees during the time course study

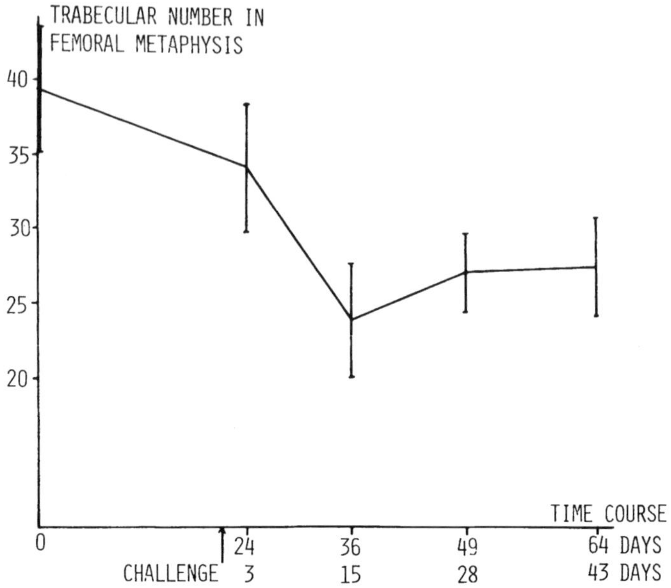


**Figure 63.6** Mean and standard deviation of the trabecular number in the femoral metaphysis, in the right knees during the time course study

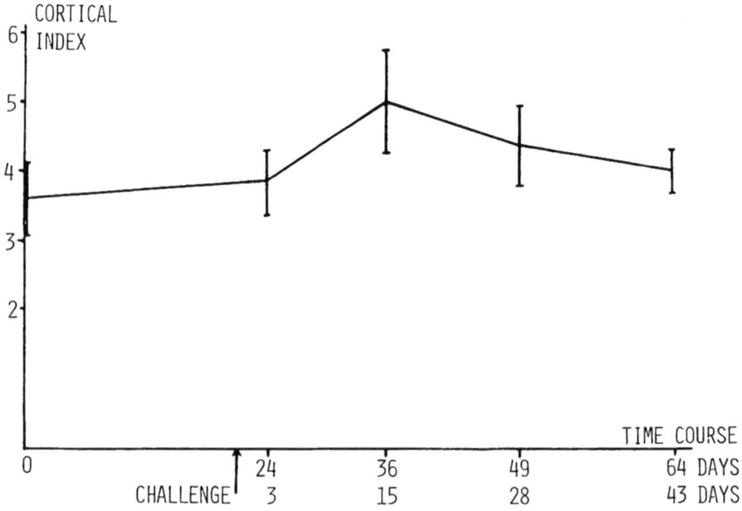


**Figure 63.7** Mean and standard deviation of the cortical index of the right knees during the time course study

*Radiography and measurements*

These were the same as described above in the time course study.

**Results**

Statistical analyses were carried out to assess the difference between the drug treated animals and the arthritic controls using non-parametric analysis by the Wilcoxon rank sum test for groups of unequal size[4]. It is immediately obvious that all radiographic parameters measured distinguished clearly between normal and arthritic knees. None of the drugs displayed a therapeutic effect. Osteoporosis was worse in the D-penicillamine group and was significantly different ($p < 0.02$) from the arthritic controls (Figure 63.8) suggesting that this drug exacerbates the condition. A not unexpected result, as several investigators have reported the enhancement of cell mediated inflammation in animals treated with this drug[5–7].

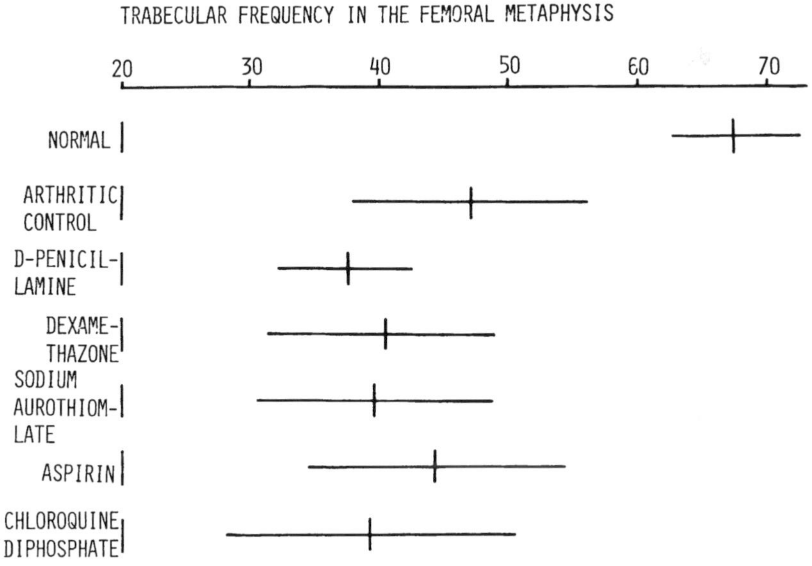


**Figure 63.8** Mean and standard deviation of the trabecular number in the femoral metaphyses, showing the levels of osteoporosis in the different drug treated groups

**Conclusion**

The failure of the anti-rheumatic drugs to be active in this model may be due to a number of factors.

(1) The arthritis induced in the knee of the guinea pigs was too severe for the

drugs to have any effect.

(2) The inflammatory arthritis may not involve those characteristics sensitive to the drug.
(3) The species may be unsuitable.
(4) The antigen may be inappropriate.
(5) The drug dosage may be incorrect.

Nevertheless, these experiments clearly demonstrate the usefulness of microfocal radiography in determining joint damage and the activity of drugs in small animals. Recently the X-ray unit had been modified to obtain magnification radiographs for examining and to quantify joint damage in patients.

## Acknowledgments

Gratitude is tended to Mr C. Hallett for assistance with the statistical evaluation, to the University of London Central Research Fund for support in purchasing the MS 27 stereoscope and to Mr K. Fitzpatrick for preparing the photographs.

## References

1 Ely, R. V. (1972). X-ray microscopy. In Weissberger, A. and Rossiter, B. W. (eds.) *Physical Methods of Chemistry*, Part IIIA, pp. 715–779. (New York: Wiley)
2 Buckland-Wright, J. C. (1976). The microfocal X-ray unit and its application to bio-medical research. *Experientia*, **32,** 1613
3 Buckland-Wright, J. C. (1977). The microfocal X-ray unit: a demonstration of its potential. *Med. Biol. Illus.*, **27,** 163
4 Wilcoxon, F. and Wilcox, R. A. (1964). *Some Rapid Approximate Statistical Procedures*. (Pearl River: Lederle Laboratories)
5 Arrigoni-Martelli, E., Bramm, E. and Binderup, L. (1977). Immunopharmacological investigations on sulphydryl compounds: Comparative study of D-penicillamine, 5-mercaptopyridoxine and 4-mercaptopropionylglycine. *Riv. Farmacol. Ter.*, **8,** 335
6 Cunningham, F. M., Ford-Hutchinson, A. W., Oliver, A. M., Smith, M. J. H. and Walker, J. R. (1978). The effects of D-penicillamine and levamisole on leucocyte chemotaxis in the rat. *Bri. J. Pharmacol.*, **63,** 119
7 Dieppe, P. A., Willoughby, D. A., Huskisson, E. C. and Arrigoni-Martelli, E. (1976). Pertussis vaccine pleurisy: a model of delayed hypersensitivity. *Agents Actions*, **6,** 618

64

# Glutathione in erythrocytes: a parameter of change in disease activity and response to drugs in rheumatoid arthritis

E. MUNTHE, E. KÅSS AND E. JELLUM (NORWAY)

## INTRODUCTION

Several thiols have been shown to have anti-rheumatic activity. Rheumatoid factor molecules are split *in vitro* by the thiol penicillamine. This was the rationale behind the use of penicillamine in the treatment of rheumatoid arthritis (RA)[1]. Later studies showed, however, that this mechanism did not operate *in vivo*, and it is still unknown how penicillamine works in RA. Other thiols and anti-oxidants, for example, the vitamin $B_6$ derivatives 5-thiopyridoxine[2] and its disulphide pyrithioxine[3], and also thiola (thiopronine or 2-mercapto-propionyl glycine)[4,5] are all found effective as slow-acting, 'second-line' anti-rheumatic drugs. The immunopotentiating drug levamisole has also an anti-oxidant effect, probably through a sulphydryl metabolite[6]. Gold salts used in the treatment of RA are usually given as thio-compounds[7]. It has also been claimed that the action of chloroquine in RA is due to interference with mercaptides[8]. No convincing relation between a known biological effect of these drugs and clinical response to them in RA has yet been demonstrated.

It has been our working hypothesis that the action of these drugs has a common mechanism involving SH-groups. For this reason, we decided to study their possible interference with naturally-occurring thiols *in vivo*. Many investigators have used the finding of decreased serum sulphydryl groups as a parameter of increased disease activity in RA[9,10]. Gold salts, penicillamine[11,12], levamisole[13] and corticosteroids[14] have been found to increase the extracellular SH-levels *in vivo*. No longitudinal studies of *intracellular* sulphydryl groups in RA have, however, been performed. Such studies should deserve interest, also in relation to the unbalanced redox state with high levels of reduced NADP which were observed in rheumatoid cells by investigators at the Kennedy Institute, London[15,16]. Therefore we examined how thio-drugs and spontaneous changes in rheumatic disease activity could interfere with the levels of intracellular, reduced glutathione (GSH), the most important intracellular source of SH, apart from protein-SH. In this paper we report an *in vivo* increase in erythrocyte GSH (E-GSH) after treatment of RA with penicillamine and other 'second-line' anti-rheumatic drugs, and a rapid, but slight, increase after intramuscular injection of corticosteroids. Spontaneous, diurnal changes of E-GSH in RA were also found.

## MATERIALS AND METHODS

### Blood sampling

Consecutive blood samples were collected by venous puncture from healthy individuals and patients with various rheumatic diseases, mostly RA (Table 64.1), for determination of reduced, free GSH in erythrocytes. Some patients were followed with regular weekly or monthly tests. Determinations were performed just before and during the use of 'second-line' anti-rheumatic drugs.

**Table 64.1** E-GSH ($\mu$mol/g) in healthy individuals and patients with rheumatic diseases

| *Diagnosis* | *Number* | *Mean* | *Range* |
|---|---|---|---|
| Healthy individuals | 10 | 1.98* | 1.64 – 2.38 |
| Rheumatoid arthritis | 163 | 2.06 | 1.41 – 3.17 |
| Juvenile chronic arthritis | 9 | 2.19 | 1.60 – 2.53 |
| Ankylosing spondylitis | 12 | 2.21 | 1.75 – 2.78 |
| Psoriatic arthritis | 3 | 2.00 | 1.75 – 2.46 |
| Secondary amyloidosis | 4 | 2.36 | 1.94 – 3.00 |
| Systemic lupus erythem. | 5 | 2.17 | 1.66 – 2.73 |
| Dermatomyositis | 3 | 2.06 | 1.86 – 2.34 |

*Based on 40 tests, 4 from each individual

In 10 RA patients who complained of morning stiffness, all anti-inflammatory and anti-rheumatic drugs were withdrawn between 12 am the day before, until 12 am on the day of sampling. Blood was taken at 7.00 am and 12.00 am. Similar samples were taken from healthy individuals who used no drugs.

In patients treated with intramuscular injection of 1–2 ml of a 'two-phase' corticosteroid (Celeston Chronodose = 3 mg betamethasone phosphate + 3 mg betamethasone acetate per ml), blood was taken sometimes 3, 2, or 1 day before, as well as always immediately prior to the injection and at regular intervals thereafter.

All samples were collected in heparinized tubes, immediately cooled to 4 °C on ice cubes and erythrocytes were isolated by centrifugation and washed with saline before being analysed for intracellular GSH within 1–2 h after sampling. Some samples were stored at −70 °C until analysed, but no longer than 4–5 days, due to some decline in GSH levels after longer storage (storage at −20 °C caused considerable degradation of GSH).

**GSH determinations**

E-GSH was determined by an enzymatic method using GSH reductase after oxidation of GSH[17]. The values obtained with this method corresponded to values obtained using an amino acid analyser. Standard samples were included in all test series. Mean value in healthy blood donors was 1.98 ± 0.5 μmol/g (Table 64.1), in accordance with the literature.

Glutathione present as mixed disulphides was determined after prior reduction with dithiothreitol (DTT). To separate between protein-bound and non-protein mixed disulphides of glutathione, the haemolysate of the erythrocytes was first gel-filtered on a Sephadex G-25 column prior to reduction.

**'Second-line' drug treatment**

D(-)penicillamine (D-PCA) was given as Cuprimine MSD capsules 250 mg according to a 'go low, go-slow' schedule starting with 250 mg daily and increasing with 250 mg every month up to a maximum of 1000 mg daily. Cysteine supplement was given as tablets of 250 mg L-cysteine in doses identical to the penicillamine dose. Treatment with this amino acid was initiated either from the first stage of D-PCA treatment or from the time when no clinical effect and no increase in GSH were observed after the use of 1000 mg penicillamine for more than one month. D-PCA and cysteine were not taken simultaneously (to avoid mixed disulphide formation).

Levamisole was given as one single weekly oral dose of 150 mg. *Gold salt* was given as weekly intramuscular injections of 50 mg auro sodium thiomalate (Myocrisin, Pharma Rhodia). Treatment with *sodium thiomalate* alone was given as one daily oral dose of 200 mg. The alkylating agent chlorambucil was given as Leukeran tablets (Wellcome) up to 0.2 (mg/kg)/day.

**Patients and measurements of disease activity**

All RA patients had definite or classical disease according to the ARA-criteria and were in anatomical stages II-III. All patients were followed with a series of clinical and laboratory parameters for disease activity, including regular counting of diseased joints, measurement of grip strength, grading of morning stiffness and pain by visual analogue scale and routine haematological, renal and liver tests etc.

## RESULTS

### Spontaneous E-GSH variations

When E-GSH in the rheumatic patients was measured before exposure to penicillamine or other 'second-line' drugs, no significant differences were found between patients with RA and other rheumatic diseases, compared to levels in 10 healthy individuals over a period of 10–14 months (Table 64.1). The spontaneous variation in E-GSH. in healthy individuals did not exceed ± 20% of the primary values, when measured in consecutive samples over 10 months (Figure 64.1). Each individual seemed to have his own range of E-GSH and there were considerable variations between individuals. Patients with little or no change in disease activity showed only minor changes in E-GSH, comparable to those seen in healthy controls. In contrast, patients with active RA had more labile levels, sometimes with rapid changes over a few days, which could be related to changes in disease activity. E-GSH tended to decrease during relapse and increase before remissions. Exceptions to this rule were only rarely observed.

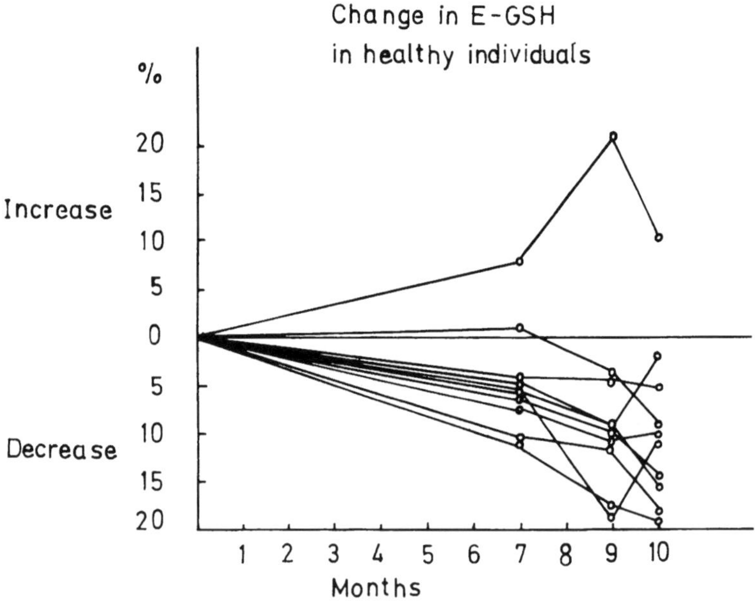


**Figure 64.1** Percent change in erythrocyte glutathion (E-GSH) over 10 months in relation to the first measured values in ten healthy individuals

In patients with pronounced morning stiffness (for example case 2 and 6 in Table 64.2), a lower E-GSH was found in the morning than in the middle of the day. This was a trend in all patients where anti-inflammatory drugs were withdrawn, but the difference was small (Table 63.2). No similar trend was seen in healthy individuals. Introduction of corticosteroids abolished the difference.

**Table 64.2** E-GSH (μmol/g) measured in 10 RA patients at 7 and 12 a.m.

| *Patient* | *1* | *2* | *3* | *4* | *5* | *6* | *7* | *8* | *9* | *10* |
|---|---|---|---|---|---|---|---|---|---|---|
| Hour | | | | | | | | | | |
| 07.00: | 1.70 | 1.39 | 1.90 | 1.43 | 1.96 | 1.84 | 1.68 | 2.27 | 2.49 | 2.55 |
| 12.00: | 1.75 | 1.56 | 1.91 | 1.56 | 1.97 | 1.97 | 1.75 | 2.31 | 2.50 | 2.57 |

## Corticosteroid-induced E-GSH variations

During the first 24 h after an intramuscular injection of betamethasone, E-GSH levels increased up to 8–13% above the pre-injection values (Figure 64.2). A decline was then usually seen already after 36–48 h. After 4–5 days, pre-injection values were again reached and sometimes even lower values were found, indicating a rebound effect.

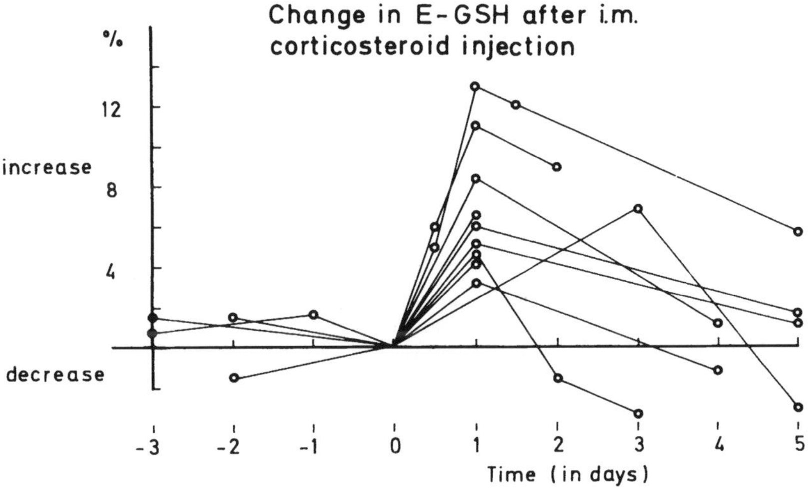


**Figure 64.2** Relative values of E-GSH before and after an intramuscular corticosteroid injection given at time 0. Values calculated as percent of the E-GSH concentration immediately before the injection

## Penicillamine-induced increase in E-GSH

Good responders to penicillamine showed a 20–35% increase in E-GSH already after 2–8 weeks of treatment. Usually this rise was seen long before any clinical effect became apparent. The clinical response to the treatment in the responders, for example G.A., L.R. and L.K. in Figure 64.3, was first seen after 1 to 4 months. Non-responders to D-PCA showed either a minor increase (5% or less) or sometimes even a decrease, particularly in cases of RA whose condition deteriorated despite the treatment (Figure 64.3). In responders, a short, initial fall could sometimes precede the increase in E-GSH. A rise to more than 20% of the pre-treatment values predicted a remission.

In patients where penicillamine treatment induced long-lasting and almost complete remission of RA (for example L.K., Figure 64.3), E-GSH showed a tendency to decline slowly towards the pre-treatment values.

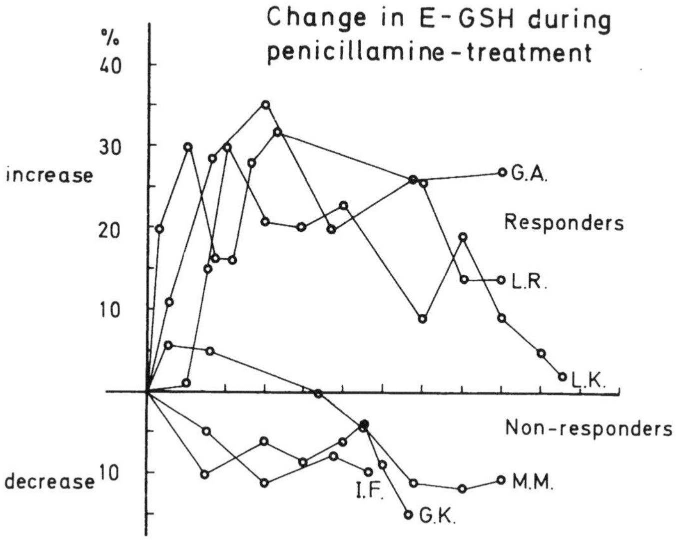


**Figure 64.3** Percent change of E-GSH in relation to the pre-treatment concentration during penicillamine treatment of three good responders (G.A., L.R. and L.K.) and three non-responders (I.F., G.K. and M.M.), all with active RA

## Cysteine supplementation to D-PCA

The addition of cysteine to the penicillamine treatment enabled us to demonstrate an increased cysteine concentration in the serum of these patients. Intracellular cysteine would rapidly be utilized for the synthesis of GSH, and we therefore studied the influence of cysteine supplement on E-GSH. In some patients with a moderate response to D-PCA, cysteine supplement could cause a further increase up to 50% higher than the pre-D-PCA values, followed by a marked clinical improvement 2–4 weeks after reaching the peak E-GSH level (Figure 64.4). In other cases, cysteine supplementation was followed by a transitory or permanent deterioration, corresponding to a decline

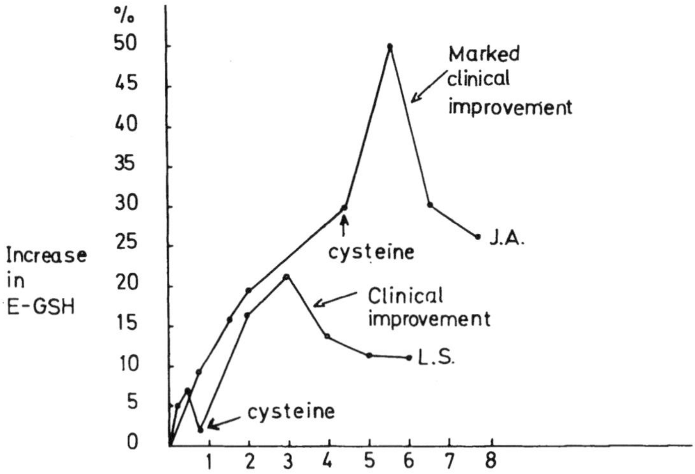


**Figure 64.4** Percent increase in E-GSH in relation to pre-penicillamine (PCA) values observed after giving cysteine in addition to PCA in two RA patients who did not respond satisfactorily to PCA alone (L.S. was a previous non-responder to PCA)

in E-GSH (Figure 64.5). Sometimes an initial decrease was followed by a marked increase in E-GSH (K.B., Figure 64.5). In two patients where cysteine was given without D-PCA, no changes in disease activity or E-GSH were observed.

**State of glutathione in RA erythrocytes**

Only about 1% of the glutathione was found to be protein-bound in RA erythrocytes. Up to approximately 10% of the total glutathione was present in the form of non-protein glutathione mixed disulphide. A minimum of about 90% of the total glutathione was therefore present in the free, reduced form. The decline in the mixed disulphide was 8–10% in cases with 30–50% increase in reduced E-GSH.

**E-GSH during other 'second-line' drugs**

Three RA patients were treated with levamisole, but only one responded clinically. Only in the responder did the E-GSH level increase more than 20% from the pre-treatment values, while the other two only had transiently increasing levels up to 15% during the first 4–6 weeks. Thereafter a decline was found.

Three seropositive RA patients were treated with Myocrisin, but none of them showed significant response to the treatment after 9 months. The increase in E-GSH was up to 10–12% of the initial value, maximum being reached after 4–6 weeks, followed by a decline in two of the patients. In the

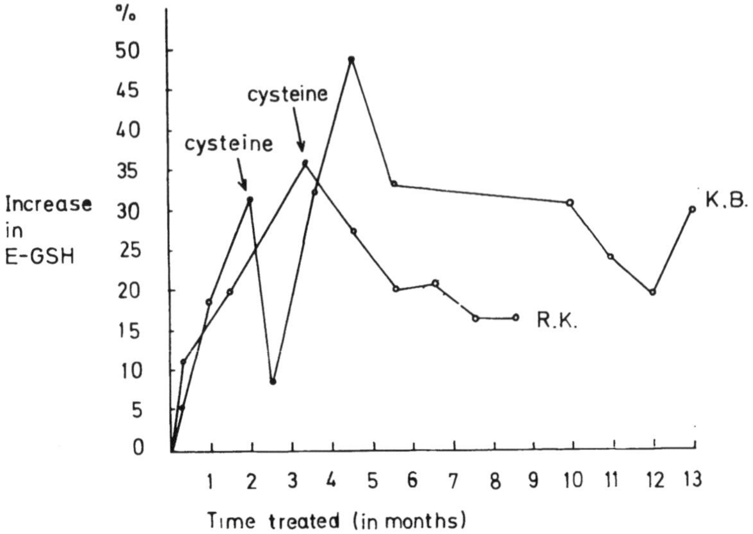


**Figure 64.5** Percent change in E-GSH in relation to pre-penicillamine values in an RA-patient with a temporary deterioration (K.B.) and in one who steadily deteriorated after cysteine (R.K.). In R.K. cysteine had to be withdrawn after 4 months

third, levels were lower than the initial values during the whole period, down to 15% lower. This patient showed a clear deterioration, and all three were later transferred to other treatment. We have not yet had the opportunity to follow E-GSH in a responder to Myocrisin.

Three patients were treated with sodium thiomalate without gold. During the first 4–6 weeks after the start of thiomalate, increasing E-GSH levels were observed in two, but not up to more than 10 to 15%. The third patient showed no increase. However, only one of the patients showed signs of deterioration, while one showed definite improvement and another modest improvement during 3–4 months of observation. None had severe disease.

One patient treated with Leukeran showed more than 20% increase already 4 weeks after start of treatment and a definite clinical improvement after 8 weeks.

## DISCUSSION

Our observations indicate that a 20–50% increase of E-GSH levels compared with the pre-treatment values predicts a remission, which usually occurs 2–6 weeks later. This reaction is, however, *not* specific for penicillamine, as was suggested in our previous reports[18,19].

A decrease in E-GSH was frequently accompanied by a deterioration, but not in all cases. Decrease was common in drug responders after some months with high values.

Decrease in reduced GSH may lead to decreased efficacy of glutathione peroxidase and a decreases detoxification mechanism. A gradual accumulation of superoxide radicals ($\cdot O_2$), hydrogen peroxide ($H_2O_2$) and possibly hydroxyl radicals ($\cdot OH$) could be the result and disastrous for the cell[20–22]. Gluthathione seems to have a direct anti-inflammatory activity. This has been demonstrated by GSH-induced inhibition of acute, experimental inflammation in animals after footpad and peritoneal injection[23]. This inhibition may be due to the ability of GSH to increase PGE/PGF ratio[24], to inhibit prostaglandin formation and to act as a scavanger of free radicals.

It is not likely that E-GSH concentrations in RA patients were low enough to account for any erythrocyte pathology. Whether a relationship exists between low E-GSH values and the slight haemolysis and reduced survival time of erythrocytes[25] in active RA, has to be studied.

The increased levels observed in drug responders were not due to increase of reticulocytes in the peripheral blood, as these cells were counted and found normal. The sometimes pronounced change of E-GSH in RA is likely to be a secondary event following alterations in other tissues, as for example in the joints. Granulomatous localized sub-dermal inflammation in the rat has been shown to depress GSH, catalase and ascorbic acid in liver cells, possibly by some kind of humoral factor released from the inflamed site[26]. A factor from the rheumatoid inflamed tissues could hypothetically interact with erythrocytes and cause a decrease of GSH.

The increase in E-GSH could in part be a direct drug action, for example by liberation of GSH from its mixed disulphides. Such mechanism could, however, not explain all of the observed increase. The increase is probably an *in vivo* phenomenon, as no changes in E-GSH were observed when D-PCA or dexamethasone were incubated with erythrocytes *in vitro*.

Two observations seem to contradict the importance of low GSH in chronic inflammation:

(1) Children and adults with congenital deficiency of glutathione synthetase[21,22] have sometimes no detectable GSH in erythrocytes and other tissues, and they have not been reported to suffer from chronic, inflammatory disease. They are, however, susceptible to recurrent infections and neutropenia which can be cured by vitamin E treatment[22].

(2) During fasting conditions, the GSH-content of the liver has been shown to decline. However, rheumatoid arthritis patients are reported to improve during periods with no food intake[27].

Chayen and co-workers found that the intracellular redox disturbance in rheumatoid synovial cells could be restored *in vitro* and *in vivo* with corticosteroids, moving the balance towards the oxidized form of NADP[16]. This could mean consumption of NADPH by increased reduction of glutathione (increased activity of the GSH reductase). A similar mechanism could explain the steroid-induced increase in E-GSH.

Although the explanation of the observed increase of E-GSH is unclear and the role of GSH in RA is not yet understood, the present studies show that determination of E-GSH might be useful for the early detection of therapeutic responses in rheumatoid arthritis.

**Acknowledgment**
The skilful technical assistance of Mrs Gro Guldal is acknowledged. This work was supported by grants from Norsk Hydro, Norske Kvinners Sanitetsforeining, Det Norske Revmatismeråd and Trondheim Revmatikerforening.

## References

1 Jaffe, I. A. (1976). Penicillamine treatment of rheumatoid arthritis – rationale, pattern of clinical response, and clinical pharmacology and toxicology. In Munthe, E. (ed.) *Penicillamine Research in Rheumatoid Disease*. (Norway: Fabritius/MSD)
2 Jaffe, I. A. and Huskisson, E. C. (1979). 5-Thiopyridoxine in rheumatoid arthritis. Abstract No. 216, W10, IXth European Congress Rheum., Wiesbaden, F.D.R. (2–8/9), 60
3 Camus, J. P., Massias, P., Chaouat, Y., Lechewallier, P.-L., Crouzet, J. and Prier, A. (1979). Pyrithioxine in rheumatoid arthritis – a pluricentric trial on 150 patients. Abstract 171. W7 IXth European Congress Rheum., Wiesbaden, F.D.R. (2–8/9), 52
4 Pasero, G., Ciompi, M. L., Barbieri, P. and Mazzoni, M. R. (1979). Thiopronine therapy in rheumatoid arthritis. Abstract 143, W7, IXth European Congress Rheum., Wiesbaden, F.D.R. (2–8/9), 47
5 Amor, B., Mery, C. and de Gery, A. (1979). Tiopronine – a new long acting drug in R.A. Abstract 170. W7 IXth European Congress Rheum., Wiesbaden, F.D.R. (2–8/9), 52
6 Sree Kumar, K., Chirigos, M. A. and Weiss, J. F. (1979). Protection of rat liver microsomes from NADPH-, ascorbate-, and X-irradiation – induced lipid peroxidation by levamisole. *Int. J. Immunopharmacol.*, **1**, 85
7 Jellum, E., Munthe, E., Guldal, G. and Aaseth, J. (1979). Gold and thiol compounds in the treatment of rheumatoid arthritis. *Scand. J. Rheumatol. Suppl.*, **28**, 28
8 Gerber, D. A. (1964). Effect of chloroquine on the sulphydryl group and the denaturation of bovine serum albumin. *Arthritis Rheum.*, **7**, 193
9 Lorber, A., Bovy, R. and Chang, C. (1971). Sulphydryl deficiency in connective tissue disorders: Correlation with disease activity and protein alternations. *Metabolism*, **20**, 446
10 Haataja, M. (1975). Evaluation of the activity of rheumatoid arthritis. A comparative study on clinical symptoms and laboratory tests with special reference to serum sulphydryl groups. *Scand. J. Rheumatol Suppl.* **4**, 7
11 Haataja, M., Nissilä, M. and Ruutsalo, Helka-Marjatta (1978). Serum sulphydryl levels in rheumatoid patients treated with gold thiomalate and penicillamine. *Scand. J. Rheumatol.*, **7**, 212
12 Pavelka, K., Susta, A. and Sobeslavsky, C. (1971). A contribution to the mechanism of action of D-penicillamine in the treatments of rheumatoid arthritis. Müller, W., Harwerth, H.-G. and Fehr, K. (ed.) *Rheum. Arthritis*, p. 665. (Basle: Colloquia Geigy)
13 Hall, N. D. and Gillan, A. H. (1979). Effects of antirheumatic drugs on protein sulphydryl reactivity of human serum. *J. Pharm. Pharmacol.*, **31**, 676
14 Larsen, B. and Bent-Hansen, K. (1957). Changes in serum sulphydryl and serum glycoprotein in rheumatoid arthritis during treatment with adrenocortical steroids. *Scand. J. Clin. Lab. Invest.*, **9**, 89

15 Chayen, J., Bitensky, L., Butcher, R. G. and Poulter, L. W. (1969). Redox control of lysosomes in human synovia. *Nature* (London), **222,** 281

16 Chayen, J., Bitensky, L., Butcher, R. G. and Cashman, B. (1973). The effect of experimentally induced redox changes on human rheumatoid and non-rheumatoid synovial tissue *in vitro*. *Beitr. Path.*, **149,** 127

17 Tietze, S. (1969). Enzymatic method for quantitative determination of nanogram amounts of total unoxidized glutathione: application to mammalian blood and other tissues. *Analyt. Biochem.*, **27,** 502

18 Munthe, E., Guldal, G. and Jellum, E. (1979). Effect of slow-acting antirheumatic drugs on the intracellular glutathione level in rheumatoid arthritis. Abstract 178, W7, IXth European Congress Rheum., Wiesbaden, F.D.R. (2–8/9), 53

19 Munthe, E., Guldal, G. and Jellum, E. (1979). Increased intracellular glutathione during penicillamine treatment for rheumatic arthritis. *Lancet*, **2,** 1126

20 Christophersen, B. O. (1968). The inhibitory effect of reduced glutathione on the lipid peroxidation of the microsomal fraction and mitochondria. *Biochem. J.*, **106,** 515

21 Marstein, S., Jellum, E., Halpern, B., Eldjarn, L. and Petty, T. L. (1976). Biochemical studies of erythrocytes in a patient with pyroglutamic acidemia (5-oxoprolinemia). *New Engl. J. Med.*, **295,** 406

22 Boxer, L. A., Oliver, J. M., Spielberg, S. P., Allen, J. M. and Schulman, J. D. (1979). Protection of granulocytes by vitamin E in glutathione synthetase deficiency. *New Engl. J. Med.*, **301,** 901

23 Torrielli, M. V., Franzone, J. and Natale, T. (1980). Interference of antioxidants with prostaglandin biosynthesis. This volume, Chap. 46

24 Lands, W., Lee, R. and Smith, W. (1971). Factors regulating the biosynthesis of various prostaglandins. In Ramwell, P. and Shaw. J. (eds.) *Prostaglandins. Ann. N.Y. Acad. Sci.*, **180,** 107

25 Mowat, A. G. (1971). Hematologic abnormalities in rheumatoid arthritis. *Semi. Arthritis Rheum.*, **1,** 195

26 Bragt, P. C., Bransberg, J. I. and Bonta, I. L. (1979). Depletion of hepatic antioxidants during granulomatous inflammation in the rat and local anti-inflammatory effects of free radical scavengers. *Agents Actions Suppl.* (In press)

27 Sköldstam, L., Larsson, L. and Lindström, F. D. (1979). Effects of fasting and lacto-vegetarian diet on rheumatoid arthritis. *Scand. J. Rheumatol.*, **8,** 249

# 65

# Effect of drugs on serum copper and its correlation with other humoral factors in rheumatoid arthritis

M. CUTOLO, S. ROVIDA, E. SAMANTA AND S. ACCARDO
(ITALY)

## INTRODUCTION

It was decided to study serum copper levels (sCu) in patients with rheumatoid arthritis (RA) in the light of accumulating experience of an abnormal copper metabolism in rheumatoid arthritis as well as other diseases 4, 8, 11, 12, 18, 20, 24.

The effect on serum copper levels by non-steroid anti-inflammatory drugs (NSAID) alone and associated with D-penicillamine (DPA) during the treatment of RA was evaluated; moreover observed changes were correlated with other bio-humoral signs such as erythrocyte sedimentation rate (ESR), C reactive protein (CRP), rheumatoid arthritis factor title (RF) and haemoglobin concentration (Hbc).

## SUBJECTS

A healthy control group (*n* 44; mean age 51.20 ± 2SD 18.5 years) and an RA patient group with 'classical' or 'definite' form selected by ARA (American Rheumatism Association) criteria (*n* = 66; mean age 52 ± 22.2 years; 44 females and 22 males) were evaluated.

Sixty-six patients were divided into three groups as follows:

Group A ($n = 20$; mean age; 53.41 ± 22.6 years) consisted of RA patients not yet treated with non-steroid anti-inflammatory drugs (NSAID) and/or long acting anti-rheumatic drugs.

Group B ($n = 30$; mean age 52.41 ± 22.4 years) was constituted by RA patients in NSAID treatment only (aspirin, indomethacin, phenylbutazone and derivatives, arilalcanoic derivatives) from 4 to 8 months.

Group C ($n = 16$; mean age 54.63 ± 24.2 years) was formed by RA patients treated with NSAID plus d-penicillamine (DPA 400–900 mg/dl daily) from 6 to 10 months.

None of the women in these groups was taking oral contraceptives[25] nor were other diseases alterating serum copper levels present[20] (see Table 65.1).

**Table 65.1** Subjects examined and their type of treatment

| | *n* | *mean age± 2SD* | *Treatment* | *Term* (months) |
|---|---|---|---|---|
| Healthy control group | 44 | 51.20±18.5 | none | — |
| RA group A | 20 | 53.41±24.6 | untreated | — |
| RA group B | 30 | 52.41±22.4 | NSAID* | 4/8 |
| RA group C | 16 | 54.63±24.2 | NSAID** + DPA | 6/10 |

* aspirin, indomethacin, phenilbutazone and derivatives, arilalcanoic derivatives
**D-penicillamine= 400–900 mg daily.

## METHODS

Sera samples were all collected in early morning. Copper (sCu) was measured by a colorimetric method (test-combination Boehringer): top sera after deproteinization were treated with specific chromogen (bathocuproin) then from the optical density (OD) the concentration copper in the sample was calculated. Erythrocyte sedimentation rate (ESR) was evaluated by Westergrens's method.

C reactive protein (CRP) was evaluated by latex test (Sclavo): the title was expressed by the highest dilution capable of producing agglutination. The RA factor (RF) was determined by latex test (Sclavo) and the title was expressed as for the CRP. Haemoglobin concentration (Hbc) (Sclavo) was evaluated by a colorimetric method.

## RESULTS

### Serum copper levels

Serum copper level found in the healthy control group was of 157.36±2SE μg/dl (24.7 ± 2 μmol/l), slightly higher than the one showed by the literature previously examined[20,18]. Serum copper in group A (untreated) and group B (treated with NSAID) was raised, while it was decreased in group C (treated with NSAID plus DPA). The altered serum copper levels found in the three groups of RA patients are summarised in Table 65.2.

**Table 65.2** Copper levels in serum from healthy control group and from three groups of RA patients

| | *n* | *sCu* (μg/dl±SE) |
|---|---|---|
| Healthy control group | 44 | 157.36±13 |
| RA group A (untreated) | 20 | 294.44±26.10 |
| RA group B (NSAID) | 30 | 200.82±26.22 |
| RA group C (NSAID+DPA) | 16 | 129.13±16.22 |

Conversion: traditional units to SI.
Copper, 6.37 μg/dl = 1 μmol/l.

The analysis of variance between all tested groups pointed out a strongly significant difference ($p < 0.001$).

**Correlation between copper and other humoral factors in RA**

The correlation between serum copper and C reactive protein (CRP) showed a positive significance ($p < 0.01$) in group A (untreated) and group B (NSAID) (see Table 65.3)

**Table 65.3** The relationship of sCu to erythrocyte sedimentation rate (ESR), C reactive protein (CRP), rheumatoid factor title (RF) and haemoglobin concentration (Hbe)

| | | *sCu/ESR* | *sCu/CRP* | *sCu/RF* | *sCu/Hbc* |
|---|---|---|---|---|---|
| RA group A (untreated) | 20 | $r$=0.34<br>NS | $r$=0.55<br>$p$ <0.01 | $r$=0.19<br>NS | $r$=−0.43<br>$p$ <0.05 |
| RA group B (NSAID) | 30 | $r$=0.37<br>NS | $r$=0.54<br>$p$ <0.01 | $r$=0.14<br>NS | $r$=0.29<br>NS |
| RA group C (NSAID+DPA) | 16 | $r$=0.31<br>NS | $r$=0.17<br>NS | $r$=0.08<br>NS | $r$=0.4<br>Ns |

NS= not significant

In group C (NSAID plus DPA) this relationship was not significant probably because D-penicillamine is able to further decrease the metal level by its well-known potent activity of copper chelator[14–16,24]. None of the tested groups (A,B or C) showed a significant correlation between copper and erythrocyte sedimentation rate (ESR). No one significant correlation was found in all three groups between serum copper and the rheumatoid factor title (RF).

A significant inverse correlation ($p< 0.05$) between serum copper and haemoglobin concentration (Hbc) was noted in group A, which comprised untreated rheumatoid patients.

## DISCUSSION

As is well known, serum copper under normal conditions is bound by 80/90% to ceruloplasmin; the remnant is bound loosely to albumin and firmly to low molecular weight plasma proteins[7,26]. Copper, in fact, is an essential trace element that is a constituent, as substratum co-factor of certain metalloenzymes engaged in biological reduction–oxidation (redox) processes. Copper is a constituent of cythocrome oxidase, ascorbic acid oxidase, superoxide dismutase, lysyl oxidase, ceruloplasmin or ferro oxidase[28], monoamino oxidase, etc.

As previously mentioned, raised copper levels shown in RA patients were also found during various pathological conditions[9,13,18,20]. Apart from hepatic disorders in which cholestasis is a prominent feature and the failure of biliary excretion of copper causes hepatic accumulation and raised serum levels[22,24] hypercupraemia is usually observed during acute and chronic infections, thyrotoxicosis, various lymphomas, particularly Hodgkin's disease, collagen diseases including SLE, acute rheumatic fever and also in pregnancy[4,8,9,11–13,20,25].

During the pathologic conditions mentioned above, when the biological redox reactions are increased, presumably the engaged copper-containing enzymes are also over-active. It may be that the rise of serum copper, indispensable co-factor as catalyst for the oxidase activity, occurs as a positive feedback to make the metal more available to the body. It was observed that the treatment of RA patients with NSAID, resulting in a decrease of the inflammatory condition and obviously of the related enzymatic activities, is capable of lowering serum copper concentration. It is suggested that the effect of anti-inflammatory and anti-rheumatic drugs on serum copper and the correlation show between sCu and CRP, the most sensitive acute phase protein on inflammation[19,26], could be made useful to test serum copper levels during RA as a further datum for monitoring the course of the disease[1,3].

As far as it is concerned, the non-significant correlation between sCu and ESR may be understood because the ESR depends on many factors, some of them independent of the inflammatory response; moreover NSAID and long-acting anti-rheumatic drugs (gold, levamisole, d-penicillamine) held greater and stronger effect on serum CRP and sCu than ESR[26]. The significant inverse correlation ($p<0.05$) found between sCu and Hbc was previously shown by other researchers testing sCu and serum iron[2,18] during RA and various disorders broadly categorized as inflammatory processes, including infections and malignancy[25]

In fact, since hyposideraemia is present during these diseases, the ceruloplasmin concentration (copper containing enzyme-protein) and obviously sCU are increased owing to their function as ferro-oxidase enzyme during the conversion of iron from its ferrous state to the ferric form, aiding in the gastroenteric absorption and in the mobilization of iron from storage sites[6,17,25]

## References


1 Amos, R. S., Crockson, R. A., Crockson, A. P., Walsch, L. and McConkey, B., (1978). Rheumatoid arthritis: C-reactive protein and erythrocyte sedimentation rate during initial treatment. *Br. Med. J.*, **1**, 1936

2 Brown, D. H., Buchan, W. W., El-Gobary, A. F., Smith, W. E. and Teape, J. (1979). Serum copper and its relationship to clinical symptoms in R.A. *Ann. Rheum. Dis.*, **38**, 174

3 Constable, T. J., Crockson, R. A., Crockson, A. P. and McConkey, B. (1975). *Lancet*, **1**, 1176

4 Dresch, C., Nayean, Y., Bouchet, J. and Bernard, J. (1972). Anomalies hematologiques des polyarthrites chroniques evolutives. *Nouv. Presse Med.* **1**, 163

5 Fridovich, I. (1970). Superoxide dismutase. *Ann. Rev. Biochem.*, **44**, 147

6 Frieden, E. (1973). The ferrous to ferric cycles in iron metabolism. *Nutr. Rev.* **31**, 41

7 Harper, H. A. (1977). Review of Physiologic Chemistry. (Los Altos Cal. Medical Publications)

8 Hyrgovic, M., Tessmer, C. F., Thomas, E. B., Fuller, L. M., Gamble, J. F. and Shullermberger, C. C. (1974). Significance of serum copper levels in adult patient with Hodgkin's disease. *Scand. J. Haematol.* **1**, 63

9 Jayson, M. I. V., Davies, P., Whicher, J. T. and Walkers, G. (1976). Serum copper and caeruloplasmin in ankylosing spondylitis, systemic sclerosis and morphea. *Ann. Rheum. Dis.*, **35**, 443

10 Aeseth, J., Munthe, A., Farre, Ø. and Steinnes E. (1978). Trace elements in serum and urine of patients with rheumatoid arthritis. *Scand. J. Rheumatol.*, **7**, 237

11 Jensen, K. B., Thorling, E. B. and Anderson, C. J. (1964). Serum copper in Hodgkin's diseases. *Scand. J. Haematol.* **1**, 63

12 Kolaric, K., Roguljic, A. and Fuss, V. (1975). Serum copper levels in patients with solid tumors. *Tumori*, **61**, 173

13 Koskelo, P., Kekki, M., Virkkunem, M., Lasus, A. and Somer, T. (1969). Serum caeruloplasmin concentration in RA, ankylosing spondylitis, psoriasis and sarcoidosis. *Acta Rheum. Scand.* **12**, 261

14 Marcel, E. Nimni (1979). Penicillamine and collagen metabolism. *Scand. J. Rheumatol. Suppl.*, **28**, 71

15 Munthe, E., Jellum, E. and Aeseth, J. (1979). Some aspects of the mechanism of action of Penicillamine in RA. *Scand. J. Rheumatol.* **128**, 6

16 Munthe, E. (1976). *Penicillamine Research and Rheumatoid Diseases, p. 198 (Oslo: Fabritius & Sønner)*

17 Osaki, S., Johnson, D. A. and Frieden, E. (1966). The possible significance of the ferrous oxidase activity of caeruloplasmin in normal human serum. *J. Biol. Chem.* **241**, 2746

18 Scudder. P. R., Al-Timini, D., McMurray, W., White, A. G., Zoob, B. C., and Dormandy, T. L. (1978). Serum copper and related variables in Rheumatoid Arthritis. *Ann. Rheum. Dis.* **37**, 67

19 Scudder, P. R. McMurray, W., White, A. G. and Dormandy, T. L. (1978). Synovial fluid copper and related variables in rheumatoid and degenerative arthritis. *Ann. Rheum. Dis.* **37**, 71

20 Sinha, S. N. and Gabrieli, E. R. (1970). Serum copper and zinc levels in various pathologic conditions. *Am. J. Clin. Pathol.* **54**, 570

21 Sorenson, J. R. J. (1976). *J. Med. Chem.* **19**, 135

22 Smallwood, R. A., Williams, H. A. Rosenoer, V. M. and Sherlock, K. S.: *Lancet*, 1203

23 Sternlich, I., Sandson, J. I., Morell, A. G., Korotkin, E. and Sheinberg, I. (1978). Non-caeruloplasmin copper in RA. *Arthritis Rheum.* **12**, 458

24 Tanner, H. S. *et al.* (1979). Increased hepatic copper concentration in Indian Childhood Cirrhosis. *Lancet*, 1203

25 Todd, Sanford, Davidsohn (1979). Clinical diagnosis and management by laboratory methods, 298

26 Walsh, H. A., Davies, P. and McConkey, B. (1979). Relationship between ESR and CRP in RA. *Ann. Rheum. Dis.* **38,** 362

27 Williams, D. R. (1971). *The metals of life: the solution chemistry of metal ions in biological systems*. London VNR

28 Oriente, P., Scarpa, R., Cutolo, M., Riccio, A. and Pucino, A. (1980). Serum copper and $d_2$-ceruloplasmin as further index of inflammation. *International Symposium on Rheumatoid Arthritis*, Verona. Abstract 15

# 66

# The effect of therapeutic agents on serum copper levels and serum oxidase activities in the rat adjuvant model compared to analogous results from studies of rheumatoid arthritis in humans

W. E. SMITH, D. H. BROWN, J. DUNLOP, R. HAZELTON, R. D. STURROCK AND A. J. LEWIS (UK)

## INTRODUCTION

Among the many biochemical changes observed in rheumatoid arthritis and other inflammatory disorders has been a pronounced elevation in serum copper[1–3]. A similar rise in serum copper has also been observed in the adjuvant arthritic rat[4–7]. Since ceruloplasmin is the major copper-carrying protein in serum, it seemed likely that there should be a relationship between total serum copper and ceruloplasmin in the diseased and normal states. Recent studies would support this[8,9], but there are also claims that non-ceruloplasmin copper may be the major source of additional copper in rheumatoid arthritis[3,10]. Furthermore, in studies of cancer in animals, the ratio of the amount to the activity of ceruloplasmin, the main oxidase in serum, varies with the severity of the disease[11]. We decided to investigate the copper–ceruloplasmin relationship in adjuvant arthritis in the rat and to relate this to copper levels in patients with rheumatoid arthritis and normal human controls. These studies were intended to give some insight into the activity of serum copper as well as the amount of the copper and consequently the relationship of these parameters to drug therapies was also studied.

## METHODS

Adjuvant arthritis was induced in male Wistar rats (160–180 g) using 0.05 ml *Mycobacterum butyricium* (10 mg/ml) in liquid paraffin injected into the left hind paw. Control rats received an equal volume of sterile saline solution. Drugs or drug vehicle (5% mulgofen GAF international) were daily administered orally to groups of 8 animals from the day of adjuvant injection (day 0) until day 20. Groups of 8 animals were treated with either aspirin (BDH Ltd.), auranofin (S, K and F D-39162 Smith, Kline & French Ltd.), indomethacin (Merck) D-penicillamine (Aldrich) or prednisolone (Diosynth BV) at a dose of 10–20 mg compound /kg in each case.

Samples from patients undergoing treatment for rheumatoid arthritis were from patients who had been receiving the drugs indicated for at least 2 to 3 weeks. For the second line drugs myocrisin, penicillamine, levamisole and prednisolone, an anti-inflammatory or analgesic preparation was also administered. Controls were of as wide an age distribution as could be obtained. Female subjects using oral contraceptive pills, which are known to change serum copper levels substantially, were excluded from the study.

Analysis for ceruloplasmin oxidase activity[12] using *p*-phenylene diamine and for total serum copper[13] and ultrafilterable copper[13] by atomic absorption spectrometry was by published methods. All serum samples were separated immediately after sampling and cooled to 4 °C. Analyses were carried out as soon as possible thereafter and within 24 h of sampling. Ceruloplasmin concentration was also determined in one study using Hoescht M. Partigen immunodiffusion plates and Hoescht antisera.

## RESULTS

A plot of the ratio of total serum copper to ceruloplasmin oxidase activity against total serum copper for non-arthritic control rats ($n = 47$) and control rats ($n = 44$) indicated that markedly different zones were obtained in the two cases. In Figure 66.1, 50% and 90% contour lines are indicated in both cases. These correspond to 45% and 82%, respectively, of the points plotted falling with the ellipses.

In drug-treated animals ($n = 12$), indomethacin (I) and auranofin (Au) appreciably affected the copper level and activity and produced a change towards the normal. Aspirin (As), penicillamine (Pe) and prednisolone (Pr) gave no significant effect. These results do not correlate completely with measurements of hind-paw swellings[14] in which indomethacin and predni-

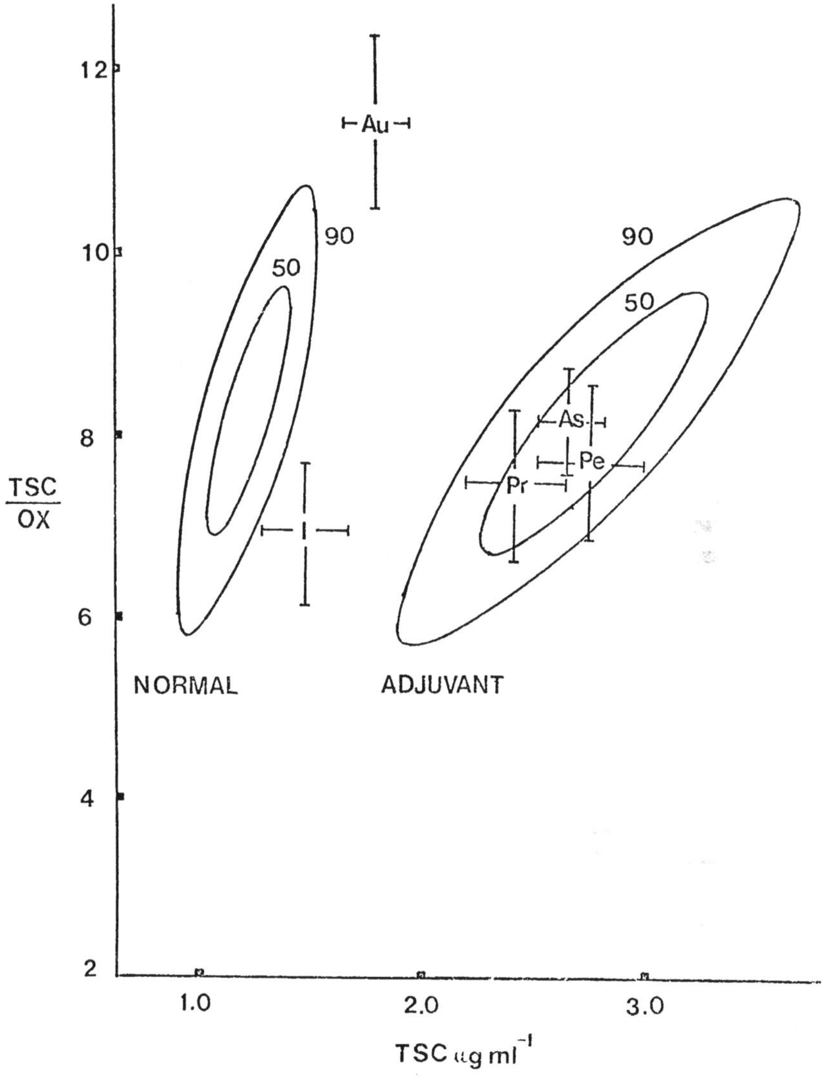


**Figure 66.1** Plot of the ratio of total serum copper level (TSC) to ceruloplasmin oxidase activity (OX) against total serum copper level, indicating the effect of adjuvant arthritis and of therapeutic agents. For details see text

solone were the most effective agents.

A study of 233 patients with rheumatoid arthritis and 39 normals (36 male, 3 female) demonstrated that both total serum copper and ceruloplasmin levels were raised in rheumatoid arthritis (Table 66.1). There was a correlation between these parameters for each drug group investigated but correlation coefficients were highest for normals and for patients whose treatment had not commenced. There were differences in mean values between each drug group, in agreement with previous studies[8,9], but the differences are rather smaller and the standard deviations are too high to enable a more precise analysis of the data. However, it would appear that drug therapy does have some effect on copper and ceruloplasmin levels.

**Table 66.1** Correlation between total serum copper and ceruloplasmin oxidase activity

| *Group* | *n* | *TS Cu mean ± SD (μg/ml)* | *CP Oxid. (Optical density) Mean ± SD* | *Correlation coefficient* |
|---|---|---|---|---|
| Normal Control | 30 | 0.95 ± 0.21 | 0.174 ± 0.038 | 0.820 |
| No treatment | 15 | 1.60 ± 0.45 | 0.252 ± 0.056 | 0.945 |
| Anti-inflammatories analgesics | 82 | 1.60 ± 0.32 | 0.268 ± 0.043 | 0.659 |
| Indomethacin | 14 | 1.74 ± 0.39 | 0.276 ± 0.063 | 0.706 |
| Myocrisin | 16 | 1.56 ± 0.32 | 0.261 ± 0.052 | 0.769 |
| Prednisolone | 28 | 1.49 ± 0.36 | 0.242 ± 0.054 | 0.710 |
| Penicillamine | 34 | 1.52 ± 0.34 | 0.258 ± 0.056 | 0.702 |
| Levamisole | 44 | 1.46 ± 0.34 | 0.252 ± 0.047 | 0.704 |
| All rheumatoids | 233 | 1.58 ± 0.37 | 0.261 ± 0.051 | 0.714 |

In all groups a significant correlation is obtained ($p < 0.001$)

In a separate study of 134 patients with rheumatoid arthritis and 49 normals (21 male and 28 female), ceruloplasmin concentrations measured by immune diffusion and ultrafilterable copper levels were also determined (see Table 66.2). It is clear that ceruloplasmin concentration as well as activity is raised in rheumatoid arthritis. A lower fraction of serum copper is present as ceruloplasmin in patients with high total serum copper levels and the activity per microgram of copper is also reduced. There may also be a difference between activity and concentration in patients with rheumatoid arthritis with different serum copper levels, but the spread of the results is too wide to enable a reliable conclusion to be drawn.

## DISCUSSION

Ceruloplasmin, as well as being an acute inflammatory indicator, is also a major oxidase in serum and the elevated levels observed in patients with rheumatoid arthritis, coupled with the length of time for which the rise is sustained, suggest that other biochemical processes may be affected. Although little is known about the action of ceruloplasmin, other parameters which also describe or reflect the state of oxidation of serum and synovial tissues are also abnormal in patients with rheumatoid arthritis. For example,

**Table 66.2** Concentrations, distribution and activity of copper-containing species in the serum of patients with rheumatoid arthritis compared to controls

| | Copper level | *TS Cu* (μg Cu/ml) *mean ± SD* | *CP Oxid: Optical density* *mean ± SD* | *CP concentration* (μg protein/ ml) *mean ± SD* | *Ultrafilterable Copper* (μg Cu/ml) |
|---|---|---|---|---|---|
| Normal | | 0.91 ±0.15 | 0.192 ±0.034 | 31.7 ±6.4 | 0.07 ±0.03 |
| Rheumatoid arthritis | 1.40 | 1.27 ±0.07 | 0.274 ±0.030 | 43.2 ±6.7 | 0.06 ±0.03 |
| | 1.40–1.80 | 1.64 ±0.13 | 0.305 ±0.034 | 51.4 ±6.1 | 0.09 ±0.05 |
| | >1.80 | 2.04 ±0.38 | 0.302 ±0.042 | 53.9 ±7.3 | 0.13 ±0.10 |

free thiol levels are consistently lower than levels found in controls[15] and rheumatoid factor is a polymerized globulin containing reducible disulphide bonds. If this tendency to have fewer thiol groups extends to the surface of circulating white cells, vital enzyme-production rates and transport functions will be affected. Furthermore, many patients with rheumatoid arthritis suffer from anaemia, which is probably not due to faulty absorption, but to an iron overload in the iron storage protein ferritin present in synovial tissue[16,20]. Release of iron present as iron III from ferritin is believed to involve a reduction process. Thus, although the exact function of ceruloplasmin as an enzyme is in some doubt, there is reason to believe that it may play some role in the aetiology of rheumatoid arthritis.

The amount of copper contained in ceruloplasmin has been disputed but it is now generally believed to contain 6 or 8 copper atoms per molecule[17], all of which are tightly bound. It may also be able to absorb extra, more loosely bound copper[18]. The difference in ratio of total serum copper to ceruloplasmin in the diseased state as compared to controls is demonstrated unequivocably for adjuvant rats (Figure 66.1) and parallel, although necessarily less precise effects can be seen in rheumatoid arthritis in man. Since ceruloplasmin concentrations do not rise in line with total serum copper in man, it would appear that a significantly greater fraction of the serum copper is due to non-ceruloplasmin copper in patients with high copper levels. Part of this increase may be due to small copper molecules, but ceruloplasmin is not believed to be in direct equilibrium with other circulating copper species and we have shown previously that total serum copper does not correlate well with ultrafilterable copper levels. Therefore, both the amount of the difference between total serum copper levels and ceruloplasmin concentration and the size and spread of ultrafilterable copper levels suggest the presence of a new copper species or a much increased level on another species such as albumin. High copper levels on albumin were found with effective treatments of animal inflammation using copper salts[14,19].

Thus, at this point in time, the fact that a change in the copper balance in serum involving changes in biologically active molecules occurs in adjuvant and rheumatoid arthritis is well established and defined. The effect of these changes on the course of these diseases is by no means understood but potential exists for further studies that may, hopefully, lead either to a more precise diagnosis of the disease or to more effective therapy. In this respect, the clear changes in copper levels and activities produced by some drugs in the rat adjuvant model and the less precise but definite changes produced by drug therapies in rheumatoid arthritis would seem to be encouraging signs.

## References


1 Niedermeir, W. (1965). Concentration and chemical state of copper in synovial fluid and blood serum of patients with rheumatoid arthritis. *Ann. Rheum. Dis.*, **24,** 544

2 Plantin, L. O. and Strandberg, P. O. (1965). Whole blood concentrations of copper and zinc in rheumatoid arthritis studied by activation analysis. *Acta Rheum. Scand.*, **11,** 30

3 Lorber, A., Cutler, L. S. and Chang, C. C. (1968). Serum levels in rheumatoid arthritis: relationship of elevated copper to protein alterations. *Arthritis Rheum.*, **11,** 65

4 Gralla, E. J. and Wiseman, E. H. (1968). The adjuvant arthritic rat: Inflammatory parameters during the development and regression of gross lesions. *Proc. Soc. Exp. Biol. Med.*, **128,** 493

5 Jacques, R., Maijer, H., Riesterer, L. and Rüegg, M. (1971). Mast cell count in the peritoneal fluid of rats with adjuvant-induced polyarthritis. *Pharmacology*, **5,** 81

6 Hirschelmann, R., Bekemeier, H. and Stelzner, A. (1977). Acute-phase reactants of the blood in rat adjuvant arthritis as indicators of the degree of inflammation and of 'specific' and unspecific anti-inflammatory effects. *Z. Rheumatol.*, **36,** 305

7 Lewis, A. J., Cottney, J., Teape, J., Dunlop, J., Smith, W. E. and Brown, D. H. (1980). Copper and its involvement in the inflammatory process. *Eur. J. Rheumatol. Inflamm.* (In press)

8 Scudder, P. R., Al-Timmini, D., McMurray, W., White, A. G., Zoob, B. C. and Dormandy, T. L. (1978). Serum copper and related variables in rheumatoid arthritis. *Ann. Rheum. Dis.*, **37,** 67

9 Brown, D. H., Buchanan, W. W., El-Ghobarey, A. F., Smith, W. E. and Teape, J. (1979). Serum copper and its relationship to clinical symptoms in rheumatoid arthritis. *Ann. Rheum. Dis.*, **38,** 174

10 Pruzanski, W., Russel, M. L., Gordon, D. A. and Ogryzlo, M. A. (1973). Serum and synovial fluid proteins in rheumatoid arthritis and degenerative joint disease. *Am. J. Med. Sci.*, **265,** 485

11 Linder, M. C., Bryant, R. R., Lunn, S., Scott, L. E. and Moor, J. E. (1979). Ceruloplasmin elevation and synthesis in rats with transplantable tumours. *Enzyme,* **24,** 85

12 Boiano, J. M., Menden, E. E., Murthy, L. and Petering, H. G. (1977). Modification of a p-phenylene diamine oxidase method to permit non automated ceruloplasmin determinations in batches of rat serum or plasma. *Anal. Lett.*, **10,** 197

13 Teape, J., Kamel, H., Brown, D. H., Ottaway, J. M. and Smith, W. E. (1979). An evaluation of the use of electrophoresis and carbon furnace atomic absorption spectrometry to determine the copper level in separated serum protein fractions. *Clin. Chim. Acta.*, **94,** 1

14 Lewis, A., Brown, D. H., Dunlop, J. and Smith, W. E. (unpublished results)

15 Dunlop, J. and Hazelton, R. (unpublished results)

16 Crichton, R. R. (1973). Ferritin Structure and Bonding. **17,** 67

17 Ryden, L. and Björk, I. (1976). Reinvestigation of some physiochemical and chemical properties of human ceruloplasmin (Ferroxidase). *Biochemistry*, **15,** 3411

18 Frieden, E. and McKee, D. J. (1971). Binding of transition metal ions by ceruloplasmin. *Biochemistry*, **10,** 3880

19 Brown, D. H., Dunlop, J., Smith, W. E., Teape, J., Cottney, J. and Lewis, A. J. (1979). Copper distribution following administration of cuprous oxide to rats and guinea pigs. *Agents Actions*, **9**,
20 Blake, D. R., Eastham, E. J., and Thomson, M. (1980). Serum and synovial fluid ferritin in rheumatoid arthritis. This volume, Chap. 67

# 67

# Serum and synovial fluid ferritin in rheumatoid arthritis

D. R. BLAKE, E. J. EASTHAM AND M. THOMPSON (UK)

## INTRODUCTION

Anaemia commonly follows any chronic inflammatory condition. The causes are complex and centred around alterations in iron kinetics[1,2]. In patients with rheumatoid arthritis, studies using $^{59}$Fe-labelled transferrin suggest that intravenously injected iron is utilized in a normal manner and incorporated into circulating erythrocytes[3]. However, in chronic inflammatory states, defective utilization of iron from senescent erythrocytes has been shown using $^{59}$Fe-labelled cells[4] and studies with $^{59}$Fe-labelled dextran implicates reticuloendothelial cell dysfunction as the cause[5]. The excess iron stored within the RE cell is reflected by a rise in the serum ferritin.

Ferritin is an iron containing protein predominantly found within the cytoplasm of the hepatic and reticuloendothelial cells. In normal people and in those with uncomplicated iron deficiency states, serum ferritin reflects the total iron stores of the body[6]. However, in liver diseases and in inflammatory states serum ferritin is elevated to a degree disproportionate to that of bone marrow iron stores[2].

The objective of this study was to investigate the relationship between ferritin and other laboratory parameters of inflammatory activity. As the synovial membrane in patients with rheumatoid arthritis shares many histological features of a reticuloendothelial organ[7] we were prompted to measure both serum and synovial fluid ferritin in this disorder and to study their interrelationship with both the local (intra-articular) and more systemic aspects of this inflammatory condition.

## PATIENTS AND METHODS

Serum and synovial fluid samples were collected from rheumatology outpatients who required joint aspiration or injection with intra-articular steroids. Two separate groups of patients were studied: (1) 50 patients fulfilling the American Rheumatism Association criteria for the diagnosis of classical, definite or probable rheumatoid arthritis (RA), and (2) 15 patients with non-inflammatory effusions. Ferritin was estimated on an aliquot of both serum and synovial fluid, which had been allowed to clot, centrifuged and stored at −20 °C, using an immunoradiometric assay (Gammadab $^{125}$I Ferritin Kit, Travenol Laboratories).

Disease activity was assessed by the duration of morning stiffness, and an articular pain index, both for the joint aspirated and cumulative index for all joints with evidence of active synovitis (Ritchie index[8]). The duration of the disease and the presence or absence of extra-articular features of the rheumatoid process (vasculitis, nodule formation, etc.) was recorded. Laboratory markers of disease activity within blood and serum included, (a) haemaglobin, (b) erythrocyte sedimentation rate, (c) Rose–Waaler titre, (d) C reactive protein, (e) complement components (C3 and C4) and immune complex levels ($^{125}$I C1q binding[9]). Local assessment of activity within the synovial fluid included, (a) absolute polymorph count, (b) Rose–Waaler Titre, (c) fasting serum/synovial fluid glucose ratio, (d) total protein, (e) IgG, (f) complement components (C3 and C4) and (g) immune complexes ($^{125}$I C1q binding). In addition, record was made whether the joint aspirated was weight or non-weight bearing.

The data was analysed between groups by the Man–Whitney non-parametric U test and within groups by the Spearman rank correlation coefficient test.

## RESULTS

The ferritin levels in serum and synovial fluid are shown in Table 67.1. Although there was no significant difference in serum levels between the two groups, the highest and lowest values were in those patients with RA. No sig-

**Table 67.1** Ferritin levels ($\mu$g/l) in patients with rheumatoid arthritis and osteoarthrosis (mean ± SD)

| | *Rheumatoid arthritis* $n = 50$ | *Osteoarthrosis* $n = 15$ |
|---|---|---|
| Serum ferritin | 158 ± 241 | 104 ± 97 |
| Synovial ferritin | 855 ± 1289 | 106 ± 33 |

nificant correlation existed between serum ferritin and any clinical or laboratory index of disease activity. However, when considering those patients with seropositive rheumatoid arthritis, (Rose–Waaler titre $\geq$ 1:32), with evidence of extra-articular features of the disease, in contrast to those patients with such features, the serum ferritin was significantly raised ($p < 0.001$) (Table 67.2).

**Table 67.2** Serum ferritin levels ($\mu$g/l) in patients with or without extra-articular features of rheumatoid disease (mean ± SD)

| | *Without* | *With* |
|---|---|---|
| Serum ferritin | 86 ± 15 | 200 ± 213 |

In every case, ferritin levels were higher within the synovial fluid than in the serum. A significant correlation existed between fluid and serum ferritin for the patients with rheumatoid arthritis ($r = 0.4$, $p < 0.001$) but not for the patients with osteoarthrosis.

Ferritin was found in all synovial fluid samples but was on average eight times higher in those patients with RA and in three attained values greater than 5000 μg/1. All patients with osteoarthrosis had values below 200 μg/1 compared to 74% of patients with RA who exceeded this value. There was a highly significant difference between the groups ($p < 0.001$). The correlation coefficients and corresponding significance values between synovial ferritin and the various laboratory parameters of disease activity are shown in Table 67.3. There was no correlation between joint fluid ferritin and the duration of joint symptoms or the duration of morning stiffness, although fluid ferritin correlated weakly with the local articular pain index ($r = 0.3$:$p < 0.05$). Synovial ferritin levels were similar in weight and non-weight bearing joints.

**Table 67.3** Relationship between synovial fluid ferritin and synovial fluid indices of disease activity in rheumatoid arthritis

| *Indices* | *Correlation (r)* | *Significance (p)* |
|---|---|---|
| Rose–Waaler | 0.41 | 0.01 |
| Absolute polymorph count | 0.30 | 0.05 |
| Synovial fluid glucose | −0.30 | 0.05 |
| Serum/synovial fluid glucose ratio | −0.60 | 0.001 |
| Immune complexes | 0.58 | 0.001 |
| C3 ($n = 36$) | −0.57 | 0.001 |
| C4 ($n = 36$) | −0.34 | 0.05 |
| IgG | 0.57 | 0.001 |
| Total protein | 0.37 | 0.01 |

$n = 50$ unless otherwise stated

## DISCUSSION

Deposits of iron have been found in up to 96% of excised rheumatoid synovial membranes[10]. Much of this iron was found to be in the form of ferritin within the cytoplasm and lyosomes of synovial cells and therefore the finding of ferritin within synovial fluid was to be anticipated. Muirden suggests that the explanation for the presence of iron within synovial cells is local microbleeding induced by trauma[10]. An alternative hypothesis is that the cells of the synovial membrane actively break down effete circulating red cells in direct competition with other organs of the reticuloendothelial system. Our data would support this hypothesis as we did not find higher levels of ferritin within the weight bearing joints which would have been expected if trauma was the explanation. The significant correlation between synovial fluid ferritin and immune complex levels and IgM rheumatoid factor, both considered to be derived from cells within the synovial membrane, supports the view that ferritin is (a) locally derived, and (b) acting as an index of reticuloendothelial activity. The observation of Bentley and Williams[11] that certain patients had raised serum ferritin levels without stainable marrow also supports this hypothesis – the iron is selectively concentrated within actively diseased synovial membrane.

The significant association between serum ferritin levels and the presence of extra-articular manifestations and the lack of association with other systemic indices of inflammatory activity is of interest. Whereas it is generally considered that the systemic manifestation of the rheumatoid process develops in patients with more active joint disease, this view does not accord with clinical experience, where patients are noted to 'polarize' towards one extreme. Recent evidence suggests that the 'polar extremes' might have different immunological markers[12] and our data might support this view.

We suggest that the estimation of synovial fluid ferritin directly reflects activity of the reticuloendothelial cells in the synovial membrane and as such may be of use in the assessment of this disease. Serum ferritin levels did not correlate closely with other indices of inflammatory activity in this cross-sectional study but appears to be a useful laboratory marker of the presence of extra-articular features of the disorder. These observations are the basis of further longitudinal studies.

### References

1 Hershko, C., Cook, J. D. and Finch, C. A. (1974). Storage iron kinetics. VI. The effect of inflammation on iron exchange in the rat. *Br. J. Haematol.*, **26**, 67

2 Lipschitz, D. A., Cook, J. D. and Finch C. A. (1974). A clinical evaluation of serum ferritin as an index of iron stores. *N. Engl. J. Med.*, **290**, 1213

3 Raymond, F. D., Bowie, M. A. and Dugan, A. (1965). Iron metabolism in rheumatoid arthritis. *Arthritis Rheum.*, **8**, 233

4 Haurani, F. I., Burke, W. and Martinez, E. J. (1965). Defective reutilisation of iron in the anaemia of inflammation. *J. Lab. Clin. Med.*, **65**, 560

5 Beamish, M. R., Davies, A. G., Eakins, J. D., Jacobs, A. and Trevett, D. (1971). The measurement of reticuloendothelial iron release using iron dextran. *Br. J. Haematol.*, **21**, 617

6 Jacobs, A., Miller, E., Worwood, M., Beamish, M. R and Wardrop, C. A. (1972). Ferritin in the serum of normal subjects and patients with iron deficiency and iron overload. *Br. Med. J.*, **4,** 206

7 Allison, N. and Chorley, R. K. *Diagnosis in Joint Disease. A Clinical and Pathological Study of Arthritides*. 193. (New York: Wood)

8 Ritchie, D. M., Boyle, J. A., McInnes, J. R., Jasani, K. M., Dalabos, T. C., Grieveson, P. and Buchanan, W. W. (1968). Clinical studies with an articular index for the assessment of joint tenderness in patients with rheumatoid arthritis. *J. Med.*, **147,** 393

9 Zubler, R. H., Lange, G., Lambert, P. H. and Miescher, P. A. (1976). Detection of immune complexes in unheated sera by modified $I^{125}$ C1q test. *J. Immunol.*, **116,** 232

10 Muirden, K. D. (1970). The anaemia of rheumatoid arthritis: The significance of iron deposits in the synovial membrane. *Aust. Ann. Med.*, **2,** 97

11 Bentley, D. P. and Williams, P. (1974). Serum ferritin concentration as an index of storage iron in rheumatoid arthritis. *J. Clin. Pathol.*, **27,** 786

12 Papadimitriou, G., Bacon, P. A., Carter, S. D. and Hall, N. D. (1980) Rheumatoid immunoblasts and the effect of gold and cytotoxic drugs. This volume, Chap. 80

# 68

# Circulating and intra-articular immune complexes in rheumatoid arthritis: their relationship with disease activity

D. R. BLAKE AND I. GRIFFITHS (UK)

## INTRODUCTION

Whereas immunopathologists are agreed that the maintenance of chronic inflammation in the rheumatoid joint is at least partly the result of persistent local formation of immune complexes, there is little agreement on how closely either serum or synovial fluid immune complex levels correlate with either the severity, the activity, the occurrence of systemic features of the disease, or the duration of the disease.

We have measured both serum and synovial fluid immune complexes, using an $^{125}$I Clq binding assay, and correlated our results with a battery of clinical and standard laboratory indices of disease activity.

## METHOD

### Patients

Paired serum and synovial fluid samples were obtained from (1) 40 patients with classical or definite RA (sheep cell agglutination test (SCAT) serum positive $\geq$ 1:32), and (2) 15 patients with definite RA (SCAT serum negative titre $<$ 1.32). For comparison, paired samples were also taken from (3) 11 patients with osteoarthrosis with effusions, and (4) 9 patients with other sero negative inflammatory arthropathies (psoriasis, ankylosing spondylitis and Reiters).

**Clinical assessment**

From each patient we recorded:

(1) The duration of their disease.
(2) The duration of swelling of the aspirated joint.
(3) The patient's assessment of their disease (3 points scale).
(4) The duration of morning stiffness.
(5) The patient's assessment of the degree of pain within the joint aspirated.
(6) An articular pain index for the joint aspirated.
(7) A cumulative articular pain index for joints with an active synovitis (Ritchie index)[1].
(8) The presence of extra-articular features of rheumatoid disease (nodules, vasculitis, etc.).

In addition, when more than one joint could be aspirated, (1) the patient's assessment of the worst joint, (2) the Ritchie score[1] for each joint aspirated, and (3) the duration of swelling of each joint aspirated, was recorded.

**Laboratory**

Immune complexes were measured in both serum and synovial fluid using the $^{125}I$ C1q binding assay as described by Zubler[2]. The synovial fluid samples were allowed to clot at room temperature, centrifuged and stored within 90 min of collection at −90°C. Both serum and synovial fluid samples were batch assayed at the end of the study. Using standard clinical laboratory techniques, the haemaglobin, platelet count and ESR were measured and absolute white cell count and polymorph count measured in synovial fluid. The following parameters were measured in both serum and synovial fluid: glucose, protein, albumin, globulin and IgG. All tests were performed in the fasting state. Complement levels (C3 and C4) were measured in both serum and synovial fluid by Mancini immunodiffusion plates.

All the data were non-parametric and consequently analysed between groups using the Man–Whitney U test and within groups by the Spearman rank correlation coefficient test.

## RESULTS

**Between groups**

Figure 68.1 shows the distribution of serum and synovial fluid immune complex levels for the four groups. In all cases, synovial fluid immune complex levels were greater than the corresponding serum samples. The upper limit of normality (serum) for this assay is indicated, and was established from 20 healthy volunteers.

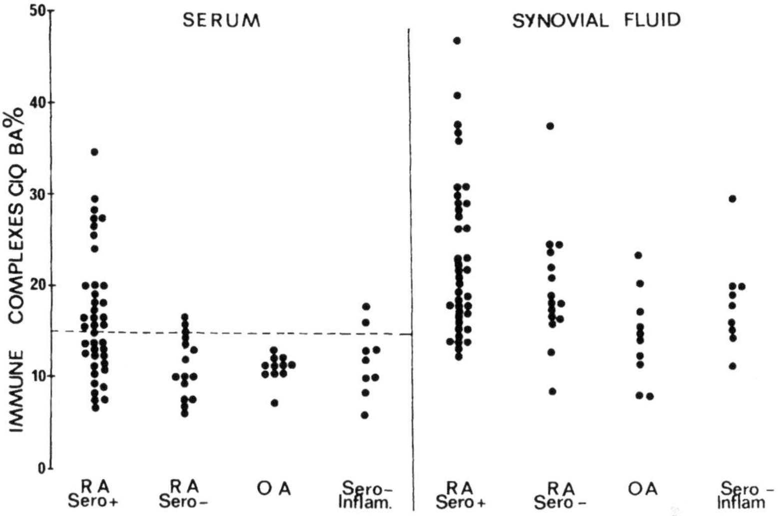


**Figure 68.1** Paired serum and synovial fluid immune complex levels

Within the synovial fluid, both sero-positive and sero-negative rheumatoid arthritis patients had significantly greater immune complex levels than the OA patients ($p<0.01$:$p<0.05$), although within the serum, only the sero-positive RA group had significantly higher levels than the control group ($p<0.0001$). A significant correlation ($r=0.5$:$P<0.01$) existed between synovial fluid and serum immune complex levels for the patients with seropositive RA, but for no other group.

## Within groups

*Clinical assessment*

Both serum and synovial immune complexes correlated with the duration of morning stiffness ($p<0.05$:$p<0.05$) for the patients with sero-positive rheumatoid arthritis. However, no significant correlation existed between immune complex levels, either serum or synovial fluid, and any other clinical measurement, when considering the groups either separately or together. In addition, no correlation existed with disease duration or duration of swelling of the individual joints. In four patients, 2 joints were available for aspiration. In each case, immune complex levels were found to be similar, as were the majority of other laboratory parameters of disease activity. However, both the patients' and physicians' assessment made clear reference to a more active joint which bore no relationship to the eventual immune complex (SF) level.

A significant positive association was observed between both serum and synovial fluid immune complex levels and the presence of extra-articular features of rheumatoid disease (rheumatoid nodules, digital vasculitis) (serum $p<0.05$: synovial fluid $p<0.001$). No other systemic manifestation of rheumatoid arthritis was noted in this group of patients.

*Laboratory tests*

Table 68.1 details the correlation coefficients and associated significance values between immune complex levels in both serum and synovial fluid and the various laboratory parameters measured for the patients with rheumatoid arthritis (both sero-positive and sero-negative).

**Table 68·1** Correlations between serum and synovial fluid immune complex levels and parameters of inflammatory activity in serum (S) and synovial fluid (SF)

| | *Immune complexes* Clq | | | |
|---|---|---|---|---|
| | *Serum* | | *Synovial fluid* | |
| | *r (correlation)* | *p < (significance)* | *r(correlation)* | *p < (significance)* |
| Immune complexes (S) | — | — | 0·5 | 0.001 |
| Rose–Waaler (S) | 0·43 | 0·01 | 0·38 | 0·05 |
| Haemoglobin | −0·38 | 0·01 | — | NS |
| Platelet count | — | NS | — | NS |
| Erythrocyte sedimentation rate | 0·43 | 0·01 | 0·48 | 0·001 |
| C reactive protein (S) | — | NS | — | NS |
| Total protein (S) | — | NS | 0·48 | 0·001 |
| albumin (S) | — | NS | — | NS |
| globulin (S) | 0·3 | 0·05 | 0·48 | 0·001 |
| IgG (S) | 0·3 | 0·05 | — | NS |
| White cell count (SF) | — | NS | 0·42 | 0·001 |
| Absolute polymorph count (SF) | — | NS | 0·42 | 0·001 |
| Rose–Waaler (SF) | 0·39 | 0·01 | 0·37 | 0·05 |
| protein (SF) | — | NS | 0·48 | 0·001 |
| albumin (SF) | — | NS | — | NS |
| globulin (SF) | — | NS | 0·49 | 0·001 |
| IgG (SF) | — | NS | — | NS |
| Fall in glucose (SF) (relates to serum) | — | NS | 0·33 | 0·05 |

Significant correlations were observed between serum immune complex levels and Rose–Waaler titre, haemaglobin and erythrocyte sedimentation rate, although, interestingly, stronger correlations existed between synovial fluid immune complex levels and these parameters. Within the synovial fluid, complex levels correlated significantly with the white cell count, absolute polymorph count, total protein and globulin levels, and weakly with the Rose–Waaler titre and fall in synovial fluid glucose.

When corrected for synovial fluid globulin concentration[3], we found that

C4 levels in synovial fluid of both the sero-positive and sero-negative RA group were lower than in the OA group. Although there was a close correlation between C3 and C4 levels in synovial fluid in sero-positive rheumatoid arthritis ($p<0.001$), sero-negative rheumatoid arthritis ($p<0.05$) and the other inflammatory group ($p<0.02$), we did not observe a significant correlation between synovial fluid C1q binding and either C4 or C3 within any of the groups. Similarly, we did not find a correlation between synovial fluid complement and the polymorphonuclear white cell count of synovial fluid within any group.

Serum C4 levels correlated inversely with serum C1q binding only in sero-positive rheumatoid arthritis ($p<0.002$), there being no observed correlation between serum C3 and C1q binding in any group.

## DISCUSSION

There is now overwhelming evidence that an altered immune system plays a central role in the pathogenesis of rheumatoid arthritis. The recognition of complement fixing 1gM and 1gG rheumatoid factors[4,5], both free and complexed, in serum and more especially synovial fluid, in addition to the evidence of complement activation, particularly in synovial fluid[6], suggest that the humoral immune system is an important effector arm of the inflammatory response. This study supports and extends this concept by showing that immune complex levels, as judged by C1q binding, in synovial fluid of patients with rheumatoid arthritis correlate with the other measures of inflammation: the absolute neutrophil count and the lowering of synovial fluid/serum glucose ratios. Although an immunogenetic susceptibility to rheumatoid arthritis is becoming increasingly probable, the initiating factor or factors in the development of rheumatoid arthritis remain unknown. The observation that the majority of patients with intermittent or palindromic rheumatism eventually develop classical rheumatoid arthritis[7], suggests that in certain subjects the ability to 'turn off' the inflammatory response is lost at a certain point in the natural history of their disease. Whether this is due to a basic change in the inflammatory response or a loss of control mechanisms is unknown. One aim of this study was to assess whether the incidence and quantity of complexes within RA synovial fluid changed with duration of disease. We did not, however, find any significant associations between levels of complex in either synovial fluid or serum and disease duration but only six of the RA patients had had their disease for 1 year or less and obviously studies at an earlier stage of the disease are required.

The correlation between C4 and C3 complement levels in synovial fluid in all groups except OA suggests that the complement system is activated by the classical pathway. We, like Hasselbacher[3], did not observe a correlation between synovial fluid, white cell count and C3 levels, nor did we observe a correlation with C1q binding. These findings probably reflect the difficulty in interpreting isolated protein estimations of complement levels in synovial fluid when rates of synthesis and catabolism are unknown.

Although there are numerous pitfalls in extrapolating information obtained for fluid analysis, on either serum or synovial fluid, to tissue pathology[8], our findings would support the hypothesis that in established rheumatoid arthritis complexes in synovial fluid, acting presumably via the classical complement pathway results in chemotaxis and subsequent glucose utilisation.

The failure to find a correlation between levels of complexes within synovial fluid and clinical assessment of joint inflammatory activity at a single point in time indicates the need for prospective studies in early RA to determine the effect of immune complexes, upon the development of synovitis and subsequent joint destruction.

## References


1 Ritchie, D. M., Boyle, J. A., McInnes, J. R., Jasani, K. M., Dalabos, T. C., Grieveson, P. and Buchanan, W. W. (1976). Clinical studies with an articular index for the assessment of joint tenderness in patients with rheumatoid arthritis. *Q. J. Med.*, **147,** 393

2 Zubler, R. H., Lange, G., Lambert, P. H., Miesder, P. A. (1976). Detection of immune complexes in unheated sera by modified $1^{125}$C1q test. *J. Immunol.*, **116,** 232

3 Hasselbacher, P. (1979). Immunoelectrophoretic assay for synovial fluid C3 with correction for synovial fluid globulin. *Arthritis Rheum.*, **22,** 243

4 Zuaifler, N. J. and Schur, P. (1968). Reaction of aggregated mercaptoethanol treated gamma globulin with rheumatoid factor – precipitation and complement fixation studies. *Arthritis Rheum*, **11,** 523

5 Vaughan, J. H., Kaplan, R. A., Slovin, S. F. and Carson, D. A. (1978). Biological properties of anti-1gG antibodies. In Panayi, G. S. and Johnson, P. M. (eds.). *Immunopathogenesis of Rheumatoid Arthritis*, pp 56–59. (Reedbooks)

6 Ruddy, S. and Austen, K. F. (1970). The complement system in rheumatoid synovitis. I. An analysis of complement component activities in rheumatoid synovial fluid. *Arthritis Rheum*, **13,** 713

7 Ward, L. K. and Ohihiro, M. M. (1959). *Ard. Int. Med. Rheum.*, **2,** 208

8 Winfield, J. B., Faiferman, I. and Koffler, D. (1977). Avidity of anti-DNA antibodies in serum and 1gG glomerular eluates from patients with SLE. *J. Clin. Invest.*, **59,** 90

# 69

# $\beta_2$-Microglobulin, anti-$\beta_2$-microglobulin activity and circulating immune complexes in rheumatoid arthritis: seric and synovial studies

B. DUQUESNOY, M. ASFOUR, F. SANTORO AND B. DELCAMBRE (FRANCE)

## INTRODUCTION

The elevation of seric $\beta_2$-microglobulin ($\beta_2$m) levels is well known in inflammatory diseases[5,20]. The exact role $\beta_2$m plays is not so clear. It is present on the surface of nucleated cells and platelets, bound to HL-A, to form the light chain of it. Moreover, its amino acid sequence shows a high degree of homology with domains of human IgG ($CH_3$). These two properties are the main reasons for the interest of the detection of $\beta_2$m in autoimmune diseases. Michalski[10] and Talal[19] show the elevation of salivary and synovial $\beta_2$m levels in Sjöngren's syndrome and rheumatoid arthritis (RA), in relation with the illness. According to these authors, the elevation of $\beta_2$m indicates local production in the tissue, especially salivary tissue. Ström[18] only found such results in 38% of sicca syndrome. In systemic lupus erythematosus (SLE), Revillard[16], by using a precipitation of radio-labelled $\beta_2$m in polyethylene glycol, showed a $\beta_2$m binding activity significantly higher than in control sera. Ooi[12] detected this activity by using a double antibody assay. Finally Manicourt Brauman[8] and Orloff[13] detected high levels of seric and synovial $\beta_2$m in R.A., in correlation with joint count and the erythrocyte sedimentation rate (ESR). In a recent work, Manicourt[9] points out the fact that there is a correlation between $\beta_2$m and complement components. For these authors, the elevation of $\beta_2$m would be due to lymphocyte infiltration in synovial tissue. These levels of $\beta_2$m are much higher in RA than in some other inflammatory rheumatic diseases such as ankylosing spondylitis or Rieter's disease (Amor[1]).

In this work, we studied seric and synovial $\beta_2$m in RA and their relation with some parameters of the immune response: circulating immune complexes (CIC) complement components, anti-IgG antibodies (anti-IgG Ab).

## MATERIAL AND METHODS

### Patients

Serum samples from 225 patients of the 'Clinique de Rheumatologie' (Pr. Robert D'Eshougues) were studied. They comprised: 120 RA who satisfied the ARA criteria for classical or definite RA, 55 of which were considered as sero-positive (RA+) (rheumatoid factor titer in Waaler–Rose $\geq$ 64 or in latex test > 40) and sero-negative (RA −); 22 inflammatory chronic arthritis (IA), 10 ankylosing spondylitis; 6 psoriatic arthritis; 3 Reiter's disease; 1 relapsing polychrondritis; 2 pseudomyalgia rheumatica; 24 temporarily unclassified inflammatory arthritis (UIA), and 59 healthy blood donors (NHS). Synovial fluid samples from 15 control subjects were collected; osteoarthritis, necrosis, algodystrophy and gout, without any known inflammatory arthritis.

### $\beta_2$-microglobulin

Radio-immunoassay kits (Phadebas, Pharmacia, Sweden) were employed to measure the $\beta_2$m contents of synovial fluid and sera of patients. All the people with renal insufficiency were excluded from the study (urea and creatinin in normal range, no daily proteinuria). According to our experience, the normal values were 2.07 ± 0.9 g/ml (mean ± 2SD).

### Circulating immune complexes

The CIC were investigated by the $^{125}$I C1q binding test according to Zubler and Lambert[21]. Briefly, $^{125}$I C was mixed with test serum, previously treated with 0.2 mol/l EDTA. Free C1q was separated from C1q bound to CIC by precipitation with 3 % polyethylene glycol (PEG). All the tests were done in triplicate and the results were expressed as per cent $^{125}$IC1q precipitated compared to the radioactivity precipitated with trichloracetic acid (TCA) in control tubes.

### Complement studies

Levels C1q, C4, C3 and properdin B Factor were evaluated by radial immunodiffusion[7] on plates supplied by the Behring Institute (Harbour – Lohn, West Germany).

**[$^{125}$I]IgG**

Human unaggregated IgG Cohn fraction II (Miles laboratories, Elkhart, Indiana, USA) was radio iodinated according to Morrison, Bayse and Webster[11].

**Detection of anti-IgG antibodies**

Anti-IgG Ab were investigated by three methods: classical Waaler–Rose and latex tests (reagents from the Pasteur Institute, Paris) and the radio-immunoprecipitation PEG assay (RIPEGA)[17]. For the RIPEGA, [$^{125}$I]IgG was separated from IgG bound to anti-IgG Ab by precipitation with 7 % PEG. Results were expressed as per cent [$^{125}$I]IgG precipitated as compared with the protein-bound radioactivity precipitable with 20 % TCA.

**Inflammation**

Intensity of inflammation was mainly evaluated by two parameters: ESR and $\alpha_2$ globulin level.

**[$^{125}$I]$\beta_2$m ammonium sulphate precipitation assay**

We used a screening procedure described by OOI[12] in SLE. 100 µl of test serum, previously inactivated by heating at 56 °C for 30 min was added to tubes and diluted with 0.85 ml of phosphate buffered saline (PBS). An aliquot of 0.05 ml of [$^{125}$ I]$\beta_2$m microglobulin was then added and the mixture incubated at 37 °C for 30 min followed by overnight incubation for 16 h at 4 °C. 1 ml saturated ammonium sulphate was added and mixed in a rotator at 4 °C for 30 min. 1 ml of supernatant was taken off. Radioactivity of both fractions was determined in an automatic gamma counter. Statistical analysis was carried out using Student's *t*-test and MacNeman's discordance test.

## RESULTS

**$\beta_2$m detection**

The results of the detection of seric $\beta_2$m CIC, anti-IgG and complement activation are summarized in (Table 69.1). Elevation of seric $\beta_2$m was found between the RA patients and the healthy subjects. Significantly high levels of

**Table 69.1** $\beta_2$-microglobulin ($\beta_2$m), circulating immune complexes and anti-IgG antibodies (anti [$^{125}$ I]IgG Ab) levels in rheumatoid arthritis (RA) and control (NHS) groups

| *Patients* | *No* | $\beta_2 m$ | $^{125}IC19$ | anti[$^{125}$I]IgG Ab |
|---|---|---|---|---|
| NHS | 59 | 2.07*±0.45† | 10.01±1.5 | 9.7±1.21 |
| RA+ | 55 | 4.59±1.99 | 22.15±8.88 | 15.77±5.46 |
| RA− | 65 | 4.13±2.29 | 14.81±4.71 | 11.52±2.97 |

* Mean
† Standard deviation

$\beta_2$m were detected in 75 % of RA (81 % of RA + 69 % of RA) have higher levels than the normal subjects, mean ± 2SD (Figure 69.1). In the other groups, 47 % of IA and 50 % of UIA have high levels.

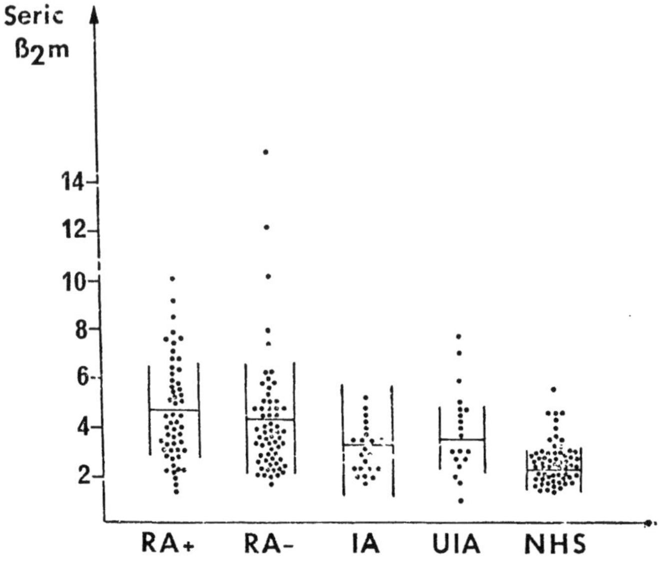


**Figure 69.1** Seric $\beta_2$m levels in rheumatoid arthritis patients (RA+ and RA−), inflammatory arthritis patients (IA), unclassified inflammatory arthritis patients (UIA) and control subjects (NHS)

The detection of synovial $\beta_2$m was carried out on synovial fluid of 27 RA (11 RA + and 16 RA −) and 15 control subjects (Table 69.2), and a quotient of synovial fluid and sera was calculated. Elevated levels were found in 22 patients (31%) (Figure 69.2). Moreover, if we study quotients, only one control subject had a quotient higher than one against 18 RA (Figure 69.3). A significant correlation was observed between seric and synovial $\beta_2$m ($r$ = 0.56, $p < 0.01$) (Figure 69.4).

**Table 69.2** Seric and synovial $\beta_2$m levels in rheumatoid arthritis (RA + and RA −) and control subjects (NHS)

| *Patients* | *No* | *Seric $\beta_2m$* | *Synovial $\beta_2m$* | *Synovial/seric $\beta_2m$* |
|---|---|---|---|---|
| RA+ | 11 | 4,83*±1.85† | 6.93±3.62 | 2.13±2.21 |
| RA− | 16 | 4.2±2.5 | 4.64±2.24 | 1.65±0.42 |
| NHS | 15 | 2.07±0.45 | 2.7±0.61 | 0.7±0.18 |

* Mean
† Standard deviation

**Detection of CIC**

The detection of CIC by using $^{125}$I C1q is similar to our previous work (Table 69.1). It was interesting to compare these two inflammatory parameters, CIC and seric $\beta_2$m. In the group of RA − patients, there is a significant correlation between CIC and $\beta_2$m (Figure 69.5) ($r = 0.52$ $p < 0.001$). On the contrary, we did not detect any correlation in the group of RA + patients ($r = 0.08$). These results led us to study the possibility of an anti-$\beta_2$m activity in the sera of RA patients by using an ammonium sulphate precipitation. We selected 52 sera from patients with high levels of CIC and complement activation.

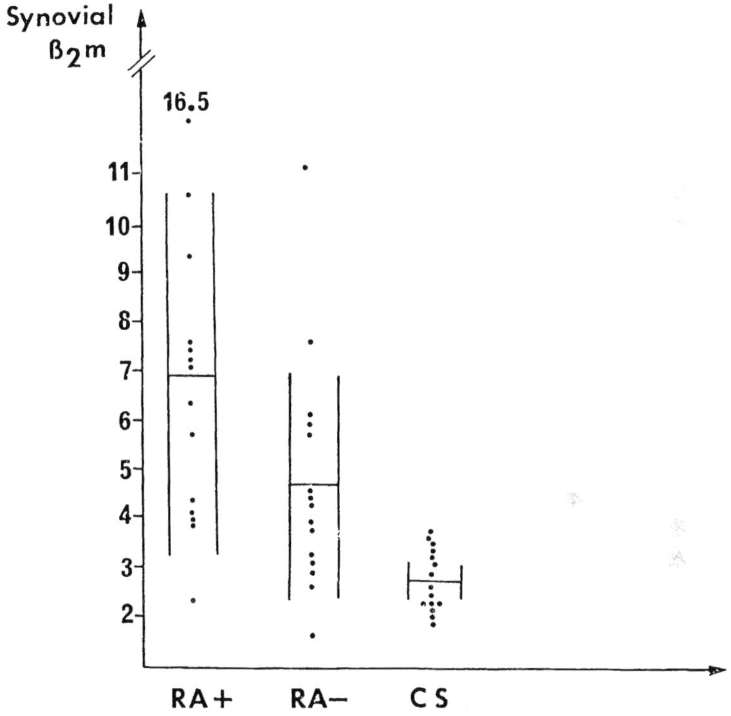


**Figure 69.2** Synovial $\beta_2$m levels in rheumatoid arthritis (RA+ and RA−) patients and control subjects (CS)

In all the sera we detected an anti-$\beta_2$m activity much greater than that of healthy subjects (mean ± 2SD). The lowest percentage of [$^{125}$I]$\beta_2$m of the RA sera (52 %) is higher than the most elevated value of the group NHS. The difference is very significant (Figure 69.6).

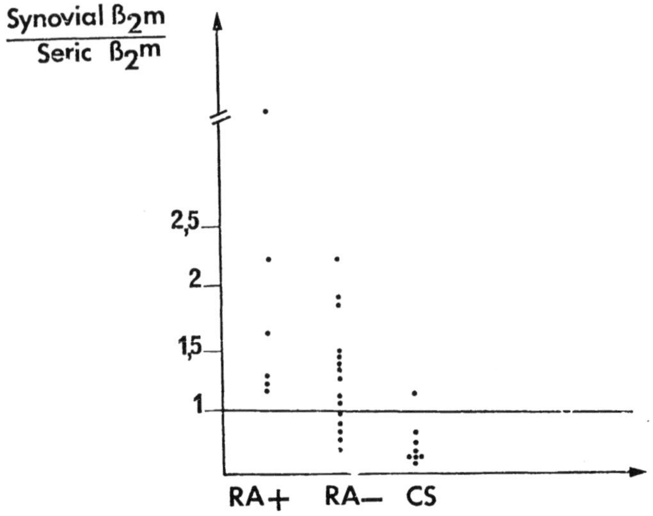


**Figure 69.3** Synovial/seric $\beta_2$m ratio in rheumatoid arthritis patients (RA) and control subjects (CS)

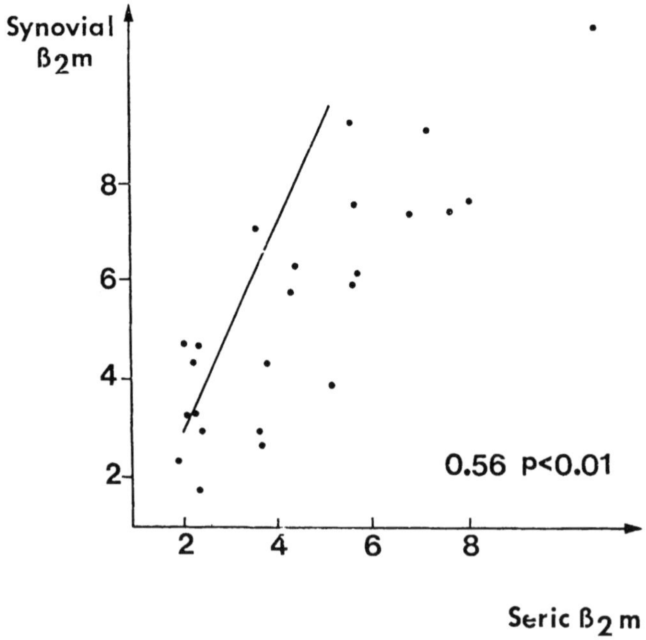


**Figure 69.4** Correlation between seric and synovial $\beta_2$m in rheumatoid arthritis

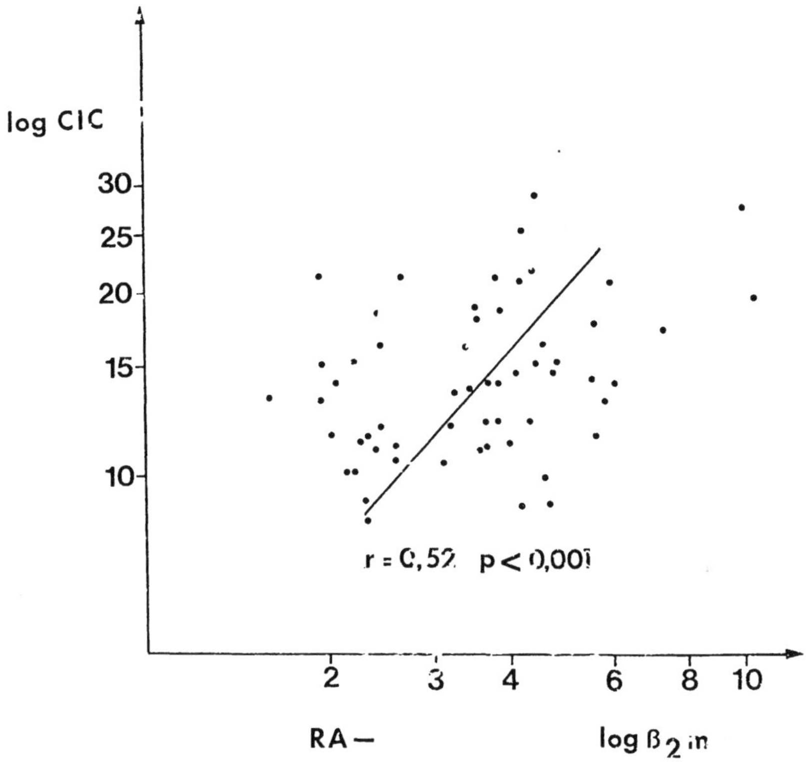


**Figure 69.5** Correlation between circulating immune complexes (CIC) and $\beta_2$m microglobulin in sero-negative rheumatoid arthritis

**Detection of anti-IgG Ab**

We found elevated levels of anti-IgG Ab with significant correlation between these parameters and CIC ($r = 0.44$, $p < 0.001$) confirming our previous work[4,16]. On the contrary, there is no correlation between seric $\beta_2$m and anti-IgG Ab ($r = 0.26$) in RA+ or RA−.

**Complement activation**

The mean levels of the total haemolytic complement ($CH_{50}$) and the complement components C1q, C4 C3 and B factor were within the normal range obtained with healthy people. Among all the patients with RA, seven (5 RA+ and 2 RA−) show a low C4 level (< 20 mg/100 ml) (Table 69.3). In all these patients, the illness was considered as old or severe, and twice it was an 'overlap syndrome' (isolated anti-DNA antibody). In all these cases there was CIC four of them in very high levels(> 20% $^{125}$I C1q precipitation), and even one at 52 % and anti-IgG Ab in large amounts. It is interesting to notice

**Table 69.3** Circulating immune complexes, anti-IaG antibodies and seric $\beta_2$-microglobulin levels in seven patients with C4 low levels

| Patients | | *C4* (mg/100 ml) | *CIC* | *anti-IgG Ab* | $\beta_2 m$ (mg/ml) |
|---|---|---|---|---|---|
| 2.70.209 | RA+ | 9 | 52 | 22 | 4.45 |
| 2.75.249 | RA+ | 5 | 21 | 16.5 | 7.54 |
| 2.79.021 | RA+ | 5 | 17.5 | 32 | 7.57 |
| 2.75.122 | RA+ | 14 | 33 | 30 | 2.20 |
| 2.74.089 | RA+ | 8.4 | 13.5 | 32 | 8 |
| 1.78.358 | RA− | 10 | 27 | 10 | 10.15 |
| 1.79.004 | RA− | 15.6 | 28 | 25.5 | 4.46 |

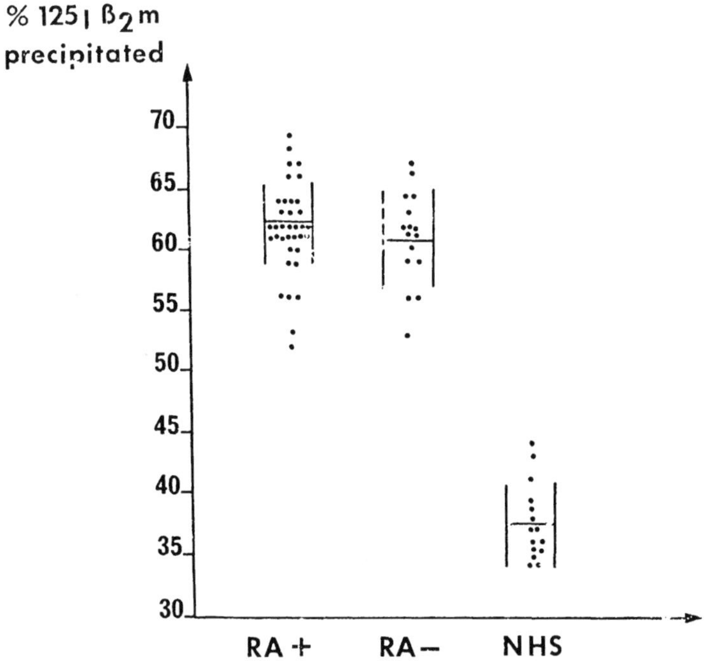


**Figure 69.6** Levels of [$^{125}$I]$\beta_2$m ammonium sulphate precipitation in rheumatoid arthritis patients (RA+ and RA−) and control subjects (NHS)

that in six cases seric $\beta_2$m was high (> 4.45 mg/ml). Only in one case (number 275122) was seric $\beta_2$m at a low level with elevated CIC, however, synovial $\beta_2$m was very high (16.53 g/ml).

A comparison between seric $\beta_2$m and ESR showed a weak correlation between these two parameters ($r = 0.32, p < 0.01$) (Figure 69.7) or ESR and synovial-$\beta_2$m/seric-$\beta_2$m ratio ($r = 0.518$, $p < 0.05$).

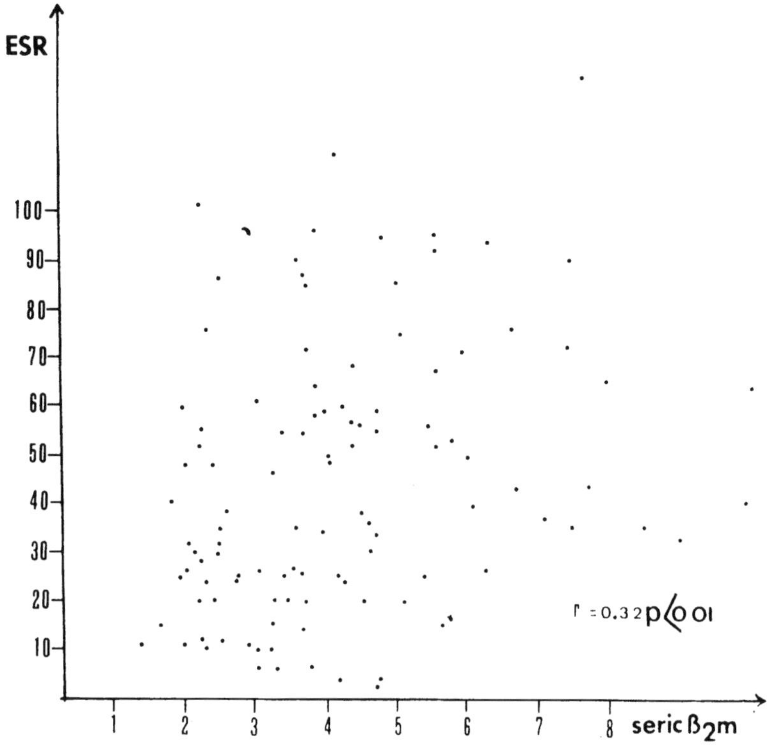


**Figure 69.7** Correlation between ESR and $\beta_2$m in rheumatoid arthritis group

## DISCUSSION

In this work, we found in sero-positive or sero-negative RA patients, whatever the form, elevated seric and synovial $\beta_2$m in comparison with control subjects. Moreover, synovial-$\beta_2$m/seric $\beta_2$m-ratio is superior to 1 in 82 % with regard to the control group (only one ratio superior to one). These results are in agreement with several studies[2,8] A positive correlation between seric $\beta_2$m and C1q binding CIC was found in the sero-negative RA group. In contrast, this correlation does not exist in the sero-positive RA group. These results let us discuss the exact place of $\beta_2$m in the immune response. We tried to pinpoint this action by using a $[^{125}I]\beta_2$m ammonium sulphate precipitation assay. There is an increased anti-$\beta_2$m activity in either sero-positive or sero-negative RA (the lowest level in RA is superior to the mean + 3SD in the NHS group). This abnormal activity could be due to RF reacting against the amino acid sequence of $\beta_2$m homologous with domains of human IgG. The absence of correlation between seric $\beta_2$m and anti-IgG Ab or between anti-$\beta_2$m activity and anti-IgG Ab are not suggestive of that hypothesis. This activity could represent anti-$\beta_2$m antibodies. Plesner[15] discusses hypothesis: application of rabbit antibodies to immunoglobulin light in intermediate gels using the crossed radio-immunoelectrophoresic method failed to depress the abnormal $\beta_2$m precipitate. However, in SLE, Ooi[12] showed such an anti-$\beta_2$m activity by using an ammonium sulphate precipitation assay. Sucrose density gradient ultracentrifugation demonstrate the 7S material complexes to [$^{125}$I]$\beta_2$m[12]. Moreover, Revillard[16] found such an anti-$\beta_2$m activity in PEG precipitation. Chromatography of SLE sera on polyacrylamide agarose gel Ac A 3/4 showed that most of the $\beta_2$m binding activity was recovered in the IgG peak.

In our experiments, we found positive correlation between $\beta_2$m and CIC in RA−. Previously, we have noticed a difference between the two groups of RA[4] If there was a positive correlation between C1q binding CIC and anti-IgG Ab detected by RIPEGA, this correlation was better in RA+. These data may suggest that CIC are made with IgG–anti-IgG Ab in RA+; on the contrary, in RA– a certain amount of $\beta_2$m–anti-$\beta_2$m complexes could be present.

## References


1 Amor, B., Georgiadis, A., Kahan, A. and Delbarre, F. (1978). La $\beta_2$-microglobuline dans la spondylarthrite ankylosante et le syndrome de Fiessinge Leroy–Reiter. *Pathol. Biol.*, **26**, 377

2 Brauman, H., Manicourt, D. and Orloff, S. (1978). $\beta_2$-microglobuline dans le liquide synovial. *Pathol. Biol.*, **26**, 373

3 Cunningham, B. A., Wang, J. L., Berggard, I. and Peterson, P. A. (1973). The complete amino acid sequence of $\beta_2$-microglobulin. *Biochemistry*, **12**, 4811

4 Duquesnoy, B., Santoro, F., Wattre, P. and Delcambre, B. (1978). Complexes immuns circulants et anticorps anti IgG dans la polyarthrite rhumatoïde. *Rev. Rhum.*, **45**, 417

5 Evrin, P. E. and Wibell, L. B. (1973). Serum $\beta_2$-microglobulin in various disorders. *Clin. Chim. Acta*, **43**, 183

6 Falus, A., Meretey, K., Bohm, U. and Bozsoky, S. (1978). High synovial fluid/serum ratio of beta$_2$-microglobulin and simultaneous occurence of hidden rheumatoid factors in R.A. *Rheumatology*, **8**, 287

7 Mancini, G., Carbonara, A. O. and Heremans, J. F. (1965). Immunochemical quantitation of antigens by single radial immunodiffusion. *Immunochemistry*, **2**, 235

8 Manicourt, D., Brauman, H. and Orloff, S. (1978). Plasma and urinary $\beta_2$-microglobulin in patients with rheumatoid arthritis. *Ann. Rheum. Dis.*, **37**, 328

9 Manicourt, D. (1977). $\beta_2$-microglobuline et affections rhumatismales. *Acta Rheumatol. Belg.* **1**, 263

10 Michalski, J. P., Daniels, D. T., Talal, N. and Grey, H. M. (1975). $\beta_2$-microglobulin and lymphocytic infiltration in Sjöngren's syndrome. *N. Engl. J. Med.*, **293**, 1228

11 Morrisson, M., Bayse, G.S. and Webster, R. O. (1971). Use of lacto peroxidase catalyzed iodination immunochemical studies. *Immunochemistry*, **8**, 289

12 Ooi, B.S., Ooi, Y.M., Pesce, A. J., and Pollak, V. E. (1977). Antibodies to $\beta_2$-microglobulin in the sera of patients with systemic lupus erythematosus. *Immunology*, **33**, 535

13 Orloff, S. (1977). Some new criteria for the evaluation of disease activity in rheumatoid arthritis. *Acta Rheumatol. Belg.* **1**, 263

14 Perrin, L. H., Lambert, P. H. and Miescher, P. A. (1975). Complement breakdown products in plasma from patients with systemic lupus erythematosus and patients with membrane proliferative or other glomerulonephritis. *J. Clin. Invest.*, **56**, 165

15 Plesner, T. and Wiik, A. (1979). Demonstration of electrophoretic heterogeneity of serum $\beta_2$-microglobulin in systemic lupus erythematosus and rheumatoid arthritis: evidence against auto antibodies to $\beta$-microglobulin. *Scand. J. Immunol.*, **9**, 247

16 Revillard, J. P., Vincent, C. and Rivera, S. (1979). Anti $\beta_2$-microglobulin lymphocytotoxic auto antibodies in systemic lupus erythematosus. *J. Immunol.*, **122,** 614

17 Santoro, F., Duquesnoy, B., Wattre, P., Delcambre, B. and Capron, A. (1977). The use of the radioimmuno precipitation – PEG Assay (RIPEGA) to detect anti-IgG antibodies. *Biomedicine*, **27,** 230

18 Ström, T., Evrin, P. E. and Karlson, A. (1978). Serum $\beta_2$-microglobulin in Sjögren's syndrome. *Scand. J. Rheumatol.*, **7,** 97

19 Talal, N., Grey, H. M., Zvaifler, N., Michalski, J. P. and Daniels, T. E. (1975). Elevated salivary and synovial fluid $\beta_2$-microglubulin in Sjögren's syndrome and rheumatoid arthritis. *Science*, **187,** 1196

20 Wibell, L. B. (1976). Studies on $\beta_2$-microglobulin in patients and normal subjects. *Acta Clin. Bel.*, **31,** (Suppl.) 14

21 Zubler, R. H., Nydegger, U., Perrin, L. H., Fehr, K. and Mc.Cormick, J. (1976). Circulating and intraarticular immune complexes in patients with rheumatoid arthritis. Correlation of $^{125}$I-C1q binding activity with clinical and biological features of the disease. *J. Clin. Invest.*, **57,** 1308

# 70

# Technetium-99m labelled leukocytes: preparation, animal studies and potential application

N. LINHART, B. BOK, M. MEIGNAN
AND M. GOUGEROT (FRANCE)

## INTRODUCTION

Several authors have used labelled phagocytes to detect inflammatory foci in cases of infection[2,3]. $^{51}Cr$ was the first marker used but its high photon energy and long physical half-life are obvious drawbacks[4]. Other gamma emitters such as $^{67}Ga$ have also been suggested for human leukocyte labelling[5] and for direct intravenous administration in abscess detection.

The criteria of a good labelling technique are the following: (a) high labelling efficiency; (b) high stability (activity should remain within the labelled cells); (c) high cell specificity (only polymorphonuclear phagocytes should be labelled), and (d) normal viability especially as regards cell chemotaxis. In other words, labelled cells should be able to move to infectious foci as easily as unlabelled cells.

We have developed a new leukocyte labelling technique, used earlier for red cell labelling. In this method, 'cold' tin pyrophosphate is used as a first step since $^{99m}Tc$ in pertechnetate form does not label any type of blood cells[1].

## MATERIALS AND METHODS

### Preparation of labelled leukocytes

A leukocyte-rich suspension is required for labelling. 20 ml human venous blood was collected in a 60 ml sterile heparinized syringe (2% heparin Choay) containing 25 ml dextran (high molecular weight 500 000*). The blood was allowed to settle for 70–90 min at 20 °C with the syringe in a vertical position. The remaining red cells were removed from this supernatant by adding 80 ml $NH_4Cl$ 0.87% solution. After centrifugation and washing with 9% NaCl, a leukocyte-rich suspension was thus obtained.

The suspension was then incubated for 15 min at 37 °C with a stannous pyrophosphate solution (59.4 mg pyrophosphate and 1.3 mg stannous chloride in a 3 ml solution), using 150 µl per 20 000 leukocytes. The resulting sediment was ready for labelling by incubation for 10 min at 20 °C together with 1 ml of high specific activity pertechnetate solution (20–30 mCi/ml). The suspension was again centrifuged for removal of supernatant and free pertechnetate. In order to perform animal studies, beagle dogs were chosen because they show a high recovery rate of white blood cells after dextran sedimentation. Then the labelling procedure is the same.

**Quality control methods**

Quality controls consist in verifying the stability of the label and functional value of labelled cells. Stability is tested by usual methods. The value of the leukocytes was estimated by morphological study, chemotaxis and metabolic tests: cell morphology was examined by electron microscopy after the cells had been fixed with 2.5% glutaraldehyde and put in epoxy resin (EPON). These microscope studies were made before and after incubation of the cells with stannous pyrophosphate, and after $^{99m}Tc$ labelling. They were also performed after hypotonic lysis.

Chemotaxis was measured by the Cutler and Nelson technique[6,7]. Leukocyte migration was observed using a light microscope, after 2½ h incubation at 37 °C. This test was also performed after each labelling step simultaneously with the stability test described above.

There are many metabolic tests for the study of the biochemical phenomena associated with phagocytosis and the death of pathogenic agents caused by polymorphonuclear cells. Some results are shown in Table 70.1. In order to perform animal studies, the same tests were again controlled on one normal and one abscessed animal.

**Animal studies**

Twelve beagle dogs were used. The mean weight was about 10 kg. Six were normal controls. In the six others an abscess was induced using a 0.2 ml turpentine subcutaneous injection at the internal side of the knee. A blood sample was taken 24 h after the turpentine injection and was followed by the labelling procedure and reinjection. 5 ml blood samples were taken at 15 min, 30 min, 60 min, 2 h, 3 h, 4 h, 5 h, 6 h, 11 h, 19 h and 24 h, to study the half-life of blood radioactivity disappearance.

External counting was performed during 24 h. Moreover, in two abscessed dogs, $^{113m}In$-labelled iron-free transferrin was administered at 6 h to show the distribution of an intravascular tracer. Organ biopsy or autopsy samples were

**Table 70.1** Metabolic test results

| | *Ingestion* (number of *Klebsiella* associated with the granulocytes after 10 min) | *$O_2$ consumption* (nanoatoms of $O_2$ consumed per $10^6$ granulocytes/min) | | *$H_2O_2$** | Iodination† |
|---|---|---|---|---|---|
| | | *Spontaneous* | *Stimulated* | | |
| Labelled cells | 4.8 | 3.3 | 11.8 | 5 | 8.6 |
| | 4.8 | 1.9 | 11.7 | 3.9 | 7.7 |
| | 4.5 | 1.5 | 8.7 | 3.1 | 12.3 |
| Normal | 7.6 | 2 | 16 | 6.2 | 16 |
| Control cells | ±2.5 | ±1 | ±2.5 limit 11 | ±2 | ± 4 |

Three assays were performed with labelled cells. Results which are considered abnormal are those which fall at least within a 5% significance limit. *nmol of $H_2O_2$ produced per $10^6$ granulocytes/min. † nmol of iodide per $10^7$ granulocytes

taken in two normal and two abscessed dogs, then washed and counted, the results being expressed as a per cent of the administered activity/g. In four abscessed dogs, multiple samples of the abscess content were also taken out and counted.

## RESULTS

### In vitro studies

In general 40–45% of the human leukocytes in the initial blood sample were recovered in the final suspension, corresponding to $50\times10^6$ leukocytes but only $5\times10^6$ red cells. Labelling efficiency was therefore 30–35% in normal blood. The label released at 24 h was about 25%. Therefore the preparation should be used immediately after labelling. The high affinity of pyrophosphate for the red cells constitutes a serious problem. It is therefore imperative in this technique to remove the red cells before labelling. The same chemotaxis was observed before and after labelling (Table 70.2).

Electron microscope examination revealed no major abnormality in the nuclei or the cytoplasm of most granulocytes. The only abnormality observed was a relative degranulation of neutrophils, although eosinophils were normal (Figure 70.1). The metabolic test values were at the lower limit of normal, and the viability of these labelled white cells was thus obvious.

### Animals studies

*In vitro* controls show dog leukocytes to be normal, as concerns metabolic activity and chemotaxis. The morphological appearance on the electron micro-

**Table 70.2** Chemotaxis tests results

| | *A* *Stimulated migration* | *B* *Spontaneous migration* | *A/B* *Chemotactic index* | *A–B* *Chemotactic differential* |
|---|---|---|---|---|
| Normal control cells | 5.85 | 2.31 | 2.75 | 3.54 |
| (8) $X \pm$ SD | ± 0.75 | ± 0.85 | ± 0.78 | ± 0.72 |
| Labelled cells | 5.69 | 2.48 | 2.37 | 3.21 |
| $X \pm$ SD | ± 0.76 | ± 0.54 | ± 0.43 | ± 0.58 |

Normal: index = 2.9 ± 0.73 (2 < index < 4).

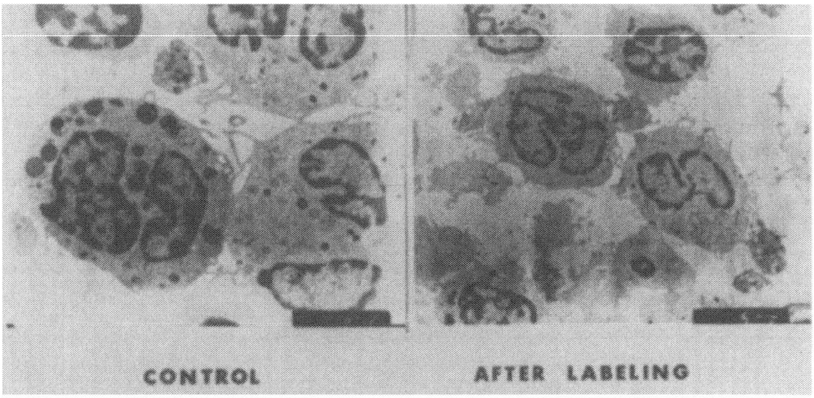


**Figure 70.1** Morphological appearance of PMN before and after labelling

scope is satisfactory. In normal dogs, blood sample analysis showed a progressive disappearance of the radioactive label, following a biexponential pattern. The half-life of the first one was not calculated since it is very short. The half-life of the second exponential is about 12 hr.

In abscess bearing dogs the same data are noted concerning blood, urine and organ accumulation. Abscess accumulation of radioactivity is clearly identified after 3 h but increases to a maximum after 6 h. The abscessed-leg/normal-leg activity ratio varies from 3.0 to 4. Hyperactivity is not related to hyperemia since the [$^{113m}$In]siderophillin study shows a decreased surface activity on the abscessed leg, the ratio being 1/12 (Figure 70.2). Abscess dissection shows significant necrosis. Abscess fluid radioactivity is always higher than blood or muscle tissue activity, and the ratios vary between 1.5 and 3.

## DISCUSSION

### Cell specificity

The separation technique used resulted in a final product rich in granulocytes but the monocytes were not eliminated. Several methods of removing red

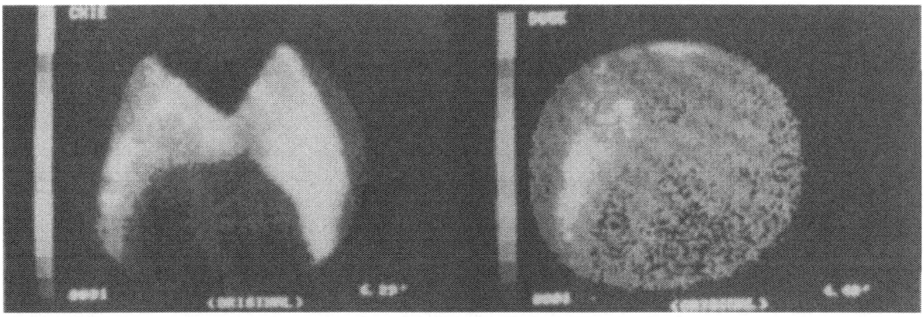

**Figure 70.2** Tc abscessed leg visualization, compared with hypoactivity using [$^{113m}$In]transferrin injection

cells without damaging white cells have been described in the literature. The most satisfactory was the $NH_4Cl$ method, as described by Gray[8], which was the technique chosen for this study.

**Viability tests**

The results obtained for labelled cells are satisfactory but not completely normal. Chemotaxis of the labelled cells was positive, but raises an important question. Are the cells which are observed to move, labelled or not? Another possibility is that they might not be labelled homogeneously, in which case unlabelled cells still move towards the attractant, but labelled cells could not. We are now trying to verify these facts.

**Comparisons to other labelling techniques**

The oxin-In method, as described by Thakur[9] is now widely used. Uptake of the labelling agent is high and it remains strongly bound to the cells[2,3]. The chemical pattern of the uptake is well understood[9]. However, this technique means placing the living cells for quite a long period in an acid medium, corresponding to very unphysiological conditions. The results will be soon published.

The $^{99m}$Tc method chosen here is not completely atoxic[10], but toxicity to labelled cells seems low, and the functional behaviour of the leukocytes does not seem to be affected.

**In vivo utilization**

Polymorphonuclear cells viability cannot be assessed completely using only *in vitro* tests. *In vivo* studies remain, of course, necessary to fully appreciate the functional value of these cells. Moreover, results may be different from normal and for blood from infected patients or patients with haematological diseases.

**Abscess visualization**

The most important point remains abscess visualization, with an abscess/

normal ratio between 3.0 and 4.0 to 1. The blood supply to the abscessed region, as assessed by [$^{113m}$In]transferrin immediate accumulation, is low (Figure 70.2). This is unusual but can be related to the large amount of necrosis in this poorly delineated aseptic abscess, the appearance of which is very peculiar. This low blood supply might prevent leukocytes from getting to the lesion and the fair value of the uptake.

There is no significant accumulation of radioactivity in the central region of the abscess. Therefore, counting rates on the pus itself are low. The major part of the activity actually lies in the peripheral region. The results might be different in other kinds of abscesses, especially septic ones. They may also be related to the duration between the turpentine injection and the scan.

## CONCLUSION

The method we propose may permit in man, as in dog, production of high activity labelled white cells. Functional properties and chemotaxis *in vitro* are maintained. This method is easy to perform, needs only 20 ml blood samples, and uses as a marker $^{99m}$Tc.

In aseptically provoked abscesses there is an obvious increase in local radioactivity in spite of a decreased local blood supply. Therefore, scintigraphic demonstration of such foci is easy. Cellular microscopic autoradiograms are now being used in order to identify which white cells are labelled and the labelling site.

This suspension can be used not only to detect infections or inflammatory foci using scintigraphic techniques, but also to quantify inflammatory processes and other phenomenon including cell migration. It would be possible, coupling cellular countings with radioactive countings, to study leukocyte pools or quantify cell migration through skin windows.

### References


1 Linhart, N., Bok, B., Gougerot, M., Gaillard, M. T., Meignan, M. (1979). Tc 99m labelled human leukocytes: an *in vitro* functional study, *Acta Haematol.*

2 Mc Afee, J. G. and Thakur, M. L. (1976). Survey of radioactive agents for *in vitro* labeling of phagocytic leukocytes. I. Soluble agents. *J. Nucl. Med.* **17**, 480

3 Mc Afee, J. G., and Thakur, M. L. (1976). Survey of radioactive agents for *in vitro* labeling of phagocytic leukocytes. II, Particles. *J. Nucl. Med.*, **17**, 488

4 Dresch, C. and Najean, Y. (1967). Étude de la cinétique des polynucléaires après marquage 'in vitro' par le radiochrome. Étude critique de la méthode et résultats obtenus chez les sujets normaux. *Nouv. Rev. Fr. Hematol.*, **7**, 17

5 Biello, D. R, Levitt, R. G. and Leland Melson, G. (1979). The roles of Gallium – 67 Scintigraphy, Ultrasonography, and computed tomography in the detection of abdominal abscesses. *Semin. Nucl. Med.*, **9**,

6 Cutler, J. E. (1974). A simple *in vitro* method for studies on chemotaxis. *Proc. Soc. Exp. Biol. Med.*, **147**, 471

7 Feliu, E. Gougerot, M. A., Hakim, J., Cramer, E., Auclair, C., Rueff, B., and Boivin, P. (1977). Blood polymorphonuclear dysfunction in patients with alcoholic cirrhosis. *Eur. J. Clin. Invest.*, **7**, 571

8 Gray, H. W., Tsan, M. F. and Wagner, H. N., Jr (1977). A quantitative study of leukocyte cohesion. Effects of divalent cations and pH. *J. Nucl. Med.*, **18**, 147
9 Thakur, M. L., Segal, A. W., Louis, L., Welch, M. J. and Peters, T. J. (1977). Indium 111 labeled cellular blood components: mechanism of labeling with special reference to studies with human neutrophils. *J. Nucl. Med.*, **18**, abstract 619
10 Parmentier, C., Chavaudra, J. and Meignan, M. (1978). Dose received by lymphocytes in the course of labeling techniques using Tc 99m. *J. Nucl. Med.*, **19**, 223

# 71

# Knee rheumatoid synovitis (KRS) successfully treated with intra-articular rifamycin SV (Abstract)

I. CARUSO, F. MONTRONE, M. FUMAGALLI,
D. DELL'ACQUA AND E. LORA (ITALY)

The effects of intra-articular rifamycin SV on rheumatoid synovitis were evaluated in two studies, open and double-blind versus saline solution. All together, 35 patients were treated with 250–500mg weekly (maximum 10 weeks). Synovial fluid analysis (SFA), clinical activity assessment (CA) and needle biopsy (NB) were performed before, during (SFA and CA) and after (NB) treatment; the latter at various time periods (1–28 months). 34 out of 35 patients experienced a complete disappearance of effusions and marked clinical improvement (lowering of pain and morning stiffness of 55–65%). Only 1 of 10 patients treated with saline solution showed disappearance of effusion and amelioration of clinical condition. The side effects consisted of painful local reaction (20%). In 4 patients (11%) reactions were accompanied by increase of synovial fluid and temperature rose to 38 °C; these reactions subsided within 12–24 h after infiltration. A direct correlation ($p<0.01$) was found between number of infiltration and the activity grade of synovitis. Synovial membrane showed a reduction of cellular infiltrate and an increase of newly formed connective tissue. Some experimental studies in progress suggest that rifamycin exerts an anti-mitotic effect on synovial membrane and an inhibitory action on synthesis of inflammatory mediators. The striking success of KRS suggested that rifamycin may be beneficial in PIP and MCP rheumatoid arthritis; the preliminary results of these trials are very encouraging.

# 72

# HLADR typing and rheumatoid arthritis (RA) (Abstract)

P. MERCIER, R. DALLEST AND H. ROUX (FRANCE)

31 RA patients were studied, 15 of them were sero-positve and 20 of them were women. HLADR typing was realised by using 43 antisera to identify DW 1,2,3,4,5,6,7 specificities. DW 4 specifity was identified using 7 sera, 3 of them monospecific. Results are given in the following table.

| *HLADR* | *RA* (*n*) | *n* = 31 (%) | *Controls* (*n*) | *n* = 116 (%) |
|---|---|---|---|---|
| DRW 1 | 7 | 22.58 | 23 | 19.83 |
| DRW 2 | 7 | 22.58 | 22 | 18.96 |
| DRW 3 | 4 | 12.9* | 27 | 23.27 |
| DRW 4 | 10 | 32.26*† | 15 | 12.93 |
| DRW 5 | 9 | 29.03 | 39 | 33.62 |
| DRW 6 | 7 | 22.58 | 31 | 26.72 |
| DRW 7 | 12 | 38.71 | 37 | 31.9 |
| DRW | 6 | 19.35 | 38 | 32.76 |

This work confirms the increase of DRW 4 in RA, but the level is lower than in other studies. The increase seems to correlate with a lowering of non-identified specificities. Relative risk according to Woolf is 3.206 for DRW 4 in this study. DRW 2 is not lowered and DRW 1 and DRW 7 are not increased. In the group of male RA the increase of DW 4 remains significant.

DRW 4/RA men 5/11 = 45.45 % $\chi^2 = 8.01$ $p < 0.005$ RR = 5.61
DRW 4/RA women 5/20 = 25 % $\chi^2 = 1.980$ $p$ NS RR = 2.24

# 73

# Preliminary studies comparing $^{67}Ga$ uptake with $^{99m}Tc$ uptake and clinical score in rheumatoid arthritis (Abstract)

C. B. CLAYTON, W. C. DICK, I. HOLLOWAY,
D. RAMAN, AND M. THOMPSON (UK)

Radiosotope investigations are being used increasingly in clinical rheumatology for initial diagnosis and as a means of achieving objective indices of changes in disease activity. Uptake appears to occur non-specifically both in terms of the radio-isotope selected and of the underlying cause of inflammatory disease. While the use of $^{99m}Tc$ has received some attention, the potential value of the preferential uptake of $^{67}Ga$ in inflammatory tissue has not been exploited in the study of inflamed joints. $^{67}Ga$ images of shoulders, elbows, hands and knees obtained 24 h, 48 h and 72 h after injection show marked accumulation of the isotope over the involved joints. Gallium has a different biochemical behaviour from technetium and may provide a means of detecting and studying a separate, although overlapping, aspect of the total inflammatory response.

All patients in this study had 'classical' rheumatoid arthritis, and were seropositive for IgM rheumatoid factor. Clinical assessment, $^{99m}Tc$ uptake and $^{67}Ga$ uptake profiles were obtained and repeat studies were performed 7 days later (week to week variability). In some cases data were obtained before and after an intra-articular injection of corticosteroid (required for clinical reasons) with a 1-week interval between studies. Results were compared with those obtained in normal volunteers. Patients were assessed clinically in a standard manner at the same time each day. After general medical and full rheumatological examination the following assessments were made: articular index of joint tenderness, grip strength, and clinical knee score summing pain, tenderness, swelling and stiffness. Radio-isotope measurements involved injecting 200 μCi $^{99m}$Tc pertechnetate intravenously on the morning of day one. The activity in the vicinity of each knee joint was recorded continuously for the first 30 min following injection and a thigh count was obtained immediately thereafter. 1.24 mCi [$^{67}$Ga]citrate (2.5 mCi when imaging was intended) was injected intravenously on the afternoon of day one. Knee uptakes were recorded for 30 min thereafter as for $^{99m}$Tc. 5 min counts over the knees and thighs were obtained on each of the next three days. It was concluded that:

(1) $^{67}$Ga count rates were elevated over inflamed joints and fell in parallel with clinical indices during therapeutically-induced amelioration in the activity of the inflammatory process.

(2) $^{67}$Ga plateau count rate reflected changes in clinical index better than did the early rate of uptake.

(3) $^{67}$Ga uptake profiles reflected a function distinct from $^{99m}$Tc studies and from clinical assessment.

(4) There was wide dispersal of measured values and heterogeneity among patients. Therefore it was important to examine the results for individual patients separately.

(5) The role of $^{67}$Ga in the assessment of joint disease deserves further study based upon a more complete knowledge of the intermediary metabolic process involved.

# Discussion

**Dr E. C. Huskisson (Chairman)** invited Dr Buckland-Wright to describe his X-ray studies of arthritis.

**Dr J. C. Buckland–Wright (UK)** had used a microfocal X-ray unit to produce high definition radiographs of guinea pig knee joints which were then used as a model for experimentally induced arthritis following the methods of Dumonde and Glynn. The procedure allowed direct measurement from the radiograph with quantification of changes over time, both erosive changes and measurement of osteoporosis. Erosive changes were measured by following the increase in intercondylar distance; the latter were monitored by following the loss of trabeculae. Having established the time course of inflammatory changes, attempts were then made to study the influence of drugs on the process, but such investigations were of limited success, possibly because the model produced too marked an arthritis for the drugs to be effective.

**Dr C. Cashin (UK)** said that the drugs used included chloroquine, aspirin, dexamethasone and D-penicillamine, all in what would be considered normal therapeutic doses for the guinea pig. Dosing was commenced 5 days before challenge with the antigen and continued for 28 days. The most significant changes observed had been exacerbation of the X-ray picture with penicillamine and to a lesser extent with aspirin. Such changes were not observable using conventional measurements of knee swelling or joint flexion. They were perhaps not surprising since the literature contained reports of potentiation of T cell mediated hypersensitivity reactions occasioned by penicillamine. So far they had not studied the effects of anti-inflammatory drugs which had been reported to stop erosive changes in adjuvant arthritis.

**Dr F. Wong (USA)** had used alizarin red staining rather than X-rays to study bone changes in adjuvant arthritis and had found that such bone changes could be decreased by appropriate period of drug treatment.

**Dr Buckland–Wright** accepted that this was so. However, their own particular model had not been successful for showing drug responses. Possibly the drugs might not have had any effect in the guinea pig. The antigen might have been inappropriate, the dosage wrong, or the experimentally induced arthritis might have induced so severe a response that the drugs were ineffective. He had established radiographically that guinea pigs which had been sensitized but had not received a subsequent challenge dose still showed such erosive changes. This argued for early development of the arthritis but they had examined it only at a much later stage.

**Dr E. Munthe (Norway)** was invited to continue this theme by describing his own work on penicillamine. He said that early investigations had shown that labelled penicillamine slowly penetrated into red cells *in vitro*. This led them to examine the *in vitro* effects of the drug during the treatment of rheumatoid arthritis. Since it was a thiol and since glutathione was the most important non-protein thiol found intracellularly, they speculated that penicillamine might undergo some reductive change during treatment. They therefore measured the *in vitro* concentrations of reduced glutathione in blood from patients before and during treatment with penicillamine. In patients responding well to penicillamine they observed an increase of 20–30% in glutathione levels in the red cells after 3 weeks of treatment, although the clinical effect usually became apparent only after 2–3 months. Patients not responding to penicillamine showed no similar increase. Patients deteriorating on penicillamine treatment often showed decrease in red cell glutathione levels. The effect could not be observed *in vitro* when red cells were incubated with penicillamine and so it was apparently an *in vitro* phenomenon. It did not however, appear to be specific for penicillamine. In a few cases it had also been observed after 4–6 weeks of treatment with levamisole and a rise of 10–15%, 24 h after intramuscular injection of corticosteroids, had also been observed. This latter rise normalized after 2–3 days. They were pursuing this work as a possible means of separating responders and non-responders to penicillamine. He agreed with the Chairman that so few phenomena correlated with the drug response that these results were particularly interesting. Unfortunately, however, no other biochemical parameters appeared to correlate. He could not explain the phenomenon. Perhaps it was due to liberation of glutathione from protein binding or perhaps to some other biochemical disturbance. The real challenge, of course, was to examine glutathione in cells other than erythrocytes and they had so far been able to correlate these changes in leukocytes and red cells from one patient. The fact that there tended to be a fall in glutathione levels during active disease phases implied that each individual had his own normal range of glutathione levels and one had to use each individual as his own control.

**Dr Winter (USA)** said that this raised the question of cause and effect. It was possible that one was overcoming disease activity through some other mechanism and as the patient's disease became less active his glutathione level increased to normal. However, he agreed that this was probably not likely because the rise preceded the clinical improvement.

**Dr M. Cutulo (Italy)** described his studies of serum copper levels in rheumatoid arthritis. He had taken three groups of patients, the first untreated, the second treated with non-steroidal anti-inflammatory agents and the third treated with non-steroidal drugs plus d-penicillamine. A healthy control group was also examined, and serum copper levels were assessed in all of them. Levels in the untreated patients were greater than those in patients on non-steroidal anti-inflammatory drugs which in turn were greater than for those on non-steroidals plus penicillamine. Levels in this third group were lower than those in the healthy controls. Significant correlation were found between serum copper levels and sero-reactive proteins in the untreated and non-steroidal treated groups but no such correlation was found in the group on combined treatment, probably because penicillamine was a potent chelator which would decrease serum copper levels. In the untreated rheumatoid group there was an inverse correlation between copper and haemoglobin concentration, a fact consistent with other data which showed an inverse correlation between serum levels of copper and iron. Increases in serum copper were also known to occur in other conditions such as infectious disease, rheumatic fever and thyrotoxicosis.

**Dr W. E. Smith (UK)** was invited to describe his related work on total serum copper levels in rheumatoid arthritis. Using a rat model of adjuvant arthritis they had then found not only that copper levels were raised but that the activity of the copper in plasma did not bear a constant relationship to its amount. They believed that this effect might involve ceruloplasmin, an active oxidase, sometimes described as a peroxidase. On transferring their studies to human patients it became clear that at high copper levels there was a fall in the percentage of ceruloplasmin in the serum. They also measured the ultrafilterable copper levels. However, the difference between the amount of ceruloplasmin present and the total serum copper did not seem to be fully accounted for by ultrafilterable copper. Some other factors seemed to be present, the nature of which was not, so far, clear. However, this and other considerations suggested that the blood and associated cells appeared to be in a more oxidized configuration in rheumatoid arthritis than in normal cases.

**Dr Wong** had had difficulty in showing any effect of auranofin in the adjuvant arthritis model and he wondered whether Dr Smith had succeeded in finding an appropriate therapeutic dose.

**Dr Smith** said that the amounts that they had been using, 10–30 mg/kg, had been considerably higher than the levels used in clinical cases.

**Dr D. R. Blake (UK)** described his work on serum ferritin and its relationship to disease activity in rheumatoid arthritis. He said that the role of ferritin as an index of iron stores had been the subject of much debate. Although serum ferritin might accurately reflect iron stores in normal individuals, its level had been found to be disproportionately raised in relation to such stores in patients with rheumatoid arthritis, especially when serum ferritin was compared with bone marrow ferritin. They had been interested in studying the relationship between synovial fluid ferritin and various disease parameters. The finding of ferritin within synovial cells had been made in Australia more than 5 years ago and it was therefore no surprise to find ferritin within the synovial fluid. Such levels correlated very well with various laboratory parameters of disease but no similar correlation could be found with serum ferritin. However, ferritin levels were found to be particularly high in patients with extra-articular features of rheumatoid disease compared to those without such features. Immune complex levels were also high in these patients. Iron derived from red cells was in the ferrous form. It was taken up by the reticulo-endothelial system and oxidized to the ferric form, a reaction believed to liberate either the peroxide or the superoxide. His group would suggest the liberation of either of these oxides caused further reticulo-endothelial cell dysfunction, which would account for the inability of these cells (synovial cells among them) to catabolize the immune complexes detected in C1q binding assays, i.e. high molecular weight complexes also associated with the presence of extra-articular features.

**Dr V. Duquesnoy (France)** reported on his investigations which were intended to detect $\beta_2$-microglobulin ($\beta_2$m) and to study its correlation with other parameters. They had found high levels both in sera and synovial fluid in rheumatoid patients compared with controls. In particular, the ratio of synovial to serum $\beta_2$m was much higher in the rheumatoid patients. This raised level showed a weak correlation with ESR. There was also a correlation with the circulating immune complexes detected by the C1q binding test but only in the sero-negative rheumatoid arthritis group. Other studies showed the existence of anti-$\beta_2$m activity in both sero-positive and sero-negative patients. The possible role of this activity in the inflammatory response required further investigation.

**Dr M. C. Linhart (France)** described his investigations with labelled polymorphonuclear leukocytes (PMN). He said that such cells were often used in the detection of infectious foci, but their viability had been questioned. He had used a new labelling technique involving $^{99m}$Tc in which viability and functional activity of the cells was assessed by metabolic and EM studies and shown to be normal. The most important question was whether the labelled cells would move to infectious foci as easily as unlabelled ones. *In vitro* chemotaxis was therefore assessed in agarose and was positive. Cell migration *in vivo* was also examined and radioactive accumulation in abscesses in dogs was seen after 3 h. In this respect, the method was superior to labelling with radioactive indium. $^{99m}$Technetium-labelled cells appeared to retain both their functional and their migratory capacities.

**Dr I. Caruso (Italy)** described his work with rifamycin in the treatment of rheumatoid synovitis of the knee. 72 patients had been treated with 250–500 mg weekly and synovial fluid analysis together with clinical assessment, was carried out before, during and after treatment. All patients treated with rifamycin showed complete disappearance of effusions and marked clinical improvement although only one of 10 patients treated with a saline control solution showed similar effects. Side effects of rifamycin consisted of a painful local reaction in 20%. The synovial membrane in treated patients showed a reduction of cellular infiltrate and an increase of newly formed connective tissue.

**Dr W. C. Dick (UK)** gave an account of his investigations attempting to follow the changes occurring in rheumatoid arthritis using different markers. They had found that uptake of $^{67}Ga$ was elevated in inflamed joints and subsequently reduced, although not to normal values, when the condition improved either naturally or in response to treatment. Subsequently they had performed simultaneous investigations using $^{99m}Tc$ and $^{67}Ga$. The two markers reflected different aspects of the process of chronic inflammation, and it was futile to debate which was the better. In addition however, the possibility existed of using anions, monovalent cations and various other markers and so such studies should be regarded as part of a comprehensive programme and not simply a series of individual investigations. Gallium uptake was a complex process. It could be found free, bound to transferrin, albumin or lactoferrin. In each case it moved at a different rate and their task at present was to carry out distributional studies to understand this complexity. Some gallium was localized in leukocytes but it was oversimplistic to imagine that all of it was. In conclusion, he wished to make the general point that the role of many individual molecules had been discussed, but in his view real progress would only be made when it was possible to measure them dynamically and simultaneously, and hence obtain an overall picture of the changes that were occurring.

# Section VII

# Immune Aspects

CHAIRMAN: T. L. Vischer
CO-CHAIRMAN: M. Glatt

# 74

# Macrophage activation by *Listeria*-specific T cell sub-populations (Abstract)

S. H. E. KAUFMANN, M. M. SIMON
AND H. HAHN (W. GERMANY)

Specific interaction of inflammatory T cells with intracellular bacteria (or bacterial antigens) and macrophages *in vivo* results in macrophage activation and granuloma formation, parallelled by delayed-type hypersensitivity reactions. Using the listeriosis model in mice, we have studied the Lyt phenotype(s) of inflammatory T cells involved in macrophage activation both *in vitro* and *in vivo*. Specific inflammatory T cells from *Listeria*-infected mice were purified on nylon wool columns and selected for sub-populations by treatment with anti-Lyt antisera and complement. Inflammatory T cells involved in protection to Listeria organisms and in delayed-type hypersensitivity to listerial antigens were of the Lyt 123 phenotype. Participation of other Lyt T cell sub-sets *in vivo* could not be ruled out. *In vitro* interaction of *Listeria*-specific inflammatory T cells with listerial antigen and macrophages resulted in macrophage activation, as assessed by the production of mitogenic protein. These *in vitro* data indicate that macrophage activation is accomplished by Lyt 1 T cells rather than Lyt 123 T cells. However, participation of Lyt 123 T cells appears likely.

# 75

# Activation of mouse peritoneal macrophages and of the alternative pathway of the complement system by cartilage specific collagen type II

H. U. SCHORLEMMER, H. HANAUSKE-ABEL
AND B. F. PONTZ (W. GERMANY)

## INTRODUCTION

Chronic inflammatory reactions are of considerable medical importance all over the world. Chronic inflammation is accompanied by tissue degradation and repair. The degradation is especially important in the connective tissues of joints, where loss of articular cartilage and bone results in the pain and deformity of rheumatoid arthritis. The fibrosis associated with repair is a major factor in the pathogenesis of cirrhosis and other conditions. It is also prominent in rheumatoid synovia, especially during the later stage of the disease.

Destruction of cartilage by inflammatory processes is characteristic of several types of arthritis. To explain the pathogenesis of such destruction of cartilage it is necessary to define the cells capable of degrading the normal substrates of cartilage matrix. The macrophage is the characteristic cell type in chronic inflammatory responses[1,2]. The loose connective tissues of rheumatoid synovia are densely infiltrated with mononuclear cells, both lymphocytes and macrophages[3]. In the pannus which overlies areas of cartilage and bone destruction, macrophages are numerous. In considering the pathogenesis of rheumatoid arthritis and other diseases in which chronic inflammation is prominent, it is therefore essential to analyse the part played by macrophages.

Increased levels of lysosomal enzymes have been identified in many of chronic inflammatory lesions. The co-existence of some components generated by destruction of connective tissue in sites of inflammation suggests that they may influence the enzyme secretion. In view of the histopathology of the lesions, it was inevitable that the possibility of some auto-immune reactions should be considered in this condition.

Support for this was obtained in the case of rheumatoid arthritis by the demonstration, using specific immunofluorescent staining, of immunoglobulin and bound complement within the nodules[4]. Furthermore, the actual breakdown of collagen in the necrotic areas of the granulomata, especially conspicuous in rheumatoid nodules, draws attention to collagen itself as a possible source of the components involved. The so-called collagen diseases are the most obvious conditions in which immunological involvement of collagen itself might be expected. These immunologically mediated reactions could be amplified through the complement, clotting or kallicrein systems. Studies of collagen–complement interaction have shown that collagens from several vertebrates are able to inactivate human complement. Takahashi *et al.*[5] have presented data to show that there is a factor present in insoluble as well as soluble collagen and which depletes complement by the alternative pathway. The immunopathological significance of collagen interactions with the complement and other systems is not clear but since we have previously shown that the macrophage as a prominent cell type in chronic inflammatory lesions can be stimulated by complement components to produce enzymes, it was of interest to determine whether collagen was involved in the activation of these cells.

## RESULTS

### Influence of different collagen types on complement activation

All the collagen types investigated in this study were tested for their ability to activate complement in two different assay systems using C4 deficient guinea pig serum: (a) loss of haemolytically active C3, and (b) immunoelectrophoretic conversion of C3 and factor B of the alternative pathway. For comparison the C3 turnover was also checked in normal guinea pig serum or in some cases in human serum. Collagens have been tested over a wide range of concentrations in the haemolytic assay using normal and C4 deficient guinea pig serum. After incubation for 30 min at 37 °C remaining haemolytic C3 activity was measured. A significant C3 turnover could be induced in both sera (Figure 75.2). The dose response curves in C4 deficient guinea pig serum were very similar to those obtained in normal serum. Hence, C3 activation must have occurred mainly via the alternative pathway of the complement system.

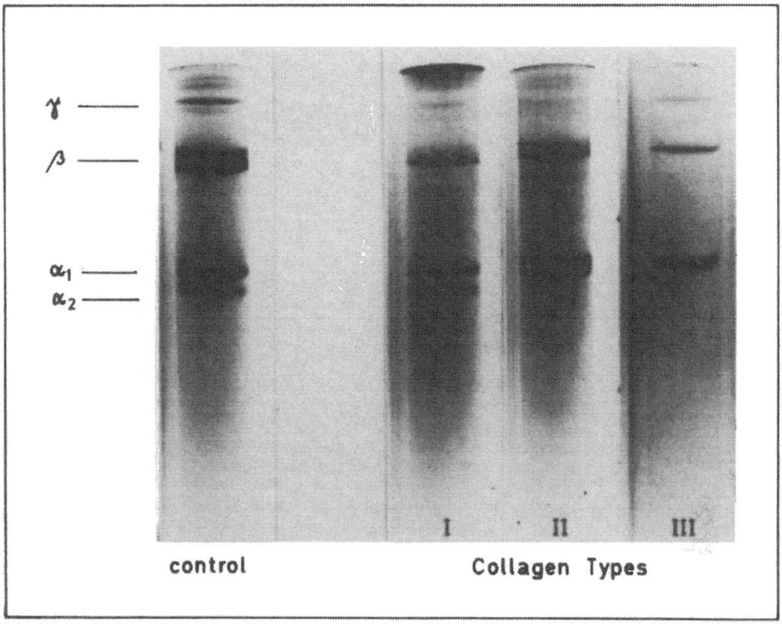


**Figure 75.1** Purity of the collagen types used. Type I, II, and III give their specific pattern with type III reduced and alkylated

As can be seen, collagen type III does not induce C3 consumption whereas both preparations, collagen type I and type II, lead to a clear C3 turnover although quantitative differences were observed. Increasing concentrations of type I and type II induced increasing C3 consumption. Comparison of the two curves showed that the amount of collagen type I necessary for maximal C3 turnover in serum differed from that of collagen type II; collagen type II required smaller amounts than type I. The minimal dose required for 50% C3 consumption in normal guinea pig serum is for collagen II about 40 μg/ml and for collagen type I about 400 μg/ml. The results reported so far strongly suggest that collagen acted via the alternative pathway of complement activation since the two collagens consume C3 in C4 deficient guinea pig serum although both collagen type I and collagen type II were clearly more effective in normal serum than in C4 deficient serum, reflecting a possible participation of antibody-C142-mediated activation of C3. As further evidence for the concept of complement activation via the alternative pathway, the conversion of C3 by collagen in normal and C4 deficient guinea pig serum was examined immuno-electrophoretically. To make sure that the reported effects of collagens are not only limited to one species we tested the substances in human serum also reaching essentially the same results. As can be seen in

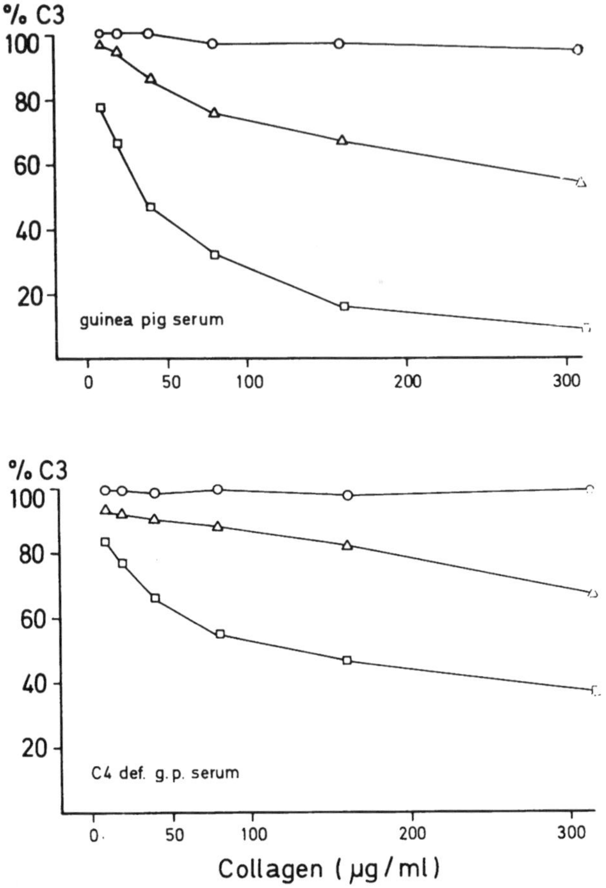


**Figure 75.2** C3 turnover in normal and C4 deficient guinea pig serum as a function of the collagen concentrations. ○ collagen type III, △ collagen type I and □ collagen type II

Figure 75.3 there was a strong conversion of C3 and also of factor B, again classifying collagen as an alternative pathway activating substance.

**The capacity of different collagens to induce the release of hydrolytic enzymes from macrophages in culture**

Marked changes in the levels and distribution of activities of acid hydrolases were induced in mouse peritoneal macrophages by collagen. Two types of experiments were performed. First, the effect of various concentrations of collagen on the levels and distribution of enzyme activity in macrophage cultures after 24 h was measured. Second, the effect of a single concentration of collagen on the time course of changes in enzyme level and distribution was

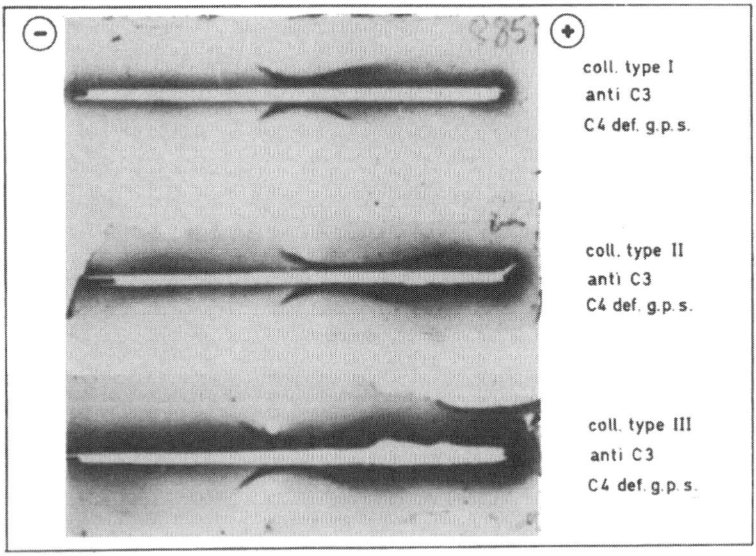


**Figure 75.3** Immuno-electrophoretic conversion of the complement component C3 in C4 deficient guinea pig serum induced by different collagen types

determined. In macrophage cultures grown in the presence of various concentrations of collagen type II for a period of 24 h, there was a dose-dependent selective release of acid hydrolases from the cells into the culture medium with a concurrent increase of the total lysosomal enzyme activity; however, the intracellular acid hydrolase content was not changed (Figure 75.4). In separate experiments it was shown that the selective release of acid hydrolases was also time dependent, with the majority of enzyme release occurring within 24 h of adding collagen type II to the cultures. In contrast, collagen type III does not cause any release of acid hydrolases from macrophages over a 48 h period at concentrations up to 200 μg/ml. Collagen type I shows intermediate activity in inducing release of acid hydrolases from mononuclear phagocytes; there is still a release of about 25%. That the release of lysosomal enzymes from macrophages induced by collagen is selective is shown in Figure 75.5. It is clear that none of the doses of collagen used result in increase in the activity of the cytoplasmic enzyme lactate dehydrogenase in the culture medium. In fact, in the presence of collagen type II slight increases in cellular levels of lactate dehydrogenase are observed, a further indication of their viability despite the selective release of a large proportion of their lysosomal enzymes.

**Induction of macrophage mediated cytotoxicity induced by collagen**

Purified collagen was added to mouse macrophages that had been recovered

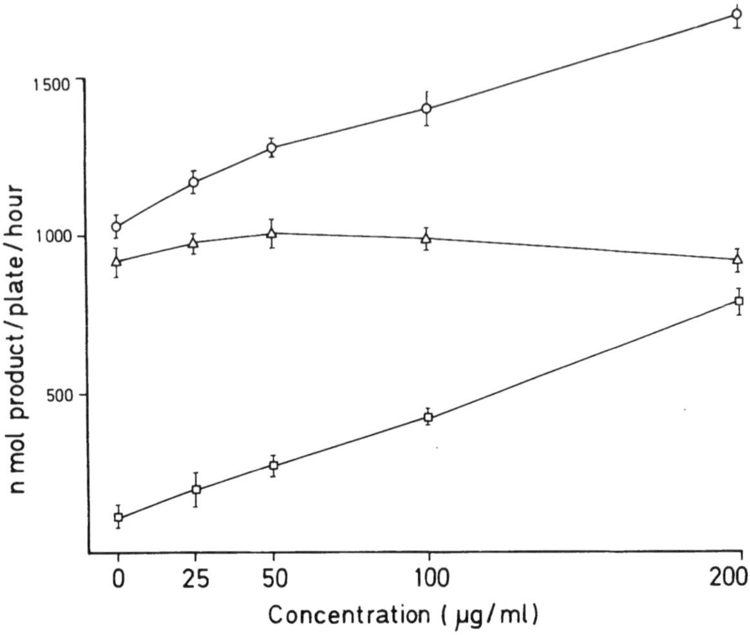


**Figure 75.4** The dose-dependent effect of collagen type II on the levels of N-acetyl-β-D-glucosaminidase in macrophage cultures. ○ Total enzyme activity, △ enzyme activity in the cells and □ enzyme activity released into the culture medium

from the peritoneal cavities without prior stimulation and cultured in serum-free medium. As can be seen, unstimulated macrophages did not kill tumour cells; however, macrophages incubated with collagen type II (100 μg/ml) lysed all or nearly all of the P815 mastocytoma cells at an effector cell to target ratio of 10:1. When the ratio of macrophages to tumour cells was reduced to 2:1 most tumour cells were still killed. Thus, stimulated macrophages could kill tumour cells by direct contact, by the release of a lytic factor or factors, or by a combination of both mechanisms. The presence of a lytic factor in the culture media of stimulated macrophages has been found in all our experiments. After cultivation of the macrophages for 48 h, the cytotoxic activity in the culture media for P815 cells was significantly greater than in the controls. Other collagens were unable to stimulate *in vitro* macrophages to be tumourolytic.

In further experiments the effect of various concentrations of collagen type II on the cytotoxic activity of macrophage cultures after 48 h was measured. The media from the activated macrophage cultures were mixed with the target cells and the mixture incubated for a further 2 h. Samples were taken for measuring the release of lactate dehydrogenase of the target cells into the

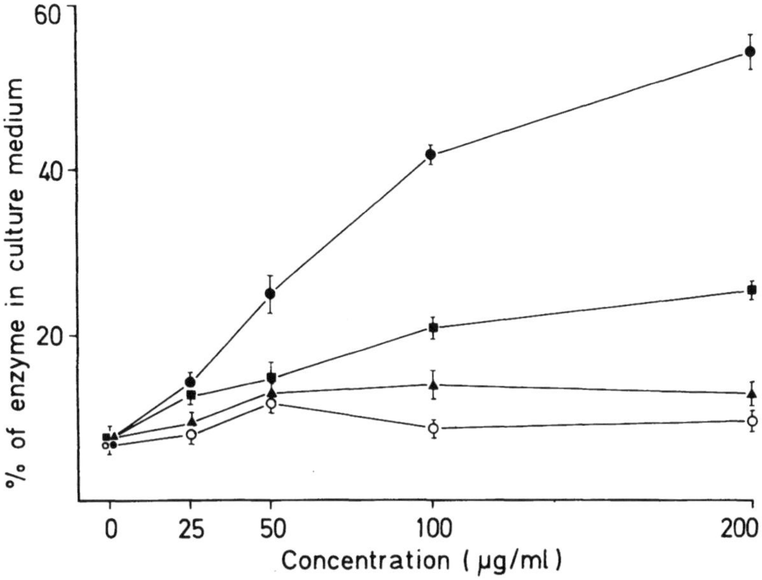


**Figure 75.5** Release of β-glucuronidase into the culture medium of mouse macrophages after exposure to increasing amounts of different collagens. ● collagen type II, ■ collagen type I, ▲ collagen type III and ○ represents release of lactate dehydrogenase into the culture medium

medium above background level. The results shown in (Figure 75.6) establish that in macrophage cultures grown in the presence of various concentrations of collagen type II for 48 h, there was a dose-dependent tumourolytic effect on the tumour target cells used. This dose-dependent activity increases such that with 100 and 200 µg/ml nearly complete release of the cytoplasmic enzyme lactate dehydrogenase is obtained.

We also examined the effect of varying the type of target cells on the degree of cytolysis obtained using macrophages treated in a constant manner. The tumour cells used were P815 mastocytoma, EL4 lymphoma, strain Raji from Burkitts lymphoma and Ml, a macrophage-like cell line. They were incubated with the culture supernatants of stimulated macrophages as described above. When these various target cells were challenged with the collagen-activated macrophage supernatants, the level of cytolysis varied markedly. The mastocytoma P815 cell could be lysed impressively to about 95%. Raji and EL4 also exhibited a significant lysis (about 85% and 75%, respectively) whereas the macrophage cell line Ml tested under the same conditions could be killed to only 55% (Figure 75.6).

## DISCUSSION

It is postulated that the central event in chronic inflammation is recruitment

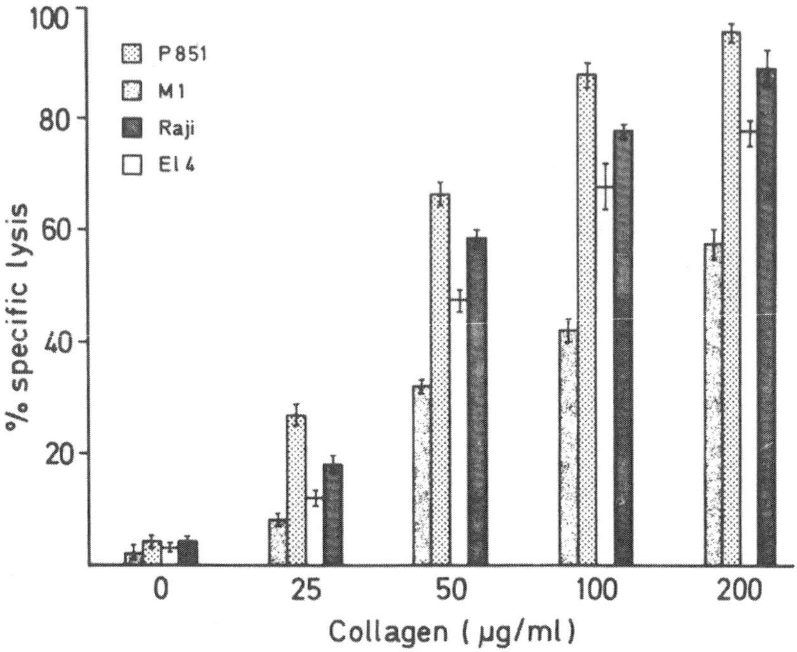


**Figure 75.6** Lysis of different tumour cell types by macrophages activated *in vitro* by various concentrations of collagen type II

of macrophages into lesions and their activation locally to become secretory cells[6,7]. Products of activated macrophages include mediators of inflammation and enzymes able to degrade tissues as well as factors promoting collagen synthesis by fibroblasts. Hence factors recruiting and activating macrophages, and the mediators and enzymes they produce, are central to understanding the pathogenesis of chronic inflammation.

The chronic inflammatory lesion characteristic of rheumatoid arthritis includes infiltration of the synovial connective tissues by mononulcear phagocytes. The presence of immune complexes as well as of collagen in these lesions is well documented[8,9] and mononuclear phagocytes interact with certain kinds of immune complexes, since they have receptors for the Fc region of the antibody molecules[10] It is well known that immune complexes can induce the selective release of hydrolases from polymorphonuclear leucocytes and mononuclear phagocytes[11] The role of macrophages in the immune response to collagen is not yet known, but they might be crucial for processing the antigen. Active participation of macrophages in resorption of tissue collagen strongly suggests the involvement of these cells in phagocytozing soluble collagen antigens.

More recent information on the possible degradation of collagen by a macrophage collagenase is based on studies by Wahl *et al.*[12] Interestingly, this collagenase can be induced by lymphokines which are released *in vitro* upon interaction with lectin. It is tempting to speculate that this type of collagenase induction also occurs *in vivo* after interaction with collagen. Binding of native or denatured collagen onto macrophages provided the first hints of a possible role in cell interaction[13]

In the study described here we tested different collagen types in their native and denatured form to see their effect of macrophage activation. Collagen type II induced the release of hydrolytic enzymes from normal mouse peritoneal macrophages cultured in a serum-free medium. This release is time- and dose-dependent and is not associated with loss of the cytoplasmic enzyme lactate dehydrogenase. In the same dose range collagen type I and type III were inactive. Collagen type II also efficiently activates complement by the alternative pathway. This is consistent with a report from Takahashi *et al.*[5] that a factor present in insoluble as well as soluble collagen depletes complement by the way of the alternative pathway. Unfortunately, no data were presented in this report relevant to the purity of the collagen preparations. This is important because several glycosaminoglycans which are likely contaminants in collagen preparations have been shown to fix complement[14]

A few remarks should be made about ways of measuring the capacity of different agents to elicit chronic inflammatory reactions. A simple method is to inject the agent into the footpad or high muscle and into knee joints of mice. After a special time the injection site is sectioned and histological examination shows the magnitude and composition of the infiltrate. The lysosomal enzyme content of the tissue at the injection site (a measure of leukocytic infiltration) gives quantitative results. An example is the demonstration by Keystone *et al.*[15] that zymosan particles elicit inflammatory responses, whereas polystyrene latex particles do not. Similar effects are seen with particles of asbestos, but not when their surface magnesium groups are removed[16] In a series of studies we have shown that a variety of agents able to elicit inflammatory responses *in vivo* increase the secretion of lysosomal enzymes in cultures of mouse peritoneal macrophages. Macrophage cultures are also known to secrete several neutral proteinases that can degrade connective tissue constituents. Horwitz and Crystal[17] found that macrophages secrete collagenase and the enzyme resembles the specific collagenase, producing two typical fragments with collagen types I, II and III. The cultured mononuclear phagocytes rapidly degrade $^{35}S$-labelled live or killed explants of ear or articular cartilage of young rabbits[18] Among the enzymes secreted by activated macrophages are neutral proteases able to degrade proteoglycan, collagen and elastin, to activate plasminogen and to cleave the native complement component C3. These enzymes are important in the pathogenesis of chronic inflammation, including the destruction of cartilage in joints and of lung substance in emphysema.

Normal macrophages synthesize and secrete intact complement components including C3 and factor B of the alternative pathway. As already discussed[19] the culture media of activated macrophages contain enzyme activity able to cleave C3. Highly purified guinea pig C3b was found to elicit a dose-dependent release of several hydrolases but not of lactate dehydrogenase with macrophages cultured in a serum-free medium[20]. We have suggested[21] that a common factor in macrophage stimulation is activation of complement by the alternative pathway. An early consequence of the activation is cleavage of the complement component C3 into a small fragment C3a and a large fragment C3b. Macrophages have a surface receptor for C3b[22] and attachment of C3b to the receptor is followed by activation of the cells. When the macrophages are stimulated by a variety of agents that induce chronic inflammation *in vivo*, the cells release proteolytic enzymes that cleave their own C3 to produce more C3b, so that serial activation can occur. The C3b formed is able to activate other macrophages whereas the C3a released appears to be important in the tumourolytic effects of macrophages as well as having some microbicidal functions[23,24] As an anaphylatoxin triggering the release of mast cell granule contents, C3a also plays a role in the pathogenesis of inflammation. The C3b formed not only activates macrophages further, but also could trigger the cascade of reactions of the terminal complement sequence. Activated complement components (C3a, C5a, C567) are chemotactic for macrophages, recruiting more cells into the lesions. It seems that three mechanisms for activating complement must be distinguished: activation of the classical pathway through C1, C4, and C2 to cleave C3; activation of the alternative pathway via C3b, factor B, factor D and properdin to cleave C3; and activating macrophages to cleave C3. The C3b released can combine with factor B of the alternative pathway to produce C3bBb which cleaves more C3 in a humoral amplification system. Moreover, since C3b can activate macrophages to release further C3b, a cellular amplification system also exists.

Here we have found that mouse peritoneal macrophages in culture can be activated by collagen to secrete lysosomal enzymes. Looking for a common factor among the variety of agents that induce chronic inflammation *in vivo* and enzyme secretion *in vitro* our attention has been drawn to the fact that they activate complement by the alternative pathway. Enzyme secretion by macrophages may be important in the pathogenesis of chronic inflammation for several reasons. The first is the degradation of connective tissue constituents, including proteoglycan matrix of cartilage, collagen and elastin. The possible role of these processes in erosion of cartilage in arthritis, breakdown of connective tissue fibres in the lung and other types of degradation in and around inflammatory sites, is obvious. The role of proteinase interactions in sequential activation is again evident; neutral proteinases activating collagenase, plasminogen activator activating plasminogen and so forth. Analogous activation occurs in the complement system: once C3 is cleaved C3bBb forms a cleavage complex amplifying the system. A second role for lysosomal enzymes is the generation of inflammatory mediators, including activated complement components.

From the evidence reviewed in this paper, it is clear that complement activation, macrophage activation and secretion induced by collagen plays a central role in the pathogenesis of chronic inflammation.

**Acknowledgment**
The authors wish to thank Miss A. Börner for her excellent technical assistance.

**References**

1 Allison, A. C. (1978). Macrophage activation and nonspecific immunity. *Inter. Rev. Exp. Pathol.,* **18,** 303
2 Davies, P. and Allison, A. C. (1976). Secretion of macrophage enzymes in relation to the pathogenesis of chronic inflammation. In Nelson, D. S. (ed.) *Immunobiology of the Macrophage*, pp. 428. (New York: Academic Press)
3 Ishikawa, H. and Ziff, M. (1976). Electron microscopic observations of immunoreactive cells of the rheumatoid synovial membrane. *Arthritis Rheum.*, **19**, 1
4 Nowoslawski, A. and Brzosko, W. J. (1967). Immunopathology of rheumatoid arthritis. II. The rheumatoid nodule. *Pathol. Eur.*, **2,** 302
5 Takahashi, M., Kawachi-Takahashi, S., and Matsnura, M. (1975). Interaction of collagen with serum complement: inhibition of complement-mediated hemolysis. *Int. Arch. Allergy Appl. Immunol.,* **48,** 642
6 Page, R. C., Davies, P., and Allison, A. C. (1974). Participation of mononuclear phagocytes in chronic inflammatory diseases *J. Retic. Soc.,* **15,** 413
7 Allison, A. C., Ferluga, J., Prydz, H., and Schorlemmer, H.U. (1978). The role of macrophage activation in chronic inflammation. *Agents Actions,* **8,** 27
8 Ziff, M. (1973). Pathophysiology of rheumatoid arthritis. *Fed. Proc.*, **32,** 131
9 Spector, W. G. and Heesom, N. (1969). The production of granulomata by antigen-antibody complexes. *J. Pathol.,* **98,** 31
10 Huber, H. and Weiner, M. (1974). Binding of immune complexes to human macrophages: the role of membrane receptor sites. In Wagner, W. H. and Hahn, H. (eds.) *Activation of Macrophages,* p. 54, *(Amsterdam: Excerpta Medica)*
11 Cardella C., J., Davies, P. and Allison, A. C. (1974). Immune complexes induce selective release of lysosomal enzymes. *Nature (London),* **247,** 46
12 Wahl, L. M. Wahl, S. M., Mergenhagen, S. E. and Martin, G. R. (1974).Collagenase production by endotoxin-activated macrophages. *Proc. Natl. Acad. Sci. (USA)* **71,** 3598
13 Hopper, K. E., Adelmann, B. C., Gentner, G., and Gay, S. (1976). Recognition by guinea pig peritoneal-exudate cells of conformationally different states of the collagen molecule. *Immunology*, **30,** 249
14 Gewurz, H. and Ertel, N. (1973). Non-immune activation of complement: two new phenomena. In *Non-specific Factors Influencing Host Resistance*, p. 340
15 Keystone, E. C., Schorlemmer, H. U., Pope, C. and Allison, A. C. (1977). Zymosan-induced Arthritis. *Arthritis Rheum.*, **20,** 1396
16 Schorlemmer, H. U., Davies, P., Hylton, W., Gugig, M. and Allison, A. C. (1977). The selective release of lysosomal acid hydrolases from mouse peritoneal macrophages by stimuli of chronic inflammation. *Br. J. Exp. Pathol.,* **58,** 315
17 Horwitz, A. L. and Crystal, R. G. (1976). Collagenase from rabbit pulmonary alveolar macrophages *Biochem. Biophys. Res. Commun.*, **69,** 296
18 Hauser, P. and Vaes, G. (1978). Degradation of cartilage proteoglycans by a neutral proteinase secreted by rabbit bone marrow macrophages in culture. *Biochem. J.*, **172,** 275
19 Schorlemmer, H. U. and Allison, A. C. (1976). Effects of activated complement components on enzyme secretion by macrophages. *Immunology,* **31,** 781
20 Schorlemmer, H. U., Davies, P. and Allison, A. C. (1976). Ability of activated complement

components to induce lysosomal enzyme release from macrophages. *Nature (London)*, **261**, 48

21 Schorlemmer, H. U., Fergula, J., and Allison, A. C. (1977). Interactions of macrophages and complement components in the pathogenesis of chronic inflammation. In Willoughby, D. A., Giroud, J-P. and Velo, G. P. (eds.) *Perspectives in Inflammation*, p.191. (Lancaster: MTP Press)

22 Griffin, F. M., Bianco, C. and Silverstein, S. C. (1975). Characterization of the macrophage receptor for complement and demonstration of its functional independence from the receptor for the Fc protein of immunoglobulin G. *J. Exp. Med.*, **141**, 1269

23 Schorlemmer, H. U., Hadding, U., Bitter-Suemann, D. and Allison, A. C. (1977). The role of complement cleavage products in killing of tumour cells by macrophages. In James, K., McBride, B. and Stuart, A. (eds.) *The Macrophage and Cancer*, p. 68. (Edinburgh: Econoprint)

24 Taylor-Robinson, D., Schorlemmer, H. U., Furr, P. and Allison, A. C. (1978). Macrophage secretion and the complement cleavage product C3a in the pathogenesis of infections by mycoplasmas and L-forms of bacteria and in immunity to these organisms. *Clin. Exp. Immunol.*, **33**, 486

76

# Interaction of macrophages and synthetic polyanions in the inflammatory response

H. U. SCHORLEMMER, U. HADDING AND
D. BITTER-SUERMANN (WEST GERMANY)

## INTRODUCTION

Polyanions are, within the immunological field, of considerable interest. They exert a variety of functions on both humoral and cellular levels. Dextran sulphate (DS), for example, is known to activate the alternative pathway of complement[1,2] and interacts with components of the classical pathway[3,4]. It is known to replace T cell function and to trigger B cell activation[5,6]. In addition, polyanions gained interest because of their macrophage activating effect[7,8] and their anti-viral and anti-tumour activity[9,10]. In previous publications we described a relationship of the capacity of some polyanions such as carrageenins or dextran sulphates of different molecular weights and degrees of sulphation to induce chronic inflammatory responses *in vivo*, to activate macrophages so that they secrete enzymes and kill tumour cells[7,11,12].

To analyse this process further it is useful to have a series of related compounds of known chemical composition and biological activity. Utilizing DS as a model substance it was demonstrated that the capacity of polyanions for activation of the alternative pathway of the complement system and for activation of macrophages depends on the degree of substitution with sulphate groups, but also requires a certain minimum molecular weight of the inducing polyanion[2,7]. Polyanions with a molecular weight below 10 000 did not activate either the alternative pathway of the complement system or macrophage cultures to secrete lysosomal enzymes. In previous studies soluble polyanions were used. It is the purpose of this communication to describe the interaction of insoluble polyanions with cultured macrophages and to show an inhibitory effect of low molecular weight polyanions on the activation of macrophages by high molecular weight polyanions.

## RESULTS

### The capacity of insoluble synthetic polyanions to induce the release of lysosomal enzymes from mouse peritoneal macrophages in culture

Here we describe the interaction of insoluble polyanions, namely, sulphated Sephadex with cultured macrophages. Mouse peritoneal macrophages exposed to Sephadexsulphate show marked changes in levels and distribution of acid hydrolase activities. The magnitude of these changes depends on the time of incubation and the concentration of the sulphated Sephadex. Figure 76.1 compares the extent of the release of a representative lysosomal enzyme, β-glucuronidase with the amount of the cytoplasmic enzyme LDH in the culture medium from macrophages exposed to sulphated Sephadex G-200. The dose-dependent release of acid hydrolases from macrophages induced by these particles is shown to be selective. The level increases from a base line amount of approximately 10% of total culture activity to nearly 70% in the presence of 800 μg/ml of sulphated Sephadex G-200. Similar findings were made when two other lysosomal enzymes, namely *N*-acetyl-β-D-glucosaminidase and β-galactosidase, were assayed. There was no evidence of any cytotoxic effect of Sephadexsulphate as indicated by measurement of lactate dehydrogenase levels in cells and culture media.

Comparison of several sulphated Sephadex preparations from different G-types and differing in sulphur content, showed that the amount of Sephadex-sulphate necessary for maximal release of lysosomal enzymes differed for these preparations. As seen in Figure 76.2, some of the preparations induced selective enzyme release. Increasing Sephadexsulphate concentrations induced increased hydrolase secretion. The experiment revealed sulphated Sephadex G-200 to be the most powerful inducer. The Sephadexsulphate preparations of lower G-types proved to be less effective; sulphated Sephadex G-25, which had also the lowest sulphur content, was inactive. Non-substituted Sephadex had no effect at the same and higher concentrations.

### The time course of acid hydrolase secretion from macrophages in culture exposed to sulphated Sephadex G-200

The time course of enzyme production and release was studied in mouse macrophage cultures maintained for various times up to 72 h in the presence of a single dose of 100 μg/ml of Sephadexsulphate G-200. This time dependence of the selective release of acid hydrolases caused by the stimulus is shown in Figure 76.3. Macrophage cultures exposed to Sephadex sulphate show a change compared to control cultures in the distribution of *N*-acetyl-β-D-glucosaminidase, between cells and culture medium. By 9 h a significant

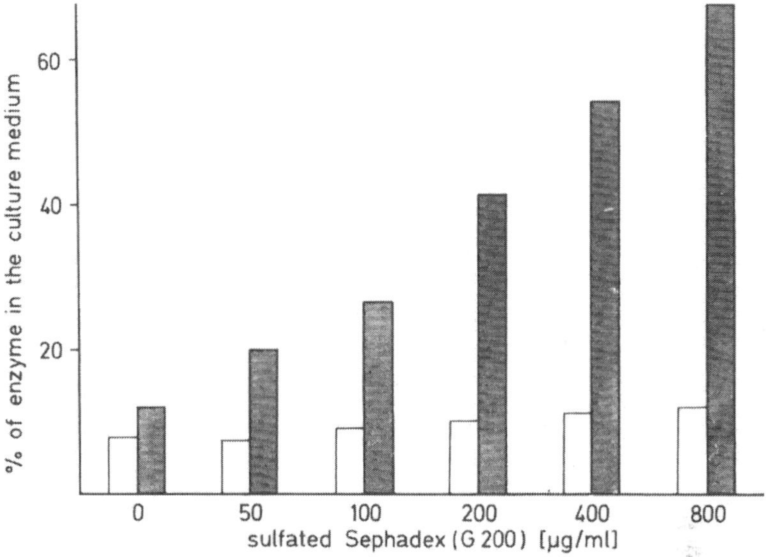


**Figure 76.1** The release of β-glucuronidase (▩) and lactate dehydrogenase (□) from macrophages cultured in a serum-free medium with increasing concentrations of sulphated Sephadex G-200. The cultures of mouse peritoneal macrophages were assayed after incubation with Sephadex sulphate G-200 for 24 h

increase in the amount of *N*-acetyl-β-D-glycosaminidase in the medium is seen. Subsequently a rapid rise in the release of enzyme into the culture medium occurs so that by 72 h approximately 60% of the total enzyme activity is found in the culture medium. This release of acid hydrolases occurs with no detectable loss of cellular lactate dehydrogenase into the culture medium and there is no decrease of cell viability at 72 h even in the absence of serum in the culture medium.

**Requirement of a minimal molecular weight for macrophage activation and the effect of low molecular polyanions on macrophage activation by various activators**

Prior to inhibition experiments, the macrophage activating capacity of the utilized batches of the various, well-known activators of polyanionic character was confirmed. Soluble dextran sulphates (400 μg/ml) of various molecular weights, polyethylene-sulphonic-acid (400 μg/ml) of different molecular weight, pentosanpolysulphate (1000 μg/ml), various preparations of carrageenin (400 μg/ml) with different numbers of sulphate groups per molecules (9.6%; 8.9% and 7.1% sulphur) and several sulphated Sephadexes of various G-types were tested. For comparison the interaction of cultured macrophages with zymosan (100 μg/ml) has been investigated. Incubation of macrophages with the activators in the given concentrations induced a selec-

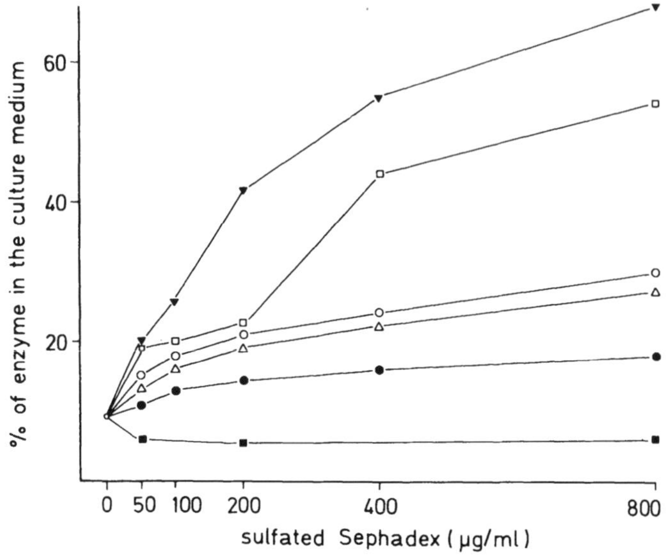


**Figure 76.2** The dose dependent effect of sulphated Sephadex preparations from different Sephadex G-types on the release of β-glucuronidase activity from macrophages into the culture medium. Sulphated Sephadex G-25 ●; G 75 △; G 100 ○; G 150 □ and G 200 ▼. Non-substituted Sephadex G-200 ■ had no effect on the enzyme secretion

tive release of lysosomal enzymes (Figure 76.4). Some polyanions, e.g., the polyethylenesulphonic-acid preparations had identical chemical composition and differed only in the molecular weight (or chain length of the molecule).

Testing the polyanion fractions listed above for their macrophage-activating capacity revealed that a certain minimum molecular weight is required for activation. Polyethylene sulphonic acid with a molecular weight of $2.8 \times 10^4$ induced enzyme secretion from macrophages. The polyanion fractions with a molecular weight below $1 \times 10^4$ (polyethylene sulphonic acid, MW $8.2 \times 10^3$, Sp 54: MW $2.8 \times 10^3$) failed to activate macrophages. These data confirm the results obtained with dextran sulphate[7] and carrageenin[11] showing that the capacity to trigger macrophage activity requires a minimal molecular weight and depends on the degree of $SO_4$ substitution. In the case of the insoluble Sephadex–sulphate preparations the activating potency depends on the degree of the G-type and the sulphur content.

In other experiments we tested whether the low molecular weight polyanions were totally inert or whether they were able to influence the action of other polyanionic stimuli which activate macrophages. Dextran sulphate (MW 500 000) was incubated with Sp 54 or polyethylene sulphonic acid (MW 8200) or sulphated Sephadex G-25 in concentrations given in Table 76.1 together with mouse peritoneal macrophages for 24 h. After incubation

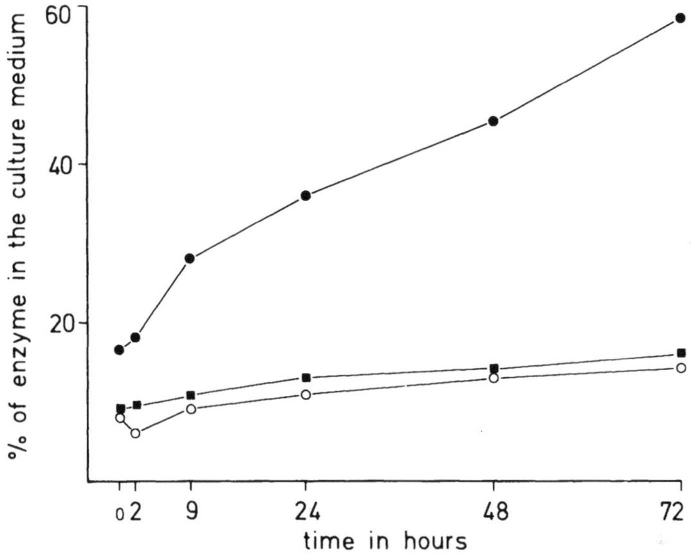


**Figure 76.3** The time dependent release of *N*-acetyl-β-D-glucosaminidase (●) and lactate dehydrogenase (○) from macrophages exposed to a single dose of 100 μg/ml of sulphated Sephadex G-200 cultivated in a serum-free medium. Controls (■) show glucosaminidase release in the absence of added particles

enzyme activity in the culture medium was determined. Dextran sulphate (MW 500 000) induced an enzyme secretion of about 45% in the absence of the low molecular weight polyanions. In the presence of the small polyanions the enzyme secretion induced by dextran sulphate (MW 500 000) was nearly completely inhibited. A similar result was obtained using sulphated Sephadex G-100 as activator and Sephadex–sulphate G-25 as inhibitor. The low molecular weight polyanions alone had no effects on macrophage activation, not even in high concentrations. The inhibitor action of the low molecular weight polyanions turned out not to be restricted to the respective homologous polyanion species but they also inhibited the inducing effect of other, different polyanions. This inhibitory action of low molecular weight polyanions is even not only restricted to act selectively on polyanionic activators but can also impair the action of non-polyanionic activators, for instance neutral polysaccharides (zymosan). Table 76.1 summarizes the data of experiments using low molecular weight polyanions as inhibitors. All activators tested were strongly inhibited in their capacity to induce enzyme secretion from cultured macrophages.

### Soluble and insoluble synthetic polyanions enable mouse peritoneal macrophages to kill tumour cells *in vitro*

Although unstimulated macrophages are not cytotoxic, macrophages stimu-

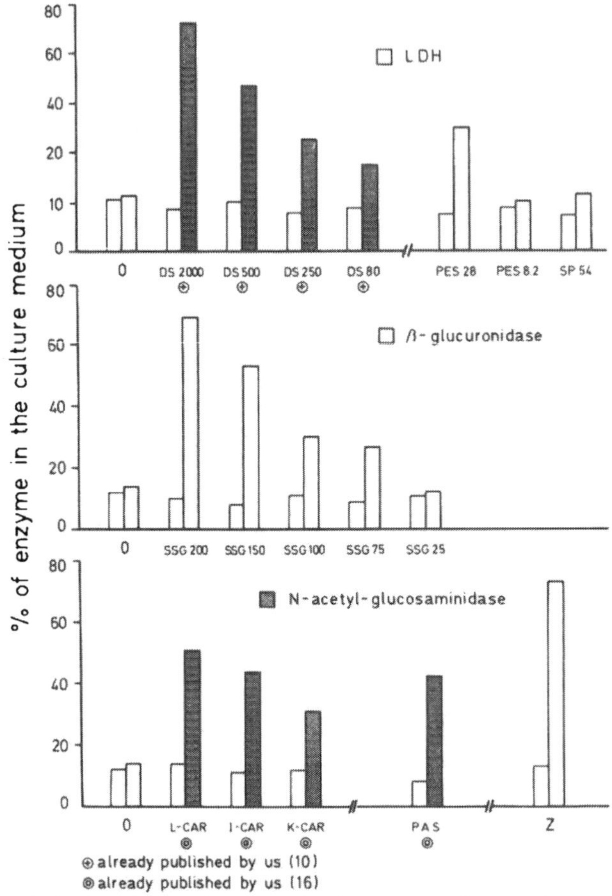


**Figure 76.4** Activation of macrophages by polyanions to secrete lysosomal enzymes depends on the degree of substitution with sulphate groups, but requires also a certain minimum molecular weight of the inducing polyanion + results already published by us O; already published in reference 11

lated *in vivo* or *in vitro* with various materials become cytotoxic. We have investigated the effect of culturing mouse peritoneal macrophages with different polyanions on the capacity of macrophages to kill tumour cells. Macrophages were recovered from the peritoneal cavities of NMRI or athymic nude (nu/nu) mice without prior stimulation and cultured in a serum-free medium to which was added, in the respective cases, the synthetic soluble or insoluble polyanions. As shown in Table 76.2, unstimulated macrophages did not increase release of LDH from the target cells into the medium above background level. However, macrophages incubated with dextran sulphate (MW 500 000) or sulphated Sephadex G-200 lysed all or nearly all the tumour

**Table 76.1** Inhibition of macrophages by low molecular weight polyanions to secrete acid hydrolases induced by various activators.

| *Macrophage activation with* | *% of the enzyme activity in the culture medium* | *Inhibited by low molecular weight polyanions* | |
|---|---|---|---|
| 0-contr | 9.8 ± 0.7 | | NT* |
| DS (500) (400 μg/ml) | 42.4 ± 2.1 | SP54 (1000 μg/ml) | 12.3 ± 0.9 |
| | | PES (8.2) (400 μg/ml) | 10.1 ± 0.4 |
| | | SS (G25) (400 μg/ml) | 18.4 ± 1.3 |
| SS (G200) (400 μg/ml) | 39.2 ± 1.7 | SS (G25) (400 μ/ml) | 10.8 ± 0.6 |
| Z (100 μg/ml) | 73.5 ± 3.2 | SS (G25) (400 μg/ml) | 38.6 ± 1.2 |

* NT: not tested

**Table 76.2** Lysis of P815 mastocytoma cells by the culture supernatants from macrophages activated *in vitro* with soluble and insoluble polyanions

| | % specific LDH release | | | |
|---|---|---|---|---|
| *Stimulating agent* | *NMRI macrophages* | | *nu/nu macrophages* | |
| | *mean* | σ | *mean* | σ |
| 0 | 12.5 | 1.7 | 7.6 | 1.7 |
| SS (G 200) (400 μg/ml) | 91.2 | 7.7 | 80.9 | 4.2 |
| SS (G 25) (400 μg/ml) | 4.3 | 0.6 | 21.7 | 0.8 |
| DS (500) (400 μg/ml) | 75.0 | 2.6 | NT* | |
| Seph (G 200) (1000 μg/ml) | 4.1 | 0.8 | NT* | |
| Z (100 μg/ml) | 83.7 | 3.0 | 81.4 | 2.1 |

* NT: not tested

cells. Stimulated macrophages could kill tumour cells by direct contact or by the release of a lytic factor (or factors). The presence of a lytic factor in the culture media of stimulated macrophages has been found in all our experiments. Macrophages from nude mice were slightly less cytotoxic than macrophages from normal mice, but they still were stimulated and the culture supernatants could kill about 80% of the tumour target cells used. Various other substances (sulphated Sephadex G-25, polyethylene sulphonic acid MW 8200 and Sephadex G-200) were unable to stimulate macrophages *in vitro* to secrete tumourolytic factors into their culture media (Table 76.2 and Figure 76.5). In an attempt to show the special molecular requirements of polyanions we have tested soluble components of different molecular weight and sulphated Sephadex preparations from different G-types and varying in sulphur content. Testing these fractions for their macrophage activating capacity to kill tumour cells revealed that a certain minimum molecular weight is required for activation and is dependent on the number of sulphate groups per molecule. Dextran sulphate (MW 500 000) and sulphated Sephadex G-200 induced a powerful cytotoxicity in cultured macrophages, whereas polyethylensulphonic-acid with a molecular weight of 8200 and the sulphated Sephadex preparations of a lower G-type proved to be less effective; Sephadex sulphate G-25 which had also the lowest sulphur content was inactive. In contrast, these low molecular weight polyanions were found to have an inhibitory effect on the inducing activity of high molecular weight polyanions (Figure 76.5).

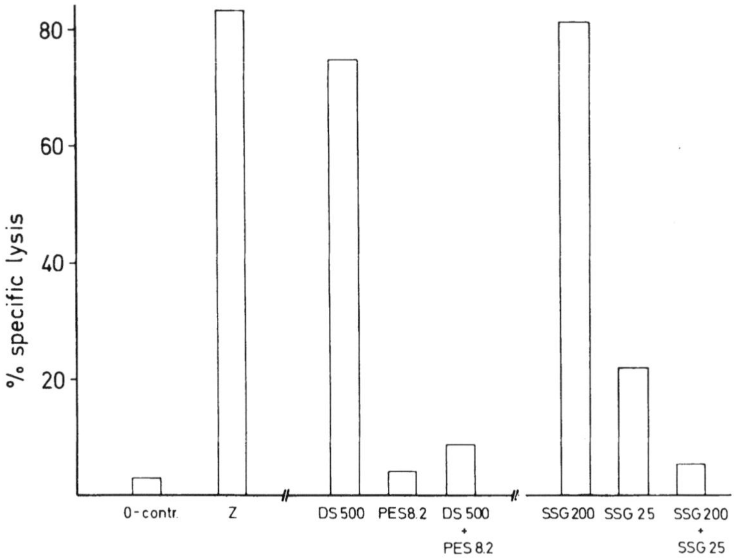


**Figure 76.5** Influence of low molecular weight polyethylene sulphonic acid (MW 8200) and sulphated Sephadex G-25 on the *in vitro* induction of macrophage mediated cytotoxicity stimulated by soluble and insoluble polyanions

As shown also in other publications from our laboratory[13,14], the media of macrophages cultured with dextran sulphate (MW 500 000) or sulphated Sephadex G-200 but not in the absence of these agents were found to contain material with anaphylatoxic activity, inducing contraction of guinea pig terminal ileum. The tachyphylaxis and cross-desensitization and also the selective release of serotonin from guinea pig platelets with reference samples of C3a identify the active agent in media of stimulated macrophages as C3a. Further evidence that the lytic activity is due to C3a comes from experiments using specific antiserum against C3a. The lytic activity of culture media was virtually abolished by anti-C3a. These results focus attention to the fact that macrophages stimulated by various polyanions secrete a lytic factor indistinguishable pharmacologically and immunologically from C3a.

## DISCUSSION

Mackaness[15] introduced the term 'macrophage activation' to describe morphological changes in mononuclear phagocytes. Subsequently the terms 'activation' and 'stimulation' have been used to describe the responses of macrophages to a large number of stimuli both *in vivo* and *in vitro*. As indicated elsewhere[16] the use of these terms should always be made with reference to both the stimulus being studied and the cellular response which is measured. The analysis of responses of mononuclear phagocytes to various agents *in vivo* is difficult since inflammatory lesions in which macrophages are present contain also other cells.

Extensive use has been made of *in vitro* culture methods for studying biochemical responses of macrophages to various stimuli. This biochemical response of macrophages to an endocytic stimulus is characteristic of many other responses of macrophages to agents brought into their environment. The simplest way to characterize these responses is by direct morphological observation, but macrophage responsiveness also can be defined by a large number of functional criteria which develop or are enhanced after a given stimulation. These include increase in pinocytosis and the development of the capacity to kill viruses, infectious agents and tumour cells. We have reviewed elsewhere various functional and biochemical responses of macrophages[12,14] as well as their secretory activities[7,11,17]. To illustrate how the biochemical responses of mononuclear phagocytes vary according to the state of stimulation of the cells and the nature of the stimulus, we will discuss here only the selected example of the polyanions as a stimulus. Many of these polyanionic agents injected parenterally elicit chronic inflammatory reactions. One widely used by experimental pharmacologists and immunologists is carrageenin, a mixture of sulphated D-galactose and 3,6-dehydro-D-galactose extracted from seaweed. Because of the heterogeneous nature of carrageenin we prefer dextran sulphate, which has a uniform polysaccharide structure and offers the chance of varying independently the degree of substitution with sulphate groups as well as the molecular size of the carrier. As shown by ourselves[7] and others[10], there is a conversion of the resting macrophage to an activated state by soluble polyanions which constitutes a highly effective surveillance and potent antitumour mechanism. Once activated, macrophages can regulate cell proliferation[18] and destroy cells with abnormal growth properties[19].

In previous studies soluble substances, e.g. sulphated polysaccharides, were always used. Insoluble polyanions have the advantage of being separable from the reaction mixture (supernantants of activated macrophages) by centrifugation. In order to persue this experimental approach, chlorosulphonic acid was used to substitute insoluble Sephadex with sulphate groups. The resulting centrifugable polyanion, sulphated Sephadex, was found to be an activator of macrophages, similar to the soluble dextran sulphate. The results which are presented establish that sulphated Sephadex is an efficient inducer of lysosomal enzyme secretion from cultured macrophages. The release is time- and dose-dependent and is not associated with loss of the cytoplasmic enzyme lactate dehydrogenase or any other sign of cell death.

The mechanisms for macrophage activation, expressed as selective enzyme secretion and target cell lysis, are still far from being understood. There is growing evidence that the agents which induce chronic inflammation share the capacity to activate macrophages[11,17]. Looking for a common factor among the variety of agents that induce chronic inflammation *in vivo* and hydrolase secretion *in vitro*, our attention has been drawn to the fact that they all activate complement by the alternative pathway[11]. An early consequence of the activation is cleavage of the complement component C3 into a smaller fragment C3a and a large fragment C3b. Normal macrophages are known[20] to synthesize and secrete several intact complement components including C3 and factor B of the alternative pathway[21]. However, when the macrophages are activated[22] by C3b, dextran sulphate[7] or in other ways, they release the cleavage products C3a and C3b. The C3b so formed can activate other macrophages, so that serial activation can result[12]. Incubation of macrophages with polyanions or C3b in a serum free medium resulted in the appearance of a substance with anaphylatoxic activity[13]. When added to a guinea pig terminal ileum preparation, it produced contraction and tachyphylaxis and specific desensitization toward a reference sample of C3a identified by material in the supernatant as C3a. We have found C3a of guinea pig origin to be highly lytic for tumour cells or transformed lymphocytes[23]. Formation of C3a appears to make a major contribution to the tumourolytic effect of macrophages. Antibodies against C3a markedly inhibit the tumourolytic effects of activated macrophages. C3a also lyses mycoplasmas and L forms of bacteria[24]. The factors in stimulated macrophages described by Currie and Basham[25], Sethi and Brandis[26], and Sharma *et al.*[27] may also be C3a.

We suggest that a common factor in macrophage stimulation is activation of complement by the alternative pathway. Attachment of C3b, which is formed to the complement receptor on macrophages, is a powerful activator resulting in acquisition of the capacity to secrete lysosomal enzymes and to lyse tumour cells in culture[12,14]. Likewise, we have found that peritoneal macrophages from normal mice cultured with polyanions like dextran sulphate or sulphated Sephadex (activators of complement by the alternative pathway) become activated to secrete enzymes and become lytic for tumour cells. There is a striking parallelism with the capacity of various soluble and insoluble polyanions to activate the alternative pathway of the complement system, to induce enzyme secretion from cultured macrophages and to stimulate macrophages to be cytolytic *in vitro*. The low molecular weight polyanions show an inhibitory effect on the activation of macrophages to secrete acid hydrolases and to be cytolytic induced by high molecular weight polyanions. These effects are important in the pathogenesis of chronic inflammation.

## ACKNOWLEDGMENT

The authors wish to thank Miss A. Börner and Mrs M. Maruhn for their excellent technical assistance. This work was supported by grants of the SFB 107 Mainz, Germany.

### References

1 Hadding, U., Dierich, M., König, W., Limber., M., Schorlemmer, H. U. and Bitter-Suermann, D. (1973). Ability of the T-cell-replacing polyanion dextran sulfate to trigger the alternative pathway of complement activation. *Eur. J. Immunol.*, **3,** 527

2 Burger, R., Hadding, U., Schorlemmer, H. U., Brade, V. and Bitter-Suermann, D. (1975). Dextran-sulphate: a synthetic activator of C3 via the alternative pathway. *Immunology*, **29,** 549

3 Loos, M., Volanakis, J. E. and Stroud, R. M. (1976). Mode of interaction of different polyanions with the first, the second and the fourth component of complement. III. *Immunochemistry*, **13,** 789

4 Loos, M. and Bitter-Suermann, D. (1976). Mode of interaction of different polyanions with the first, the second and the fourth component of complement. IV. *Immunology*, **31,** 931

5 Diamantstein, T., Vogt, W., Rühl, H. and Borchert, G. (1973). Stimulation of DNA synthesis in mouse lymphoid cells by polyanions *in vitro*. I. *Eur. J. Immunol*, **3,** 488

6 Persson, U. C. J., Hammarström, L. L. G. and Smith, C. J. E. (1977). Macrophages are required for the dextran-sulfate induced activation of B-lymphocytes. *J. Immonol.*, **119,** 1138

7 Schorlemmer, H. U., Burger, R., Hylton, W. and Allison, A. C. (1977). Induction of lysosomal enzyme release from cultured macrophages by dextran sulfate. *Clin. Immunol. Immunopathol.*, **7,** 88

8 Gemsa, D., Seitz, M., Kramer, W., Till, G. and Resch, K. (1978). The effect of phagocytosis, Dextran sulfate, and cell damage on $PGE_1$ sensitivity and $PGE_1$ production of macrophages. *J. Immunol.*, **120,** 1187

9 Schultz, R. M., Papamatheakis, J. D. and Chirigos, M. A. (1977). Interferon: An inducer of macrophage activation by polyanions. *Science*, **197,** 674

10 Schultz, R. M., Papamatheakis, J. D., Luetzeler, J. and Chirigos, M. A. (1977). Association of macrophage activation with antitumor activity by synthetic and biological agents. *Cancer Res.*, **37,** 3338

11 Schorlemmer, H. U., Bitter-Suermann, D. and Allison, A. C. (1977). Complement activation by the alternative pathway and macrophage enzyme secretion in the pathogenesis of chronic inflammation. *Immunology*, **32,** 929

12 Schorlemmer, H. U., Ferluga, J. and Allison, A. C. (1977). Interactions of macrophages and complement components in the pathogenesis of chronic inflammation. In Willoughby, D. A., Giroud, J. P. and Velo, G. P. (eds.) *Perspectives in Inflammation*, pp. 191. (Lancaster: MTP Press)

13 Ferluga, J., Schorlemmer, H. U., Baptista, L. C. and Allison, A. C. (1978). Production of the complement cleavage product C3a by activated macrophages and its tumorolytic effects. *Clin. Exp. Immunol.*, **31,** 512

14 Schorlemmer, H. U., Hadding, U., Bitter-Suermann, D. and Allison, A. C. (1977). The role of complement cleavage products in killing of tumour cells by macrophages. In James, K., McBride, B. and Stuart, A. (eds.) *The Macrophage and Cancer*, pp. 68. (Edinburgh: Econoprint)

15 Mackaness, G. B. (1970). Cellular immunity. In van Furth, R. (ed.) *Mononuclear Phagocytes*, p. 461. (Oxford: Blackwell Scientific)

16 Allison, A. C., Ferluga, J., Prydz, H., and Schorlemmer, H. U. (1978). The role of macrophage activation in chronic inflammation. *Agents Actions*, **8,** 27

17 Schorlemmer, H. U., Edwards, J. H., Davies, P., and Allison, A. C. (1977). Macrophage responses to mouldy hay dust, Micropolyspora faeni and zymosan, activators of complement by the alternative pathway. *Clin. Exp. Immunol.*, **27,** 198
18 Keller, R. (1977). Mononuclear phagocytes and antitumour resistance. In James, K., McBride, B. and Stuart, A. (eds.) *The Macrophage and Cancer*, p. 31. (Edinburgh: Econoprint)
19 Hibbs, J. B. (1974). Discrimination between neoplasia and non-neoplastic cells in vitro by activated macrophages. *J. Natl. Cancer Inst.*, **53,** 1487
20 Lai A Fat, R. F. M. and van Furth, R. (1975). In vitro synthesis of some complement components (C1q, C3 and C4) by lymphoid tissues and circulating leucocytes in man. *Immunology*, **28,** 359
21 Bentley, C., Bitter–Suermann, D., Hadding, U., and Brade, V. (1976). In vitro synthesis of factor B of the alternative pathway of complement activation by mouse peritoneal macrophages. *Eur. J. Immunol.*, **6,** 393
22 Schorlemmer, H. U., Davies, P., and Allison, A. C. (1976). Ability of activated complement components to induce lysosomal enzyme release from macrophages. *Nature (London)*, **261,** 48
23 Ferluga, J., Schorlemmer, H. U., Baptista, L., and Allison, A. C. (1976). Cytolytic effects of the complement cleavage product, C3a. *Br. J. Cancer*, **34,** 626
24 Taylor–Robinson, D., Schorlemmer, H. U., Furr, P. M. and Allison, A. C. (1978). Macrophage secretion and the complement cleavage product C3a in the pathogenesis of infections by mycoplasmas and L-forms of bacteria and in immunity to these organisms. *Clin. Exp. Immunol.*, **33,** 486
25 Currie, G. A. and Basham, C. (1975). Activated macrophages release a factor which lyses malignant cells but not normal cells. *J. Exp. Med.*, **142,** 1600
26 Sethi, K. K. and Brandis, H. (1975). Cytotoxicity mediated by soluble macrophage products. *J. Natl. Cancer Inst.*, **55,** 393
27 Sharma, S. D., Piessens, W. F., and Middlebrook, G. (1980). *In vitro* killing of tumour cells by soluble products of activated guinea pig peritoneal macrophages. *Cell. Immunol.*, **49,** 379

# 77

# Activation of complement by metal compounds that induce chronic granulomatous inflammation

V. D. RAMANATHAN, P. BADENOCH-JONES AND J. L. TURK (UK)

## INTRODUCTION

A number of compounds that are known to induce chronic granulomatous inflammation have been shown to activate the complement system[1]. In a previous report from this laboratory[2], certain aluminium and zirconium compounds that are known to induce chronic granulomas were shown to activate complement. It was found that these compounds were able to consume total haemolytic complement, generate anaphylatoxins and split C3 in normal human serum independent of the formation of the classical and the alternative pathway convertases. Furthermore, some of the compounds were shown to be dependent on plasminogen to activate the complement system. The mechanics of this complement activation were further investigated and the relevance of these findings to the induction of granulomas will be discussed in this communication.

Some of these aluminium and zirconium compounds are widely used in deodorant, anti-perspirant and antacid preparations. A few of their known properties are listed in Table 77.1.

## MATERIALS AND METHODS

Normal human serum was obtained from healthy laboratory volunteers. C4 deficient guinea pig serum was a gift from Dr I. McConnell, Medical Research Council, Cambridge. Purified plasminogen and purified C3 were

**Table 77.1** Summary of some of the known properties of the metal compounds

| | *Physical State* | *Haemolysis*[9] | *Enzyme release from macrophages*[10] | *Granuloma formation* | *Activation of complement* | *Other activities* |
|---|---|---|---|---|---|---|
| Kaolin | particulate | + | not done | foreign body[11] granuloma | + | activation of the Hageman factor[14] |
| AGH | particulate | + | + | foreign body[12] granuloma | + | |
| $Al(OH)_3$ | particulate | + | + | foreign body granuloma | + | |
| ZAG | particulate | + | + | foreign body granuloma | + | |
| $Zr(OH)_4$ | particulate | – | – | — | – | |
| NaZrl | soluble | – | not done | hypersensitivity[13] granuloma | + | |

obtained from Kabi, Stockholm, Sweden and Cordis Laboratories, Miami, Florida, USA, respectively. Haemolytic C3 was titrated as described by Bitter-Suermann and his co-workers[3].

A modification of the method of Brade *et al.*[4] was used to detect the solid-phase activation of complement by the metal compounds. 1 ml of normal human serum was treated with an equal volume of the various particulate compounds for 15 min at 37 °C. It was then centrifuged and the pellet was washed and resuspended to 1.0 ml in buffer. In the second stage, 0.1 ml of this suspension was incubated with 100 $CH_{50}$ units of C3 at 37 °C for 10 min and the percentage conversion of C3 was determined by two-dimensional electrophoresis[5].

## RESULTS

### Consumption of haemolytic C3

The metal compounds were able to consume C3 in C4 deficient guinea pig serum when the latter was treated at dilutions of 1 in 2 and 1 in 100 (Figure 77.1). Sensitized red red cells (EA) which activate the classical pathway were unable to consume complement in this serum. Zymosan was active at a serum dilution of 1 in 2 but not at 1 in 100. This shows that the consumption of complement by the metal compounds is independent of the involvement of the classical and the alternative pathway convertases.

### Pathway of activation

The dependence of some of these metal compounds on plasminogen for activating C3 was demonstrated using plasminogen-depleted serum (Table 77.2). Aluminium chlorhydrate, aluminium hydroxide and zirconium aluminium glycinate were dependent on plasminogen for their activation of C3.

**Table 77.2** Conversion of C3 in human serum by ACH, $Al(OH)_3$ and ZAG in the presence or absence of plasminogen

| | *Plasminogen depleted serum* | *Plasminogen depleted serum + plasminogen** |
|---|---|---|
| GVBS | 5.6 ± 2.3 | 3.6 ± 2.1 |
| Zymosan (2 mg/ml) | 57.7 ± 3.0 | 60.2 ± 5.9 |
| ACH (10 mg/ml) | 0 | 36.4 ± 6.3 |
| $Al(OH)_3$ (10 mg/ml) | 0 | 33.2 ± 4.6 |
| ZAG (10 mg/ml) | 0 | 36.5 ± 1-7 |

*100 μg of plasminogen was added to 1.0 ml of plasminogen depleted serum. Conversion of C3 was demonstrated by two-dimensional electrophoresis. Each value represents mean ±SE of four experiments.

Kaolin was able to activate C3 in plasminogen depleted serum; the addition of 10 mol/l EDTA to this serum inhibited the activation of C3 (Table 77.3).

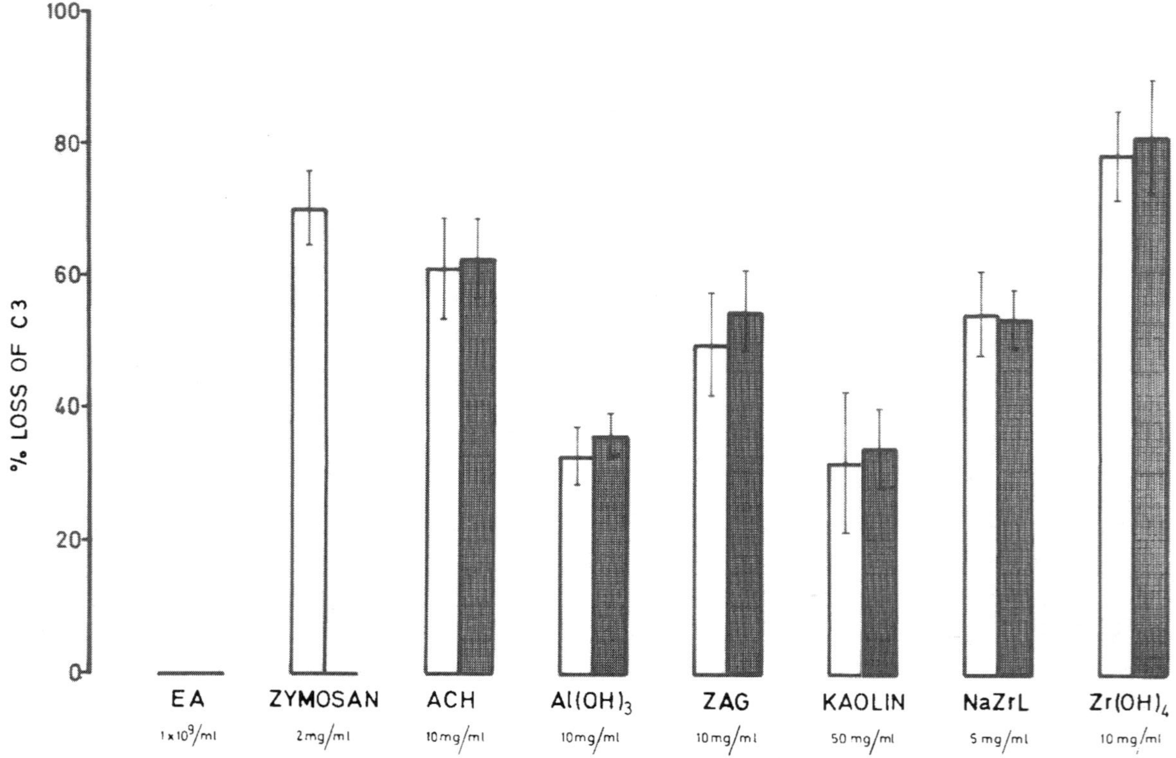


**Figure 77.1** *Consumption of haemolytic C3 by the metal compounds from C4 deficient guinea pig serum at 1 in 2 (□) and 1 in 100 (■) dilutions*. C4 deficient guinea pig serum was treated with the metal compounds and controls at 1 in 2 dilution and 1 in 100 dilution (which blocks the alternative pathway), at 37 °C for 15 min. Residual haemolytic C3 was titrated. Results are expressed as percentage loss of complement compared with serum treated with buffer. Each value represents the mean ± SE of four experiments

The addition of either 100 μg/ml of plasminogen or 5 mol/l $Ca^{2+}$ and $Mg^{2+}$ restored the ability of kaolin to activate C3. This indicates that kaolin activates complement through a pathway resembling the classical pathway and through a plasminogen-dependent pathway.

**Table 77.3** Conversion of C3 by kaolin in normal human serum and plasminogen depleted serum (PDS) in the presence of buffer, 10 mol/l EDTA and 10 mol/l Mg EGTA

| | *% C3 conversion* |
|---|---|
| NHS + kaolin | 27.5 ± 12.7 |
| NHS + EDTA 10 mol/l + kaolin | 40.9 ± 11.1 |
| PDS + kaolin | 34.9 ± 6.5 |
| PDS + EDTA 10 mol/l + kaolin | 0 |
| PDS + Mg EGTA 10 mol/l + kaolin | 0 |
| PDS + $Ca^{2+}$ 10 mol/l + Mg EGTA + kaolin | 39.8 ± 5.6 |
| PDS + plasminogen* + 10 mol/l EDTA + kaolin | 42.5 ± 3.7 |

* 100 μg of plasminogen was added to 1.0 ml of plasminogen depleted serum. Conversion of C3 was demonstrated by two-dimensional electrophoresis. Each value represents mean ± SE of four experiments.

## Activation of purified C3

Of the metal compounds tested, sodium zirconium lactate alone was able to cleave purified C3 directly (Table 77.4). The other metal compounds required serum factors for this activation.

**Table 77.4** Conversion of purified C3 by the metal compounds*

| *C3 treated with* | *% C3 conversion* | *C3 treated with* | *% C3 conversion* |
|---|---|---|---|
| buffer | 0 | buffer | 0 |
| zymosan | 0 | zymosan X† | 53.9 ± 4.06 |
| AGH | — | AGH X | 49.3 ± 8.8 |
| $Al(OH)_3$ | — | $Al(OH)_3$X | 49.15 ± 2.5 |
| ZAG | — | ZAG X | 57.60 ± 6.3 |
| kaolin | 0 | kaolin X | 31.72 ± 6.22 |
| $Zr(OH)_4$ | 0 | $Zr(OH)_4$ X | 0 |
| NaZrl | 44.0 ± 5.2 | — | — |

*Conversion of C3 was demonstrated by two-dimensional electrophoresis. Mean ± SE of four experiments.

† Zymosan or the metal compounds were incubated with normal human serum at 37 °C for 15 min and centrifuged. The pellet was washed and resuspended in buffer.

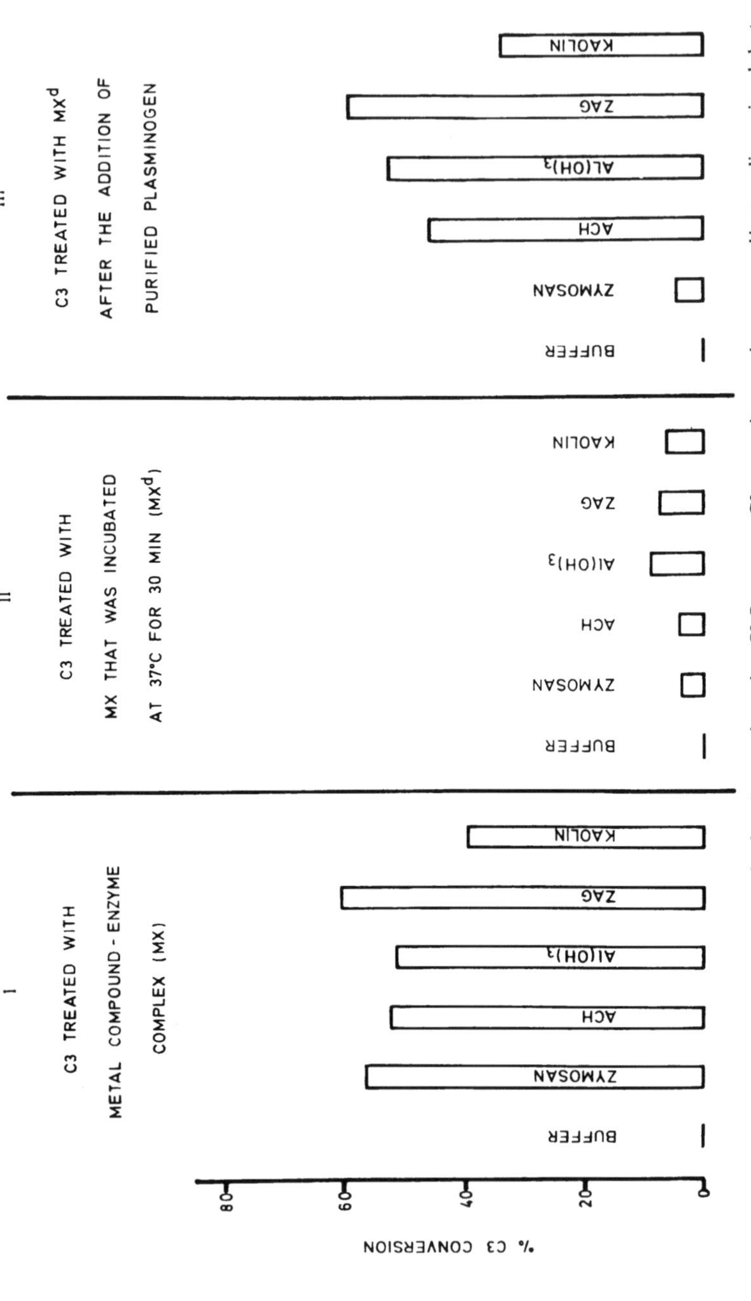


**Figure 77.2** *Formation, decay and regeneration of a plasminogen-dependent C3 Convertase.* C3 conversion was demonstrated by two-dimensional electrophoresis. Each point represents the mean of four experiments

**Activation of C3 in the solid phase**

Particulate activators of the alternative pathway like zymosan or anti-tumour polysaccharides have been shown to assemble the alternative pathway C3 convertase on their surface[4,6]. This C3 convertase was found to decay rapidly when incubated at 37 °C and could be regenerated by purified factor B.

The particulate metal compounds were found to assemble a similar C3 convertase on their surface (Figure 77.2 column 1). This convertase decayed rapidly when incubated at 37 °C for 30 min (Figure 77.2 column 2). The addition of purified plasminogen was able to restore the activity of the C3 convertase assembled on the surface of the metal compounds but not that assembled on zymosan (Figure 77.2, column 3).

## DISCUSSION

All the metal compounds except zirconium hydroxide were able to activate complement. Zirconium hydroxide consumed haemolytic C3 but this did not result in the activation of complement. Concanavalin A has also been shown to bind C3 without activating it[7].

It had earlier been shown that aluminium chlorhydrate, aluminium hydroxide and zirconium aluminium glycinate were unable to activate C3 in serum depleted of plasminogen[2]. The addition of purified plasminogen to this serum restored the ability of the three metal compounds to activate C3 (Table 77.2).

Lachmann[8] suggested that kaolin, like latex, aggregates immunoglobulins on its surface and thereby activates C1q. The results of the present investigation suggested that kaolin activates complement through a pathway resembling the classical pathway as well as through a plasminogen-dependent pathway (Table 77.3).

It was interesting to note that sodium zirconium lactate, a soluble metal compound that induces granulomatous hypersensitivity, was able to cleave purified C3 directly (Table 77.4). The particulate metal compounds, on the other hand, required other serum factors for this activation.

The behaviour of the plasminogen-dependent C3 convertase assembled on the metal compounds was similar to that of the alternative pathway convertase C3bBb. The exact molecular composition of this C3 convertase is unknown but is likely to involve the Hageman factor and plasminogen.

The importance of the local activation of complement in granulomatous inflammation has been emphasized by the findings of Schlorlemmer and his co-workers[1]. They reported that a variety of agents that induce chronic inflammation are able to activate complement and release lysosomal enzymes from macrophages. The released lysosomal enzymes can further activate macrophages and thus perpetuate the inflammatory state. The metal compounds that induce granuloma formation were found to activate complement in the solid phase (particulate compounds) or directly (sodium zirconium lactate). It is thus possible that the ability of the metal compounds to induce granuloma is directly related to their complement activating property.

## References


1 Schorlemmer, H. U., Bitter-Suermann, D. and Allison, A. C. (1977). Complement activation by the alternative pathway and macrophage enzyme secretion on the pathogens of chronic inflammation. *Immunology*, **32,** 929

2 Ramanathan, V. D., Badenoch-Jones, P. and Turk, J. L. (1979). Complement activation by aluminium and zirconium compounds. *Immunology*, **37,** 881

3 Bitter-Suermann, D., Hadding, U., Melchert, F. and Wellensiek, H. J. (1970). Independent and consecutive action of the complement components C5, C6 and C7 in immune hemolysis-I. Preparation of EAC 1–5 with purified guinea pig C3 and C5. *Immunochemistry*, **7,** 955

4 Brade, V., Lee, G. D., Nicholson, A., Shin, H. S. and Mayer, M. M. (1973). The reaction of zymosan with the properdin system in normal and C4-deficient guinea pig serum. *J. Immunol.*, **111,** 1389

5 Hudson, L. and Hay, F. C. (1976). *Practical Immunology*, 1st Edn., p. 139. (London: Blackwell Scientific)

6 Hamuro, J., Hadding, U. and Bitter-Suermann, D. (1978). Solid-phase activation of alternative pathway of complement by β-1, 3 glucans and its possible role for tumour regressing activity. *Immunology*, **34,** 695

7 Bitter-Suermann, D., Hadding, U., Schorlemmer, H. U., Limbert, H., Dierich, M. and Dukor, P. (1975). Activation by some T-independent antigens and B cell mitogens of the alternative of the complement system. *J. Immunol.*, **115,** 425

8 Lachmann, P. J. (1975). Complement. In Gell, R. R. A., Coombs and Lachmann P. J. (eds.) *Clinical Aspects of Immunology*, 3rd Edn., p. 333. (London: Blackwell Scientific)

9 Ramanathan, V. D. (1980). Activation of complement by agents inducing chronic granulomatous inflammation. Ph. D. thesis. University of London

10 Badenoch-Jones, P., Turk, J. L. and Parker, D. (1978). The effects of some aluminium and zirconium compounds on guinea pig peritoneal macrophages and skin fibroblasts in culture. *J. Pathol.*, **124,** 51

11 Lord, G. H. and Wilson, J. E. (1968). *J. Am. Vet. Med. Assoc.*, **153,** 910

12 Turk, J. L. and Parker, D. (1977). Granuloma formation in normal guinea pigs injected intradermally with aluminium and zirconium compounds. *J. Invest. Dermatol*, **68,** 336

13 Turk, J. L. and Parker, D. (1977). Sensitization with Cr. Ni and Zr salts and allergic type granuloma formation in the guinea pig. *J. Invest Dermatol*, **68,** 341

14 Ogston, D., Ogston, O. M., Ratnoff, D. and Forbes, C. D. (1969). *J. Clin. Invest.*, **48,** 1786

# 78

# Different susceptibilities to 4-hydroperoxycyclophosphamide of T cell sub-sets involved in delayed-type hypersensitivity of mice to sheep red blood cells

S. H. E. KAUFMANN, H. HAHN AND T. DIAMANTSTEIN

## INTRODUCTION

It has been amply shown that cyclophosphamide (Cy), in addition to its immunosuppressive properties, enhances the cellular immune response to heterologous red blood cells, and both elimination by Cy of B cells and suppressor T cells ($T_S$ cells) have been postulated as the underlying mechanism[1-3]. 4-hydroperoxycyclophosphamide (4-HPCy) is a derivative of Cy which in contrast to Cy acts on lymphocytes *in vitro* since the compound in aqueous solution is converted to 4-hydroxycyclophosphamide, the naturally occurring metabolite of Cy[4].

The experiments reported below were undertaken in order to establish the relative sensitivities to Cy of T cell sub-sets involved in delayed-type hypersensitivity (DTH) to sheep red blood cells (SRBC) in mice.

## MATERIAL AND METHODS

### Mice and sensitization

$(B6D2)F_1$ mice were used at 6–12 weeks of age. Mice were sensitized by the i.v. injection of various doses of SRBC as described elsewhere[5]. Cy (Endoxan, Asta Werke, Brackwede, FRG) was dissolved in sterile water immediately before use and 200 mg/kg were injected i.v. DTH was tested as described elsewhere[5]. Results are expressed in 0.1 mm units and represent the mean differences between SRBC-injected and sham-injected contralateral footpads.

**Transfer of spleen cells**

For transfer of DTH, $2 \times 10^7$ spleen cells were mixed with $1.25 \times 10^8$ SRBC and injected s.c. in a volume of 0.05 ml into one hind footpad of non-sensitized recipients. For transfer of suppression, $5 \times 10^7$ spleen cells were injected i.v. into mice which had been pretreated with 200 mg/kg Cy i.v. 2 days previously. Immediately after cell transfer, DTH was induced and 5 days later DTH reactions elicited as described previously[3].

**Treatment of spleen cells with 4-HPCy**

4-HPCy was a generous gift of Dr Burkert, Asta-Werke, Brackwede, FRG. The compound was dissolved in RPMI 1640 medium immediately before use. $1 \times 10^7$ spleen cells/ml were incubated with graded amounts of 4-HPCy for 60 min at 37 °C in 5% $CO_2$ in air. After incubation, cells were washed three times, counted, and their viability determined by trypan blue exclusion.

## RESULTS

**Susceptibility to 4-HPCy of antigen activated $T_{DTH}$ cells**

Prospective donor mice were optimally sensitized for DTH with $10^8$ SRBC given under Cy-modulation[5] and on the day of the optimal immune response their spleens were removed. Spleen cells were incubated with graded doses of 4-HPCy, and, after washing, injected into normal recipient mice together with SRBC. Table 78.1 (experiment 1) shows that $T_{DTH}$ cells proved resistant to 4-HPCy up to a concentration of 3 μg/ml.

**Susceptibility to 4-HPCy of antigen- activated $T_s$ cells**

Prospective donor mice were injected with a suppressive dose of $10^9$ SRBC[3] and spleen cells collected 4 days later. Spleen cells were incubated with graded doses of 4-HPCy, and, after washing, transferred to Cy-pretreated recipients in which DTH was induced immediately thereafter. As seen in Table 78.1 (experiment 2), suppression was susceptible to treatment of cells with doses of 4-HPCy exceeding 1 μg/ml.

**Selective elimination of $T_S$ cells, but not of $T_{DTH}$ cells, from spleen cell preparation of unresponsive mice**

It has been shown that spleens of mice made unresponsive by high doses of SRBC contain both $T_{DTH}$ cells and $T_S$ cells[6]. If so, it might be possible to selectively eliminate $T_S$ cells from spleen cell suspensions of unresponsive mice by

**Table 78.1** Relative susceptibilities of antigen activated $T_{DTH}$ cells and $T_S$ cells to 4-HPCy

| *4-HPCy* ($\mu$g/ml) | *Experiment 1: transfer of DTH* *Mean DTH* (0.1 mm)* | *Experiment 2: transfer of suppression* *Mean DTH* (0.1 mm)† | *Experiment 3: selective elimination of $T_s$ cells* *Mean DTH* (0.1 mm)‡ |
|---|---|---|---|
| 0 | 6.8 | 2.1 | 3.9 |
| 0.1 | 6.0 | 2.4 | 4.4 |
| 0.3 | 6.2 | 3.3 | 4.1 |
| 1.0 | 6.2 | 4.2 | 6.2 |
| 3.0 | 5.8 | 8.3 | 7.9 |
| 10.0 | 3.9 | 9.7 | 6.5 |
| control | 3.0 | 12.1 | 3.6 |

* (B6D2) F1 mice were sensitized with $10^6$ SRBC, 4 days later their spleens were removed, and $1 \times 10^7$ cells/ml incubated with graded amounts of 4-HPCy. After washing, $2 \times 10^7$ spleen cells, together with $1.25 \times 10^8$ SRBC, were transferred locally into one hind footpad of syngeneic recipients. DTH reactions were measured 24 h later. Control mice received equal amounts of untreated spleen cells.

† (B6D2) F1 mice were sensitized with $10^9$ SRBC, 4 days later their spleens were moved, and $1 \times 10^7$ cells/ml incubated with graded amounts of 4-HPCy. After washing, $5 \times 10^7$ spleen cells were injected i.v. into syngeneic recipients which had been pretreated with 200 $\mu$g/kg Cy i.v. 2 days previously. Recipients were sensitized with $10^8$ SRBC immediately after cell transfer and 5 days later challenged using $1 \times 10^8$ SRBC. DTH reactions were measured 24 h later. Control mice received equal amounts of untreated spleen cells.

‡(B6D2) F1 mice were sensitized with $10^8$ SRBC, 4 days later their spleens were removed, and $1 \times 10^7$ cells/ml incubated with graded amounts of 4-HPCy. After washing, $2 \times 10^7$ spleen cells, together with $1.25 \times 10^8$ SRBC, were transferred locally into one hind footpad of syngeneic recipients. DTH reactions were measured 24 h later. Control mice received equal amounts of untreated spleen cells.

4-HPCy *in vitro* without affecting $T_{DTH}$ cells. Indeed, 4-HPCy treatment *in vitro* caused $T_{DTH}$ cells in otherwise unreactive spleen cell preparations to become demonstrable (Table 78.1, experiment 3). Thus, using 1–3 $\mu$g 4-HPCy/$10^7$ cells, $T_{DTH}$ cells were detectable by adoptive transfer experiments.

**Susceptibility to 4-HPCy of precursors of $T_S$ cells**

*In vivo* pretreatment of mice with Cy reverses unresponsiveness induced by $10^9$ SRBC to a state of reactivity and this Cy effect in turn can be reversed by transfer of normal splenic T cells indicating the T cell nature of precursors of suppression (Kaufmann, Hahn, and Diamantstein, manuscript submitted for publication). In order to determine their sensitivity to 4-HPCy *in vitro*, spleen cells from normal mice were incubated with graded doses of 4-HPCy. As shown in Table 78.2, reconstitution of Cy pretreated mice was abrogated by treatment of spleen cells with as little as 0.3 $\mu$g 4-HPCy/$10^7$ cells, demonstrating the high susceptibility to 4-HPCy of precursors of suppression.

## DISCUSSION

Studies to define the mode of action of Cy as an immunomodulating agent have thus far been hampered by the fact that Cy is active *in vivo* only. This situ-

**Table 78.2** Relative susceptibility of precursors of $T_S$ cells to 4-HPCy

| *4-HPCy* (μg/ml) | *Mean DTH* (0.1 mm)* |
|---|---|
| 0 | 2.6 |
| 0.1 | 4.1 |
| 0.3 | 11.3 |
| 1.0 | 8.2 |
| 3.0 | 9.8 |
| control | 10.7 |

* $1 \times 10^7$ spleen cells/ml from normal (B6D2)F1 mice were incubated with graded amounts of 4-HPCy, and, after washing, $5 \times 10^7$ cells transferred i.v. to syngeneic recipients. Recipient mice had been pretreated with 200 mg/kg Cy 2 days prior to cell transfer. 1 day after cell transfer, mice received $10^9$ SRBC i.v., and after another 4 days it was attempted to induce DTH using $10^6$ SRBC (i.v.). DTH reactions were elicited 4 days later using $1 \times 10^8$ SRBC and measured after 24 h. Control mice received no cells.

ation has been changed as a result of the availability of 4-HPCy which in aqueous solution spontaneously yields a compound acting on lymphocytes *in vitro*[4]. Using 4-HPCy we have characterized T lymphocyte sub-sets involved in DTH to SRBC in mice and their precursors with respect to their relative susceptibilities to 4-HPCy. Our data allow the following ranking order of the T cell sub-sets with respect to their relative susceptibilities: $T_S$ cell precursors > antigen activated $T_S$ cells > antigen activated $T_{DTH}$ cells.

Our results confirm and extend previous observations on DTH to heterologous erythrocytes[1,2,7,8] derived from *in vivo* models which suggest that T cell sub-populations with different functions differ in their susceptibilities towards Cy. It is now possible to explain the multitude of different, if not contradictory, effects of Cy on the immune system on a cellular basis. Furthermore, these data provide additional criteria for distinguishing different T cell sub-sets.

## References

1 Lagrange, P. H., Mackaness, G. B. and Miller, T. E. (1974). *J. Exp. Med.*, **139,** 1529
2 Ramshaw, I. A., Bretscher, P. A. and Parish, C. R. (1976). *Eur. J. Immunol.*, **6,** 674
3 Kaufmann, S. H. E., Ahmed, J. S., Chahin, M., and Hahn, H. (1979). *Immunology*, **38,** 613
4 Shand, F. L. and Howard, J. G. (1979). *Eur. J. Immunol.*, **9,** 17
5 Hahn, H., Kaufmann, S. H. E., Miller, T. E. and Mackaness, G. G. (1979). *Immunology*, **36,** 691
6 Hahn, H., Kaufmann, S. H. E., Falkenberg, F., Chahin, M. and Horn, W. (1979). *Immunology*, **38,** 51
7 Askenase, P. W., Hayden, B. J. and Gershon, R. K. (1975). *J. Exp. Med.*, **141,** 697
8 Ramshaw, I. A., Bretscher, P. A., and Parish, C. R. (1977). *Eur. J. Immunol.*, **7,** 180

# 79

# RES impairment in NZB/W mice

Y-H. CHANG, C. M. PEARSON, D. CHIA,
AND K. R. AOKI (USA)

## INTRODUCTION

NZB/W mice develop a murine lupus very similar to human systemic lupus erythematosus (SLE). The pathogenesis of both diseases remains poorly understood. There is, however, extensive evidence that antigen–antibody complexes play a central role[1,2]. Much of the tissue damage in these diseases appear to result from deposition of immune complexes in the kidney and other tissue[3,4] and the attendant initiation of inflammatory events. Tissue localization may occur from a failure to clear immune complexes from the circulation due to (1) an excessive rate of antibody production and the consequent overloading of the reticuloendothelial system (RES), (2) a subnormal rate of catabolic removal of immune complexes due to impaired RES function, or (3) a combination of these two phenomena. Investigations in the past have placed much emphasis on the hyperactivity of autoantibody production whereas possible impairment of the disposal system for the immune complexes has not received due attention. This investigation was conducted to ascertain whether an impairment in the disposal of soluble immune complexes underlies, or at least contributes to, the pathogenesis of murine lupus in NZB/W mice.

## MATERIALS AND METHODS

### Preparation of mouse IgG

IgG was isolated from pooled sera of normal Swiss Webster mice by 50% saturated ammonium sulphate (SAS) precipitation followed by column chromatography with DEAE Sephadex (Pharmacia, Piscataway, NJ, USA). IgG was concentrated to 12.0 mg/ml by ultrafiltration and stored at −20 °C in 0.05 mol/l phosphate buffered saline, pH 7.4 (PBS). Protein concentrations are determined by optical absorption at 280 nm using an extinction coefficient ($E^{1\%}_{1cm}$) of 14.5.

**Preparation of $^{125}$I-labelled soluble aggregates of mouse IgG([$^{125}$I]A-IgG)**

[$^{125}$I]A-IgG was kindly provided by Dr David W. Knutson. It was prepared as follows. IgG was radiolabelled with $^{125}$I to a specific activity of 0.1 mCi/mg by the chloramine T method[5]. Concentrations of proteins were determined by optical absorption at 280 nm using an extinction coefficient ($E^{1\%}_{1cm}$) of 14.5. Aggregations were performed by heating a solution (10 mg/ml) of [$^{125}$I] IgG in 0.1mol/l phosphate-buffered saline (pH 7.4) for 20 min at 63 °C. Soluble aggregates of different sizes were separated by ultracentrifugation for 4 h at 260 000 × *g* in 12.0 ml 10–30% w/v sucrose gradients. Self-aggregation of isolated aggregates was prevented by separating A-IgG in gradients made with Tris-buffered Hank's solution, pH 7.4 (TBH), containing 0.5% bovine serum albumin and then storing A-IgG at −20 °C in the same protein-containing buffer. Isolated aggregates were dialysed before use against TBH to reduce the concentration of sucrose and all preparations were greater than 97% trichloroacetic acid (TCA) precipitable at the time of their use. Aggregates were always centrifuged at 3000 rev/min for 15 min immediately before use to insure that only soluble material was present. The size distribution, homogeneity and stability of the various A-IgG isolates were checked by periodic ultracentrifugation which showed that no appreciable self-aggregation or dissociation into free IgG had occurred.

**Peritoneal Macrophages**

Resident peritoneal macrophages were obtained from freshly killed mice by washing the peritoneal cavity with two 3.0 ml portions of Tris-buffered Hank's balanced salt solution (pH 7.4). The cells were washed three times and resuspended in tris-buffered Hank's balanced salt solution containing 0.5% BSA and 100 mg/100 ml glucose (TBH–BSA) to a concentration of $2 \times 10^7$ cells/ml. 75–85% of the large granulated cells counted were esterase positive with benzidine.

**Degradation of [$^{125}$I]A-IgG by peritoneal macrophages**

A 0.2 ml volume of a suspension of peritoneal macrophages in TBH–BSA–G ($2 \times 10^7$ cells/ml) was added into a 16 × 125 mm plastic tube containing 0.1 ml of a solution of [$^{125}$I]A-IgG in TBH–BSA (approximately $1 \times 10^5$ ct/min/ml) and incubated at 37 °C for 4 h unless otherwise indicated. The incubation was terminated by adding 0.7 ml of cold (4 °C) saline containing 0.5% EDTA. The cells were then separated by centrifugation at 700 *g* for 6 min and washed once with 1.0 of EDTA saline. A 2.0 ml of a 10% trichloroacetic acid (TCA) solution was then added to the combined supernatant and the TCA precipitable (unaltered complexes) and TCA soluble (metabolized complexes) radioactivity determined. The cell pellet was similarly treated with 2.0 ml of 5% TCA solution. Greater than 95% of the TCA soluble products were found to be dialysable, of which 13% was free iodine. The rest were amino acids and small peptides based on Sephadex G-25 chromatography.

**Degradation of [$^{125}$I]A-IgG by liver slices**

A 0.1 ml volume of a [$^{125}$I]A-IgG solution 4 pmol/ml was injected into the tail vein. The mouse was then sacrificed by cervical dislocation at 5 min after intravenous injection. The liver was excised, gall bladder removed along with other non-hepatic tissues, and placed in ice-cold medium (TBH–BSA). The liver was sliced into approximately 1 mm thick slices. The slices were divided into four samples and weighed. Two of the samples were homogenized in 6.0 ml of TBH–BSA immediately and the amounts of TCA soluble and TCA precipitable radioactivity determined. The TCA soluble radioactivity is considered as products of [$^{125}$I]A-IgG resulting from *in vivo* degradation. The other two samples were placed in incubation vials containing 6.0 ml of TBH–BSA and incubated with shaking for 4 h. The total and the TCA soluble radioactivity was determined exactly as with the other two samples.

## RESULTS

**Degradation of [$^{125}$I]A-IgG by peritoneal macrophages obtained from the young and the old NZB/W mice**

The ability of macrophages obtained from the young (6 weeks of age) and the old (32 weeks of age) animals were determined. The [$^{125}$I]A-IgG used had an average size of 54 IgG molecules per aggregate. The amounts of TCA soluble products found were expressed as percentages of the total of [$^{125}$I]A-IgG introduced at the beginning of incubation (Figure 79.1). Macrophages obtained from old NZB/W mice degraded [$^{125}$I]A-IgG at a rate of 0.18 fmol/min/4 × $10^6$ cells versus 0.09 fmol/min/ 4 × $10^6$ cells for the old animals.

In a second experiment, six groups of NZB/W mice (6–10 per group) of different age (2–8 months) were studied. The macrophages were incubated in the presence of [$^{125}$I]A-IgG for 4 h at 37 °C. The functional impairment appeared between 3 and 4 months of age, and deteriorated progressively with age (Figure 79.2).

**Degradation of [$^{125}$I]A-IgG by peritoneal macrophages obtained from the young and the old Swiss Webster mice**

A group of 6-week-old and a group of 32-week-old female Swiss Webster mice were used in this experiment. The ability of macrophages obtained from each animal to degrade [$^{125}$I]A-IgG (54.4 molecules/aggregates) was determined. [$^{125}$I]A-IgG (1.35 μg) was added to 0.2 ml of a suspension of macro-

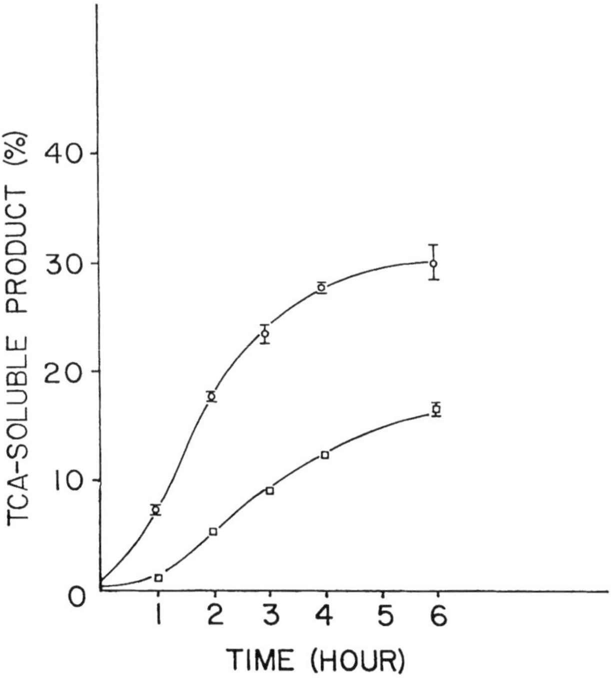


**Figure 79.1** Degradation of soluble A-IgG by young (○) and old (□) NZB/W mice. Ten animals were used for each group. Standard errors of the means are indicated

phages ($2 \times 10^7$ cells/ml) and incubated at 37 °C for 4 h. The macrophages ($4 \times 10^6$ cells) obtained from the young animals degraded 0.707 μg of [$^{125}$I]A-IgG and the macrophages obtained from the old animals degraded 0.760 μg of [$^{125}$I]A-IgG (Figure 79.3).

**Hepatic uptake and degradation of [$^{125}$I]A-IgG by the young and the old NZB/W mice**

A group (5) of 6-week-old female NZB/W mice and a group (5) of 28-week-old female NZB/W mice were used in this experiment. Each animal received an intravenous injection of 0.1 ml of a [$^{125}$I]A-IgG solution ($1 \times 10^6$ ct/min/ml). The animal was sacrificed 5 min after the intravenous injection and the liver was immediately removed. A portion of the liver was weighed and used to determine the amounts of TCA soluble and TCA precipitable radioactivity present in the liver. The combined TCA soluble and TCA precipitable radioactivity represents the uptake of [$^{125}$I]A-IgG. The TCA soluble radioactivity represents the amounts of degradation products present in the liver at the time of sacrifice (Table 79.1). On an equal weight basis, there was no difference between the uptake of [$^{125}$I]A-IgG of the young and the old animals.

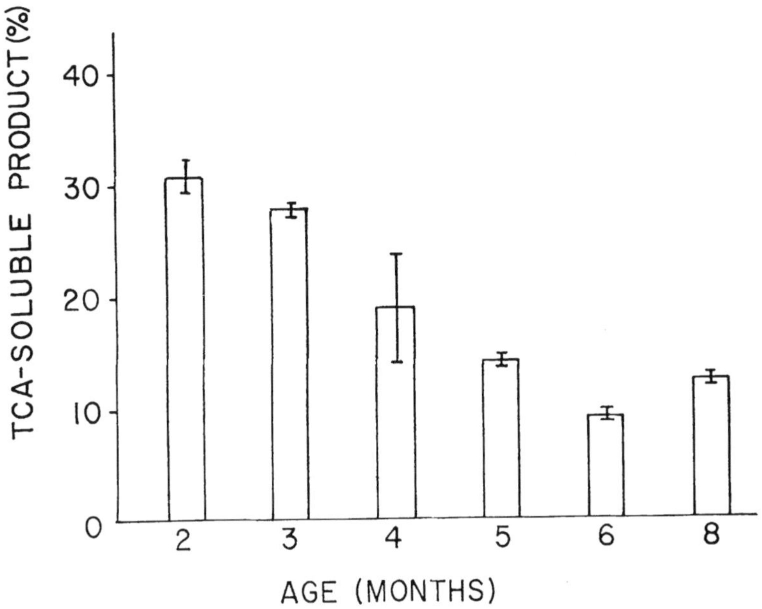


**Figure 79.2** Degradation of soluble A-IgG by peritoneal macrophages obtained from female NZB/W mice at different ages. Six to ten animals were used per group. Standard errors of the means are indicated

There appeared to be slightly less degraded [$^{125}$I]A-IgG per milligram of liver from the old animals than that from the young animals at the time of sacrifice, but the difference was not statistically significant ($p > 0.05$).

Another portion of the liver was cut into 1.0 mm thick slices, weighed and then incubated at 37 °C for 4 h and the amounts of TCA soluble and TCA precipitable radioactivity determined (Table 79.2). On an equal weight basis, livers from the young animals degraded more [$^{125}$I]A-IgG during the 4 h incubation period than those of the old animals.

**Table 79.1** Hepatic uptake of [$^{125}$I] A-IgG by the young and the old female NZB/W mice

| | *Radioactivity (ct/min) per mg of liver* | | |
|---|---|---|---|
| | *TCA precipitable* ±*SE* | *TCA soluble* ±*SE* | *Total* ±*SE* |
| Young | 26.23±2.06 | 3.36±0.12 | 25.44±2.14 |
| Old | 24.97±0.49 | 2.98±0.18 | 25.83±0.52 |

**Table 79.2** *In vitro* degradation of [$^{125}$I]A-IgG by slices of liver from the young and the old female NZB/W mice

| | Radioactivity (ct/min) per mg of liver | | | |
|---|---|---|---|---|
| | *TCA precipitable* ±*SE* | *TCA soluble* ±*SE* | *[$^{125}$I]A-IgG solubilized* in vitro *±*SE* | *Degradation* (%) |
| Young | 15.72±1.56 | 10.96±.122 | 9.52±0.58 | 39.9±1.30 |
| Old | 17.31±0.63 | 9.96±0.33 | 7.56±0.31 | 33.1±1.20 |

*Corrected for TCA soluble radioactivity present at the beginning of incubation.

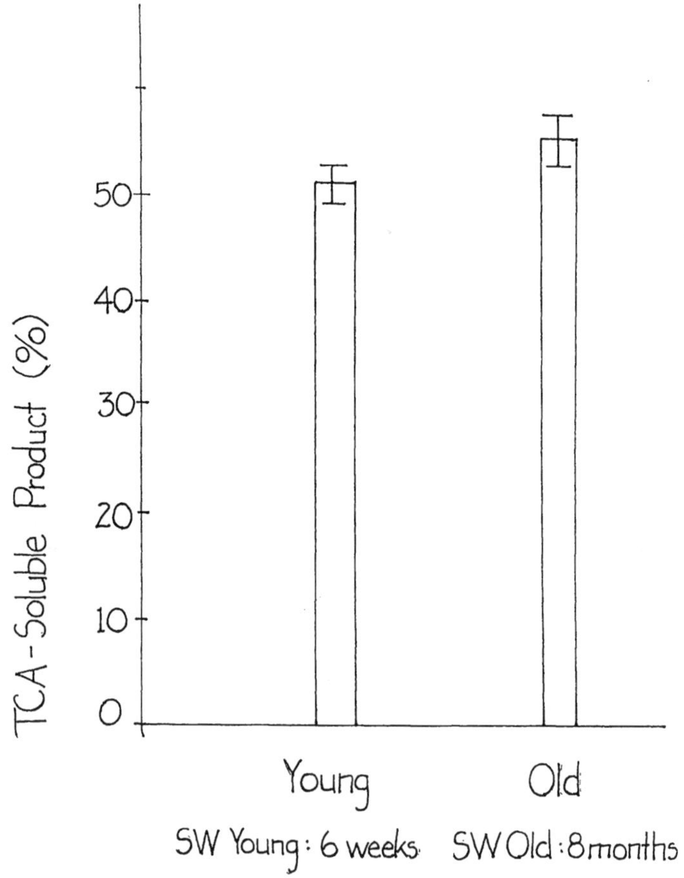


**Figure 79.3**

## DISCUSSION

Murine lupus that develops in NZB/W mice is quite similar to human systemic lupus erythematosus and is believed to result from deposition of immune complexes in tissues such as joints and kidney and the attendant initiation of inflammatory events. A major condition necessary for such tissue deposition is the persistence of the complexes in the circulation for sufficient periods of time[6]. Tissue localization may occur from a failure to clear immune complexes from the circulation due to (1) an excessive rate of antibody production and the consequent overloading of the reticulo-endothelial system (RES), (2) a subnormal rate of catabolic removal of immune complexes due to impaired RES function, or (3) a combination of these two phenomena. Hyperactive humoral immunity in terms of autoantibody production in old NZB/W female mice[1], and in patients with SLE[7], has been well established. Although there is no longer any doubt that the high levels of circulating immune complexes in animals with murine lupus and in patients with SLE or rheumatoid arthritis reflect brisk synthesis of antibodies, there are observations which suggest that an impairment in the RES disposal of immune complexes also play a significant role. For example, a reduced clearance rate of polyvinylpyrolidone has been observed in NZB/W female mice just prior to the development of renal disease implicating a pathogenic role for reduced RES function.[8]

Soluble heat-aggregated IgG (A-IgG) fixes complement[9], binds to macrophages and is rapidly removed from the circulation by the RES and catabolized by macrophages in a manner similar to immune complexes[10,11]. We chose to use soluble A-IgG instead of immune complexes in the present study because stable, highly purified A-IgG of known size and composition (IgG content) can be readily prepared.

Under our experimental conditions, macrophages obtained from old (8 month) NZB/W mice were found to degrade A-IgG *in vitro* at a much slower rate than those from the young (2 month) animals (Figure 79.1). This functional impairment first occurred at 3 months of age, prior to the appearance of clinical signs of murine lupus or detectable anti-DNA antibody, and deteriorate progressively with age (Figure 79.2). The data suggest that this phenomenon is not secondary to the disease development. Since macrophages from old (8 month) female mice of the Swiss Webster strain (who do not develop lupus-like disease with age) degrade A-IgG as efficiently as those of the young (2 month) animals (Figure 79.3), the progressive deterioration of macrophage function seen in NZB/W mice would not seem to be a part of the normal ageing process.

Since the liver is quantitatively the most important organ for the disposal of macromolecules including aggregated albumin[12] and DNA[13] possible difference in the hepatic uptake and degradation of [$^{125}$I]A-IgG between the young and the old NZB/W mice was investigated. On an equal weight basis, there was no difference between the hepatic uptake of [$^{125}$I]A-IgG of the young and the old animals (Table 79.1), but livers from the young animals degraded significantly more [$^{125}$I]A-IgG *in vitro* during a 4 h incubation period than those of the old animals (Table 79.2). It thus appears that a deterioration of the disposal system for immune complexes may be involved in the pathogenesis of murine lupus in NZB/W mice.

## ACKNOWLEDGMENTS

We thank Dr David W. Knutson for providing us with a generous supply of [$^{125}$I]A-IgG. The valuable technical assistance of Miss Shirley Lo and Mrs Fran Beck is gratefully acknowledged. This work was supported in part by Grant no. 79–00077, Department of Health Services, State of California, USA.

### References

1 Goldblum, R., Pillarisetty, R. and Talal, N,(1975). Independent appearance of antithymocyte and anti-RNA antibodies in NZB/NZW Fl mice. *Immunology,* **28,** 621

2 Cochrane, C. G. and Koffler, D. (1973). Immune complex disease in experimental animals and man. *Adv. Immunol.*, **16,** 185

3 Baldwin, D. S., Lowenstein, J., Rothfield, N., Gallo, G. A. and McCluskey, R. (1970). The clinical course of the proliferative and membranous forms of lupus nephritis. *Ann. Intern. Med.,* **73,** 929

4 Cooke, T. D., Hurd, E. C., Jasin, H. E., Bienenstock, J. and Ziff, M. (1975). Identification of immunoglobulins and complement in rheumatoid articular collagenous tissue. *Arthritis Rheum.*, **18,** 541

5 McConahey, P. J. and Dixon, F. J. (1966). A method of trace iodination of protein for *in vivo* studies. *Int. Arch. Allergy Appl. Immunol.,* **29,** 185

6 Cochrane, C. G. and Hawkins D. (1968). Studies of circulating immune complexes. III. Factors governing the ability of circulating complexes to localize in blood vessels. *J. Exp. Med.,* **127,** 137

7 Kunkel, H. G., Muller-Eberhard, H. J., Fudenberg, H. H. and Tomase, T. B. (1961). Gamma globulin complexed in rheumatoid arthritis and certain other conditions. *J. Clin. Invest.*, **40,** 117

8 Morgan, A. G. and Steward, M. W. (1976). Macrophage clearance function and immune complex disease in New Zealand Black White $F_1$ hybrid mice. *Clin. Exp. Immunol.*, **26,** 133

9 Christian, C. L. (1960). Studies of aggregated gammaglobulin I. Sedimentation, electrophoretic and anticomplementary properties. *J. Immunol.*, **84,** 112

10 Kijlstra, A., Knutson, D. W., Daha, H. R. and van Es, L. A. (1977). Glomerular localization of preformed immune complexes. Abstract presented at the Spring Meeting of the British Society for Immunology, April 1977

11 Shinomiya, T. and Koyama, J. (1976). *In vitro* uptake and digestion of immune complexes containing guinea-pig $IgG_1$ and $IgG_2$ anti-bodies by macrophages. *Immunology,* **30,** 267

12 Benacerraf, B., Biozzi, G., Halpern, B. N., Stiffel, C. and Mouton, D. (1957). Phagocytosis of heat denatured human serum albumin labeled with $^{131}$I and its use as a means of investigating liver blood flow. *Br. J. Exp. Pathol.,* **38,** 35

13 Chia, D., Dorsch, C., Barnett, E. V. and Levy, L. (1977). Metabolism of exogenous single strand of DNA in normal and NZB/W mice. *Immunology,* **32,** 351

# 80

# Rheumatoid immunoblasts and the effect of gold and cytotoxic drugs

G. PAPADIMITRIOU, P. A. BACON, S. D. CARTER AND N. D. HALL (UK)

## INTRODUCTION

The successful clinical use of thoracic duct drainage[1] has confirmed the important role of the lymphocyte in the pathogenesis of rheumatoid arthritis. It is impractical to translate these experimental manoeuvres into a clinical procedure unless the important subgroups of pathogenic lymphocytes can be identified. Activated lymphocytes deserve special attention in this context in view of their known characteristics. Activated lymphocytes with the morphological appearance of immunoblasts have previously been identified in increased numbers in rheumatoid arthritis[2] and shown to be large cells with an increased thymidine uptake.

Sub-populations of lymphocytes can be separated by fractionation on Ficoll density gradients[3], which is a particularly convenient way to separate large less dense cells from small denser cells[4]. This methodology has been applied to peripheral blood lymphocytes from rheumatoid arthritis and the less dense cells have been shown to be activated lymphocytes with the morphological characteristics of the previously defined 'immunoblasts'[4]. This work has now been extended to cross-sectional studies of patients either before or after treatment and to serial studies of treatment with either gold or cyclophosphamide. They confirm the suggestion that the less dense cells are indeed a marker of active rheumatoid synovitis.

## METHODS

Peripheral blood lymphocytes separated on Ficoll–Hypaque were carefully layered on to 8-step discontinuous Ficoll gradient as previously described[4]. Cells from each interface were collected and counted. The numbers in the low density fractions are small and so in the present study the results have been pooled to give three groups of cells. The first four steps were pooled as low density (LD) fraction; the next two gradients were pooled as the medium density cells (MD), and the highest density band, together with any cells in the bottom of the tube, were pooled as the high density (HD) fraction. The LD fraction contained the activated cells, including those with the morphological characteristics of immunoblasts, with enlarged nuclei and more prominent cytoplasm. The HD fraction contained normal small resting lymphocytes and compact nuclei and very little cytoplasm. In six healthy controls the mean ($\pm$ 2 1SD) for these groups were:

| | |
|---|---|
| LD | $4.0 \pm 1.1$ |
| MD | $14.0 \pm 2.9$ |
| HD | $81.9 \pm 5.5$ |

These figures are in accord with the larger group of healthy controls previously studied[4]

Patients with classical or definite rheumatoid arthritis were studied. In spot studies, 11 patients with active untreated synovitis were compared with 11 patients on established gold therapy. A further four patients with active rheumatoid disease including active synovitis were followed through a course of cyclophosphamide given as intermittent intravenous bolus doses as previously described[5]

## RESULTS

Cross-sectional studies (Table 80.1) showed that patients with active rheumatoid arthritis prior to initiation of any second line therapy had increased numbers of LD and MD cells compared to the healthy controls and compared to 11 patients on established gold therapy, many of whom had already made a clinical response to the treatment.

**Table 80.1** Comparison of the results of patients with active rheumatoid synovitis with those patients on established gold therapy

| | *Active RA* $n = 11$ ($\pm$ 1SD) | *RA – gold* $n = 11$ ($\pm$ 1SD) |
|---|---|---|
| LD | 17 ($\pm$ 4) | 9 ($\pm$ 3) |
| MD | 43 ($\pm$ 11) | 21 ($\pm$ 4) |
| HD | 40 ($\pm$ 16) | 70 ($\pm$ 8) |

EFFECT OF GOLD AND CYTOTOXIC DRUGS ON IMMUNOBLASTS

Serial studies on four patients during gold therapy confirmed the fall in the numbers of LD cells and concomitant increase in HD cells during therapy. There was considerable individual variation, as illustrated in Figure 80.1,

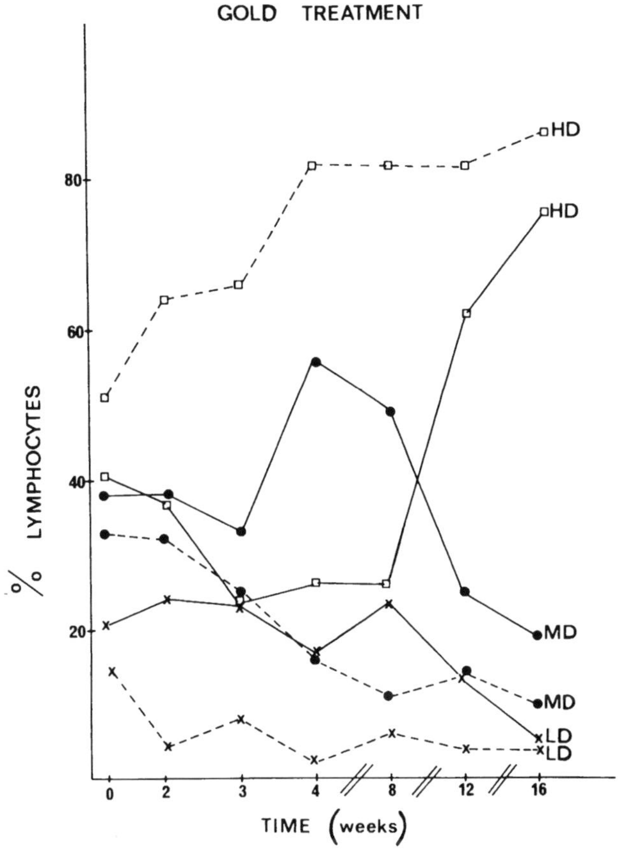


**Figure 80.1** (See text)

with the fastest and slowest response contrasted. Patient 1 showed an immediate fall in LD cells and a rapid fall in MD cells, so that by 4 weeks his proportions in the three fractions were within the normal range. This patient made a rapid clinical response to the gold therapy. In contrast, patient 2 responded very poorly and slowly to the gold therapy. This is reflected in her lymphocyte sub-populations. Her initial levels of LD cells were higher than patient 1, were still grossly elevated at 8 weeks and abnormal at 12 weeks. It was not until 16 weeks that her cell distribution pattern was normal. Clinical improvement commenced at about this time and continued slowly but steadily thereafter.

Six observations were made on two of the patients immediately before and 24 h after a gold injection to observe any direct effect of gold on the circulating lymphocytes. A small fall in the LD and MD fractions were seen in each case but this was considerably less than the overall fall seen during the treatment period.

4 patients with active rheumatoid synovitis were followed during an intermittent cyclophosphamide regime. All 4 patients had elevated levels of LD and MD cells before therapy (Table 80.2). Clinically, this regime was not as effective in treating synovitis, producing little fall in articular index or objective thermographic index of joint inflammation. At the end of the 10 week study period, only 1 of these 4 patients had a normal distribution of lymphocytes on his Ficoll gradient. 2 out of 4 still had increased numbers of LD cells. 3 out of 4 had increased MD cells.

**Table 80.2** Serial response to IV cyclophosphamide. Table shows the percentage of lymphocytes in each group of the Ficoll gradient fractions in four patients followed serially during an intermittent bolus cyclophosphamide regime

| | *LD* | *MD* | *HD* |
|---|---|---|---|
| Week 1 | 13 | 30 | 57 |
| Week 4 | 16 | 22 | 62 |
| Week 7 | 8 | 18 | 74 |
| Week 10 | 7 | 56 | 37 |

The immediate effect of cyclophosphamide was studied by repeat samples on the same patients within 48 h of the bolus dose (Figure 80.2). There was a significant immediate fall in LD and MD cells with a return to a normal pattern in three out of the four patients. This immediate effect is in contrast to the lack of any long term effect of this regime, either lymphocyte subpopulations or the synovitis by clinical or thermographic criteria.

## DISCUSSION

The use of Ficoll density gradients has confirmed and extended the previous studies using morphological criteria to show that activated lymphocytes are circulating in increased numbers in the peripheral blood of patients with rheumatoid arthritis. The less dense cells on the Ficoll gradient had the morphology of activated cells or 'immunoblasts' and have been shown to have an increased spontaneous uptake of [$^3$H]thymidine[4]. The Ficoll gradient is a con-

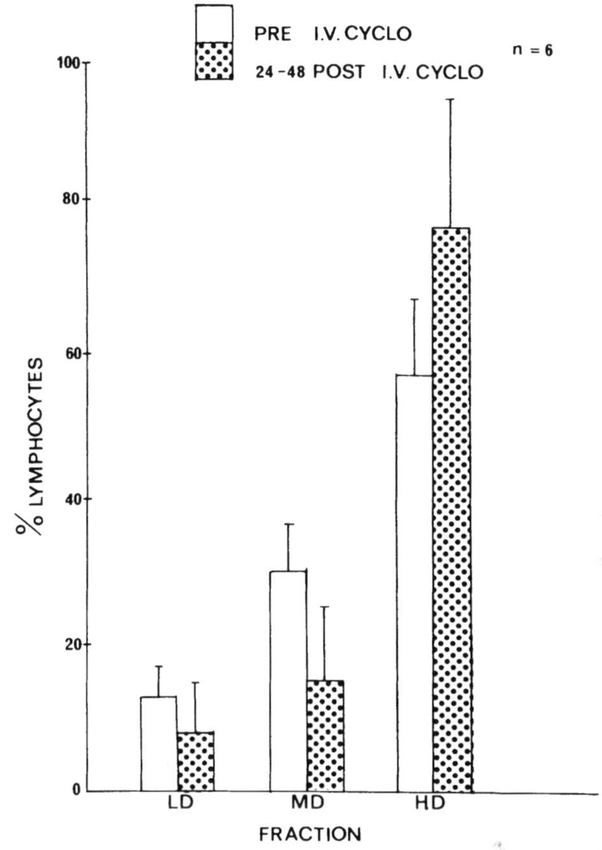


**Figure 80.2** Immediate response to bolus cyclophosphamide from the mean of 6 studies immediately before therapy, as contrasted with the results of the same patients within 48 h of the cyclophosphamide injection

venient and reproducible way of making serial assessments of the incidence of these cells in rheumatoid arthritis during treatment.

Spot studies comparing untreated active patients with those on established gold therapy show that there are higher numbers of less dense cells in the former group. Serial studies of gold therapy have confirmed that the numbers fall during therapy. The rate of fall appears to correlate with, but usually to precede, the appearance of clinical improvement. The one patient who made a poor and delayed response to gold showed the most persistent abnormality in her Ficoll gradient pattern. The immediate effect of a single gold injection on the lymphocyte density distribution was not very marked, suggesting that the gold does not act directly on the circulating cells but may influence their formation. This is in contrast to intravenous cyclophosphamide where an immediate marked but transient effect on circulating cells is seen. However, this intermittent bolus regime, although effective in rheumatoid vasculitis[5] has little effect on the synovitis of rheumatoid arthritis. The pattern of lymphocyte distribution at the end of such a course of cyclophosphamide was still abnormal in three out of four patients studied, correlating with their poor clinical response. It appears that cyclophosphamide, in contradistinction to gold, is immediately effective on the circulating cell levels. However, this regime of cyclophosphamide does not appear to influence the underlying production of abnormal cells in rheumatoid arthritis.

These results suggest that increased numbers of less dense cells in rheumatoid arthritis are a marker of active synovial inflammation. Further evidence of this has come from a study of patients with systemic rheumatoid disease. A group of patients with active synovitis alone has been compared with patients with rheumatoid disease characterized by vasculitis and multiple nodules in the absence of active synovitis[6] The expected increase in less dense cells was seen in the synovial group but did not occur in those with systemic rheumatoid disease. We have already shown that activated cells are found in synovial fluid in rheumatoid arthritis more frequently and in higher numbers than in the peripheral blood[7]. Whether these cells are formed in rheumatoid synovium or are migrating from the peripheral blood into the synovium is not clear. However, in view of the known altered migratory patterns of activated cells[8,9] it is likely that the less dense cells found in the peripheral blood in rheumatoid arthritis have an important role in perpetuating and perhaps spreading the immune inflammation characteristic of rheumatoid synovitis.

## Reference


1 Pearson, C. N. Palus, H. E. and Mackleder, H. I. (1975). The role of the lymphocyte and its products in the propagation of joint disease. *Ann. NY Acad. Sci.*, **256,** 150

2 Bacon, P. A., Sewell, R. L. and Crowther, D. (1975). Reactive lymphoid cells (immunoblasts) in autoimmune and haematological disorders. *Clin. Exp. Immunol.*, **19,**201

3 Gorczynski, R. M., Miller, R. C. and Phillips, R. H. (1970). Homogeneity of antibody-producing cells as analysed by their buoyant density in gradients of Ficoll. *Immunology,* **19,** 817

4 Carter, S. D. (1979). Density distribution of peripheral blood lymphocytes in health and rheumatoid disease. PhD. thesis, University of Bath

5 Scott, D. G. I., Allen, C., Papadimitriou, G. and Bacon, P. A. (1979). Effect of immunosuppression on rheumatoid synovitis and vasculitis. The Heberden Society, November, London

6 Papadimitriou, G. and Bacon, P. A. (1980). Lymphocyte subpopulations by Ficoll gradient in rheumatoid synovitis and rheumatoid disease. (In preparation)

7 Eghtedari, A. A., Bacon, P. A. and Collins, A. J. (1980). Immunoblasts in synovial fluid and blood in the rheumatic diseases. *Ann. Rheum. Dis.* (In press)

8 Hall, J. G. and Smith, M. E. (1970). Homing of lymph-borne immunoblasts to the gut. *Nature* (London), **226,** 262

9 Parrott, D. M. V. and Ferguson, A. (1974). Selective migration of lymphocytes within the mouse small intestine. *Immunology*, **26,** 571

# 81

# Immunological and clinical effects of human placenta-eluted gammaglobulins (PEGG) in rheumatoid arthritis

J. SANY, J. CLOT, M. BONNEAU AND M. ANDARY (FRANCE)

## INTRODUCTION

The human foetus is considered as an allograft which is accepted by the pregnant mother for still unknown reasons, since humoral and cell mediated responses have been demonstrated against the paternal haplotype[2]. Alloantibodies to transplantation antigens have been shown in the placenta. After elution at acid pH, Voisin and Chaouat[26] have reported that placenta eluates were able specifically to enhance an incompatible graft from paternal tissue. The pioneering work of Revillaed *et al.*[17] showed that maternal sera contained antibodies that effectively inhibited the mixed lymphocyte reaction (MLR) of maternal cells against paternal lymphocytes. Bonneau *et al.*[3,4] demonstrated that purified IgG eluted from human placenta were able to inhibit the MLR by blocking HLA-DR antigens carried on stimulating cells[18]. In addition, these fractions or the $F(ab)'_2$ fragments thereof were shown to prevent the binding of erythrocyte-IgG antibody (EA) complexes to human mononuclear cells.

Rheumatoid arthritis (RA) is a chronic systemic rheumatic disease in which immunological aspects have recently dominated research endeavours. Among them, MLR abnormalities[1], the presence of 'high avidity' Fc-receptor bearing circulating cells[22,23] and the clinical observation of frequent pregnancy-associated remissions lead us to treat RA patients with human placenta-eluted gammaglobulins (PEGG).

## MATERIALS AND METHODS

### Patients

Five patients (3 women, 2 men; mean age 56.4 years; range 47–68 years) with classical severe sero-positive (Waaler–Rose reaction) rheumatoid arthritis (RA) according to the American Rheumatism Association criteria[20] were studied. According to Steinbrocker's classification[25], radioclinical stages were III in all the cases; functional stages were III in 4 patients, IV in one case. RA was clinically active in all patients; 3 cases had rheumatoid nodules. The mean duration of the disease was 7.8 years (2–12 years).

Treatments included analgesic drugs (paracetamol), anti-inflammatory drugs (indomethacin 150 mg daily) in four cases, anti-malarial drugs (hydroxychloroquine 600 mg daily) in two cases. One patient received delta-cortisone per os 10 mg daily and another hydrocortisone per os 40 mg daily because of a chronic suprarenal failure. In all cases, the treatment was continued without any modification for more than 6 months; new drugs were not associated during the therapeutic period with PEGG.

### Obtainment of placenta-eluted gammaglobulins (PEGG)

Placental trophoblast-bound gammaglobulins were eluted, fractionated and purified according to a general protocol (Figure 81.1) already reported[3].

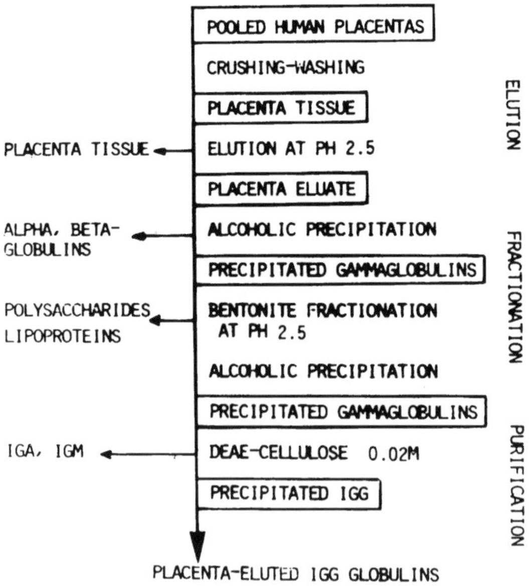


**Figure 81.1** General protocol used for preparation of placenta-eluted gammaglobulins

Briefly, placenta eluates were prepared by elution at acid pH 2.5 from large pools of human placenta tissues previously washed and without retroplacental blood. Gammaglobulins were recovered after alcoholic precipitations and fractionation on bentonite and aerosil gels. Purified IgG fractions were obtained by chromatography on QAE Sephadex A-50 (Pharmacia). The final solution of PEGG (batch SO658 and S0800) contained 47.7 g/l of proteins and 36.8 g/l of IgG.

### Therapeutic protocol

Each ampoule of 5 ml contained 250 mg of PEGG. In four patients, we used batch S0658, in one case batch S0800. In all cases, the same batch was used during all the therapeutic period. Each patient received a slow intravenous perfusion (5 h) of 1500 mg of PEGG diluted in 250 ml of isotonic sodium chloride. This treatment was done according to different procedures.

(1) In one case (number 1), treatment was given in an discontinuous way, 1500 mg once a week during 4 weeks (total dose 6000 mg).

(2) In two cases (numbers 2 and 3), treatment was given continuously; 1500 mg daily during 6 days (number 2, 9000 mg) or 7 days (number 3, 10 500 mg).

(3) In two cases (numbers 4 and 5), there were two steps in the treatment. In a first period, patients received a continuous treatment of 1500 mg daily during 7 days (10 500 mg). In one case (number 4) a second continuous therapeutic period with the same dose was performed 3 months after the first therapeutic trial. The second step was constituted by a discontinuous therapeutic period including 1500 mg of PEGG every fortnight. Patient number 4 received one perfusion twice at a 15-day interval and then two perfusions (2 following days) every fortnight 7 times. Patient number 5 received one perfusion 15 days after the end of the continuous treatment and then three perfusions (3 following days) 15 days later.

### Clinical survey

Clinical evaluation of patients was made before the treatment, after an 8 day period of treatment and after each perfusion for discontinuous treatments. Clinical assessment was always done in the morning at the same hour and included pain evaluation (by graphic method and scoring method: 0 = no pain; 1 = mild pain; 2 = moderate pain; 3 = severe pain), morning stiffness in minutes, time needed for a 15 metre walk (in seconds), and Lee's[16] and Ritchie's[19] indexes. Clinical evaluation was carried out by the same investigator without any preceding clinical data. Patients were followed after the end of the treatment during 16 months (number 1), 22 months (number 2), 12 months (number 3), 6 months (number 4), 1 month (number 5)

Results were expressed as good if an improvement $\geq 50\%$ of the above parameters was noted, very good if the improvement reached 75%. Other cases in which clinical improvement was $< 50\%$ were considered as failure. Local and general tolerance (especially renal tolerance) of PEGG was carefully studied in each case.

**Biological parameters**

We studied in all cases before and after treatment: erythrocyte sedimentation rate (ESR), red blood cell, white blood cell and platelet counts, Waaler–Rose reaction, blood uraemia, creatininaemia, total complement and fractions C3 and C4, total blood proteins, protein electrophoresis, serum IgG, IgA, IgM levels, antinuclear and anti-DNA antibodies, proteinuria.

**Immunological studies**

Several immunological parameters were investigated before treatment with PEGG and at days 8, 30, 60 and 90 after the intravenous injections. Circulating immune complexes (CIC) were detected by the polyethylene-glycol (PEG)-C4 assay[14], in which endogenous complement component C4 precipitated with CIC was determined by laser nephelometry[12].

Lymphocyte membrane markers were studied according to methods previously published in detail[10,11]. T cells were assessed by E-rosette forming cells (E-RFC), active E-RFC and heterologous specific anti-human T lymphocyte antigens serum[6]. B cells, bearing surface membrane immunoglobulins (SmIg) were enumerated by surface immunofluorescence. Fc-receptor bearing cells were detected by rosette formation in the presence of ox erythrocyte-IgG antibody (OEA) complexes. Monocyte contamination was judged by peroxidase staining.

Mitogen responsiveness was studied by *in vitro* lymphocyte cultures[9,11]. Three mitogens were used: phytohaemagglutinin (PHA), Concanavalin A (Con A) and pokeweed mitogen (PWM). The results were expressed as stimulation index corresponding to the ratio: disintegrations per minute of quadruplicate cultures in the presence of mitogen/disintegrations per minute of quadruplicate unstimulated cultures.

Mixed lymphocyte cultures (MLC) were always performed with unrelated lymphoid cells from a same donor for each patient under study. Both normal and RA lymphocytes were used as responding and stimulating (mitomycin-treated) cells. A leukocyte migration inhibition test (LMIT) was performed according to a previously reported method[8] in the presence of streptokinase (250 U/ml) as positive control and human purified slightly aggregated IgG (250 μg/ml)[7].

## RESULTS

### Clinical data

Two failures were observed (patients number 1 and 2). Patient 1 received a discontinuous therapy (1500 mg weekly); in patient 2 the continuous treatment had to be stopped after 6 days because of renal side effects. In one case (number 3), a very good and prolonged (8 months) result was obtained but only 3 months after the end of the treatment. In two patients we noted a very good (number 4) and a good result (number 5) after 5 days of a daily treatment in case number 4 and 7 days of the same therapy in case number 5. Improvement was impressive in both cases with a marked decrease of all clinical indexes; in one patient (number 4), a decrease of some rheumatoid nodules of more than 50% of their initial volume with total disappearance of other nodules was noted 7 days after the beginning of treatment. In patient 4 (Figure 81.2(a)), the improvement obtained after the first therapeutic period lasted 3 months and then the disease flared up; the second therapeutic period gave also a very good result but of a shorter duration (5 weeks). In patient 5, the result lasted 3 weeks. Discontinuous treatment was a failure in case 5. In patient 4 an improvement was noted by this therapeutic method, but it was not considered as significant (because of a slight decrease of indexes).

### Tolerance and side effects

Local tolerance was excellent in all cases. General tolerance was good in four out of five cases. Benign side effects such as transitory nausea (three cases), headache (one case), oedema of the upper lip, at the end of the first perfusion were noted; all these side effects disappeared in spite of the repetition of perfusions. In a 47-year-old woman, not yet in menopause, an increased volume of breast and a weight augmentation (3 kg) was noted; this side effect spontaneously disappeared in 21 days. In only one case (number 2), treatment had to be interrupted because of nausea, obnubilation and proteinuria of 1.40 g daily with an increase of blood urea (0.80 g/l) and a slight increase of creatininaemia (17 mg/1); the nephropathy occurred on the fifth day of treatment which was stopped after 6 perfusions of 1500 mg (total dose: 7500 mg of PEGG). This side effect totally disappeared without sequella in 15 days.

### Immunological data

Some immunological parameters were shown to be unmodified after treatment with PEGG compared to the results recorded before the intravenous perfusions. It was the case for cell-mediated immune responses to IgG, assessed by LMIT. Rheumatoid factor levels were not significantly modified. The proportions of monocytes, of SmIg-bearing B cells (Figure 81.3) of E-RFC (Figure 81.4) and of human T lymphocyte antigen-positive cells remained similar before and after treatment.

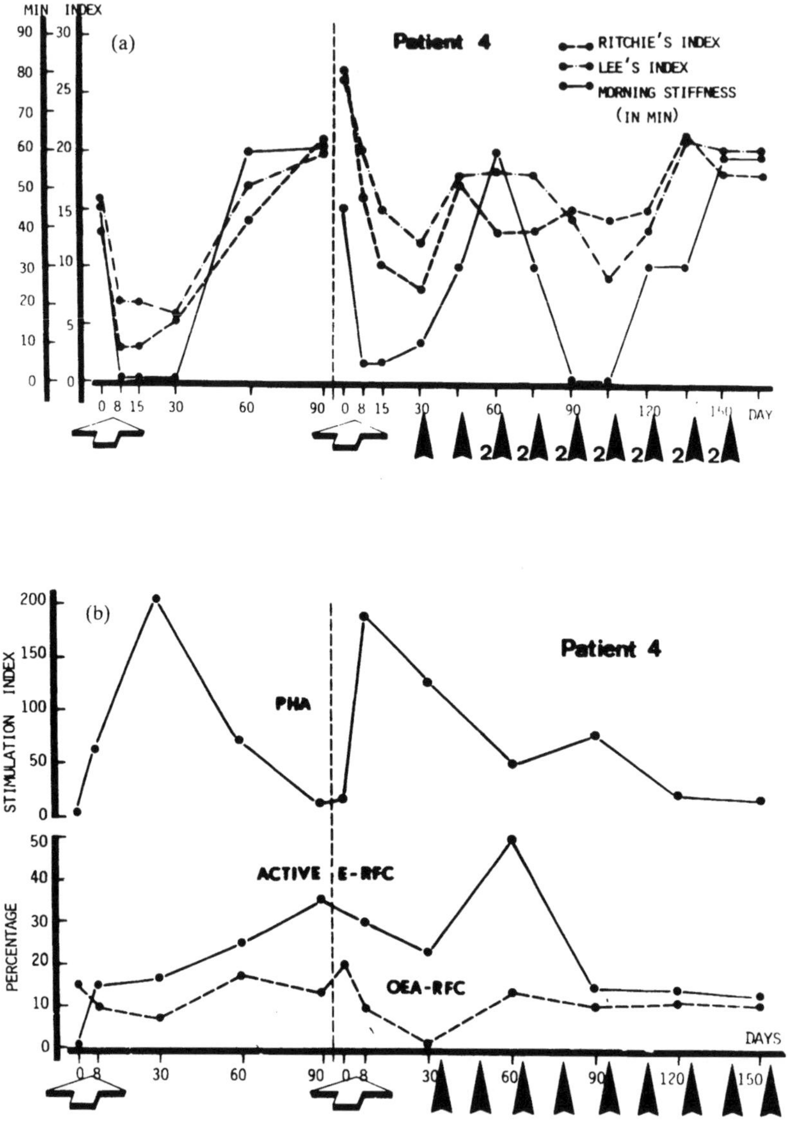


**Figure 81.2** Data obtained from patient number 4. (a) Clinical data. The large arrows represent 7 day perfusions with PEGG. The black arrows represent 1 day perfusion or 2 day perfusions (number 2 before the arrow). (b) Immunological data

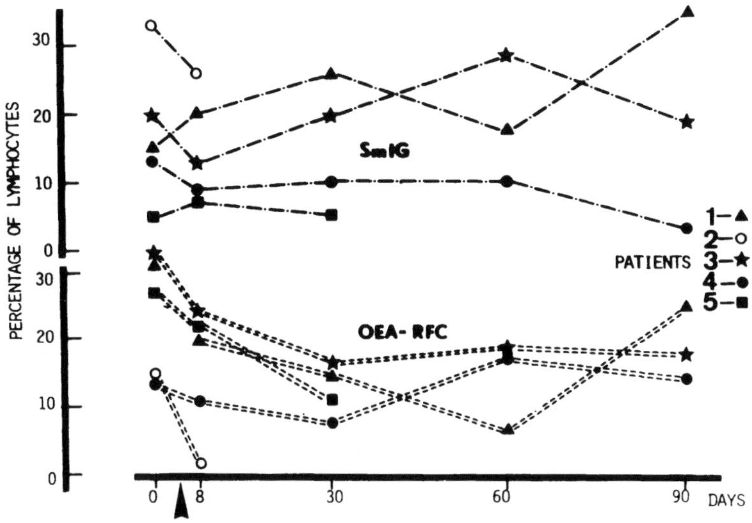


**Figure 81.3** Modifications of surface membrane Ig bearing cells (SmIg) and of OEA-rosette forming cells (OEA-RFC) in patients before (day 0) and after PEGG perfusions. The black arrow indicates 7 day perfusions

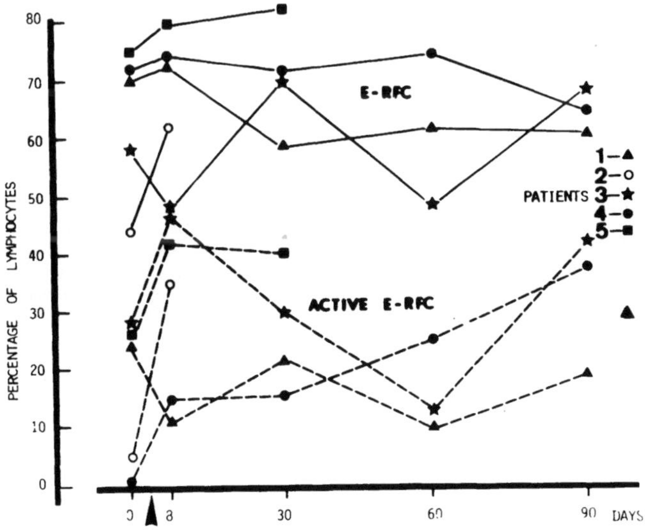


**Figure 81.4** Modifications of E-rosette forming cells (E-RFC) and active E-RFC in patients before (day 0) and after PEGG perfusions. The black arrow indicates 7 day perfusions

In contrast, the following parameters were significantly modified as early as just after the last PEGG injection (day 8). CIC decreased in all patients (from 50 to 95% decrease) within the month following the perfusions. They remained in a normal range during 3 months (cases 1, 3 and 5) or returned to pathological values (case 4). The percentage of increase of active E-RFC (Figure 81.4) was 40 to 100% in all cases but one (patient receiving discontinuous PEGG-perfusions) within the first week. Two patients (numbers 2 and 4) had very low active E-RFC percentages before therapy. OEA-RFC, detecting Fc-receptor bearing lymphocytes, were always decreased during the first month (Figure 81.3), then returned to normal values.

Studies on mitogen responsiveness (Figures 81.5 and 81.6) showed that mainly PHA stimulation, and, to some extent, Con A stimulation were enhanced in all cases (from 30% to 99% of increase). Such a phenomenon lasted 2 months, then mitogen stimulation returned to abnormally low levels as before therapy. An increase of PWM stimulation was noted in patients 2, 3 and 4 (Figure 81.6). The responses to allogenic cells assessed by MLC were found to be normal in cases 4 and 5 after treatment, whereas they were lacking before.

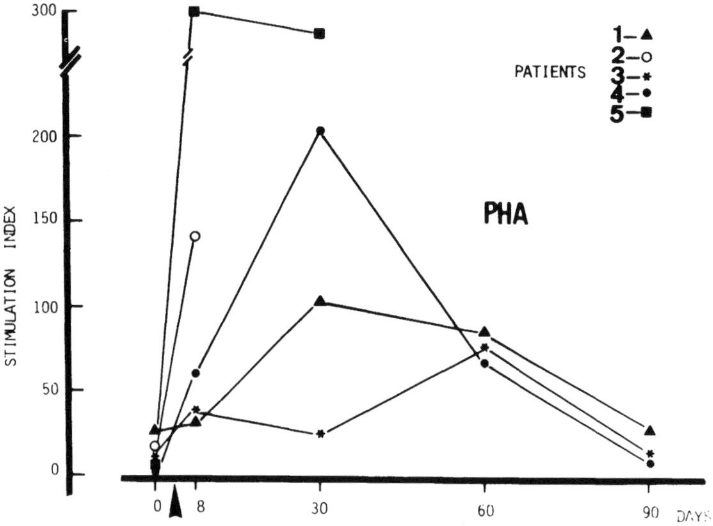


**Figure 81.5** Modifications of PHA stimulation of lymphocytes from patients before (day 0) and after PEGG perfusions (on the right side of the black arrow)

Sera were collected in patients receiving discontinuous perfusions. As it was demonstrated that PEGG *in vitro* inhibited mixed lymphocyte reaction, we performed MLC with lymphoid cells from two unrelated blood donors in the presence of such sera. A 50% inhibition of MLC was noted and due to sera

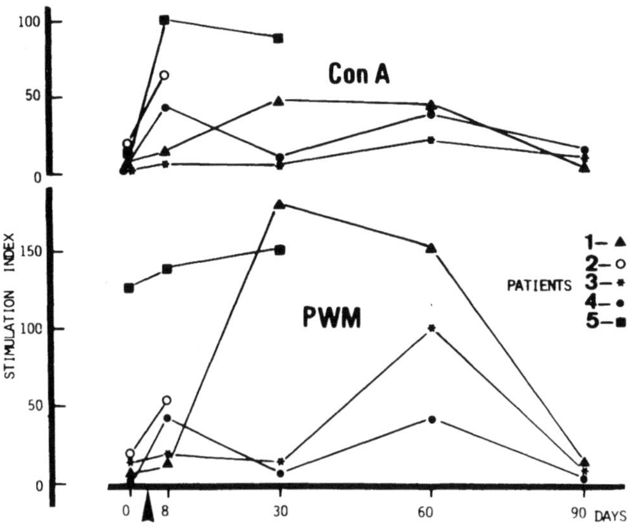


**Figure 81.6** Modifications of Con A and PWM stimulation of lymphocytes from patients before (day 0) and after PEGG perfusions (on the right side of the black arrow)

collected up to 8 days after the last intravenous injection. Such an inhibition was not significant in sera drawn up at days $\geq 9$. Other biological data were found to be unmodified after PEGG therapy.

**Clinical and immunological correlations**

All patients had immunological modifications, but only 3 patients were significantly improved. In one of them (number 3), a spontaneous improvement cannot be excluded because the result appeared 3 months after the treatment; however, in this case, the clinical improvement occurred when active E rosettes increased and when mitogen responsiveness became normal. In patients 4 (Figure 81.2 (b)) and 5, there was a very good correlation between the clinical improvement and the increase of active E rosettes and the normalization of lymphocyte response to mitogens.

## DISCUSSION

Purified IgG fractions prepared by elution at acid pH from human pooled placentas were previously shown to inhibit mixed lymphocyte reactions by blocking mainly the stimulating cells[3,4,15]. Furthermore, $F(ab')_2$ fragments from these PEGG were able to prevent the binding of erythrocyte-IgG antibody (EA) complexes to human mononuclear cells. Such effects were accounted for by the presence in PEGG of HLA-DR antibodies[4] associated to Fc receptors on mononuclear cells[13].

The present work is the first report concerning the use of PEGG in an autoimmune disease such as RA. Previous clinical trials were carried out in renal and bone marrow transplantations; the results are as yet unclear[5].

A very significant clinical improvement was noted in 2 patients out of 5, all of them having a severe classical sero-positive RA. This effect was transient. However, the doses of PEGG and the periodicity of injections remain to be clearly established and may greatly influence the clinical effects. The MLC-inhibiting activity found in some sera could be used for such a purpose.

It must be pointed out that a quite good correlation exists between the clinical improvement and the immunological modifications (see patient number 4). Contrary to previous attempts[5], it seems that PEGG, used in patients without any other treatment acting on the immune response, has an immunostimulating effect on mitogen stimulation and on active E-RFC. This unexpected result was clearly shown in our patients with severe RA. The occurrence of T cell defect was already reported in such types of RA[27]. As demonstrated *in vitro*, PEGG injected into patients was able significantly to decrease Fc-receptor bearing cell proportions, as detected by OEA-RFC. The diminishing effect observed on CIC remains unclear.

The mechanism of action of such PEGG is unknown. Since part of the *in vitro* effects of PEGG can be accounted for by the presence of HLA-DR antibodies, one might speculate that the *in vivo* effects are mediated by HLA-DR bearing cells, like B cells[24] and some T cell sub-sets[21]. However, other mechanisms cannot be ruled out as interactions with Fc-receptor cells and cell-bound CIC.

In any case, PEGG acts as an immunomodulating agent able significantly to improve some RA patients. Although preliminary, our first results could lead to a better study of the relationship between pregnancy and RA remissions, and to a better understanding of pathogenesis of such a chronic disease.

## ACKNOWLEDGMENTS

We gratefully acknowledge the excellent technical assistance of Line Lioure, Christiane Clément and Evelyne Cadars.

### References

1 Astorga, G. P. and Williams, R. C. (1969). Altered reactivity in mixed lymphocyte culture of lymphocytes from patients with rheumatoid arthritis. *Arthritis Rheum.*, **12,** 547

2 Beer, A. E. and Billingham, R. E. (1971). Immunobiology of mammalian reproduction. *Adv. Immunol.*, **14,** 1

3 Bonneau, M., Latour, M., Revillard, J. P., Robert, M. and Traeger, J. (1973). Blocking antibodies eluted from human placenta. *Transplant. Proc.*, **5**, 589

4 Bonneau, M., Brochier, J., Revillard, J.P., Cordier, G., Ekladios, E., Dubernard, J. M., and Trager, J. (1975). Immunological properties of IgG eluted from human placenta. *Transplant. Proc.*, **7**, 461

5 Bonneau, M., Brochier, J., Robert, M., Dubernard, J. M., Fayol, A., Blanc, N., Revillard, J. P. and Traeger, J. (1977). Préparation, propriétés et essais pré-clinques de gammaglobulines éluées à pH acide de pools de placentas humains. In: Simep (ed.) *Transplanation et Immunologie clinique*, pp. 150–163 (Villeurbanne).

6 Brochier, J., Abou-hamed, Y. A., Gueho, J. P. and Revillard, J.P. (1976). Study of human T and B lymphocytes with heterologous antisera. I: preparation, specificity and properties of antisera. *Immunology*, **32**, 749

7 Clot, J., Sany, J. and Serre, H. (1973). Aspects de l'immunité à médiation cellulaire dans la polyarthrite rhumatoïde. *Pathol., Biol.*, **21**, 465

8 Clot, J., Elharrar, S. and Mandin, J. (1974). Luekocyte migration inhibition test: suppression of antigen-induced inhibition by antilymphocyte serum. *Ann. Immunol.*, **125 C**, 589

9 Clot, J., Massip, H. and Mathieu, O. (1975). *In vitro* studies on human B and T cell purified populations. *Immunology,* **29**, 445

10 Clot, J., Charmasson, E. and Brochier, J. (1978). Age dependent changes of human blood lymphocyte subpopulations. *Clin. Exp. Immunol.*, **32**, 346

11 Clot, J., Darenne, M., Brochier, J., Andary, M. and Guilhou, J. J. (1978). Evaluation of lymphocyte subpopulations and T cell functions in psoriasis. *Clin. Immunol. Immunopathol.*, **9**, 389

12 Clot, J., Guilhou, J. J., Guillot, B. and Meynadier, J. (1979). Immune complexes in psoriasis. In *Cutaneous Immunopathology, INSERM,* **80**, 341

13 Dickler, H. B. and Sachs, D. H. (1974). Evidence for identity or class association of the Fc-receptors of B lymphocytes and allo-antigens determined by the Ir region of the H-2 complex. *J. Exp. Med.*, **140**, 779

14 Digeon, M., Laver, M., Riza, J. and Bach, J. F. (1977). Detection of circulating immune complexes in human sera by simplified assays with polyethylene glycol. *J. Immunol. Meth.*, **16**, 165

15 Jeannet, M., Faulk, W. P., Crighton, W. D. and Fournier, K. (1974). Blocking of mixed lymphocyte cultures by IgG eluted from human placenta. In Lindhal-Kiessling, K. and Osoba, K. (Eds.)*Proceedings VIIIth Leukocyte Conference*, pp. 243–248. (London: Academic Press)

16 Lee, P., Jasani, M. K., Dick, W. and Buchanan, W. W. (1973). Evaluation of a functional index in rheumatoid arthritis. *Scand. J. Rheum.*, **2**, 71

17 Revillard, J. P., Robert, M., Betuel, H., Latour, M., Bonneau, M., Brochier, J. and Traeger, J. (1972). Inhibition of the mixed lymphocyte reaction by antibodies. *Transplant. Proc.*, **4**,173

18 Revillard, J. P., Brochier, J., Robert, M., Bonneau, M. and Traeger, J. (1976). Immunological properties of placenta eluates. *Transplant. Proc.*, **7**, 275

19 Ritchie, D. M., Boule, J. A., McInnes, J. M., Jasani, M., K., Dalakos, I. G., Griveson, P. and Buchanan, W. (1968). Clinical studies with an articular index for the assessment of joint tenderness in patients with rheumatoid arthritis. *Q. J. Med.*, **37**, 393

20 Ropes, M. W., Bennet, G. A. and Cobb, S. (1958). Revision of diagnostic criteria for rheumatoid arthritis. *Bull. Rheum. Dis.*, **9**,175

21 Samarut, C., Gebuhrer, L., Brochier, J., Betuel, H. and Revillard, J. P. (1977). Presence of Ia like antigens on human T lymphocytes bearing receptors for IgG. *Eur. J. Immonol.*, **7**, 908

22 Sany, J., Clot, J., Massip, H., Charmasson, E. and Serre, H. (1975). Sous-populations lymphocytaires impliquées dans le phénomène des rosettes rhumatoïdes. *Rev. Rheum.*, **42**, 309

23 Sharpin, R. K. C. and Wilson, J. D. (1977). Increased E-rosette formation by lymphocytes from patients with rheumatoid arthritis. *Clin. Exp. Immunol.*, **29**, 205

24 Snary, D., Barnstable, C. J., Bodmer, W. F., Goddfellow, P. N. and Crumpton, M. J. (1977). Cellular distribution, purification and molecular nature of human Ia antigens. *Scand. J. Immunol.*, **6**, 439

25 Steinbrocker, O., Traeger, C. H. and Batterman, R. C. (1949). Therapeutic criteria in rheumatoid arthritis. *J. Am. Med. Assoc.*, **140,** 659

26 Voison, G. A. and Chaouat, G. (1974). Demonstration, nature and properties of maternal antibodies fixed on placenta and directed against paternal antigens. *J. Reprod. Fertil. (Suppl.)*, **21,** 89

27 Williams, R. C., Deboard, J. R., Messner, R. P. and Mellbye, O. J. (1972). Studies of T and B cells in patients with rheumatoid arthritis and systemic lupus erythematosus. *Arthritis Rheum.*, **15,** 461

# 82

# Modification of antibody responses during non-specific acute inflammation (Abstract)

I. FLORENTIN, M. PELLETIER, G. MATHE
AND J. P. GIROUD (FRANCE)

It has been previously shown that non-specific acute inflammatory reactions are able to modify the activity of lymphocytes and macrophages. In the present work we investigated whether such a reaction could interfere with the development of antibody responses. For this purpose, $(C57Bl/6 \times DBA/2)F_1$ mice were immunized with sheep red blood cells (SRBC) as a thymus dependent antigen or with TNP-LPS as a thymus-independent one, from 1 h to 5 days after the intrapleural injection of calcium pyrophosphate (CaPP) microcrystals or a dextran solution (MW 40 000).

In mice developing a CaPP pleurisy, a significant potentiation of the antibody response to SRBC was observed when the animals were immunized 2 h 1 day or 3 days after application of the inflammatory stimulus, a maximum 2-fold increase in the number of plaque forming cells (PFC) per spleen being observed in the 2 h treated group. In mice immunized with TNP-LPS, the stimulatory effect (1.8-fold increase in the number of PCF/spleen) was only detected in the group given the antigen 3 days after pleurisy induction.

Similarly, dextran inflammation modifies the development of the antibody response to SRBC but in a different manner. A 2.4 and 2.7-fold increase of the PCF number/spleen was observed when the time interval between pleurisy induction and antigen stimulation was 1 h or 4 days. These results demonstrate that inflammatory processes of non-immunologic origin could markedly affect the immune reactivity of the host.

# 83

# Levamisole and thymopoietin pentapeptide (TP5) correction of E-rosette depression in man: *in vitro* and *in vivo* studies

F. LAGHI PASINI, A. AUTERI AND T. DI PERRI (ITALY)

## INTRODUCTION

Several clinical states may show a decrease of the circulating E-rosette forming cells. We observed that the lymphocytes with a reduced E-rosette forming power when incubated *in vitro* with levamisole either showed an increase in number to the normal values or the E-rosette forming cells did not change. This last group was less frequent and was found in clinical situations compatible with true thymus-dependent T cell depletion (leukaemia, Hodgkin's disease, LES). Frequently the incubation of lymphocytes with levamisole was promptly followed by a normalization of the E-rosette forming cells.

In order to verify the capacity of levamisole to modify this immunological defect *in vivo*, we have investigated the effect of single doses of 50, 100 and 150 mg of the drug on E-rosette forming cells (ERFC) in patients with rheumatoid arthritis and a low number of ERFC. The results obtained confirmed that levamisole produces a dose related sustained increase in ERFC and that a single dose of 150 mg restores ERFC to normal for about 1 week. These observations on the immunological effects of levamisole has pointed to the conclusion that this drug also enhances *in vivo* the immune response, when it is deficient, and has provided the rational basis of a clinical trial in rheumatoid arthritis patients[1-3].

Recently a pentapeptide (Arg-Lys-Asp-Val-Tyr), corresponding to position 32–36 of thymopoietin II, was synthetized by Goldstein[4]. This pentapeptide (TP5) has shown the whole hormonal properties of the thymic extracts. In fact, in experimental and human studies, TP5 in addition to differentiating effects on immature T cells, also acts on the function of peripheral T lymphocytes[5].

On the basis of these premises and according to our findings on the thymus-like activity of levamisole on peripheral E-rosette formation we have studied the thymopoietin pentapeptide. We have selected a population of rheumatoid arthrits patients with E-rosette lymphocyte reduction in order to verify whether TP5 could reverse this immunological defect *in vitro* and/or *in vivo*.

## MATERIAL AND METHODS

### *In vitro* studies

15 patients with classical or definite rheumatoid arthritis by the ARA criteria and with reduced E-rosette lymphocytes were selected.

*The E-rosette test*

Venous blood was collected on heparin and mononuclear cells (MNC) were separated according to Boyum[6]. After washing, MNC were suspended in Hank's balanced salt solution and their concentration was adjusted to $2 \times 10^6$ MNC/ml. 0.40 ml MNC suspension was mixed with 0.40 ml of 0.5% sheep red blood cells (SRBC). The mixture was incubated for 15 min at 37 °C and then centrifuged for 2 min at 200 *g*. 0.40 ml of supernatant was removed and the sediment incubated overnight at 4 °C. TP5, $1.33 \times 10^{-6}$ mol/l final concentration, was incubated with MNC before SRBC were added. After gentle re-suspension ERFC were counted in an haemocytometer with phase contrast microscopy. The results obtained were compared by Student's *t*-test for paired variates.

### *In vivo* studies

Patients with classical or definite rheumatoid arthritis by the ARA criteria were selected. 14 patients with reduced ERFC, which was restored to normal values after *in vitro* treatment with TP5, were included in the study. Treatment with penicillamine, steroidal or non-steroidal anti-inflammatory drugs and crysotherapy was discontinued 7 days before the intake of TP5.

7 patients received a single i.v. dose of 5 mg and 7 patients received a single i.v. dose of 50 mg of TP5. There were 10 females and 4 males ranging in age from 28 to 58 years (median=4 years) and in weight from 45 to 78 kg (median=58 kg).

ERFC without (basal) and with *in vitro* addition of TP5 were counted before, 12 h and daily for 1 week, after the administration of TP5. The E-rosette test was performed as described elsewhere. The statistical analysis of the results was performed with the analysis of variance (one way).

## RESULTS

The *in vitro* effects of TP5 on ERFC in rheumatoid arthritis patients are shown in Figure 83.1. TP5 seems to able to increase the number of ERFC in this group of patients from mean 37.2, SD 5.4, to mean 48.6, SD 5.4. The effect was found to be highly significant ($p > 0.001$ by Student's $t$-test for paired variations).

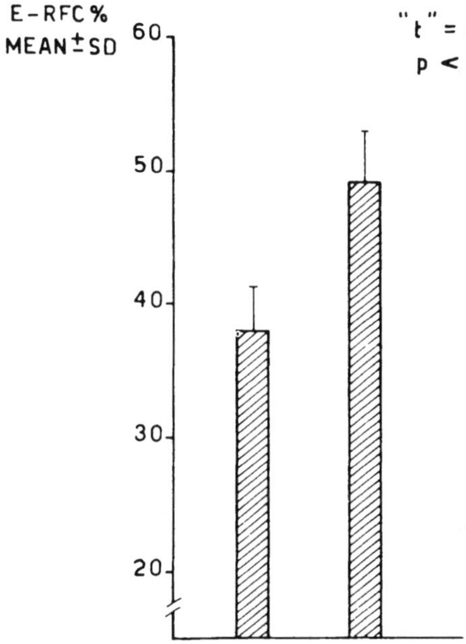


**Figure 83.1** *In vitro* effects of TP5 on ERFC of rheumatoid arthritis patients

With the administration of 5 mg of TP5 i.v. the basal values of ERFC markedly increased within 24 h and returned to the pretreatment level on the second day. The *in vitro* addition of TP5 that was able to normalize low basal values did not further increase the E-rosette forming cells during the period of treatment (Figure 83.2).

With the dose of 50 mg of TP5 the marked increase of the basal value of ERFC was more prolonged (3–4 days). In this case the *in vitro* addition of TP5 slightly increased the number of rosette forming lymphocytes (Figure 83.3). The statistical evaluation of the results showed that the two doses of the drug increased the number of ERFC in a highly significant way.

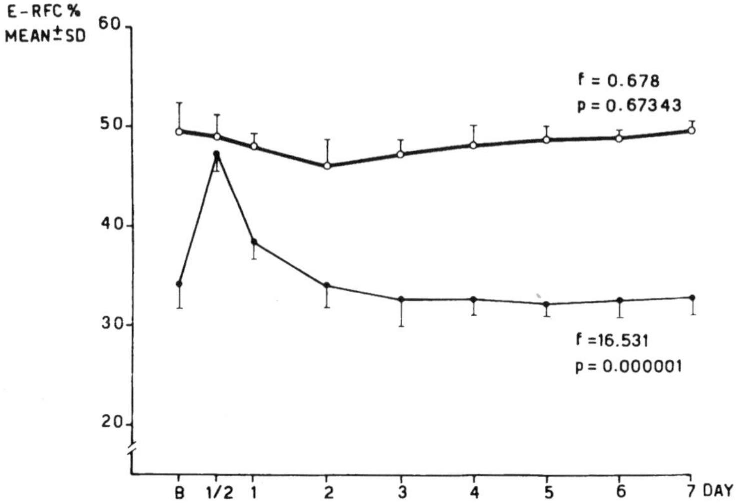


**Figure 83.2** *In vivo* effects of 5 mg of TP5 i.v. on ERFC of rheumatoid arthritis patients. ● = basal values, ○ = with *in vitro* addition of TP5

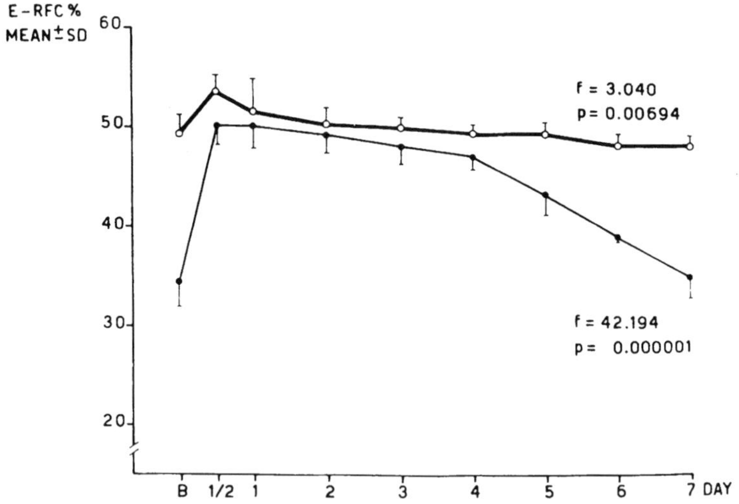


**Figure 83.3** *In vivo* effects of 50 mg of TPS i.v. on ERFC of rheumatoid arthritis patients. ● = basal values, ○ = with *in vitro* addition of TPS

## DISCUSSION

Our findings show that thymopoietin pentapeptide is able to normalize the low ERFC of rheumatoid arthritis patients when incubated *in vitro*. Its activity seems to be of the same degree of the natural thymus extracts. Although the biochemical basis of the immunological defect is not yet known it could be hypothesized that lymphocyte function is mediated by a close control of intracellular cAMP/cGMP ratio and that any relative increase of cAMP inhibits cellular function. Goldstein and co-workers demonstrated that thymopoietin pentapeptide is able to increase the intracellular level of cGMP in peripheral T lymphocytes[4]. Thereafter it is possible that the restoration to normal values of low rosetting lymphocytes in rheumatoid arthritis patients by the *in vitro* addition of TP5 could be mediated by a modulating action on cyclic nucleotide metabolism.

The *in vivo* treatment with two doses of TP5 i.v. restored the low E-rosette forming lymphocytes of the rheumatoid arthritis patients. The response of T cells to the drug depended on the injected dose. With both doses, either 5 or 50 mg, the immediate increase of the ERFC was of the same amount; the duration of the effect was less than 24 h after 5 mg of TP5 while it was still present on the fourth day after the injection of 50 mg of TP5. The increase of the ERFC was of the same degree of the increase obtained by the *in vitro* incubation of the drug of lymphocytes of not treated rheumatoid arthritis patients.

These findings led us to conclude that:

(1) A lot of rheumatoid arhritis patients show a population of lymphocytes which do not form E-rosettes; this defect can be corrected by incubation with TP5 *in vitro*.

(2) TP5 is active to restore the E-rosette forming cells *in vivo*: the duration of the *in vivo* effect appears generally to be dependent on the amount of the drug injected.

These results suggest the necessity of further investigation in a therapeutic programme to see whether the prolonged correction of T cell abnormality in rheumatoid arthritis patients can be followed by a clinical improvement.

## ACKNOWLEDGMENT

The authors gratefully acknowledge Janssen Pharmaceutica, Beerse, Belgium, for the kind gift of TP5 synthesized by G. Goldstein.

### References

1 Di Perri, T., Auteri, A., Laghi Passini, F. and Mattioli, F. (1978). A weekly oral dose of levamisole in the treatment of rheumatoid arthritis associated with E-rosette lymphocytes reduction. *Eur. J. Rheum. Inflamm.*, **1**, 155

2 Di Perri, T., Auteri, A., and Laghi Pasini, F. (1979). Immunokinetics of a single dose of Levamisole. *J. Immunopharm.*, **1**, 269

3 Di Perri, T., Auteri, A., Laghi Pasini, F. and Mattioli, F. (1979). Action of Levamisole on E-rosette forming cells and serum adenosindeaminase in Hodgkin's disease. *J. Immunopharm.*, **1**, 233

4 Goldstein, G. A synthetic pentapeptide with biological activity characteristic of the thymic hormone thymopoientin. (unpublished report)

5 Verhaegen, H. Comparison of the *in vitro* effects of thymopoietin pentapeptide and levamisole on peripheral E-rosette formation. (unpublished report)

6 Boyum, A. (1968). Isolation of mononuclear cells and granulocytes from human blood. *Scand. J. Clin. Lab. Invest.*, **21**, (Suppl. 97), 77

# 84

# Comparison between a curative and a preventive effect of an immunological therapy on an experimental gingivitis

A. DANIEL AND M. DUPONT (FRANCE)

## INTRODUCTION

In a previous work[1] it was shown that subjects with clinically healthy gingivae develop gingivitis after 14 days without oral hygiene (Figure 84.1). It was noted that the composition of the gingival connective tissue underwent marked alteration. The most important modifications were the increased size of the infiltrated connective tissue and the plasma cells' population increase. These results were in agreement with the results obtained by James and Counsell[2], Zachrisson[3] and Schroeder *et al.*[4,5].

The purpose of the present study is to double-blindly evaluate with this experimental model the effects of an oral immunological therapy on an 'established' gingivitis (curative effects) and on an 'establishing' gingivitis (preventive effects). Recent investigations have suggested that local immunity may be stimulated to contribute to protection against diseases of mucosal surfaces[6–11]. In the oral cavity locally produced immunoglobulins are found in saliva[12,13] and might play as such a protective role. It was therefore interesting to study the effects of an oral immunological therapy on gingivitis.

## MATERIALS AND METHODS

Thirty young male and female dental students in good health participated in the experiment. They were volunteers, free of active periodontal disease,

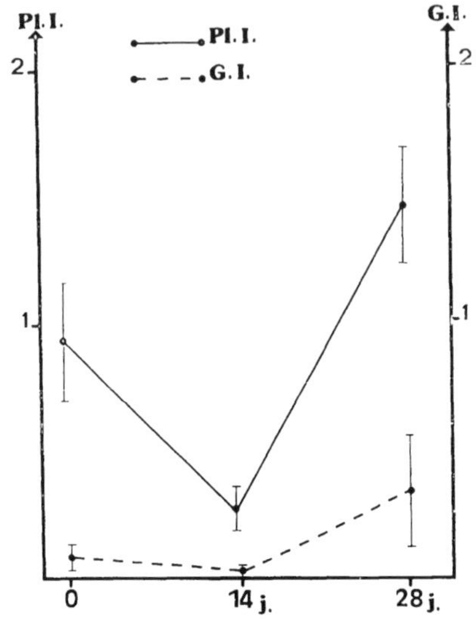


**Figure 84.1** Evolution of plaque index (●——●) and gingival index (●- - - -●) during a period of intense oral hygiene (0–14) and during the same period of plaque accumulation (14–28)

caries and defective restorations. Prior to the experiment, the subjects were instructed in oral hygiene methods and given a thorough dental prophylaxis for 14 days. Clinical examination including gingival index[14] and plaque index[15] was performed. Gingival tissue was harvested from the interdental papillae of the premolar region. Tooth cleaning was then terminated and plaque allowed to accumulate during 2 weeks (day 28). At day 28 clinical examinations were performed and gingival biopsies sampled in the same conditions as that on day 14.

During the next 2 weeks (day 42) the subjects, who were still without oral hygiene, were treated with a mixture of bacterial extracts (IRS 307) of different species usually observed during oral pathological processes (Table 84.1). The extracts were lyophilized and 6 tablets per day (0.050 g of extracts per tablet) were given to the subjects. At day 42 clinical examinations and gingival biopsies were performed in the same conditions as that on day 14 and on day 28.

At day 42 the subjects were again given a thorough dental prophylaxis for 14 days controlled by clinical examination (day 56) and during the last 2 weeks (day 70) dental plaque was allowed to accumulate, when the subjects were treated with the previously described therapy. At day 70 clinical examinations were performed and gingival biopsies sampled in the same conditions as on the other stages.

The composition of the gingival connective tissue was evaluated on three sections using a stereologic technique based on a morphometric point count-

**Table 84.1** Bacterial species used for the experiment

| | |
|---|---|
| *Lactobacillus acidophilus* | |
| *Lactobacillus helvetius* | |
| *Lactobacillus lactis* | |
| *Streptococcus A* | *(S 107* and *170)* |
| *Streptococcus H* | |
| *Streptococcus D* | *(S 226* and *19)* |
| *Staphylococcus aureus* | |
| *Corynebacterium pseudo-diphteriticum* | |
| *Fusiformis-fusiformis* | |
| *Klebsiella pneumoniae* | |
| *Candida albicans* | |

ing procedure described by Weibel *et al*[16]. The tissue sampling was carried out at three levels according to a modification of the morphometric test conditiions presented by Schroeder and Munzel-Pedrazzoli[17]

*Level I* (magnification 200 and a lattice comprising 100 light points): percentage of infiltrated connective tissue (I).

*Level II* (magnification 500 and a lattice comprising 100 light points): volume fractions occupied by collagen (Co), oedema (Oe) and vessels (V) in infiltrated connective tissue (I) and in non-infiltrated connective tissue (NI).

*Level III* (magnification 760 and a lattice comprising 100 light points): volume fractions occupied by lymphocytes (Ly), plasmocytes (P1), polymorphonuclear leukocytes (PMN), mononuclear cells (monocytes and macrophages) (Mo) and fibroblasts (Fi).

For each subject, 10 biopsies were randomly observed. Statistical analysis has been performed using Student's *t*-test and analysis of variance.

## RESULTS

### Clinical observations

During the treatment period (Figure 84.2), no difference was observed concerning the plaque index between the 'immunological therapy' group and the 'placebo' group. In contrast (Figure 84.3) the IRS group exhibited a significant decrease of the gingival index when compared with the placebo' group.

### Morphometric observations

The morphometric results confirm the clinical observations (Tables 84.2 and 84.3). The IRS group presented a decrease of the percentage of infiltrated connective tissue. This result was statistically significant at day 42. In the non-infiltrated area of the gingival connective tissue few differences were noted for the collagen volumetric density, for the oedema volumetric density and for the vessels volume fraction. Concerning the cells of the non-infiltrated

**Table 84.2** Day 42: Comparison between IRS 307 and placebo

| | *IRS 307* | *Placebo* | *t* | *p* |
|---|---|---|---|---|
| I | 45.35 ± 3.7 | 56.6 ± 7.2 | 4.52 | 0.001 |
| CoNI | 80.08 ± 3.2 | 81.62 ± 5.2 | 0.9059 | NS |
| OeNI | 6.05 ± 4.2 | 3.67 ± 1.7 | 1.3523 | NS |
| VNI | 2.44 ± 1.4 | 4.14 ± 1.6 | 2.6153 | 0.02 |
| LyNI | 0.16 ± 0.2 | 0.15 ± 0.2 | 0.1111 | NS |
| PINI | 0.05 ± 0.1 | 0.04 ± 0.1 | 0.1667 | NS |
| PMNNI | 0.37 ± 0.5 | 0.34 ± 0.5 | 0.1667 | NS |
| MoNI | 2.56 ± 1.5 | 3.3 ± 2.7 | 0.9610 | NS |
| FiNI | 7.65 ± 2 | 7.54 ± 2.3 | 0.131 | NS |
| CoI | 42.04 ± 7.7 | 35.74 ± 11.6 | 1.6579 | NS |
| OeI | 24.8 ± 3 | 24.6 ± 6.4 | 0.1053 | NS |
| VI | 4.87 ± 2 | 4.4 ± 2.2 | 0.5875 | NS |
| LyI | 3.78 ± 1.7 | 7.57 ± 3.7 | 3.4455 | 0.001 |
| PlI | 1.11 ± 1.1 | 4.93 ± 3.3 | 4.3908 | 0.001 |
| PMNT | 6.19 ± 3.2 | 5.08 ± 2.3 | 9.925 | NS |
| MoI | 10.75 ± 3.9 | 13.72 ± 2.7 | 1.7857 | NS |
| FiL | 4 ± 1.7 | 3.87 ± 1 | 0.2167 | NS |

gingival connective tissue, few remarks can be made because of their rare occurrence, especially for the inflammatory cells. Nevertheless, for the fibroblasts, which are the main cellular population, no difference was noted between the two groups.

The most interesting results concern the infiltrated gingival connective tissue, especially the cellular population. Therefore the treated group is mainly characterized at the two stages by a very significant decrease of the plasmocytes volume fraction. (Figures 84.4 and 84.5).

**Table 84.3** Day 70: Comparison between IRS 307 and placebo

| | *IRS 307* | *Placebo* | *t* | *p* |
|---|---|---|---|---|
| I | 37.9 ± 10.1 | 41.8 ± 11.1 | 0.8263 | NS |
| CoNI | 83:2 ± 6.3 | 84.5 ± 3.1 | 0.7429 | NS |
| OcNI | 4.2 ± 2.1 | 3.1 ± 1.5 | 1.5782 | NS |
| VNI | 3.1 ± 1.6 | 2.9 ± 1.2 | 0.3937 | NS |
| LyNI | 0.5 ± 0.6 | 0.5 ± 0.9 | 0 | NS |
| PINI | 0.05 ± 0.2 | 0.15 ± 0.4 | 0.8333 | NS |
| PMNNI | 0.9 ± 1 | 0.61 ± 0.7 | 0.9375 | NS |
| MoNI | 3.1 ± 2 | 2.6 ± 4.4 | 0.2488 | NS |
| FiNI | 7.6 ± 1.9 | 7 ± 1.9 | 0.75 | NS |
| OeI | 50.6 ± 10.4 | 46.6 ± 8 | 1.0256 | NS |
| DeI | 15.5 ± 7.5 | 18.5 ± 4.1 | 1.2146 | NS |
| VI | 3.2 ± 1.9 | 4.9 ± 2.3 | 2.0238 | 0.05 |
| LyI | 4.2 ± 2.2 | 3.9 ± 2.8 | 0.2941 | NS |
| PlI | 0.6 ± 0.7 | 1.3 ± 1.1 | 1.8041 | 0.05 |
| PMNI | 5.2 ± 3.9 | 6.6 ± 3.9 | 0.8805 | NS |
| Mono I | 11.8 ± 2 | 11.3 ± 2 | 0.4425 | NS |
| FiI | 5.3 ± 3.5 | 4 ± 2.9 | 1.0569 | NS |

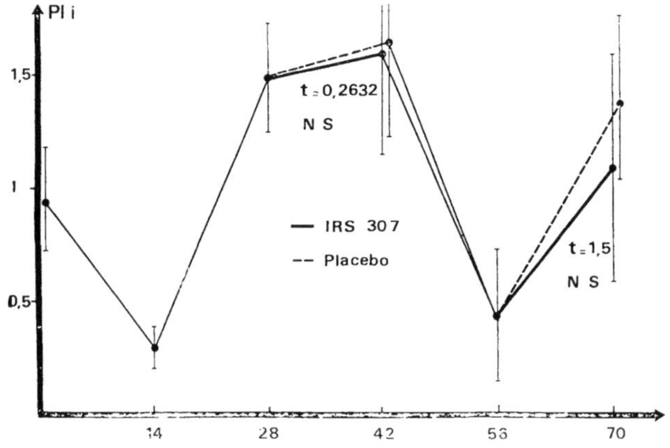


**Figure 84.2** Evolution of plaque index during the experiment

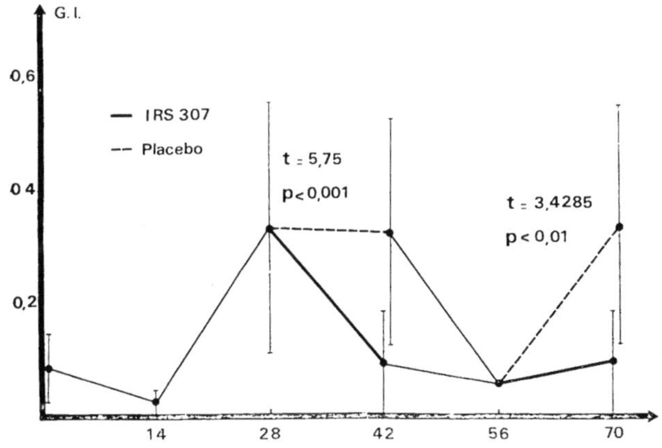


**Figure 84.3** Evolution of gingival index during the experiment

## DISCUSSION

Our results show that no modification of the plaque index is observed during the treatment phase. In contrast, we observe a significantly lower score of the gingival index for the IRS group, which proves the activity of the immunological therapy.

This clinical result is confirmed by the morphometric analysis which

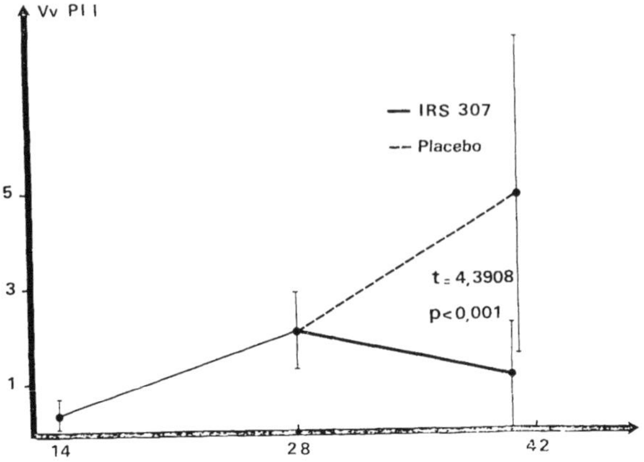


**Figure 84.4** Comparison of the Pl I volume fractions between IRS 307 group and placebo group.

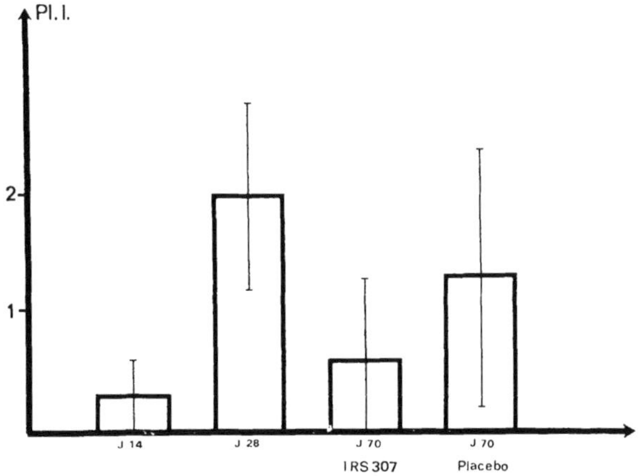


**Figure 84.5** Comparison of the Pl I volume fractions of healthy gingiva (14), gingivitis (28) and establishing gingivitis with immunological therapy (70–IRS 307 and 70–placebo

reveals a significantly smaller infiltrated gingival connective tissue for the IRS group, especially when the treatment is applied on an established gingivitis (day 42).

In order to explain the way by which this therapy can act, we think that the most interesting result is the decrease of the plasmocytes volumetric density in the IRS group when compared with the placebo group. This decrease proves there is a lower antigenic stimulation of lymphocytes by the dental plaque which is always accumulating and could be explained by the decreased penetration of dental plaque antigens into the gingival connective tissue, as shown by MacDougal[18] in rabbits.

This process, by inhibiting the intragingival immunopathological reactions, could decrease the gingival and the bony destruction observed by Guggenheim and Schroeder[19] in gnotobiotic rats sensitized by intradermal and intravenous injections of heat-killed cells of *Actinomyces viscosus*.

Our results seem to show more active effect of the therapy on established gingivitis (curative effect) than on establishing gingivitis (preventive effect).

## References


1 Daniel, A. and Dupont, M. (1978). Bacterial plaque induced gingivitis in man. Histometric analysis. *Eur. J. Rheumatol. Inflamm.*, **2,** 166

2 James, W. W. and Counsell, A. (1927). A histological investigation into "so-called pyorrhea alveolaris". *Br. Dent. J.*, **48,** 1237

3 Zachrisson, B. W. (1968). A histological study of experimental gingivitis in man. *J. Periodont. Res..*, **3,** 11

4 Schroeder, H. E. (1973). Ultrastructure of the early gingival lesion. *Rev. Fr. Odonto-Stomatol.*, **20,** 103

5 Schroeder, H. E., Munzel-Pedrazzoli, S. and Page, R. (1973). Correlated morphometric and biochemical analysis of gingival tissue in early chronic gingivitis in man. *Arch. Oral Biol.*, **18,** 899

6 Pierce, A. E. (1959). Specific antibodies at mucous surfaces. *Vet. Rev. Annotations*, **5,** 17

7 South, M., Cooper, M. D., Wollheim, F. A., Hong, R. and Good, R. (1966). The IgA system. I. Studies of the transport and immunochemistry. *J. Exp. Med.*, **123,** 615

8 South, M. A., Cooper, M. D., Wollheim, F. A. and Good, R. A. (1968). The IgA system II. The clinical significance of IgA deficiency. Studies in patients with agammaglobulinaemia and ataxiateleangectasia. *Am. J. Med.*, **24,** 168

9 Tomasi, T. B. and Grey, H. M. (1972). Structure and function of immunoglobulin A. *Prog. Allergy*, **16,** 18

10 Freter, R. (1972). Parameters affecting the association of vibrios with the intestinal surface in experimental cholera. *Infect. Immunity*, **6,** 134

11 Waldman, R. M., Cruz, J. M. and Rowe, D. S. (1972). Intravaginal immunisation of humans with Candida albicans. *J. Immunol.* **109,** 662

12 Tomasi, T. B., Tan, E. M., Solomon, A. and Prendergast, R. A. (1965). Characteristics of an immune system common to certain external secretions. *J. Exp. Med.*, **121,** 101

13 Brandtzaeg, P., Fjellanger, I. and Gjeruldsen, S. T. (1970). Human secretory immunoglobulins. I. Salivary secretion from individuals with normal or low levels of serum immunoglobulins. *Scand. J. Haematol. Suppl.*, **12,** 1

14 Loe, H. and Silness, J. (1963). Periodontal disease in pregnancy. I. Prevalence and severity. *Acta Odontol. Scand.*, **21,** 533

15 Silness, J. and Loe, H. (1964). Periodontal disease in pregnancy II. Correlation between oral hygiene and periodontal condition. *Acta Odontol. Scand.*, **22,** 112

16 Weibel, E. R., Kister, G. S. and Scherle, W. F. (1966). Practical sterologic methods for morphometric cytology. *J. Cell Biol.* **30,** 23

17 Schroeder, H. E. and Munzel-Pedrazzoli, I, S. (1973). Correlated morphometric and biochemical analysis of gingival tissue. *J. Microscopy*, **99,** 301

18 Mac Dougall, W. A. (1974). The effect of topical antigen on the gingiva of sensitized rabbit. *J. Periodant. Res.*, **9,** 153

19 Guggenheim, B. and Schroeder, H. E. (1974). Reactions of the periodontium to continuous antigenic stimulation in sensitized gnotobiotic rats. *Infect. Immun*, **8,** 565

85

# A prospective study of 17 autoantibodies (AA) in 176 cases of rheumatoid arthritis (RA) treated with D-penicillamine (DP) (Abstract)

P. YOUINOU, J.-F. MORIN, M. RAULO, N. ABUAF AND J.-C. HOMBERG (FRANCE)

176 patients (36 male/140 female; mean age, 54, range 20–87) suffering from classical or definite RA as defined by the ARA criteria were given a slowly increasing dosage of DP. The overall mean durationof DP was 22 months (6–36); the mean dose level was 16 mg/kg daily (10–25) and the mean RA duration was 92 months (11–431). 17 AA were determined before, during and after the treatment. Within 2 months of giving DP, the rheumatoid factors titre decreased, whereas antiperinuclear factor remained unchanged throughout the treatment. Between the 6th and the 12th month, various AA appeared in 12% of the patients (to ds-DNA, to skeletal muscle and to epidermal intercellular substance). Associated autoimmune disease was noted in 50% of the latter. The patients with a positive anti-nuclear factor seemed especially likely to develop a serious side effect.

# 86

# Lymphokines, monokines, leukokines: large scale production, isolation and properties of leukocyte-derived cytotaxins, cytokinesins, cytotoxins and mitogens (Abstract)

J. H. WISSLER, M. ARNOLD AND W. SCHAPER
(WEST GERMANY)

Leukocytes attracted and emigrating from the intravascular blood stream to an injured tissue site elaborate various biologically active trace components. The objective of this work is the isolation in ponderable amounts and characterization of so far chemically undefined biologically active cell-derived substances governing cellular orientation, locomotion and 'social' behaviour of different leukocyte and other dividing cell types which as tertiary messengers of tissue injury effect and regulate the multiple steps and sequences of biological functions involved in tissue repair at local and systemic cellular and humoral levels. Hence, we establish methods under sterile conditions for isolation and culture of different viable peripheral leukocyte types on large (kg amount) scales.

Peripheral leukocytes were prepared from porcine and canine blood collected in cold, siliconized sterile polypropylene or polycarbonate vessels. Blood was anticoagulated by heparin (10 U/ml) or Na-citrate (pH 7.10, 0.01 mol/l). Methocel was added (0.1% w/v) and cells collected and bulk of platelets concomitantly removed by centrifugation of supernatants (400 × $g$, 10 min, 5 °C) immediately after erythrocytes have been setted (1 × $g$, 10 °C, 20–35 min). Removal of residual erythrocytes and platelets is achieved by a single hypotonic lysis (0.2% w/v NaCl in 1 mmol/l Na, K-phosphate, pH 7.10, 0 °C, 30 s., stopped by 1.6% NaCl to restore 0.9% NaCl, pH 7.10, 0 °C, at 1/10 of initial blood volume). Cells collected by centrifugation are washed twice by 0.9% NaCl (pH. 7.10, 0°C, cells dispersed by gentle circular shaking, 1/10 of initial blood volume). Resulting white peripheral cells are the source of homogeneous populations of neutrophils, eosinophils, monocytes and lymphocytes obtained by standard techniques (Bøyum, *Scand. J. Clin. Lab. Invest.* **21,** (Suppl.) 97, 1968; Noble Cutts, 1968, *J. Lab. Clin. Med.* **72,** 533; Johnson and Garvin *Proc. Soc. Exp. Bio. Med.,* **102,** 333, 1959; Day, 1970 *Immunology,* **18,** 955,. They, or the mixed populations, are cultured in a serum-free medium without (reference) and with mitogen (5$\mu$g concanavalin-A/ml) according to Wissler and Arnold (*Z. Immun.-Forschung,* **157,** 301, 1979) at average scales of $2 \times 10^{12}$ cells/20 l (equivalent to ~1 kg of viable leukocytes at the cell differential given for mixed populations, isolated daily from 200 l of blood; yield 50%). In culture supernatants, several types of leukocyte-derived biological activities can be detected by *in vitro* assays (Wissler; Wissler *et al.*, 1972, *Eur. J. Immunol,* **2,** 73; 1980 *Z. Physiol. Chemie,* **361,**: chemotactic, positive and negative chemokinetic activities for neutrophils, eosinophils and monocytes, cytotoxic and mitogenic activities from lymphocytes. Their purification reveals discrete biologically active fractions, accounting for yet 35 proteins in the range of 10000–25000 daltons. Several other trace substances make up a low molecular weight fraction (>500 daltons). From 5000 kg porcine blood (~30 kg mitogen-stimulated viable mixed cells, ~3 mg (10% yield) of a protein with negative chemokinetic activity for monocytes can be isolated (~1mg from reference cultures) by a multistep purification procedure similar to one for serum-derived mediators (Wissler, 1972, *Eur. J. Immunol,* **2,** 73). It represents one of several different types of structural equivalents of migration inhibition activity (MIF) of crude culture supernatants. Furthermore, another trace protein represents chemotactic activity for neutrophils which is different from serum-derived chemotactic activity (Wissler, 1971, *Experientia,* **27,** 1447).

# Discussion

**Professor T. L. Vischer (Chairman)** said that the discussion would start with a consideration of T lymphocytes. He asked Dr Kaufmann whether any link existed between work on the susceptibility of T sub-sets to cyclophosphamide, the defining of surface markers and the influence which T cell sub-sets had on macrophages and inflammation.

**Dr F. H. T. Kaufmann (Germany)** said that it might be possible to correlate the susceptibility of T cell sub-sets involved in inflammation to cyclophosphamide with the Lyt phenotype. In the sheep red blood cell model it seemed clear that Lyt positive T cells were mediating delayed hypersensitivity (DTH). In particular, Lyt 1 T cells mediated DTH while Lyt 2 positive cells were suppressive and Lyt 123 T cells appeared to be regulating cells, precursors of the other T cell sub-sets. They had found that the T cells mediating DTH to sheep red blood cells were somewhat resistant to 4.hydroperoxycyclophosphamide, the cyclophosphamide derivative active *in vitro*. The suppressor T cells of DTH in this model were rather more sensitive and the precursors of the suppressor T cells were by far the most sensitive cells in their response to this derivative. Thus, there did appear to be a correlation between Lyt antiserum treatment and sensitivity to cyclophosphamide.

**Dr M. K. Jasani (UK)** noted that Dr Kaufmann had used dispersed spleen cells. He wondered what relationship this dispersed cell model had to the situation *in vivo*.

**Dr Kaufmann** said that the spleen cells incubated *in vitro* were subsequently examined *in vivo* and so the relevance of the arrangement was clear.

**Dr Jasani** said that although the relevance was obvious the question remained unresolved as to the role of the suppressor cell in the normal animal given sheep red blood cells. He wondered whether the suppressor cell would be active in the spleen or at the peripheral site.

**Dr Kaufmann** said that the existence of suppressor cells was not demonstrable when sheep red blood cells were used at concentrations optimal for DTH induction. They only appeared when the red cell concentration was $10^3$ higher than the optimal dose for DTH induction. Thus, although suppressor cell induction was possible, it was not achieved by the same means which produced DTH cells.

**Professor D. A. Horwitz (USA)** enquired about the life span of such lymphocytes. It was possible that the Lyt 1 cell might be a long-living recirculating cell, but that the Lyt 123 cell was a short-lived cell and that the effects being demonstrated were really due to the state of cellular maturation.

**Dr Kaufmann** agreed. They did not have data on the precursors of suppressor T cells but it seemed likely that they were short-lived and the effects of cyclophosphamide application *in vivo* presented a short-lived phenomenon. The precursors of suppressor T cells could be eliminated by giving cyclophosphamide prior to antigen but the effect lasted only 3–4 days, after which T suppressor cells could again be induced, suggesting a rather short life span. Antigen activated suppressor T cells could be demonstrated by adoptive transfer only on days 3–5, again indicating that they were short lived. The DTH mediating cells were somewhat more long-lived and could be demonstrated between days 4 and 10 by adoptive transfer. This pattern showed certain similarities to *in vitro* susceptibility to X-rays.

**Mr S. J. Hopkins (UK)** said that cyclophosphamide *in vivo* at a dose which would enhance the response to super-optimal levels of sheep red blood cells could also depress the response seen with sub-optimal doses of these cells. He wondered whether the same occurred with the 4-hydroxy derivative. In particular, he wondered about the response seen following pretreatment with cyclophosphamide at day −2, followed by a sub-optimal dose of sheep red cells.

**Dr Kaufmann** said that in these conditions an enhanced response was seen. Other workers had shown such a response and suggested that the enhancement occurred by *in vivo* elimination of suppressor T cell precursors. This coincided very well with his own findings that suppressor T cell precursors were sensitive to 4-hydroxycyclophosphamide in very low doses.

**Dr M. Glatt (Co-Chairman)** asked what advice should be given to pharmacologists as to the cells which they should concentrate on influencing in regard to the treatment of, for example, rheumatoid arthritis.

**Dr Kaufmann** said that the question was difficult but they had shown that different susceptibilities existed among cell populations and therefore by appropriate treatment it should be possible selectively to eliminate suppressor mechanisms, or effector or helper mechanisms.

**Professor Vischer** said that while this work on *in vitro* models was important, treatment of rheumatoid arthritis patients with cyclophosphamide in low doses was ineffective and in high doses produced a leukopenia eliminating good and bad lymphocytes together. The conference would hear later about immunoregulation which he thought was certainly a theme to be numbered among future trends.

**Professor P. Gordon (USA)** also drew attention to the non-specificity of cyclophosphamide and its derivatives. Quite apart from the fall in cell numbers in leukopenia, some days after the leukopenia had normalized, neutrophils were still under-responsive to leukotactic stimuli. This very general pattern of interference made it difficult to separate the strictly immunological phenomena from more general anti-inflammatory effects.

**Dr Kaufmann** wished in conclusion to describe some of his work on macrophages. It was generally accepted that Lyt 1 cells were mediators of delayed hypersensitivity which is why they had used the sheep red cell model. In addition, however, they had used the intracellular bacterial model using *Listeria monocytogens* and they had found that here the Lyt 123 T cells were crucially involved in hypersensitivity and protective activity. Using an *in vitro* assay in which normal macrophages were incubated with *Listeria* specific T cells and with antigen, it was clear that after interaction of T cells with macrophages and antigen the macrophage became activated and produced mitogenic protein and was capable of non-specific killing of tumour cells. Although in this assay the Lyt 1 cells were the most important macrophage activators there was also enhancement by addition of Lyt 123 cells. Thus, although the Lyt 1 were of primary importance, they also seemed to need the help of the Lyt 123 T cells for macrophage activation.

**Professor Vischer** said that macrophage activation depended, on the one hand, upon T cell factors and on the other on C3, the alternative pathway for macrophage activation. However, some substances might work either through complement or in other ways and he asked Dr Schorlemmer to review their recent work on macrophage activation.

**Professor H. U. Schorlemmer (Germany)** said that their previous findings had shown that various substances capable of inducing chronic inflammatory reactions *in vivo* were also very potent activators of *in vitro* macrophage release of lysosomal enzymes and activators of the alternative pathway of the complement system. More recently they had demonstrated the same result with collagen type II and with polyanions, either soluble polyanions or particulate substances like sulphated Sephadex beads. In both cases there was a strict parallelism between activation of macrophages and activation of the alternative pathway and they had suggested that the two mechanisms might be correlated *in vivo* in chronic inflammatory reactions.

**Professor C. M. Pearson (USA)** asked whether collagen type I or type III had been tested. Recent work had shown that incomplete adjuvant plus collagen type III but not plus types I or II could give rise to an adjuvant-like arthritis.

**Dr Schorlemmer** said that he had tested pure preparations of all three types. Only the type II was able to activate the complement system by the alternative pathway and only the type II was able to activate marcrophages to secrete lysosomal enzymes. This might be due to the polyionic character of type II collagen but this was only speculation. Using solubilized collagen he had found that it was active in both the denatured and the native forms. This was at variance with the findings of other workers who had found denatured collagen to be inactive in models of arthritis.

**Dr P. C. J. Leijh (Netherlands)** said that since macrophages were able to synthesize all complement components he wondered whether activation of the macrophage was a type of activation of the complement system on the macrophage membrane.

**Dr Schorlemmer** said there were some hints that this might be so. Because the macrophage synthesized complement components like C3 proteases and also factor B it was possible that activation of the macrophage was due to endogenous stimulation by, for example, C3b. He had found that purified C3b would lead to stimulation of macrophages to secrete other enzymes. Thus, in rheumatoid arthritis, the chronic reaction should be inhibited or regulated by the regulatory proteins which were also secreted by the macrophage.

**Dr P. Bacon (UK)** wondered whether there were any homology between collagen type II and complement components, leading to the binding of the former onto the macrophage by means of a complement receptor.

**Dr Schorlemmer** said that C1q had some similarities in structure to collagen but he did not know whether it was more like collagen type I or type II.

**Dr I. Bottcher (Germany)** asked if human macrophages had been used with human collagen in a completely homologous system.

**Dr Schorlemmer** said that activation of complement had been examined in a completely homologous system but the macrophage studied had used human collagen in mouse or guinea pig systems.

**Professor Vischer** noted recent findings that small quantities of polyanion would inhibit macrophage activation induced by the original anion molecule. He wondered if complement activation could also be clocked by small quantities of the original polyanion.

**Dr Schorlemmer** said that there was a distinct parallelism between activation of the complement system and activation of the macrophage. The same was true for inhibition of complement activation and macrophage activation by low molecular weight polyanions. On adding such low molecular weight ions to complement or serum, conversion of C3 or factor B was inhibited. Addition of high molecular weight polyanions had no effect but addition of the low and high molecular weight ions together produced inhibition, pointing to the inhibitory effects of the former.

**Dr Horwitz** wondered whether the collagen type II was providing a surface for C3 activation which then triggered the macrophage or whether it acted directly at the macrophage surface.

**Dr Schorlemmer** could not answer the question because although exogenous C3b would lead to activation of the macrophage, the nature of the C3 binding necessary to trigger the cell was not understood. Whether activation occurred via the alternative pathway or as a direct effect, was simply unknown.

**Professor S. J. Normann (USA)**, noting that the target cells used to demonstrate catalytic activity included the P815, asked whether Dr Schorlemmer was suggesting that C3a was the substance responsible for tumouricidal activity of the activated macrophage, and if so why it had been so difficult for others to demonstrate a soluble factor in the medium. In addition, he wondered why intimate contact of the tumour cell with the macrophage was essential if C3a was present in the environment.

**Dr Schorlemmer** said that the literature was confused on this point. Two groups had shown that purified guinea pig C3a was cytotoxic for several tumour cells but another had not found cytotoxic effects against P815. Possibly slightly different assay systems might have been used but now the groups planned to collaborate and exchange the relevant materials. However, it should be noted that he had demonstrated a cytolytic factor in supernatant of activated macrophages which was extremely similar to C3a and so its cytolytic role did seem likely.

**Dr S. Wong (USA)** asked whether it was established that rheumatoid arthritis was a collagen type II disease.

**Dr Schorlemmer** said that it was certainly not established. Collagen type II occurred in joint tissues and in chronic cases, where destruction occurred, Anti-collagen antibodies could be detected, but whether these features were central to the cause of the disease had not been established.

**Dr V. D. Ramanatham (UK)** in reviewing his findings on complement activation by metals, said that, in agreement with Dr Schorlemmer's findings, they had established that compounds inducing chronic inflammation were able to activate complement. Additionally, a substance such as zirconium hydroxide, which did not induce chronic inflammation or granular formation, did not activate complement. These and other findings suggested that rather than having one alternative pathway there might be several. A second general result from their work was that when searching for complement activity one should look for the presence of activation products such as C3b or the anaphylatoxin because zirconium hydroxide, which was able to consume complement, did not generate anaphylatoxin nor split C3. On being asked about the role of plasminogen, he said that he thought plasminogen was activated by the metal compounds. Although he had not examined the problem directly it was possible that metal compounds absorbed Hageman factor and activated it which in turn resulted in plasminogen activation.

**Dr Glatt** asked whether the difference between metals and zymosan would result from different activation of Hageman factor or whether the physicochemical properties of the metals simply bound more plasminogen than zymosan did.

**Dr Ramanathan** said that when he had compared zymosan with metals he had not been able to detect any significant difference in protein absorption patterns but he had not examined specific protein binding.

**Professor Pearson** reviewed his work on RES impairment in mice. It had been generally assumed that in NZB/W mice, enhancement in antibody production in immune complexes occurred. With his associate Dr Y. H. Chang they had examined NZB/W mice, 6–8 weeks and 6–8 months of age. They had discovered a progressive decrease in the ability to degrade $^{125}$I-labelled immune complexes of IgG in the older animals. This was in contrast to other strains of mouse in which the rate of degradation was comparable in both age groups. It thus appeared not only that there was an increase in production of IgG and immune complexes in this strain but also a reduced rate of degradation which allowed a build-up of such complexes. It was interesting to note that this apparent defect occurred at about 4 months, which in the NZB/W strain was somewhat earlier than the onset of the clinical signs and symptoms of nephritis and other aspects of the lupus-like syndrome. On questioning he said that no similar studies had to his knowledge been carried out on human lupus, if only because one could examine sufferers only after the onset of the disease. Nonetheless, he suspected that retarded degradation of IgG immune complexes occurred in human lupus as well.

On being asked about the relative roles of the circulating and adherent complexes he agreed that the complexes adhering to membranes probably caused more damage than those in the circulation, but the two went together.

**Dr S. C. R. Meacock (UK)** asked if the drop in phagocytic potential occurred only in the macrophages or whether it was also seen in the PMNs.

**Professor Pearson** had examined both cell types and said that the retardation occurred almost entirely in the macrophage system. He believed that some of the degradation of immune complexes occurred at the macrophage surface. In young animals, activation of surface enzymes caused the degradation but in older animals this system appeared to become defective.

**Professor J. P. Giroud (France)** then reviewed the work of his group on the potentiation of the antibody response. He said that on taking serum from animals showing an acute inflammatory reaction and injecting it into others, there were increases in both thymus-dependent and thymus-independent antibody formation. In collaboration with other groups they had tried to analyse the various components of the simple, acute non-specific inflammatory reaction, and had found that they were able to stimulate macrophages and T cells, and to vary these types of response according to the type and concentration of phytagglutinin being used. These and similar results high-lighted the marked effects which non-immunological processes could have upon the immune reactivity of the host.

**Professor Vischer** said that many chronic inflammations were known clinically to increase immunoglobulin levels. This had recently been attributed to polyclonal B cell activators and he was interested in the relationship of increased antibody levels to general immunoglobulin levels. He wondered whether Professor Giroud had observed stimulation of all antibody production in the body. He also wondered what working hypothesis was used to explain the adjuvant effect in his experiments.

**Professor Giroud** said that in acute inflammatory reactions it seemed that many different activities were being stimulated. The macrophage activating factor found in exudates had been characterized as having a very low molecular weight, but as yet he did not know whether it acted on lymphocytes, macrophages or antibody formation.

**Dr P. Bacon (UK)** described his work on rheumatoid immunoblasts. He said that the thoracic duct drainage experiments such as performed in Los Angeles had shown the importance of circulating lymphocytes in the maintenance of chronic arthritis but there were disadvantages to such an experimental procedure. His own work using Ficoll density gradients to establish cell distribution patterns showed that activated cells in rheumatoid disease appeared to be markers of active synovitis not of extravascular complications and they therefore seemed to be good targets for attack, either pharmacologically or by antibodies. The question had earlier been asked what sort of cells should be attacked in rheumatoid arthritis and in his view the circulating active cells should be a prime target. It would be of great interest to know whether such cells entered the tissues and there was need for labelling experiments to establish this point.

**Professor Vischer** noted that the immunoblasts were very dense but he wondered about their actual cell type.

**Dr Bacon** said that they were largely non-T cells. They did not correlate with Fc$\gamma$ cells, although he agreed that young T cells might not have T cell markers.

**Dr Jasani** said that Dr Bacon's group were associating disease with the presence of a particular type of cell. Dr Cats group associated it with depeletion of a particular cell type.

**Dr A. Cats (Netherlands)** believed that immunoblasts were membrane markers, so he also agreed that they were not T cells. However, in patients with rheumatoid arthritis he had found activated lymphocytes, in contrast to control individuals. He wondered whether, in individuals treated with gold, there had been a clear cut difference in immunoblasts in treated patients compared with controls.

**Dr Bacon** said that there had been a considerable overlap, an entire spectrum. He did not believe that the presence of immunoblasts was an all or none phenomenon, but rather that their numbers correlated with the degree of inflammation.

**Dr Cats** said that they had found a depression in the $T\mu$ cells which correlated with activity of the disease measured by EST and Ritchie index. He thought that when Dr Bacon had examined sufficient patients he would probably find a correlation between immunoblasts and disease activity. In his own studies, he had found varying numbers of activated lymphoblasts but it had not been possible to correlate them with disease activity.

**Dr Horwitz** said that some years previously he and Dr Ziff had examined the spontaneous proliferating active immunoblasts in lupus and rheumatoid arthritis and many of them proved to be monocyte precursors rather than lymphocytes. There was good correlation between the intensity of inflammation and cell numbers and their presence seemed to be a response to inflammation rather tham a primary factor.

**Dr Bacon** said that the immunoblasts to which he referred with non-adherent esterase negative cells but he agreed that it was difficult to rule out the possibility of them being monocyte precursors without culturing them.

**Professor J. Sany** reviewed his preliminary findings using placenta eluted gammaglobulin (PEGG). Because it was well known that remission of rheumatoid arthritis often occurred in pregnancy. He had treated 5 patients with the severe classical disease with the placental globulin. Preparation of the globulin was complicated, but basically it involved a number of extraction and separation processes leading to a mixture of pure gammaglobulins. Six ampoules of 250 mg were given i.v. daily for 7 days to 5 patients. In one patient the treatment had to be stopped on the fifth day because of proteinuria, a side effect which subsequently disappeared. 3 of the 5 patients improved, according to the usual clinical criteria, but these indices, which had fallen up to 30 days after treatment, increased again after 3 months. A second course of treatment resulted in the same responses but attempts at discontinuous treatment had failed. Thus, the results were short-lived but impressive with nodules disappearing within 7 days. E-rosette forming cells, originally low, increased to normal values after 8 days of treatment but were then again depressed. Response to mitogen, also very low in severe rheumatoid patients, increased to normal and correlated very well with the change in clinical results. All patients showed such immunological changes but clinical improvement was seen only in 3 patients out of 5. Although the drug was so short-lived it was of interest both to the clinician and the immunologist.

On being asked why patients did not respond to a chronic course of placental globulin he said that he did not know. Originally such gammaglobulins were given to patients to prevent rejection of renal grafts. Thus, they were thought to be immunodepressive. However, it was clear that they were immunomodulating, perhaps even immunostimulating, because such renal grafts survived for a shorter time than expected under this treatment. On the question of circulating immune complexes, he said that they had been measured in all patients and had decreased in all.

**Professor Gordon** wondered, in relation to PHA responses, whether a major flux in thymidine incorporation following treatment would have occurred in the absence of PHA. In other words, he wondered whether the base line would change. The question was important, because a number of studies of influenza had shown apparent effects of PHA which were strikingly related to reduction in base line values. There was a change in state, whereby the spontaneous mitogenicity of cells in the absence of PHA was reduced, thus allowing a much greater PHA response. It was important to know what the intrinsic impact of globulin injection was on mitogenicity.

**Professor A. Sfikakis (Greece)** believed that oestradiol was responsible for immunosuppression during pregnancy. It was interesting that Professor Sany had found a factor during pregnancy which was immunomodulating rather than immunosuppressive. In her own adjuvant studies in overiectomized rats treated with oestradiol they had found oestradiol itself to be immunosuppressive but they had also found a very large increase in thymus weight which might be an immunomodulating factor.

**Dr Cats** asked whether there was no antibody formation to globulins in these patients.

**Dr Sany** said that there had been no clinical problems such as anaphylaxis and the only side effect had been headache on the first perfusion. They had not so far specifically searched for antibodies in these preliminary investigations, but they planned to do so. Because the investigations were preliminary they had not used a control group. Certainly there was a need to control the patients to see whether the gamma globulin effect was specific or not, and such investigations were planned.

**Dr Glatt** asked which cells were blocked by the immunoglobulin. He wondered whether an anti-idiotypic antibody were generated which inhibited B lymphocytes.

**Professor Sany** said that they did not know how the drug acted. It might block cells bearing Fc receptors but he was not sure. Certainly it decreased E-rosette formation *in vitro* so it would act on Fc bearing receptor cells, but the specificity of this effect was not known.

**Dr A. Daniel (France)** reviewed his work on the gingivitis which occurred after 2 weeks without oral hygiene. Histologically the gingivitis was characterized by numerous plasma cells in the connective tissue. They had examined the effects of immunotherapy by giving 15 patients lyophilized bacterial extracts and giving a similar group placebo. The active group, treated with the oral bacteria, showed a decrease in gingival inflammatory index. There was a decrease in infiltrated connective tissue and in the density of plasma cells. It was possible that immunological therapy produced an increase of IgA salivary production with a subsequent influence on the passage of antigens to the gingival epithelium. Transmucosal passage of such antigens had certainly been demonstrated by Swedish workers.

On being asked about the relative significance of various contributory factors to gingivitis he said that first was the bacterial plaque. Some patients had extensive bacterial plaque, others had not. Some had a good reaction against it and others did not. For patients with bacterial plaque without severe periodontal disease he thought that the best treatment was brushing, but a drug approach nonetheless had value for the clinician. Since it was true that patients with the disease would swallow the bacteria constantly he could not readily explain the particular beneficial effects of the therapy. However, he believed that a non-specific immunological reaction was increased by salivary IgA.

**Dr. J. A. Wissler (Germany)** was asked about his procedures for preparing lymphokines in milligram quantities. He described the technique and said that it led to the separation of several different mediators. One had an activity which inhibited macrophage migration. Another had chemotactic activity for neutrophils. A third was a mitogenic factor for monocytes. Cell derived mediators from normal and mitogenic stimulated leukocytes could thus be separated as distinct molecular entities with distinct biological activities.

**Dr Glatt**, in summarizing the discussion, said that it had dealt with four main aspects. The first was the attempt to identify cell sub-groups and to establish their role in experimental models like delayed hypersensitivity. Studies on the influence of various drugs on such systems were still in progress. Secondly, they had heard very interesting results from Dr Bacon's group which had shown that differences in immunoblast sub-populations did occur in treated and non-treated rheumatoid arthritis patients. The third aspect was that of macrophage activation by macromolecules like polyanions and collagen. Complement seemed to play a central role in this process but macrophage mediated cytotoxicity and the role of C3a were still open questions. Finally, they had considered some of the factors which normally influenced the outcome of immunological processes, especially in rheumatoid arthritis. Pregnancy was one such, but gout and schizophrenia were also negatively linked with rheumatoid arthritis and he hoped that future work would help to illuminate the effects of these physiological influences on immunological networks.

# Section VIII
# Inflammation: General Aspects

CHAIRMAN: W. Dawson
CO-CHAIRMAN: J. L. Turk

# 87

# Experimental protoporphyria in hairless mice: photodermatitis

H. BAART DE LA FAILLE, R. A. WOUTERSEN, H. VAN WEELDEN AND E. H. BAART DE LA FAILLE-KUYPER (NETHERLANDS)

## INTRODUCTION

Erythropoietic protoporphyria (EPP) is an inheritable inborn error of human metabolism giving rise to an excess production and accumulation of the haem precursor protoporphyrin[1-3]. Increased concentrations of protoporphyrin can be demonstrated in, for example, erythrocytes, and to a smaller extent also in plasma. The excretion of the substance in faecal matter is often elevated; urinary porphyrins are always normal.

The main symptom is photodermatitis, an inflammatory reaction of the skin which is provoked by visible light, in particular violet (400 nm), the wavelength which is maximally absorbed by porphyrins. The reaction is characterized by a typical sensation of burning and pricking which may start during exposition to either sunlight or artificial irradiation. A distinct swelling gradually develops; frank erythema may occur but is mostly not pronounced. After large doses of light severe purpuric and bullous reactions may come into existence. In the course of years many of these acute episodes occur and they give rise to chronic alterations, namely a leathery waxy type of thickening of the skin (pseudolichenification), atrophic (seldom hypertrophic) scars and hyper- and hypopigmentations.

Microscopic and electron microscopic investigations of experimentally irradiated skin[4,5] showed severe capillary damage, primarily of the endothelium, and a cellular infiltrate. A characteristic 'foamy substance' is deposited between the capillary basement membranes. Furthermore, immunoglobulins and complement factors are observed in the same areas. The foamy material also contains lipid, which can be demonstrated 3–6 h after irradiation. Later (24–48 h) lipid is also present in abundance in the epidermal cells. Finally the irradiation induces a decrease or disappearance of the alkaline phosphatase reaction of the capillary endothelium; this has been interpreted as a sign of direct damage being done by light to the endothelial cell membrane. As a second direct target of the irradiation[6,7] lysosomes have been indicated. In the present work we have studied the photodermatitis of protoporphyric hairless mice and compared it to the response of EPP skin to light.

## MATERIALS AND METHODS

### The animals

SKH hairless -I mice (approximately 3 months of age) were fed 0.5% (w/w) DDC in standard powdered diet. With this regimen a distinct condition of protoporphyria was attained within a week; erythrocyte and plasma protoporphyrin values varied from 1500–3000 μg/100 ml packed cells, respectively, 100–500 μg/100 ml. (Protoporphyrin concentrations in EPP are as follows= erythrocytes 1000–5000 μg/100 ml packed cells, seldom higher; plasma $< 100$ μg/100 ml). However, feeding DDC uninterruptedly for a week caused a considerable intoxication manifested by weight loss, dehydration and diminished activity. The development of this condition was diminished by interrupting the application of DDC for 1 day, on the fifth day. Before the irradiation the animals were kept in subdued light.

### The irradiation

Irradiation experiments were performed with 6 Philips 40W 03RS fluorescent tubes (120 cm long), which were fixed parallel in a horizontal plane by use of a metal frame (Figure 87.1). The distance between the tubes and the table was 21 cm. The intensity of the radiation varied from 3.7–5.2 mW/cm$^2$; the emission was maximal around 410 nm (Figure 87.1). The measurement was performed with a Kipp thermopile equipped with a window of Suprasil W quartz.

During exposure the animals were placed on the table below the tubes in small transparent PVC boxes ($14.5 \times 8.5 \times 9.5$ cm) closed at the upper side by a grating. Usually 10 animals were irradiated at the same time. To obtain an impression of the skin sensitivity to light, series of increasing doses were used but after a number of experiments two standard doses were chosen, namely, 1 J/cm$^2$ and 17 J/cm$^2$. The clinical condition, especially the behaviour during irradiation, and the skin was studied during 24 h following the irradiation.

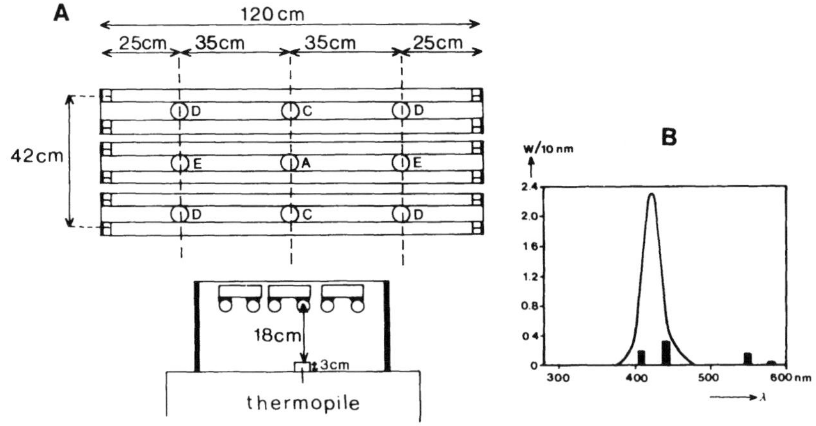


**Figure 87.1** (A) Schematic representation of irradiation apparatus. Six Philips 40W/03 RS fluorescent tubes, mounted in a metal frame, were placed horizontally at a distance of 21 cm above a table. During irradiation mice were kept separately in transparant PVC boxes, placed in row of 10 under the tubes. The intensity of the irradiation was measured at locations A, C, D and E with a thermopile. It varied from 3.7 – 5.2 mW/cm$^2$. (B) Emission spectrum shows a distinct maximum at 410 nm

**Skin thickness**

Following irradiation with 1 J/cm$^2$, skin thickness (right ear, longitudinal fold of medial part of the back skin) was measured using an OOT Oditest meter (H.C. Kroeplin, W. Germany). Measurements were performed before and 3 h and 24 h after the beginning of the irradiation.

**Electron microscopy**

Animals that had been irradiated with 1 J/cm$^2$ and 17 J/cm$^2$ were sacrificed by cervical dislocation at 1, 3, 6 and 24 h after the beginning of the irradiation. Skin specimens (medial part of the back) were either immediately snap-frozen in liquid nitrogen, fixed in formalin or fixed for 2 h in 2% glutaraldehyde in 0.1 mol/l phosphate buffer (pH 7.4). The latter specimens were post-fixed with 3% $OsO_4$ for 2 h, stained in block with aqueous uranyl acetate (10 g/l) for 20 min, dehydrated and embedded in Epon 812. Semi-thin and/or ultrathin sections were cut on an LKB ultrotome III; the former were stained with basic fuchsin and methylene blue[8]. Ultrathin sections were post-stained with lead citrate. Formalin fixed sections were routinely stained with hematoxylin eosin. Frozen tissue sections were used for lipid stains (caffeine 3:4-benzopyrene[9]), oil red 0[10], Sudan black B[11] and alkaline phosphatase (simultaneous coupling azo dye method using α naphtyl phosphate[12] or naphtol AS B I phosphate[13] as diazonium salt fast red TR salt and fast red violet LB salt were used).

**Protoporphyrin determinations**

Qualitative and quantitative porphyrin determinations were carried out as described by Woutersen *et al.*[14].

## RESULTS

**Clinical condition**

The protoporphyric mice showed a distinct hypersensitivity to violet light. 20 to 30 s after the beginning of the irradiation a very characteristic type of behaviour developed. The animals became restless, even excited, jumped against the ceilings of the boxes, scratched their skin and washed their heads vigorously. This excitation ceased after about 2 min; during the remaining period of the experiment the animals sat apathetic in their cages with their eyes closed.

Signs of photodermatitis developed during the irradiation (17 J/cm$^2$) or 15–30 min afterwards (1 J/cm$^2$). Redness and swelling were distinct at 3 h and reached their maximum at 24 h after the irradiation (see Figure 87.2). These symptoms developed sooner and appeared more severe after the large dose had been applied. Purpura was sometimes observed (edges of the ear; tail) but was never pronounced. At 24 h scratchmarks (crusts, erosions) were observed.

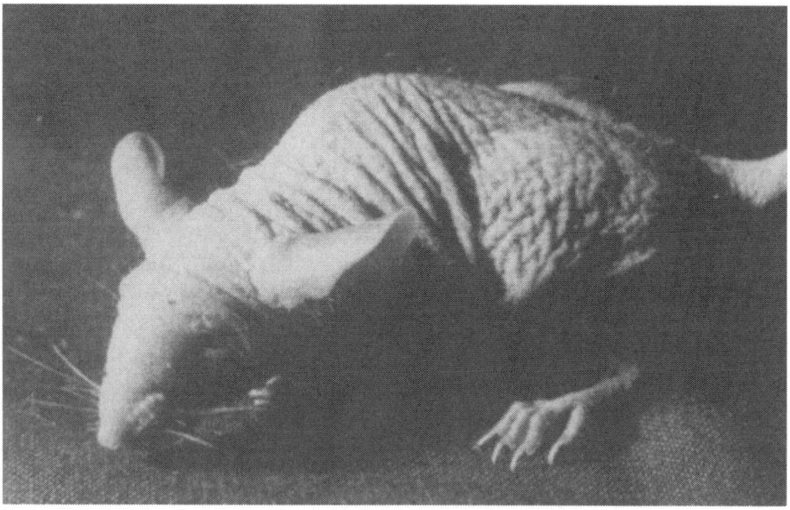

**Figure 87.2** Hairless mouse irradiated for 64 min and photographed 3 h afterwards. Oedema and erythema are evident

Most animals were ill during the first hours after the irradiation; they appeared dehydrated and intoxicated. These symptoms were pronounced in the mice who received a dose of 17 $J/cm^2$; during these experiments 0–30% died. In the 1 $J/cm^2$ irradiations a lethal course was almost never observed. We considered that death was often caused by a summation of pathogenic factors, namely the impact of the irradiation superimposed on the intoxication induced by DDC. Non-porphyric mice did not show any sign of increased sensitivity to light, i.e. neither excitation nor dermatitis occurred.

**Skin thickness**

The thickness of the skin increased considerably after irradiation (Figure 87.3). Ear measurements had practically doubled after 3 h, at 24 h a slight decrease was noted. The skin of the back showed a different pattern: here the thickness had increased after 3 h; in the following hours further progression of the thickening was observed.

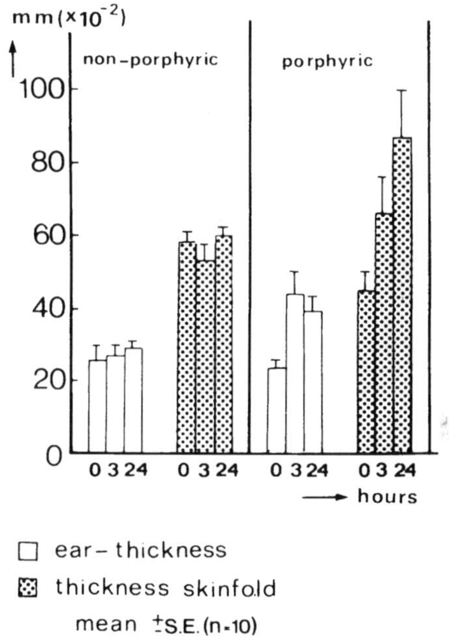


**Figure 87.3** Thickness of the right ear and of a medial longitudinal fold of the back skin of non-porphyric hairless mice measured before and 3 and 24 h after irradiation for 4 min. Protoporphyrin concentrations of erythrocytes were 3000 ± 300 μg/100 ml packed cells and of plasma 2800 ± 500 μg/100 ml. In non-porphyric mice only traces of protoporphyrin were detectable

The photosensitivity, as measured by skin thickness, appeared to be clearly dependent on the protoporphyrin concentrations in plasma and skin (Figures 87.4 and 87.5). To investigate this, porphyrin concentrations in relation to skin thickness were determined at the 7th day of DDC feeding and in similarly treated animals 24 and 48 h after DDC application had been stopped and normal diet had been resumed. In skin and plasma a significant decrease of the protoporphyrin concentrations was noted ($p < 0.01$) whereas the erythrocyte values remained practically the same (Figure 87.4).

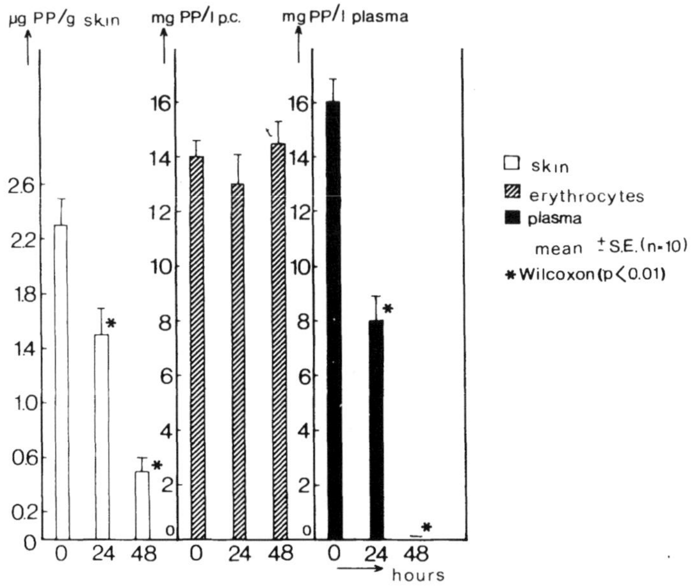


**Figure 87.4** Protoporphyrin determinations in hairless mice fed DDC for 7 days (0 h) and in mice who were initially fed similarly but then received normal diet again for 24 h and 48 h. A significant decrease of skin and plasma concentrations is observed; erythrocyte values remain practically the same

The doubling of ear thickness, which was significant ($p < 0.05$) after 7 days of DDC feeding, was not demonstrable any more 24 h or 48 h after normal diet had been resumed. Here the clinical condition of the animals, the appearance of their skin as well as their behaviour, appeared normal (Figure 87.5).

**Microscopic examinations**

The skin of non-porphyric hairless mice showed very characteristic cyst-like hair follicles which were largest in the deepest half of the dermis, where the collagen fibres were of fine texture, loosely woven. More superficially the follicles were smaller; here the collagen fibres were coarser. Sometimes the follicles contained hair remnants. Between the deep dermal layer and the muscular layer a number of fat cells were present. Furthermore, the histologic picture was identical to observations of normal mouse skin. In unirradiated protoporphyric mice the fat cells had disappeared almost entirely; the other aspects were basically the same as in non-porphyric mice.

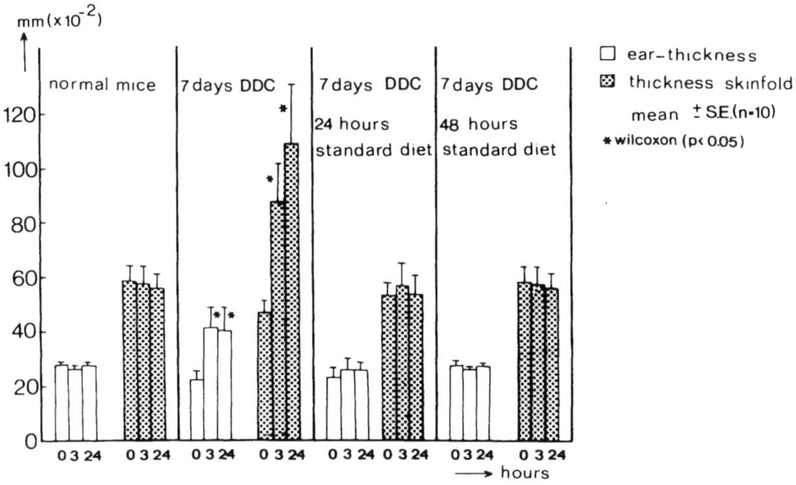


**Figure 87.5** Skin thickness in non-porphyric mice, in porphyric animals which had been fed DDC for 7 days, and in similarly treated animals 24 and 48 h after they had received standard diet again. The values in the third and fourth column are similar to those obtained in normal mice

Signs of an inflammatory response of protoporphyric skin were found 1 h after irradiation. Oedema appeared in the deep dermal level and a mixed cellular infiltrate was clearly observed at 3 h, increasing in the next few hours. It consisted of mononuclear cells, neutrophyllic granulocytes and some erythrocytes. Sometimes the mononuclear cells were present in considerable amount before granulocytes appeared; at other occasions the infiltrate was mixed from the beginning (Figure 87.6). In later stages granulocytes dominated the picture. Perivascular erythrocytes were occasionally found. In the oedematous areas large and small capillaries became dilated early and they were engorged with blood cells. The endothelial cells were swollen and diapedesis of leukocytes was evident. At 24 h many blood vessel walls were disrupted and the vessels were filled with cellular debris. In semithin sections many mast cells were found, which were often degranulated (Figure 87.7), the granules sometimes being scattered throughout the tissue. The mononuclear infiltrated cells mentioned above in part consisted of macrophages with a foamy swollen appearance evidently due to abundant phagocytosis. Fibrocytes and fibroblasts were also vacuolated. The cytoplasm of the macrophages, which was considerably vacuolated, was often studded with homogeneous droplets, suggestive of lipid (Figure 87.8). A number of lipid containing cells seemed to be shrunken fat cells. The abnormalities described also occurred, but to a smaller degree, in the superficial dermis.

Lipid was present in non-irradiated skin in the dermis, notably in the walls of the hair follicles. In the deep dermal layer considerable perifollicular

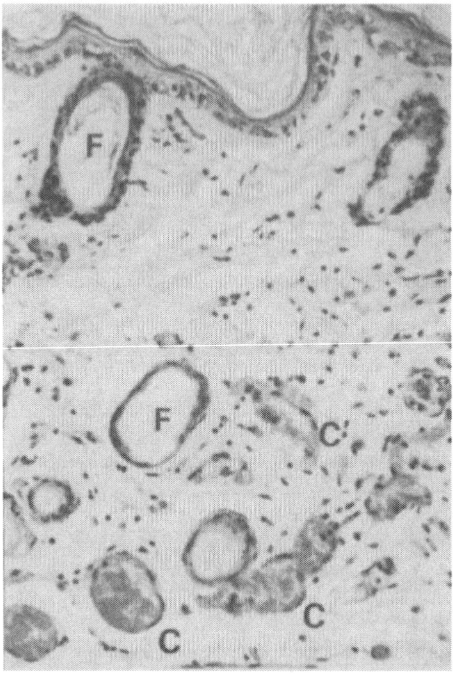


**Figure 87.6** Violet light, 64 min. Biopsy 6 h after irradiation. Capillaries (C) are dilated and studded with erythrocytes. There is oedema and an as yet moderate infiltrate of mostly mononuclear cells. The epidermal cells show vacuolization and pycnotic nuclei. F: empty follicles. C′: disrupted capillary. Haematoxylin eosin; objective 19x

deposits were observed, sometimes located in cells in the connective tissue. It appeared that after the irradiation the amount of lipid increased. This was clearly evident at 24 h when blood vessel walls and many connective tissue cells were loaded with droplets (Figure 87.9).

Finally, it was noted that the alkaline phosphatase reaction of the capillaries was consistently demonstrable in non-porphyric as well as in porphyric unirradiated skin. However, after irradiation of protoporphyric skin the enzyme reactivity had decreased. In the epidermal cells, vacuolization of the cytoplasm and inter- and intra-cellular oedema was clearly observed 6 h after the irradiation (Figure 87.6); at 24 h this had increased to a considerable degree. At this time the deposition of many lipid droplets was easily demonstrable (Figure 87.9).

**Electron microscopy**

The endothelial cells showed signs of decomposition beginning 3 h after the irradiation; oedema, vacuolization, swelling of mitochondriae, endothelial gaps and pycnosis of the nuclei were then evident. This increased into frank

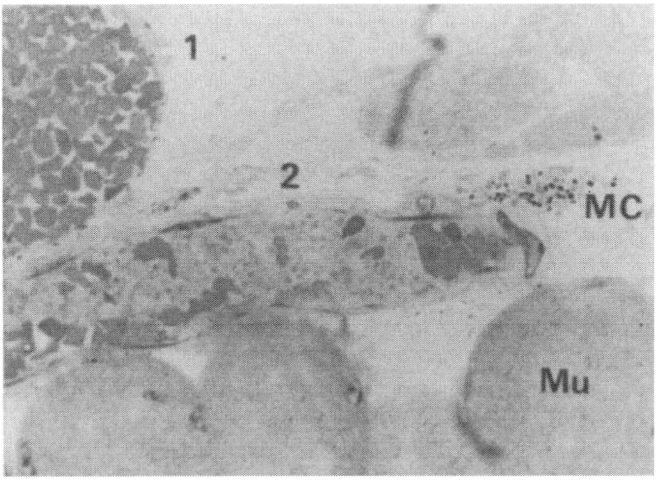


**Figure 87.7** Violet light, 64 min. Biopsy 24 h after irradiation. Two capillaries are observed. The upper vessel (1) is studded with erythrocytes and the endothelium seems to have disappeared. The other one (2) is mainly filled with debris, part of which may be a thrombocyte plug. MC: degranulated mast cell, Mu: muscle tissue, Semithin section; Huber stain, objective 75x

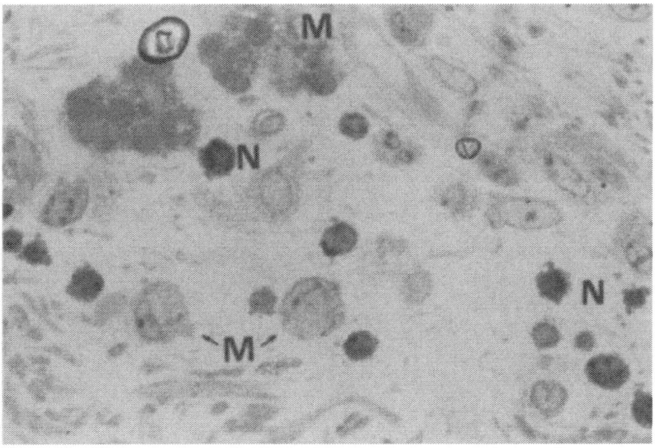


**Figure 87.8** Violet light, 4 min. Biopsy 24 h after irradiation. Oedema and mixed infiltrate consisting of neutrophils (N) and macrophages (M) showing signs of phagocytosis. Some contain round globules, probably lipid. Semithin section; Huber stain, objective 75x

necrosis and lysis of the cells; the vessel lumina were then engorged with a mixture of lytic cell remnants (Figure 87.10). Moreover, thrombocyte aggregates were sometimes observed. Many of the infiltrated cells showed similar

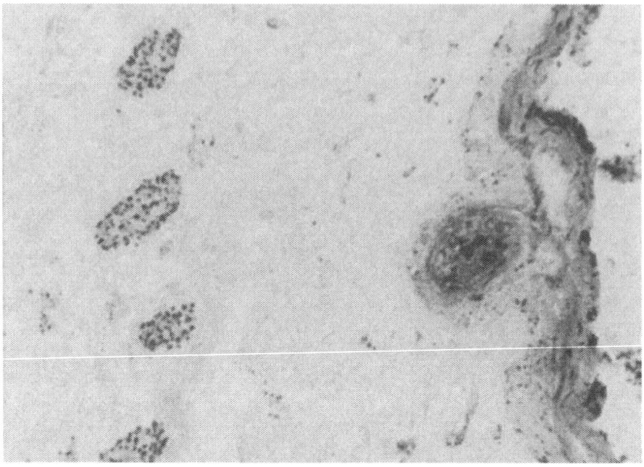

**Figure 87.9** Violet light, 64 min. Biopsy 24 h after irradiation. Capillary walls are loaded with lipid droplets, which are also present in the epidermis. Frozen section; oil red 0, objective 30x

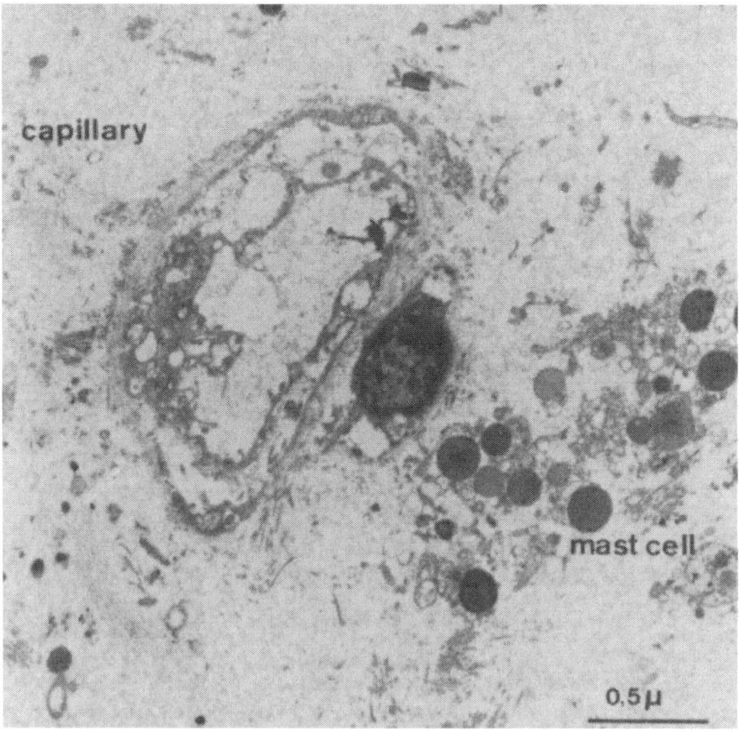


**Figure 87.10** Violet light, 64 min. Biopsy 24 h after irradiation. Capillary with vacuolated necrotic endothelium; a degranulated mast cell is also in a pronounced state of decomposition. Perivascular oedema is conspicuous 6750x

signs of decomposition. Thus there were areas in the perivascular tissue filled with foamy substance and necrotic cells. Again degranulation of mast cells was frequently observed. In the epidermis localized areas of oedema and vacuolization of the keratinocytes were seen. At 24 h after irradiation, condensation of the cell cytoplasm, necrosis, pycnosis of the nuclei and deposition of lipid droplets usually in close proximity to the nuclei were observed.

## DISCUSSION

In the present study it has been shown that a condition of increased protoporphyrin production and accumulation in hairless mice, induced by feeding them DDC, causes hypersensitivity to violet light.

Although it seems hazardous to compare inflammatory reactions of the skin of man and mouse we will try to indicate a few similarities between them. We have interpreted the typical excitement at the beginning of the irradiation as a sign of a feeling of burning. We know that in EPP patients the feeling of being burned continues for many hours or even days; handling of the animals after irradiation or bringing their skin in contact with sawdust again provoked signs of skin hypersensitivity.

The rather abundant mixed cellular infiltrate in mouse skin seems to be at variance with the scarce mostly mononuclear infiltrate in experimentally irradiated (405 nm) EPP skin. On the contrary, in EPP, erythrocyte extravasation is more evident than in the mouse. However heavy doses of sunlight induce a severe granulocytic infiltrate in EPP skin; even nuclear dust may then be observed. It should be realized, however, that in addition to visible light, sunlight also contains shortwave ultraviolet light; furthermore it has a marked heating effect. Consequently, a physiologic sunburn effect may be added to the specific protoporphyric photodermatitis.

A very characteristic phenomenon in irradiated EPP skin is the exudation of a substance of intricate composition[4,5]. This substance, which is generated in the lumina of engorged capillaries, leaks through endothelial gaps, and accumulates in an onion-skin-like pattern between the basement membranes and also perivascularly. Baart de la Faille[3,4], discussing EPP photodermatitis, stressed that it is not only composed of debris of endothelial cells and blood cells but also contains various serum proteins and lipids, as exemplified by immunofluorescence studies, lipid stains and electron microscopy. Extravasating lipid is demonstrable not only in the dermis; 1–2 days after irradiation marked lipid deposits are also demonstrable in the epidermis.

In the present investigation of protoporphyric mouse skin, the exudation of a 'foamy exudate', as described by Konrad *et al.*[15] has also been demonstrated. The exudate also contained lipid, which was deposited subsequently in the epidermis. This part of the exudative process evidently bears resemblance to the occurrences in EPP. It would be of importance to find out whether in mouse skin deposition of fibrin, immunoglobulins and various complement (indicative of complement activation) factors will take place in a similar manner as in EPP photodermatitis[4]. Immunofluorescence studies are underway to investigate these aspects of the reaction of protoporphyric mouse skin to light.

Regarding the pathogenesis of protoporphyric photodermatitis the following remarks are made. It has been proposed that various membrane structures are subject to photo-oxidative alterations in which active oxygen species, notably singlet oxygen[16] and possibly also $O_2^{-}$[14,17] or even $OH^{\bullet}$ are instrumental. According to the Grotthuss–Draper law these processes are initiated by the absorption of light by the photosensitizing substance protoporphyrin which becomes excited into a triplet state which subsequently reacts with oxygen. The available evidence indicates that it is the endothelial cells which is the main target of the irradiation. The decrease of alkaline phosphatase reactivity, which occurs in protoporphyric mice as well as in EPP skin, has been interpreted as a sign of endothelial cell membrane alteration. It is likely that endothelial lysosomes are also attacked by the irradiation; in cell cultures of fibroblasts these organelles have been shown to ingest the photosensitizing protoporphyrin and release their deleterious contents following lysosome-membrane damage caused by irradiation[7]. It has been speculated that part of the exudated lipid has been transported from the dermal capillaries to the epidermis. This may occur through lipolysis of triglycerides by the endothelial cell membrane enzyme lipoprotein lipase, which has undergone activation by the irradiation[4].

Electron microscopically we have found evidence that in addition to endothelium, other cells, for example, epidermis cells, pericytes, histiocytes, mast cells and connective tissue cells also show signs of damage after irradiation, but usually later than the endothelium. Moreover, we have found that skin explants from porphyric mice, which had been kept alive for 24 h, not only showed endothelial cell damage but also distinct vacuolization of the epidermal cells (Baart de la Faille and Woutersen, unpublished observations).

In the opinion of the authors, protoporphyric photodermatitis deserves the attention of students of inflammation. The phenomena presented call for investigations which may unravel the possible role of, for example, kininogenesis, clotting, complement activation and prostaglandin and slow reacting substance forming system. The protoporphyric hairless mice may further be of help in the search for an effective therapy of EPP photodermatitis. A subsequent paper[14] will deal with the possible mitigating influence oxygen radical scavengers will have on the hypersensitivity to light.

## ACKNOWLEDGMENTS

We are indebted to Mrs E. Blanchard-van Buuren, Miss G. C. F. de Bruin, Miss L. Smits and Mr A. H. van Veen for expert technical assistance and to Dr S. C. J. van der Putte and Dr J. B. van der Meer for giving advice regarding the microscopic and electron microscopic investigations.

## References

1 Magnus, I. A., Jarrett, A., Prankerd, T. A. J. and Rimington, C. (1961). Erythropoietic protoporphyria. A new porphyria syndrome with solar urticaria due to protoporphyrinaemia. *Lancet*, **2**, 448
2 DeLeo, V. A., Poh-Fitzpatrick, M. Mathews–Roth, M and Harber, L. C. (1976). Erythropoietic protoporphyria. 10 years experience. *Am. J. Med.*, **60**, 8
3 Baart de la Faille, H. (1979). Erythropoetische Protoporphyrie. In Korting, G. (ed.) *Dermatologie in Praxis und Klinik*, pp. 38.69–38.82 (Stuttgart: Georg Thieme Verlag)
4 Baart de la Faille, H. (1975). Erythropoietic protoporphyria. A photodermatosis. Microscopical and electron microscopical investigations of irradiated skin and a clinical study. (Utrecht: Oosthoek, Scheltema and Holkema)
5 Gschnait, F., Wolff, K. and Konrad, K. (1975). Erythropoietic protoporphyria-submicroscopic events during the acute photosensitivity flare. *Br. J. Dermatol.*, **92**, 545
6 Allison, A. C., Magnus, I. A. and Young, M. R. (1966). Role of lysosomes and cell membranes in photosensitization. *Nature (London)*, **209**, 874
7 Schothorst, A. A., Suurmond, D. and Ploem, J. S. (1977). In vitro studies on the protoporphyrin uptake and photosensitivity of normal skin fibroblasts and fibroblasts from patients with erythropoietic protoporphyria. *J. Invest. Dermatol.*, **69**, 551
8 Huber, J. D., Parker, F. and Odland, G. F. (1968). A basic fuchsine and alkalinized methylene blue rapid stain for epoxy-embedded tissue. *Stain Technol.*, **43**, 83
9 Berg, N. O. (1951). Histological studies of masked lipids. Stainability, distribution and functional variations. *Acta Pathol. Scand. Suppl.*, **90**,
10 Lillie, R. D. and Ashburn, L. L. (1943). Laboratory methods and technical notes. Supersaturated solutions of fat stains in dilute isopropanol for demonstration of acute fatty degenerations not shown by Herxheimer technic. *Arch. Pathol*, **36**, 432
11 Romeis, B. (1968). *Mikroskopische Technik*, 16th Edn. (München, R. Oldenbourg Verlag)
12 Gomori, G. (1951). Alkaline phosphatase of cell nuclei. *J. Lab. Clin. Med.*, **37**, 526
13 Burstone, M. S. (1958). Histochemical comparison of naphtol AS-phosphates for the demonstration of phosphatases. *J. Natl. Cancer Inst.*, **20**, 601
14 Woutersen, R. A., Holsteijn van, C. W. M. and Baart de la Faille, H. (1980). Experimental protoporphyria in hairless mice. II. Photohaemolysis versus photodermatitis. This volume, Chap. 88
15 Konrad, K., Hönigsmann, H., Gschnait, F. and Wolff, K. (1975). Mouse model for protoporphyria. II. Cellular and subcellular events in the photosensitivity flare of the skin. *J. Invest. Dermatol*, **65**, 300
16 Cannistraro, S., van der Vorst, A. and Jori, G. (1978). EPR studies on singlet oxygen production by porphyrins. *Photochem. Photobiol.*, **28**, 257
17 Buettner, G. and Oberley, L. W. (1979). Superoxide formation by protoporphyrin as seen by spin trapping. *FEBS Lett.*. **98**, 18

# 88

# Experimental protoporphyria in hairless mice: photohaemolysis versus photodermatitis

R. A. WOUTERSEN, C. W. M. VAN HOLSTEIJN AND H. BAART DE LA FAILLE (NETHERLANDS)

## INTRODUCTION

In 1908 Hausmann[1] proved that systemically administered haematoporphyrin might be fatal for mice if they were exposed to violet light, while a much larger dose of this substance was harmless if the animals were kept in the dark. Meyer–Betz[2] injected himself with haematoporphyrin which resulted in marked erythema and oedema of the light exposed parts of the body. In spite of this recognized relation between porphyrins and photosensitivity the pathogenesis of the dermatitis of patients who suffer from photosensitive porphyria is not fully understood.

Erythrocytes obtained from erythropoietic protoporphyria (EPP) patients[3] or protoporphyric mice[4] undergo haemolysis *in vitro* when exposed to violet light. This phenomenon is used by several investigators to study the photodynamic reactions leading to the lysis of the cell. The underlying thought of these experiments is that the reactions causing the damage of the cell membrane of the erythrocyte have aspects in common with those leading to the photodermatitis. The mechanism of the photodynamical reactions that ultimately cause the damage of the cell membrane is not fully understood.

Regarding the mechanism of the photohaemolysis some authors claimed that the cell membrane is damaged by peroxidation of unsaturated fatty acids or of cholesterol[5,6]. De Goeij *et al.*[7] and Dubbelman *et al.*[8] denied the occurrence of such a mechanism and proposed that cross-linking of membrane proteins (e.g. spectrin) is the prime cause of photohaemolysis. In spite of this controversy, however, most investigators agree that important intermediates in the photodynamic reactions leading to the damage of membrane components include PP in its excited triplet state and active oxygen species.

Cannistraro *et al.*[9] and Buettner *et al.*[10], using electron paramagnetic resonance techniques, proved that, during irradiation of PP, singlet oxygen as well as superoxide are formed (Figure 88.1). Superoxide ($.O_2$) can give rise to hydrogen peroxide ($H_2O_2$) either through the action of superoxide dismutase or spontaneously. Moreover, there is considerable evidence that in the presence of hydrogen peroxide, superoxide can give rise to the even more toxic hydroxyl radical (OH.) via the so called 'Haber–Weiss reaction'. The signifi-

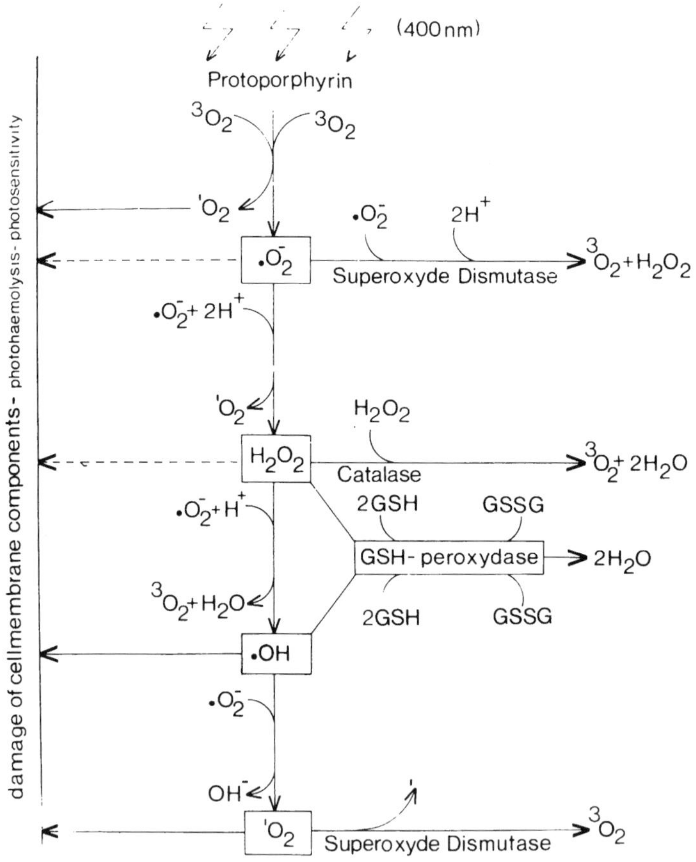


**Figure 88.1** Summary of the various types of active oxygen species, which may arise during irradiation of PP with 400 nm light. '$O_2$: singlet oxygen; $.O_2$: superoxide radical; $H_2O_2$: hydrogen peroxide; OH.: hydroxyl radical; $^3O_2$: triplet (ground) state of oxygen

cance of this reaction in biological material is still unknown[11,12]. Halliwell[13,14] suggested that trace amounts of metal ions, e.g. ferrous ions, could catalyse this reaction. Hence it is possible that hydroxyl radicals may arise during the irradiation of PP.

The photohaemolysis of erythrocytes obtained from DDC-treated mice was strongly inhibited by scavengers of superoxide (e.g. 1,2-dihydroxybenzene-3,5-disulphonic acid and diethyldithiocarbamate) and scavengers of singlet oxygen (e.g., vitamin A and beta-carotene). Scavengers of the hydroxyl radical (e.g., mannitol and benzoate) hardly protected fluorescing cells against photohaemolysis[15,16]. These results indicate that besides singlet oxygen, other active oxygen species such as superoxide and hydrogen peroxide might also be involved in the photodynamic reactions leading to the damage of the cell membrane.

We have compared the protective effects of compounds which are known, more or less specific, scavengers of active oxygen species against the photodynamically induced haemolysis with the protection of these compounds against the photodynamically induced dermatitis.

## MATERIALS AND METHODS

The hairless mice were females of the SKH I strain. They were obtained from the Central Laboratory of Animals, Academic Hospital of the University of Utrecht. The animals were made protoporphyric by feeding them 0.5% (w/w) 3,5-dicarbethoxy-1,4 dihydrocollidine (Eastman Kodak NV, Rochester, NY 14650, USA). Orgotein (Palosein) was a gift from Dr W. Huber, Diagnostic Data Inc., Mountain View, California 94043, USA. Cysteamine-HC1 (J. T. Baker) was dissolved in aqua bidestillata and neutralized to pH 7.2 by NaOH. Beta-carotene/canthaxanthin (2:3; w/w), a gift from Hoffman La Roche, was suspended in saline. Diethyldithiocarbamate and butylated hydroxy toluene were obtained from the British Drug Houses. Sterox SE (Poly-oxyethylene thioether) was obtained from Hartman-Leddon Co., Philadelphia, USA.

### The photohaemolysis experiments

To obtain blood, mice were decapitated and blood was collected in a heparinized tube. Freshly heparinized blood was centrifuged (3000 rev/min, 5 min) and washed three times with an isotonic NaCl solution. An erythrocyte suspension in saline was used with a haematocrit value of 30–40%. In most experiments, 0.2 ml of this cell suspension was added to 4.2 ml NaCl solution. All other solutes were added in advance.

Irradiation was carried out on the apparatus depicted in Figure 88.2. Using air cooling the temperature in the tubes did not exceed 35 °C. A Philips

HPW (125 W) mercury lamp was used as a light source. The light intensity varied from 22 mW/cm$^2$ (at a distance of 8 cm) to 2.6 mW/cm$^2$ (at a distance of 32 cm).

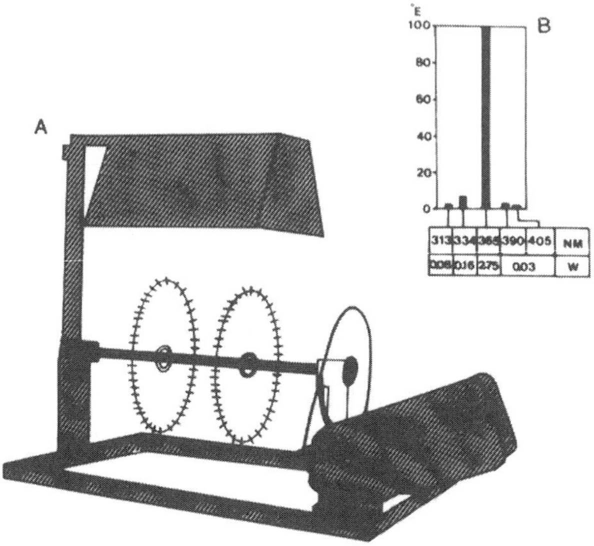


**Figure 88.2** (A) Photohaemolysis apparatus. (B) Relative spectral energy distribution of the Philips HPW lamp

The percentage haemolysis was measured according to the method described by Peterka *et al.*[3]. To obtain 100% haemolysis the cells were lysed by the addition of 4.2 ml Sterox buffer (66 mmol/l K–Na–orthophosphate buffer pH 6.6; 0.5% Sterox SE).

**Photosensitivity experiments**

The irradiation of the protoporphyric hairless mice and measuring the thickness of the ears and of a skinfold of the back was carried out as described in Chapter 87. The protoporphyrin concentrations in the blood of the protoporphyric mice were determined according to the method described by Piomelli *et al.*[17] as modified by Caffo *et al.*[18]. The protoporphyrin concentration in 1.5N HCl was determined using a Beckman model 25 spectrophotometer equipped with cuvettes with a light path of 2 cm. The calculations were carried out as described by Cripps and Peters[19].

## RESULTS

The time needed to obtain 50% haemolysis decreased with increasing PP concentration of the erythrocyte suspension (Figure 88.3). Consequently the

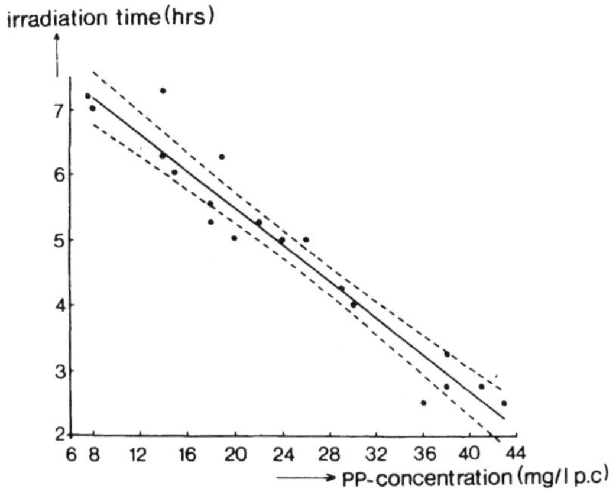


**Figure 88.3** Relation between the PP concentration of the irradiated erythrocyte suspension and the time needed to obtain 50% haemolysis. $N = 18$; correlation coefficient: 0.96. Broken lines represent the 95% reliability intervals

irradiation time needed to obtain 50% haemolysis decreased with increasing duration of the DDC feeding period. However, independent of the PP concentration, an irradiation time of about 2 h was always needed to demonstrate the first haemolysis. Using erythrocyte suspensions obtained from EPP patients with PP concentrations which were in the same range as those in protoporphyric mice, we did not find any haemolysis within 8 h of irradiation. This result shows that erythrocyte suspensions obtained from protoporphyric mice can be used as sensitive models to study the effects of scavengers of active oxygen species on haemolysis.

The effect of the anti-inflammatory drug orgotein, a protein with superoxide dismutase activity, was studied *in vitro* and *in vivo*. This protein did not protect fluorescing cells obtained from protoporphyric mice against photohaemolysis. Furthermore, intraperitoneal or intravenous administration of high (25 mg/kg body weight) or low doses (2.5 or 0.25 mg/kg body weight) of this protein to protoporphyric hairless mice did not protect them against the effects of irradiation. Figure 88.4 shows the results of one of these experiments: The thickness of the ears or of the skinfold of non-porphyric mice did not increase after irradiation. Protoporphyric animals injected with saline (control) or orgotein both were clearly affected.

Cysteamine, an antioxidant with a still unknown mechanism of action, strongly inhibited the photohaemolysis (Figure 88.5). However, intravenous administration of this compound (0.1 ml of a 2.5% solution) did not protect protoporphyric hairless mice against the effects of irradiation (Figure 88.6).

Beta-carotene/canthaxanthin, which is an effective scavenger of singlet oxygen, caused a strong inhibition of the photohaemolysis of ery-

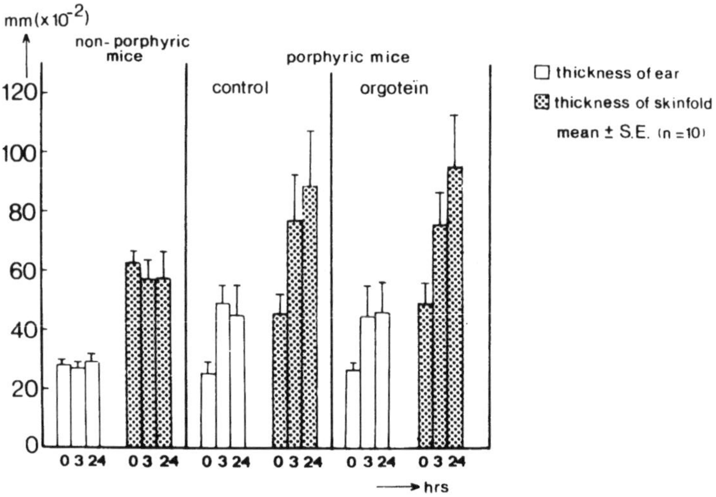


**Figure 88.4** Effect of orgotein on the photosensitivity of protoporphyric hairless mice. Orgotein (25 mg/kg body weight) was administered i.v. 1 h before and just before the irradiation of the animals for 4 min. The thickness of the ears and of the skinfolds were measured before (=0) the irradiation and 3 and 24 h after that

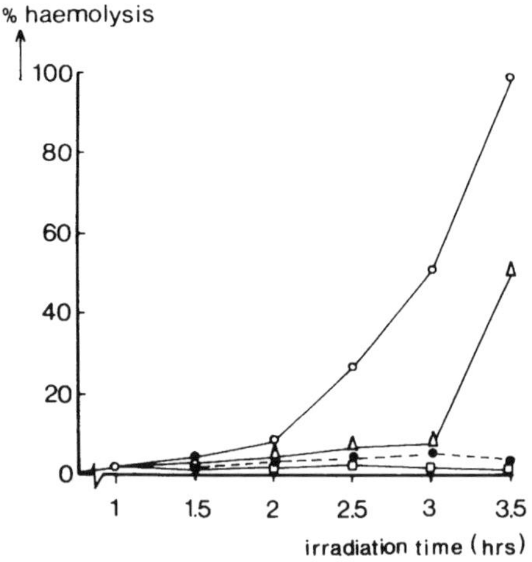


**Figure 88.5** Effect of cysteamine (15 mol/l) on the photohaemolysis of erythrocytes obtained from protoporphyric mice. The erythrocyte suspensions were irradiated for 1.5–3.5 h. After the irradiation the suspensions were kept in the dark until the % haemolysis was measured (7 h after the start of the irradiation). The erythrocyte suspensions were irradiated in the absence of cysteamine (○, △) or in the presence of this compound (□, ●). Furthermore, cysteamine was absent during the dark period (○, □) or present (△, ●)

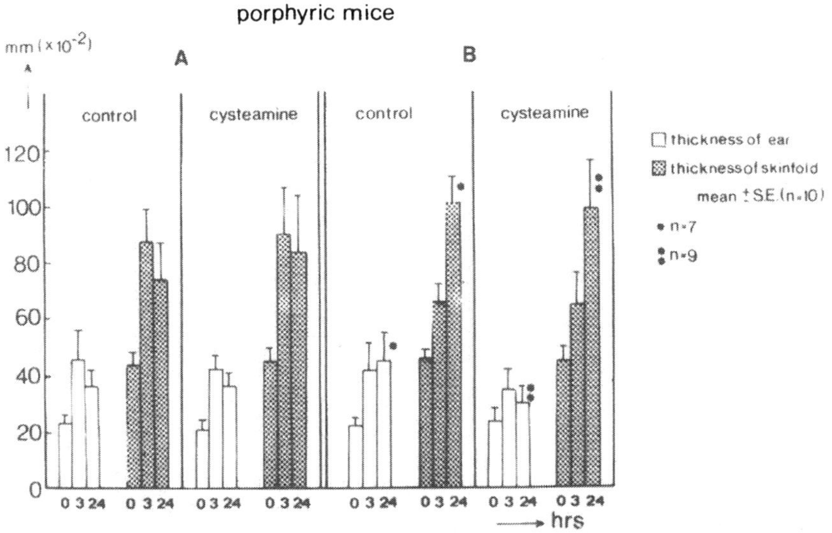


**Figure 88.6** Effect of cysteamine (0.1 ml of a neutralised 2.5% solution was administered i.v. just before the irradiation) on the photosensitivity of protoporphyric hairless mice. Irradiation time: A, 4 min; B, 64 min. The thickness of the ears and of the skinfolds were measured before (= 0) the irradiation and 3 and 24 h after that

throcytes obtained from protophyric mice (Figure 88.7(A)). To what extent this inhibition of the photohaemolysis is due to an absorption of 400 nm light by beta-carotene was studied in another experiment (Figure 88.7(B)). In this experiment two tubes with a different diameter (tube A 17.5 mm and tube B 20.5 mm) were used. This made it possible to separate the erythrocyte suspension (which is contained in compartment A) from a beta-carotene/canthaxanthin suspension (which is contained in compartment B). An inhibition of the photohaemolysis was found only if the beta-carotene/canthaxanthin suspension was in the same compartment as the erythrocyte suspension. The presence of this compound in compartment B did not protect an erythrocyte suspension obtained from protoporphyric mice, which is contained in compartment A, against haemolysis. This result indicated that the inhibitory effect of beta-carotene/canthaxanthin is not due to the absorption of 400nm light.

In spite of this very strong protection of fluorescing cells against photohaemolysis, intraperitoneal administration of this compound did not cause an impressive protection of protoporphyric hairless mice against the effects of irradiation with violet light (Figure 88.8).

The mean beta-carotene concentration in the plasma of the test animals was 7.76 μmol/l. Normal mouse plasma contained less than 0.7 μmol/l (these determinations were carried out using a HPLC-apparatus by Dr J. Schrijver from the Institute for Nutrition and Food Research TNO, Zeist, The Nether-

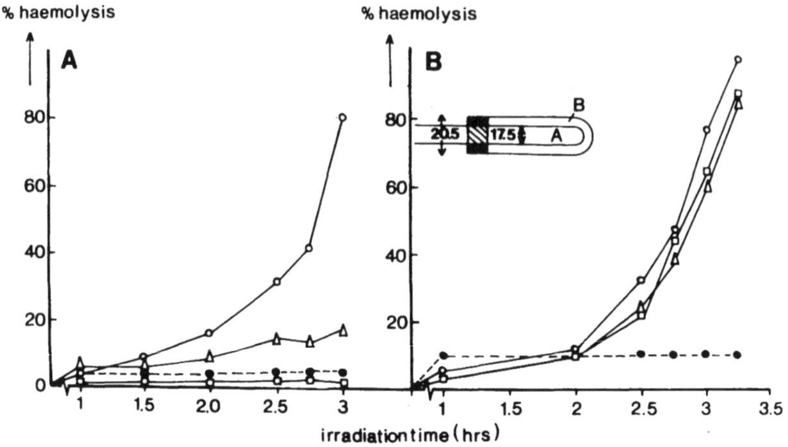


**Figure 88.7** Effect of beta-carotene/canthaxanthin (2:3; w/w 5 μmol/l) on the photohaemolysis of erythrocytes obtained from protoporphyric mice. (A) The erythrocyte suspensions were irradiated for 1 – 3 h. After the irradiation the suspensions were kept in the dark until the % haemolysis was measured (7 h after the start of the irradiation). The suspensions were irradiated in the absence of carotene (○, □) or in the presence of this compound (□, ●). Furthermore, carotene was absent during the dark period (○, △) or present (△, ●). (B) For explanation of this figure see text. The erythrocyte suspension is contained in compartment A while compartment B is absent (○), contained saline (□) or 5 μmol/l beta-carotene-canthaxanthine (△). ●: erythrocyte suspension and 5 μmol/l beta-carotene/canthaxanthin is contained in compartment A while compartment B is absent. The % haemolysis was measured directly after the irradiation

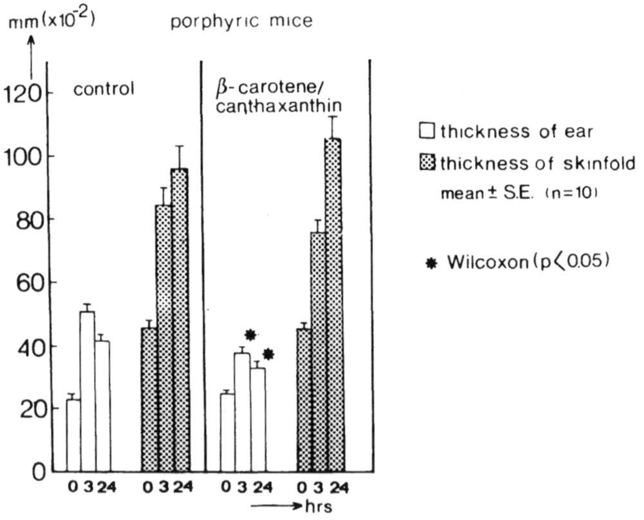


**Figure 88.8** Effect of beta-carotene/canthaxanthin on the photosensitivity of protoporphyric hairless mice. The compound was administered i.p. 24 and 3 h before the irradiation (both 1 mg). Irradiation time was 4 min, The thickness of the ears and of the skinfolds were measured before (=0) the irradiation and 3 and 24 h after that

lands). Figure 88.8 shows that beta-carotene/canthaxanthin causes a significantly smaller increase in thickness of the ears of irradiated protoporphyric hairless mice than in control-animals (protoporphyric hairless mice which were injected with saline).

In combination with other scavengers of active oxygen species (diethyldithiocarbamate, cysteamine and butylated hydroxy toluene) this compound also caused a significantly smaller increase in thickness of the skinfold (24 h after the irradiation). These results are summarized in Figure 88.9.

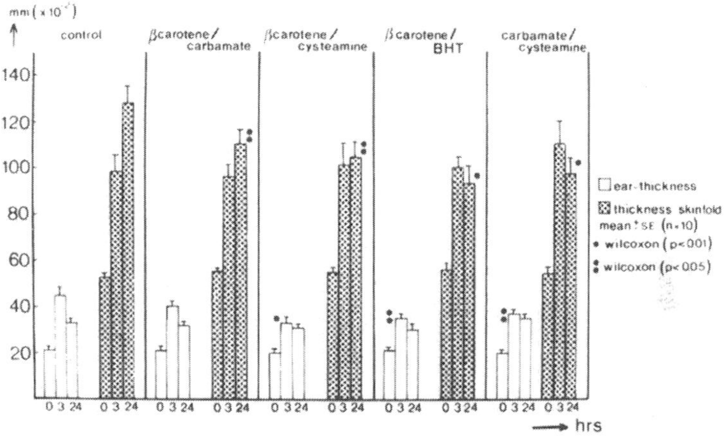


**Figure 88.9** Effects of combinations of compounds on the photosensitivity of proporphyric hairless mice. Beta carotene/canthaxanthin was injected i.p. (both 1 mg) 24 and 3 h before the irradiation. Cysteamine (0.1 ml of a 2.5% solution) was administered i.p. just before the irradiation. Carbamate (diethylidithiocarbamate; 1 mg) and BHT (butylated hydroxy toluene; 0.1 ml of a 5mg/ml suspension) were administered i.v. just before the irradiation. The animals were irradiated for 4 min. The thickness of the ears and skinfolds were measured before (= 0) the irradiation and 3 and 24 h after that

## DISCUSSION

Microscopical observations of the irradiated skin of protoporphyric hairless mice are described by Baart de la Faille *et al.* (see Chap. 87). They concluded that the photochemical reactions leading to the dermatitis seem to take place primarily in the endothelium of the dermal capillaries. The endothelial cells of the irradiated skin show swelling followed by destruction. Furthermore, perivascular infiltration of mononuclear cells and neutrophillic granulocytes, exudation of a 'foamy' appearance substance and degranulation of mast cells were observed.

Photohaemolysis experiments indicated that erythrocyte suspensions obtained from DDC treated mice are more sensitive to irradiation than blood cell suspensions obtained from EPP patients. This phenomenon seems to be due to differences in percentage of fluorescing cells in the blood. All erythrocytes in the blood of protoporphyric mice contain an elevated PP concentration, causing fluorocytosis (a typical fading orange-red fluorescence) in 100% of these cells. The blood of EPP patients contains only 10–40% of these cells. The presence of normal (non-fluorescing) cells in an erythrocyte suspension obtained from EPP patients causes an inhibition of the haemolysis[15].

The results of preliminary photohaemolysis experiments[15,16], indicated that besides singlet oxygen, superoxide might also be involved in the photodynamic reactions leading to the damage of the cell membranes (erythrocyte membranes and probably also membranes of the endothelial cells of the dermal capillaries). These results were in accordance with the electron paramagnetic resonance studies of Buettner *et al.*[10], indicating superoxide formation by PP. For these reasons the effects of orgotein were studied. Orgotein is a protein with superoxide dismutase activity which has been successfully used against various inflammatory diseases (e.g., rheumatoid arthritis[20]). The absence of an effect of this compound in our experiments may be due to the impossibility of this protein (MW = 31 000) to pass cell membranes.

Low concentrations (0.01–0.1 mmol/l) of diethyldithiocarbamate, a copper chelating agent, caused a strong inhibition of the photohaemolysis of erythrocytes obtained from protoporphyric mice[16]. This inhibition of the photohaemolysis might be caused by an interference of diethyldithiocarbamate with the superoxide dismutase activity (a copper containing enzyme), indicating that superoxide and superoxide dismutase are involved in the photodynamic reactions leading to the photohaemolysis. However, this compound showed only a very slight protection of protoporphyric hairless mice against the effects of irradiation with violet light, even in combination with beta-carotene/canthaxanthin.

Beta-carotene and canthaxanthin are well known scavengers of singlet oxygen[21]. In spite of a very strong inhibition of the photohaemolysis the protection of protoporphyric hairless mice against the effects of irradiation by this compound was not impressive. Some authors claim that high doses of beta-carotene increase the tolerance of EPP patients to sunlight markedly[21,22]. Corbett *et al.*[23], however, did not find any protection, whereas Baart de la Faille *et al.*[24] and Rossi *et al.*[25] only found a moderate improvement by this compound. Our results are comparable with those found by the latter investigators: a slight protection which is clinically not impressive.

Cysteamine is an effective protector against ionizing radiation[26]. Like glutathion, cysteamine might be able to eliminate various types of active oxygen species, e.g. hydrogen peroxide and hydroxyl radicals[27,28]. This compound showed a very strong inhibition of the photohaemolysis but hardly protected protoporphyric hairless mice against irradiation with violet light.

The observations that compounds showing a very strong inhibition of the photohaemolysis hardly protect protoporphyric hairless mice against the effects of irradiation are difficult to explain. It may indicate that the reactions leading to the photosensivivity of the skin are much more complicated than the photodynamic processes leading to the haemolysis of irradiated fluorescing blood cells.

The observation that irradiation of the skin of protoporphyric hairless mice induces a strong inflammatory reaction indicates that in addition to antioxidants (e.g., butylated hydroxy toluene), common anti-inflammatory drugs and combinations of compounds may be used. Our results demonstrate that the protoporphyric hairless mouse may serve as a sensitive animal model to increase the insight in the pathogenesis of photodynamically induced types of dermatitis.

## References


1 Hausmann, W. (1908). Ueber die sensibilisierende Wirkung tierischer Farbstoffe und ihre physiologische Bedeutung. *Biochem. Z.*, **14,** 275

2 Meyer–Betz, F. (1913). Untersuchungen über die biologische (photodynamische) Wirkung des Hämatoporphyrins und andere Derivate des Blut- und Gallenfarbstoffs. *Dtsch. Arch. Klin. Med.*, **112,** 476

3 Peterka, E. S., Runge, W. J. and Fusaro, R. M. (1966). Erythropoietic protoporphyria. III. Photohaemolysis. *Arch. Dermatol.*, **94,** 282

4 Woutersen, R. A. (1979). Experimental protoporphyria in mice and Japanese quail. Thesis Utrecht

5 Hsu, J., Goldstein, B. D. and Harber, L. C. (1971). Photoreactions associated with *in vitro* hemolysis in erythropoietic protoporphyria. *Photochem. Photobiol.*, **13,** 67

6 Lamola, A. A., Yamane, T. and Trozzole, A. M. (1973). Cholesterol hydroperoxide formation in red cell membranes and photohaemolysis in erythropoietic protoporphyria. *Science*, **179,** 1131

7 Goeij, A. F. P. M. de and van Steveninck, J. (1976). Photodynamic effects of protoporphyrin on cholesterol and unsaturated fatty acids in erythrocyte membrane in protoporphyria and in normal red blood cells. *Clin. Chim. Acta*, **68,** 115

8 Dubbelman, T. M. A. R., de Goeij, A. F. P. M. and van Steveninck, J. (1978). Photodynamic effects of protoporphyrin on human erythrocytes. Nature of the cross-linking of membrane proteins. *Biochem. Biophys. Acta*, **511,** 141

9 Cannistraro, S. A., van de Vorst, A. and Jori, G. (1978). EPR studies on singlet oxygen production by porphyrins. *Photochem. Photobiol.*, **28,** 257

10 Buettner, G. R. and Oberley, L. W. (1979). Superoxide formation by protoporphyrin as seen by spin trapping. *FEBS Let.*, **98,** 18

11 Cohen, G. (1978). The generation of hydroxyl radicals in biological systems: toxicological aspects. *Photochem. Photobiol.*, **28,** 669

12 Czapski, G. and Ilan, Y. A. (1978). On the generation of the hydroxylation agent from superoxide radical. Can the Haber–Weiss reaction be the source of OH-radicals? *Photochem. Photobiol.*, **28,** 651

13 Halliwell, B. (1978). Superoxide-dependent formation of hydroxyl radicals in the presence of iron chelates. *FEBS Lett.*, **92,** 321

14 Halliwell, B. (1978). Superoxide-dependent formation of hydroxyl radicals in the presence of iron salts. *FEBS Lett.*, **96,** 238

15 Woutersen, R. A., van Holsteijn, C. W. M. and Wit, J. G. (1979). Experimental erythropoietic protoporphyria: fluorescing blood cells in mice and Japanese quail after feeding 3,5-diethoxycarbonyl-1,4-dihydrocollidine, griseofulvin or lead. In Strik, J. J. and Koeman, J. H. (eds.) *Chemical porphyria in Man*, pp. 139–150. (Amsterdam: Elsevier/ North-Holland Biomedical Press)

16 Woutersen, R. A., van Holsteijn, C. W. M. and Wit, J. G. (1980). Experimental protoporphyria in mice: Effects of scavengers of active oxygen species on photohaemolysis (In preparation)

17 Piomelli, S. (1973). A micromethod for free erythrocyte porphyrins: the FEP-test. *J. Lab. Clin. Med.*, **81**, 932
18 Caffo, A. L. and Lubin, A. H. (1976). Modified micromethod for erythrocyte porphyrin. *Clin. Chem.*, **22**, 1412
19 Cripps, D. J. and Peters, H. A. (1967). Fluorescing erythrocytes and porphyrin screening tests on urine, stool and blood. Investigation of photosensitivity. *Arch. Dermatol.*, **96**, 712
20 Huber, W. and Saifer, M. G. P. (1977). Orgotein, the drug version of bovine Cu-Zn superoxide dismutase. I. A summary account for safety and pharmacology in laboratory animals. In Michelson, A., McCord, J. M. and Fridovich, I. (eds.) *Superoxide and Superoxide Dismutases*, pp. 517–536. (London: Academic Press)
21 Leo, V. A. de, Poh-Fitzpatrick, M. B., Mathews-Roth, M. M. and Harber, L. C. (1976). Erythropoietic protoporphyria: 10 years experience. *Am. J. Med.*, **60**, 8
22 Mathews-Roth, M. M., Pathak, M. A., Fitzpatrick, T. B., Harber, L. C. and Kass, E. H. (1977). β-Carotene therapy for erythropoietic protoporphyria and other photosensitivity diseases. *Arch. Dermatol.*, **113**, 1229
23 Corbett, M. F., Herxheimer, A., Magnus, I. A., Ramsay, C. A. and Kobza-Black, A. (1977). The long-term treatment with β-Carotene in erythropoietic protoporphyria: a controlled trial. *Br. J. Dermatol.*, **97**, 655
24 Baart de la Faille, H., Suurmond, S., Went, L. N., van Steveninck, J. and Schothorst, A. A. (1972). β-Carotene as a treatment for photohypersensitivity due to erythropoietic protoporphyria. *Dermatologica*, **145**, 389
25 Rossi, E., Curnow, D. H. and Schonberg, H. (1978). The detection of porphyria in photosensitive patients. *Pathology*, **10**, 17
26 Bacq, Z. M. (1965), *Chemical protection against ionizing radiation*. (Springfield: Charles C. Thomas)
27 Pryor, W. A. (1976). *Free radicals in biology*, Vols. I, II and III. (New York: Academic Press)
28 Armstrong, D. A. and Buchanan, J. D. (1978). Reactions of $.O_2$, $H_2O_2$ and other oxidants with sulfhydryl enzymes. *Photochem. Photobiol.*, **28**, 743

89

# Morphological studies of inflammatory reactions: the relationships between the delayed-type hypersensitivity reaction and the Arthus reaction induced in the rat with ovalbumin

L. L. RÖCKERT, M. SANDÉN AND P. M. LUNDIN (SWEDEN)

## AIM

To study the relationship between the inflammatory reaction and the immune reactivity of rats, and the participation of T and B lymphocytes in the local reaction.

## MATERIALS AND METHODS

Thymectomized and non-thymectomized Sprague–Dawley rats were sensitized intradermally with ovalbumin in Freund's complete adjuvant. The animals were divided into different groups which received different sensitizing doses of 1, 10, 100 and 500μg ovalbumin. They were challenged intradermally in the skin of the back at different times after sentitization with ovalbumin in sterile saline. Challenge doses, usually 10μg, were given 3–21 days after sensitization.

The macroscopical reactions, consisting of oedema and erythema at injection sites, were registered at 4, 8, 24 and 48 h after challenge. At the same time skin biopsies were taken for studies with light microscopy, enzymehistochemistry and immunofluorescence.

Venous blood samples were taken for determination of the specific antibody response (IgGę) with an enzyme linked immunosorbent assay (ELISA). Non-specific esterases in monocytes and neutrophil leukocytes were demonstrated with naphtol-ASD-chloroacetate method on paraffin and kryostate sectioned materials.

**Immunological methods**

T cells were demonstrated with a rabbit–anti-rat serum produced against thoracic duct cells and adsorbed with liver, erythrocytes, bone marrow cells and peritoneal macrophages.

B cells were demonstrated with an antiserum against adult spleen cells taken from neonatally thymectomized rats. The serum was adsorbed with erythrocytes and thymus cells and partly with peritoneal macrophages. An indirect fluorescence method with FITC-conjugated swine–anti-rabbit serum was used (Dako pats).

**Immunological controls**

The specificity of our serum was tested on spleen, lymph node and thymus sections from non-treated control animals. Anti-T serum showed a strong affinity to lymphocytes in thymus dependent areas (TDA) in the spleen and lymph nodes (Figure 89.1) and bindings to very few follicle cells in the spleen and lymph nodes (Figure 89.2). It also showed bindings to the majority of cells in the thymic cortex.

Anti-B serum was also tested on TDA in spleen and showed binding to very few cells (less than 5%; Figure 89.3). It also showed slight affinity to the cells in the thymic medulla and no affinity to the cells in the thymic cortex. Affinity was demonstrated to nearly 100% of the follicle cells in lymph nodes and spleen (Figure 89.4) and approximately to 50% of the cells in the red pulp of spleen.

## RESULTS

**Macroscopical reactions and light microscopy**

Macroscopical reactions with no or minimal response at 4 h after challenge and with a strong response at 24 h were called delayed-type hypersensitivity (DTH) reactions. Histologically there were no reaction at 4 h, but at 24 h a moderate or strong mononuclear infiltrate was seen (Figures 89.5 (A) and (B)), totally dominated by lymphocytes and monocytes–histiocytes.

Macroscopical reactions with early appearance, i.e. 4–5 h after challenge, which decreased at 24 h were called Arthus reactions. These reactions

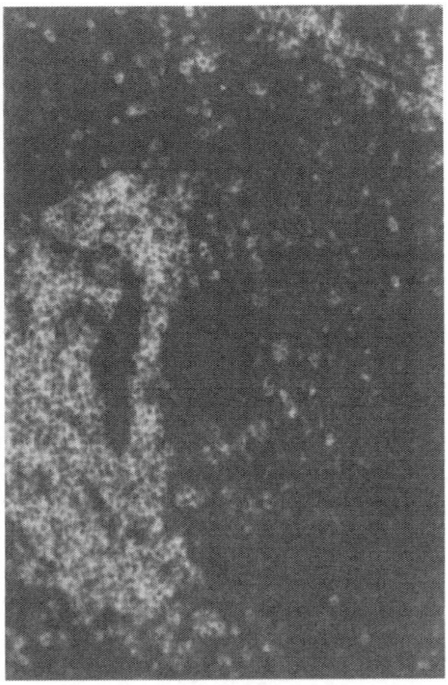

**Figure 89.1** TDA area in the spleen (left part of the figure). Strong fluorescence after treatment with anti-T cell serum

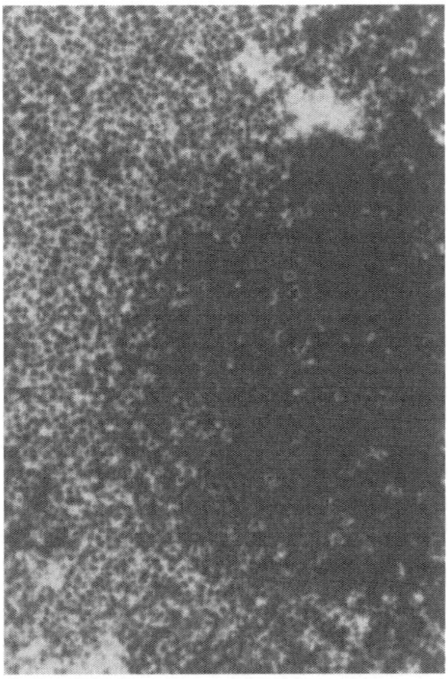

**Figure 89.2** Spleen follicle. A few positive cells after treatment with anti-T cell serum

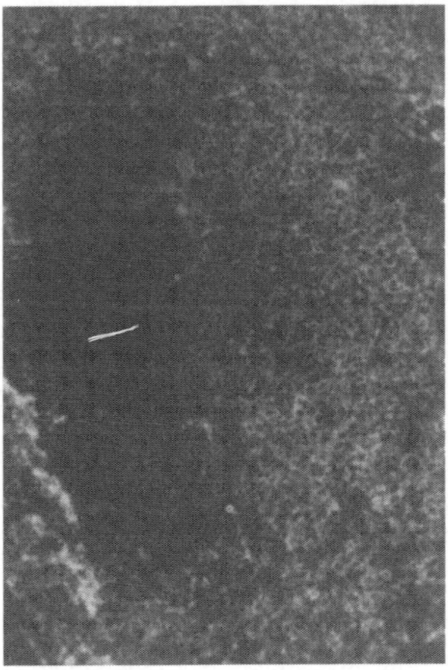

**Figure 89.3** TDA area in the spleen (left part of the figure). Dark after treatment with anti-B cell serum

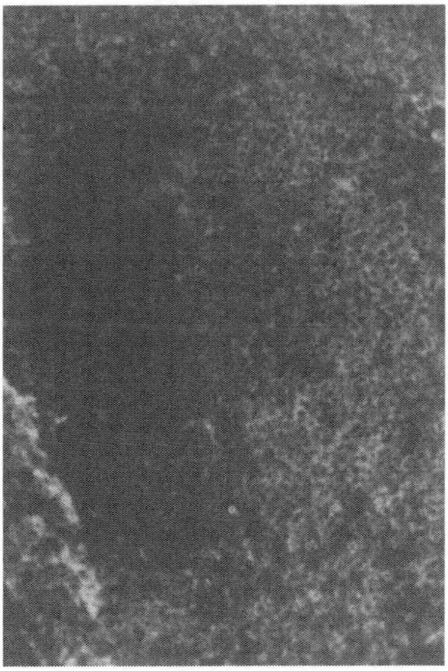

**Figure 89.4** Follicle of lymph node. Strong fluorescence of almost all cells after treatment with anti-B cell serum

(a) 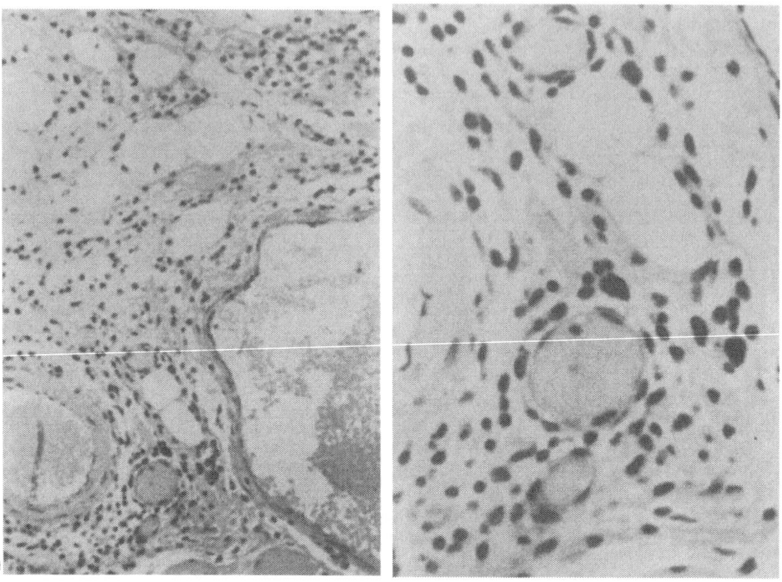 (b)

**Figure 89.5** Delayed type reaction 24 h after challenge in a non-thymectomized rat. (a) × 127 (b) × 315

showed at 4 h a histological appearance with more than 50% polymorphonuclear leukocytes (Figures 89.6 (A) and (B)). At 24 h these reactions were dominated by mononuclear cells but still contained 20–30% polymorphonuclear cells (Figures 89.7 (A) and (B)).

An intermediate type of reaction with characteristics of both DTH and Arthus reaction was called a mixed type reaction. This reaction was already observed at 4 h with a histological picture similar to that in an early Arthus reaction, but persisted and increased for 24 h or more, with a similar histological appearance to that of a late DTH reaction, i.e. a very strong predominance of mononuclear cells.

The reaction in normal non-thymectomized animals showed that low sensitizing doses gave weak and infrequent reactions and no antibody titres after shorter time intervals (3, 5 and 7 days).

Higher sensitizing doses gave earlier and stronger reactions and also higher antibody titres at earlier time intervals. This is seen in Figure 89.8 where the upper part of the diagram represents antibody titres of tested animals compared to titres from a hypersensitized animal. The lower part represent the different types of reactions.

Thymectomized animals receiving low sensitizing doses showed no consistent DTH reactions. DTH reactions were observed in animals receiving high sensitizing doses but constantly weaker than in corresponding normal animals (Figure 89.9).

(a) 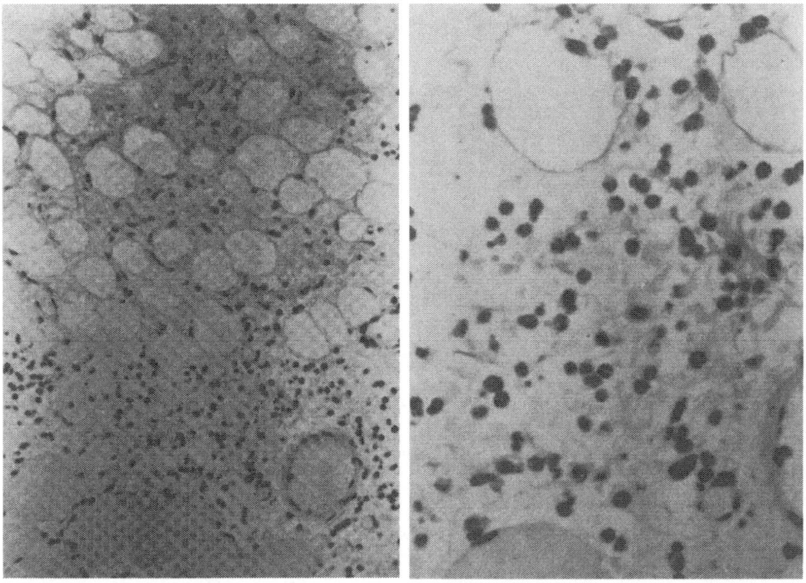 (b)

**Figure 89.6** Arthus reaction 4 h after challenge, dominated by polymorphonuclear leukocytes. (a) × 127 (b) × 315

(a) 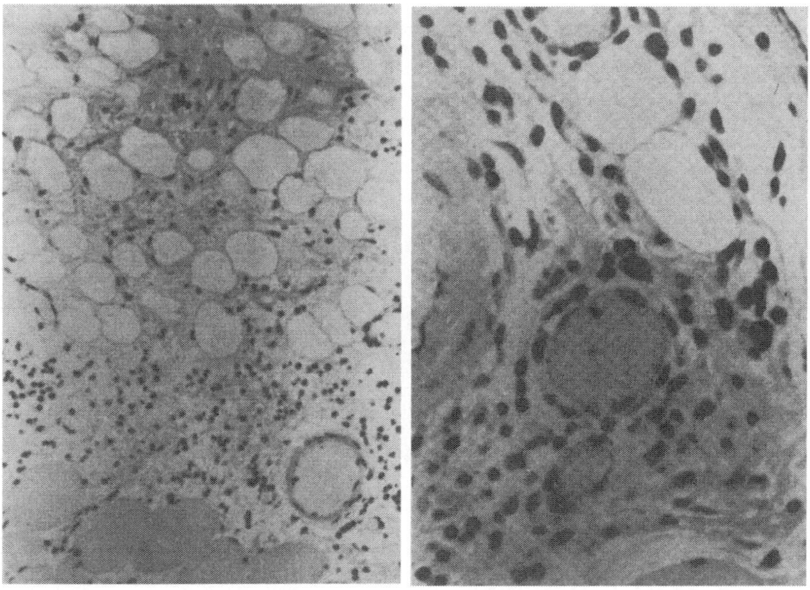 (b)

**Figure 89.7** Arthus reaction 24 h after challenge, dominated by mononuclear leukocytes, but still with about 25% polymorphonuclear cells. (a) × 127 (b) × 315

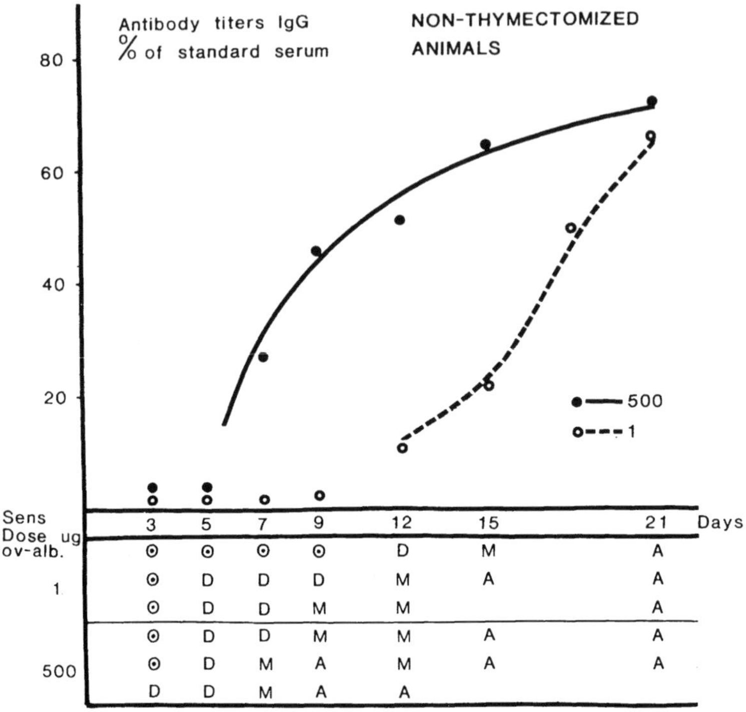


**Figure 89.8** The relationship between serum antibody titres and type of reaction in non thymectomized animals.
Key: ⊙ = no reaction; D = delayed type hypersensitivity; M = mixed reaction; A = Arthus reaction

**Table 89.1**

| *Reaction type* (number of animals) | % *T cells** *of all inflammatory cells* | % *T cells** *of lymphocytes* | % *B cells** *of all inflammatory cells* | % *B cells** *of lymphocytes* | %* *granulocytes* |
|---|---|---|---|---|---|
| DTH | | | | | |
| early, 12–15 h (8) | 14 ( 6–24) | 77 (54–100) | 2 ( 0–6) | 7 ( 0–14) | 21 (10–22) |
| late, 18–24 h (5) | 32 (15–50) | 81 (52–100) | 5 (few–13) | 19 (17–22) | 14 (13–21) |
| Mixed | | | | | |
| early, 12–14 h (8) | 27 (10–58) | 61 (25–100) | 4 ( 0–8) | 11 ( 0–25) | 30 (16–49) |
| late, 18–24 h (4) | 25 (13–50) | 81 (68–100) | 0 | 0 | 23 (10–38) |
| Arthus | | | | | |
| early, 4–8 h (10) | 6 (few–19) | | 1 ( 0–few) | | 56 (16–94) |
| 11–12 h (4) | 6 (few–13) | | 1 ( 0–few) | | 62 (42–78) |
| late, 20–24 h (7) | 7 (few–20) | | 1 ( 0–few) | | 25 (20–29) |

*mean and (range)

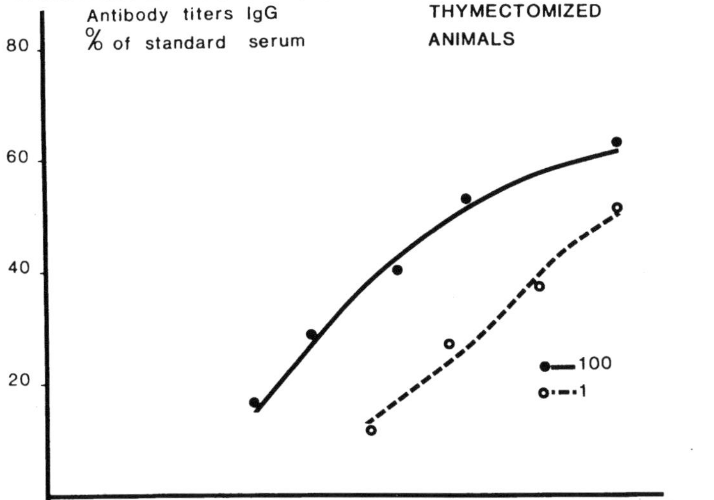


| Sens dose µg ov-alb | 3 | 5 | 7 | 9 | 12 | 15 | 21 Days |
|---|---|---|---|---|---|---|---|
| | ⊙ | ⊙ | ⊙ | M | M | M | A |
| 1 | ⊙ | ⊙ | ⊙ | A | A | M | A |
| | ⊙ | D | M | | A | | |
| | ⊙ | D | M | M | M | A | A |
| 100 | ⊙ | D | M | M | A | A | A |
| | D | D | | M | A | | |

**Figure 89.9** Same as Figure 89.8 but thymectomized animals

The Arthus reactions in thymectomized animals showed the same pattern as in normal animals but constantly weaker (Figure 89.9). The mixed type reaction (described above) was seen, at least at moderate levels of circulating antibodies, in all sensitizing groups (Figures 89.8 and 89.9).

### Immunofluorescence

The results of the determination of T and B lymphocytes are seen in Table 89.1. The majority of, or all of the cells identified as lymphocytes in both the early and late DTH reaction, were T cells (Figure 89.10). None or only few B cells could be seen (Figure 89.11). In the Arthus reaction some T cells were present (Figure 89.12) but very few B cells.

## CONCLUSIONS

In our system with sensitization of rats with ovalbumin as antigen, the essential factor determining the type of the inflammatory reaction is the time lapse between the sensitization and challenge. In both types of reactions an early influx of T lymphocytes is observed, definitely stronger in the DTH reaction than in the Arthus reaction. If these T cells are sensitized cells or not, and which sub-groups of T cells they belong to, has to be analysed further.

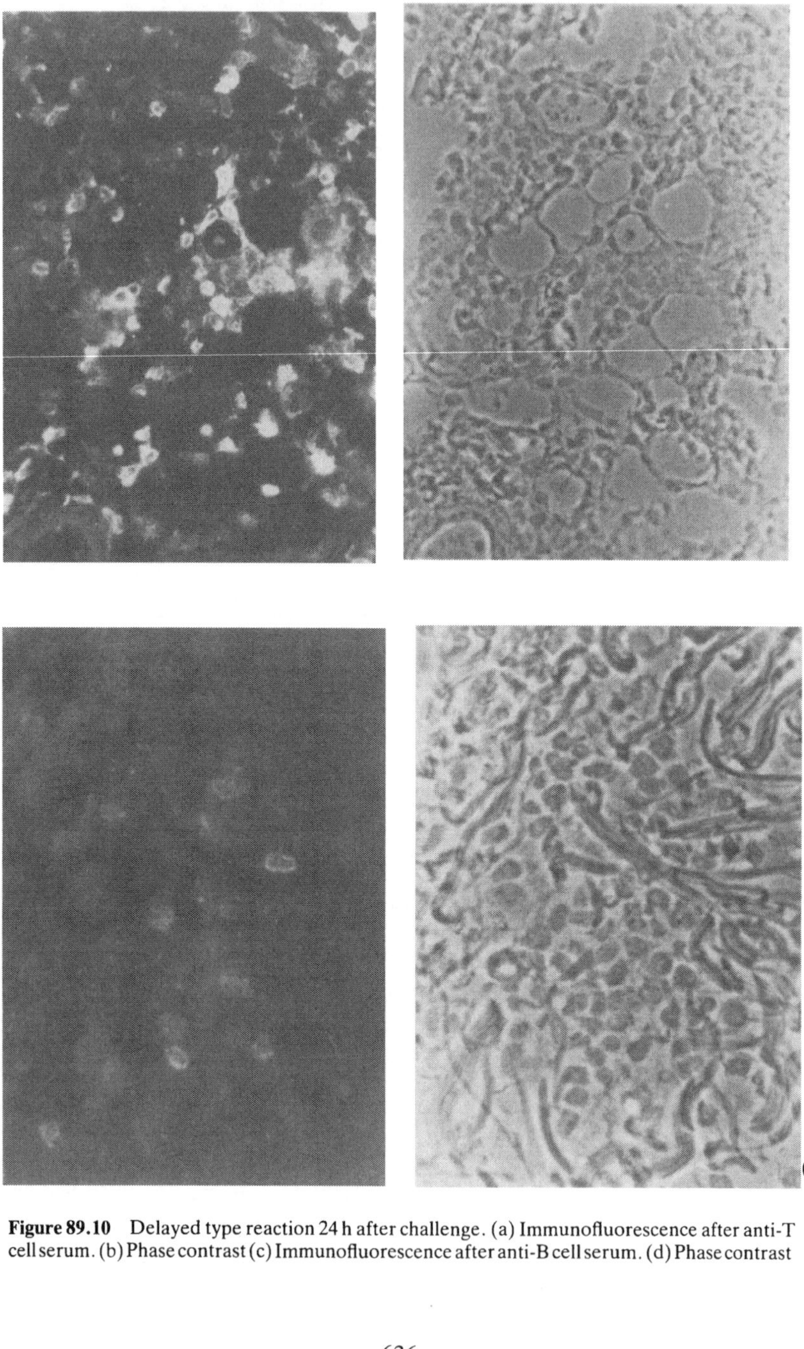

(a) (b) (c) (d)

**Figure 89.10** Delayed type reaction 24 h after challenge. (a) Immunofluorescence after anti-T cell serum. (b) Phase contrast (c) Immunofluorescence after anti-B cell serum. (d) Phase contrast

(a) 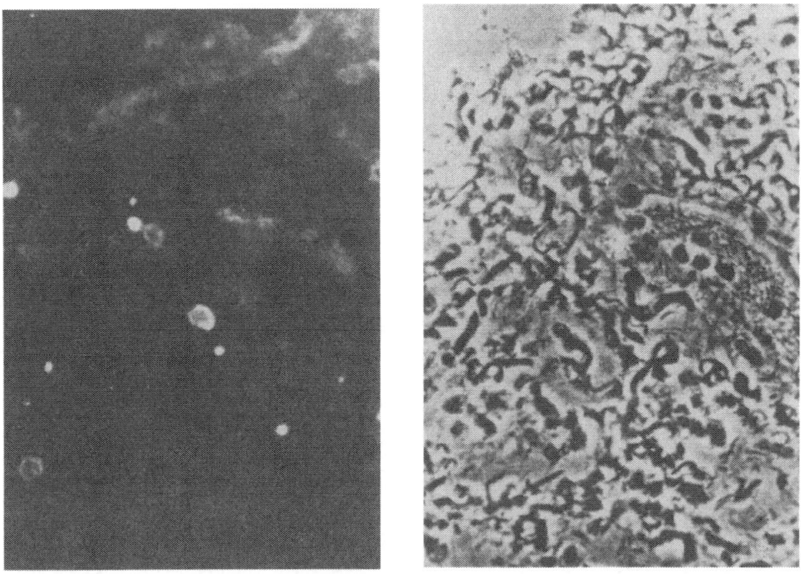 (b)

**Figure 89.11** Arthus reaction 4 h after challenge. (a) Immunofluorescence after anti-T cell serum. (b) Phase contrast

(a) 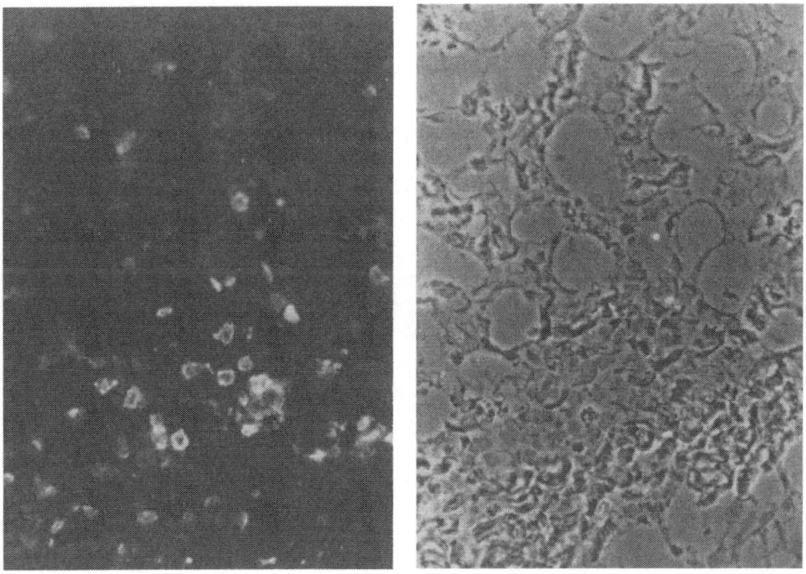 (b)

**Figure 89.12** Mixed-type reaction 12 h after challenge. (a) Immunofluorescence after anti-T cells serum. (b) Phase contrast

# 90

# Regulatory mediators in Arthus reactions: demonstration of chemotactic factor inactivator and cell directed inhibitor activity

G. TILL, M. DEBATIN AND D. GEMSA (WEST GERMANY)

## INTRODUCTION

The study of Arthus reactions has led investigators to a better understanding of the underlying pathogenic mechanism of inflammatory tissue injury evoked by local deposition of complement-activating antigen–antibody complexes. It is well accepted that neutrophils and complement are essential for the mediation of Arthus reactions. In various animal species an Arthus reaction could be inhibited by depletion of the circulating neutrophils with nitrogen mustard[1] or specific antiserum[2]. Depletion of complement with cobra venom factor pretreatment also inhibited Arthus reactions[3]. The accumulation of neutrophils, which is essential for tissue injury, is probably mediated by complement-derived chemotactic factors. In reversed passive Arthus reactions C5 chemotactic factors could be demonstrated in rat dermis[4]. Upon intradermal injection into guinea pigs of complement-derived chemotactic factors, accumulation of intravenously administered $^{51}$Cr-labelled homlogous neutrophils could be observed[5].

Although there is quite a large body of data about the onset of experimental immune complex induced vasculitis and a fairly good conception about the overall sequence of events in an early Arthus reaction, very little is known about endogenous factors and mechanisms that may control the inflammatory leukocyte infiltration. *In vitro*, neutrophil chemotaxis toward complement derived leukotactic activity can be inhibited by two means:(1) by cell directed inhibitors (CDI) such as the neutrophil immobilizing factor released from neutrophils[6] or by an activity present in human serum[7], and (2) by the chemotactic factor inactivator (CFI) present in small amounts in normal serum[8,9]. Recently it has been shown that neutrophil infiltration associated with reversed passive Arthus reaction in the rat could be suppressed by purified human CFI injected locally together with the specific antibody[10]. The authors suggested that CFI has an anti-inflammatory activity. In this communication we present evidence that increased titres of CFI and of CDI activity can be detected in the serum and in skin biopsies of rats with late Arthus reactions.

## MATERIAL AND METHODS

### Reversed passive Arthus reactions

These were induced by an intravenous application of 7 mg bovine serum albumin (BSA), followed immediately by intradermal injections of 0.5 mg of an IgG fraction of rabbit anti-BSA serum at 8 different sites on the back of 200 g male Lewis rats. Typical Arthus reactions were observed macroscopically within 4 h after antibody injection and were fully developed after 8–12 hours. The skin reactions then diminished gradually and disappeared in most cases after 72–96 h. At various time intervals after the rats were narcotized with ether, they were totally bled by heart puncture, and then skin biopsies of the injection sites were taken with a punching tool. Thereafter, the biopsies were sliced with a razor blade, and suspended for approximately 14 h in 5 ml ice-cold Tris-buffered (pH 7.4) Hanks' balanced salt solution (HBSS). Following centrifugation, the supernatants were frozen and stored at −70 °C, as were the serum samples.

### Chemotaxis assay

Lewis rat granulocytes obtained from a 0.1% glycogen-induced 4 h peritoneal exudate were washed, suspended in HBSS at a concentration of $1 \times 10^6$/ml and added to the upper compartment of a modified Boyden chemotaxis chamber. Fresh normal rat serum was incubated for 60 min at 37 °C with yeast or zymosan (50 mg/ml) to activate the complement system and to generate chemotactic activity. The reaction was terminated by an additional 30 min incubation at 56 °C. 50 $\mu$l of the chemotactically active rat serum or equivalent amounts of other test solutions were diluted in HBSS and added to the lower compartment of the chamber. Following incubation in humidified air at 37 °C for 90 min, the microporous (3 $\mu$m) cellulose nitrate filters were removed, stained, cleared with xylene and embedded in Canada balsam.

Chemotaxis of rat peritoneal neutrophils was assayed by the filter technique[11] as modified by Zigmond and Hirsch[12], i.e., the distance between the leading front of migrated neutrophils and the non-migrated cells on top of the filter was measured by light microscopy (×400) and expressed in micrometres. Measured values of triplicate filters differed by no more than 10%.

**Chemotactic factor inactivator (CFI) activity**

This was measured by pre-incubation of 50 μl of rat serum or biopsy extracts with 50 μl of yeast activated normal rat serum for 40 min at 37 °C. The reaction was terminated by heat inactivation (30 min, 56 °C) and the remaining complement derived chemotactic activity evaluated. The presence of CFI activity in the test samples diminished or abolished the chemotactic activity of yeast activated serum. Therefore, the CFI activity was expressed in per cent decrease of the migration distance of the test neutrophils.

**Cell directed inhibitor (CDI) activity**

This was determined by the following procedure: Washed rat peritoneal neutrophils were pre-incubated for 15 min at 37 °C in HBSS containing 10% of biopsy extract or serum from Arthus rats. Following incubation the cells were washed twice in HBSS and their chemotactic responsiveness tested *in vitro*. CDI activity was expressed in percent decrease of migration distance

**Complement activity (CH50)**

The complement activity of rat serum was assayed by the standard haemolysis test of Mayer[13] employing antibody-sensitized sheep erythrocytes.

## RESULTS

Reversed passive Arthus reactions were observed within 4 h of intradermal antibody injection and were fully developed after 8 h. The reactions then diminished and finally disappeared after 72–96 h. Concomitantly with the skin reactions at 4–8 h, the rats developed a granulocytosis as reflected by an increase in number of granulocytes (PMN) from 300 per μl at time 0 to 700 per μl after 4 h. (Figure 90.1). Maximum counts of PMN were observed between 4 and 8 h after onset of the Arthus reaction. After 12 h the PMN counts had dropped to background values and remained unchanged.

Measurements of haemolytic complement activity revealed that the normal CH50 values of 120 had decreased to 80 units during the first 8 h (Figure 90.1), thus indicating activation of serum complement. At the same time, a chemotactic factor (CF) activity, probably complement derived, occurred in the serum with a peak activity at 8 h (Figure 90.1), at which time the migration distance of the test neutrophils was more than 50 μm above serum background values. 4 h later the CF activity was no longer detectable,

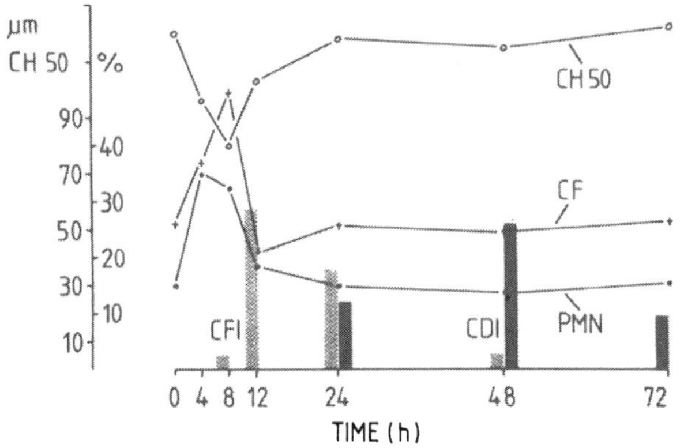


**Figure 90.1** Reversed passive dermal Arthus reaction in rats: time dependent changes in peripheral granulocyte counts (PMN) and in haemolytic complement activity (CH50). Demonstration of various serum activities such as chemotactic activity (CF), chemotactic factor inactivator activity (CFI), and cell directed inhibitor activity (CDI). Shown are representative data obtained from 4 different experiments in which at each given time 3 Lewis rats were used. PMN counts × 10 per µl. For further details see text

**Table 90.1** Chemotactic factor inactivator (CFI) and cell directed inhibitor (CDI) in reversed passive Arthus reactions

| *Time (H) after antibody injection* | *CFI** | | *CDI* | |
|---|---|---|---|---|
| | *serum* | *biopsy* | *serum* | *biopsy* |
| 4 | 0 | 24 | 0 | 0 |
| 8 | 3 | 40 | 0 | 0 |
| 12 | 29 | 50 | 0 | 0 |
| 24 | 18 | 39 | 12 | 20 |
| 48 | 4 | 34 | 26 | 61 |
| 72 | 0 | 28 | 10 | 15 |

* CFI and CDI activity expressed in percent decrease of the migration distance of test neutrophils

probably due to high titres of CFI activity now present in the serum (Figure 90.1, Table 90.1). Whereas CFI activity gradually decreased after having reached a sudden peak at 12 h, increasing amounts of CDI activity appeared in the serum with maximal activity at 48 h (Figure 90.1, Table 90.1).

To examine whether regulatory mediators of neutrophil chemotaxis were also present in Arthus lesions, biopsy extracts were tested for CFI and CDI activity. The results are depicted in Table 90.1 and are shown together with the corresponding serum values. Although the absolute amount of activity in both the serum samples and the biopsy extracts cannot be compared with each other the data clearly show that Arthus lesions contain CFI and CDI activity, and that their peak values at 12 and 48 h, respectively, are reflected in the serum. It should be added that, other than in serum, no CF activity could be detected in the extracts.

## DISCUSSION

For many years the Arthus reaction has been employed to study the pathological effects of antigen–antibody interaction in tissues as well as of inflammation in general. The overall sequence of initiating events in immune complex-induced inflammation is fairly well understood. However, very little attention has been paid to the question regarding how such inflammations could be regulated.

On the basis of experimental data from Johnson *et al.*[10] who showed that reversed passive Arthus reactions in rats could be suppressed by a local application of purified human chemotactic factor inactivator (CFI), we decided to investigate whether rats themselves may provide CFI activity as well as other inhibitors in the course of an immune complex induced inflammation. The results reported here clearly indicate that, after the development of reversed passive Arthus reactions in rats, CFI activity and also cell directed inhibitor activity (CDI) appear in Arthus lesions as well as in the serum.

The origin and nature of this CFI activity in rat serum is not yet known and awaits purification and further characterization, but it seems likely that this activity may be similar to that described in human serum[8,9]. It should be noted that the CFI activity appeared in the serum only after significant amounts of complement-derived chemotactic activity had shown up in the circulation. Because of the observation that infusion of chemotactic factors resulted in an abrupt rise in CFI activity in serum (D. Kreutzer, University of Connecticut, personal communication), we assume that complement-derived chemotactic activity generated in the course of Arthus reactions induces the abrupt rise in CFI activity observed in our experiments. As can be seen (Figure 90.1), CFI activity in turn seems to abolish the circulating chemotactic activity.

Whether the CFI activity in biopsy extracts is identical with that observed in the serum is not known. Brozna *et al.*[14] reported inactivation of complement derived chemotactic factors by lysosomal elastase and cathepsin G. As we could demonstrate high amounts of the same activities in Arthus lesions[15], the possibility exists that the CFI activity in biopsy extracts may be due to the action of elastase or other lysosomal proteases.

As with the CFI activity, the origin and nature of the DI activity in serum and biopsy extracts of late Arthus reactions is also unknown. A cell directed inhibitor of chemotaxis has been demonstrated in the serum of a patient with *Listeria* meningitis, and this inhibitor reversibly impaired the ability of both monocytes and neutrophils to respond to a variety of chemotactic factors[7,16]. Goetzl and Austen[6] described a neutrophil immobilizing factor (NIF) that is contained within the neutrophil and is released during phagocytosis. NIF is heat stable and blocks the motility and chemotactic response of the neutrophil and eosinophil. Whether one of these known inhibitors is identical with the CDI activity of late Arthus reactions remains to be elucidated.

## CONCLUSION

In the Arthus reaction the neutrophil has emerged as a cell of critical importance. Removal of neutrophils from the circulation or suppression of their accumulation in tissue by experimental inactivation of complement-derived chemotactic factors has resulted in complete or nearly complete abrogation of tissue injury.

In the search for endogenous factors that may exert inhibitory effects on the neutrophil accumulation in reversed passive Arthus reactions, we have found that after an initial phase which was characterized by complement activation, granulocytosis, and generation of chemotactic activity, a regulatory phase occurred characterized by the appearance of chemotactic factor inactivator and cell directed inhibitor activity. We believe that these activities may serve as important anti-inflammatory mediators participating in the healing process of acute immune complex induced inflammation.

**Acknowledgment**
The technical assistance of Mrs. H. Braun-Habscheid is gratefully acknowledged.

### References

1 Stetson, C. A. (1951). Similarities in the mechanisms determining the Arthus and the Schwartzman phenomena. *J. Exp. Med.*, **94,** 349
2 Cochrane, C. G., Unanue, E. and Dixon, F. J. (1965). A role of polymorphonuclear leukocytes and complement in nephrotoxic nephritis. *J. Exp. Med.*, **122,** 99
3 Cochrane, C. G., Müller-Eberhard, H. J. and Aikin, B. S. (1970). Depletion of plasma complement in vivo by a protein of cobra venom: its effect on various immunologic reactions. *J. Immunol.*, **105,** 55
4 Ward, P. A. and Hill, J. A. (1972). Biological role of complement products. Complement-derived leukotactic activity extractable from lesions of immunologic vasculitis. *J. Immunol.*, **108,** 1137
5 Jones, D. G., Richardson, D. L. and Kay, A. B. (1977). Neutrophil accumulatioon in vivo following the administration of chemotactic factors. *Br. J. Haematol.* **35,** 19
6 Goetzl, E. J. and Austen, K. F. (1972). A neutrophil immobilizing factor derived from human leukocytes. I. Generation and partial characterization. *J. Exp. Med*, **136,** 1564
7 Maderazo, E. G., Anton, T. F. and Ward, P. A. (1978). Serum associated inhibitor of leukotaxis in humans with cancer. *Clin. Immunol. Immunopathol.*, **9,** 166
8 Berenberg, J. A. and Ward, P. A. (1973). Chemotactic factor inactivator in normal human serum. *J. Clin. Invest.*, **52,** 1200
9 Till, G. and Ward, P. A. (1975). Two distinct chemotactic factor inactivators in human serum. *J. Immunol.*, **114,** 843
10 Johnson, K. J., Anderson, T. P. and Ward, P. A. (1977). Suppression of immune complex-induced inflammation by the chemotactic factor inactivator. *J. Clin. Invest.*, **59,** 951
11 Boyden, S. V. (1962). The chemotactic effect of mixtures of antibody and antigen on poly-

morphonuclear leukocytes. *J. Exp. Med.* **115,** 453
12 Zigmond, S. H. and Hirsch, J. G. (1973). Leukocyte locomotion and chemotaxis. New methods for evaluation and demonstration of a cell-derived chemotactic factor. *J. Exp. Med.*, **137,** 387
13 Mayer, M. M. (1961). Complement and complement fixation. In Kabat and Mayer (eds.) *Experimental Immunochemistry*, pp. 133. (Thoma; Springfield)
14 Brozna, J. P., Senior, R. M. Kreutzer, D. L. and Ward, P. A. (1977). Chemotactic factor inactivators of human granulocytes. *J. Clin. Invest.*, **60,** 1280
15 Debatin, K. M., Gemsa, D. and Till, G. (1980). Regulatory mediators in Arthus reactions. II. Lysosomal enzymes in biopsy and serum. This volume, Chap. 91
16 Maderazo, E. G., Ward, P. A., Woronick, C. L. and Quintiliani, R. (1977). Partial characterization of a cell-directed inhibitor of leukotaxis in human serum. *J. Lab. Clin. Med.*, **89,** 180

# 91

# Regulatory mediators in Arthus reactions: lysosomal enzymes in biopsy and serum

K. M. DEBATIN, D. GEMSA AND G. TILL (WEST GERMANY)

## INTRODUCTION

The accumulation of polymorphonuclear leukocytes (PMN) has been demonstrated as a central pathogenic event in inflammatory lesions like the Arthus reaction[1]. During the last decade, the possible role of these cells in acute inflammatory processes has been studied extensively *in vitro*. As a main focus of these investigations it has become clear that PMN, whenever they encounter immunological stimuli like immune complexes or C5a, release their granule constituents[2,3]. The various hydrolytic enzymes stored within different granules take part in the cellular bactericidal systems as well as in the digestion of ingested material (bacteria, immune complexes). However, they have also been demonstrated to degrade a wide variety of tissue substrates *in vitro* (for review see reference 3). Therefore, the release of proteolytic activities could be an important contribution to the injury which occurs in the inflamed tissue *in vivo*.

An additional aspect of neutral protease function derived from PMN has been elaborated by studies showing that human PMN elastase is not only capable of destroying basement membranes[4], but can also interact with inflammatory mediators of the complement system[5,6], or can even activate mononuclear cells (lymphocytes, monocytes[7,8]).

Furthermore, various activities of PMN granules have been detected which influence the chemotactic responsiveness of PMN[9], and the vasopermeability as well as the blood clotting. By affecting *in vitro* nearly all phenomena involved in acute inflammatory processes, the constituents of PMN granules seem to exert a many faceted function, e.g. the mediation of tissue destruction as well as modulation of the inflammatory process itself (both propagation and inhibition).

We demonstrated chemotactic factor inactivator and cell directed inhibitor activities in biopsies and serum of late Arthus reaction in rats[10]. Both inhibitors are suggested to modulate the influx of inflammatory cells, thus promoting the healing phase of acute inflammatory lesions. Since these activities may, in part, represent a direct or indirect result of the action of neutrophil lysosomal enzymes, we therefore started to study the role of enzymes released *in vivo* by PMN. In a first step, we describe the occurrence of different enzyme activities in biopsies and sera of Arthus reaction-bearing rats.

## MATERIAL AND METHODS

The details of the reverse passive Arthus model used throughout the experiments are described in detail elsewhere[10].

### Preparation of biopsy

After removing the dorsal skin bearing the reactions, the lesions were cut off in a diameter of 1.5 cm and weighed. The lesions were carefully sliced, two biopsies pooled and incubated for 24 h in 4 ml ice-cold Hanks' buffered salt solution. After this time, the extracts were centrifuged and the supernatant was decanted for further investigations. As controls, normal skin from the reaction-bearing rats as well as skin removed from rats injected with antibody alone was prepared in the same way.

### Serum

Blood was obtained by heart puncture just before the rats were sacrificed. After 1 h of clotting, serum was separated by centrifugation.

### Measurement of protein and enzyme activities

The protein content of the biopsy extracts was determined according to the Lowry method using BSA as reference. The Wroblewski[11] method was used for determination of lactate dehydrogenase activity (LDH). Lysozyme was tested according to the method of Gordon[12]. Myeloperoxidase was measured according to the method of Pütter[13] using ABTS as $H^+$ acceptor. β-glucuronidase activity was determined according to Fishmann[14]. Elastase was determined with Suc-$Al_3$-pNA as substrate[15] and cathepsin D activity was determined according to Barrett[16].

## RESULTS

Changes in the weight of biopsies are shown in Figure 91.1. The average weight of single biopsies reached a maximum at 8 h, coincident with the peak of cellular infiltration and oedema, and then rapidly decreased. The protein content in the biopsies was also measured and showed a similar pattern of time dependent changes (Figure 91.2).

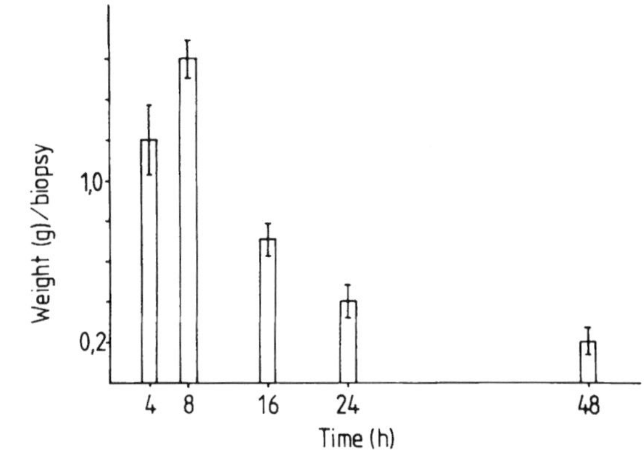


**Figure 91.1** Increase in weight of biopsies × 10 in relation to unaffected skin. Data are given as mean ± SD of three different experiments. The mean values of normal skin were 0.34 ± 0.04 g/biopsy

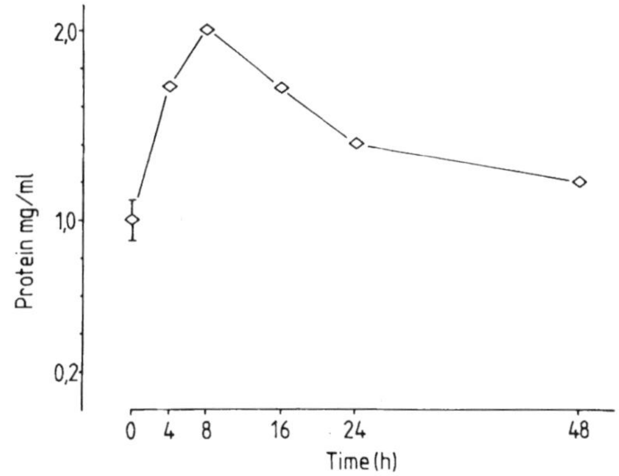


**Figure 91.2** Protein concentration in biopsy extract (2 biopsies in 4 ml medium). Values at time zero represent the mean value ± SD of normal skin. Results were expressed as milligram equivalents of BSA

The activity of LDH, an indicator of serum exudation as well as cell death, was high in unaffected skin, increased slightly with a maximum at 16 h and reached a normal range at 48 h (Figure 91.3). As a parameter of PMN infiltration, lysozyme and myeloperoxidase activities, which were completely absent in normal skin, could be detected in remarkable amounts in the early stages of reactions with a maximum at 8 h (Figure 91.3). While MPO activity decreased rapidly, lysozyme decreased in a continuous but moderate manner. This may reflect different local half-times (diffusion and inactivation) of these enzymes, but it seems more likely to be due to an infiltration with macrophages (as a source of lysozyme) at later stages during the reaction.

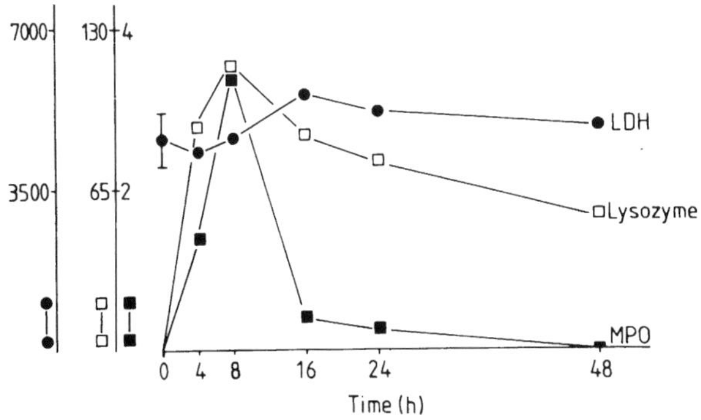


**Figure 91.3** Enzyme activities in biopsy extracts, lactate dehydrogenase (LOH) values at time zero represent mean ± SD of normal skin. Activities: LOH: U/l, MPO (myeloperoxide): U/ml, lysozyme: U/ml

A special interest of these investigations focussed on the occurrence of proteolytic activities in the biopsy extracts. Cathepsin D (acid protease) and elastase (a neutral protease) which are present in PMN granules and are demonstrated to exert potent digestive properties on various tissue substrates, could also be detected in normal skin (Figure 91.4). We expected an increase of activity during the reaction as a consequence of PMN infiltration. However, regarding the time-dependent occurrence of these enzymes we obtained a surprising result (Figure 91.4). Elastase was found with two maxima: an early peak at 4 h followed by nearly normal levels at 8 h and a second maximum at 16 h. The second increase in activity may be caused by immigrating macrophages, since these cells are known to contain and secrete considerable amounts of elastase. Cathepsin D activity decreased during the first hours of the reaction with a minimum at 8 h (Figure 91.4). After this, an increase of activity was observed with a maximum at 24 h.

In contrast to the remarkable kinetics of proteolytic activity found in the biopsy extracts, β-glucuronidase, also present in PMN granules and in normal skin, was elevated during the whole reaction time with a maximum at 16 h (Figure 91.4).

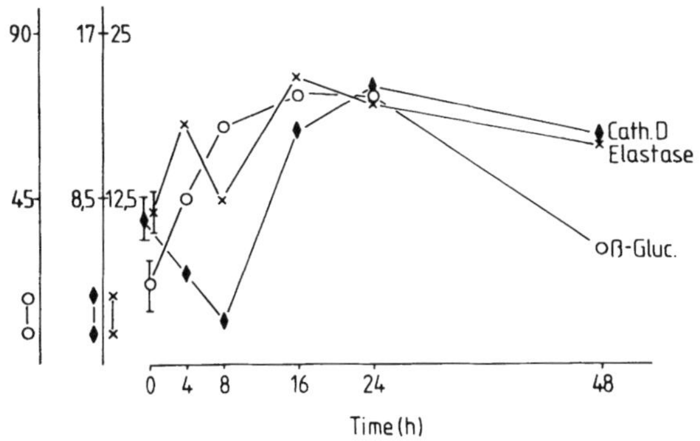


**Figure 91.4** Enzyme activities in biopsy extracts. Data given at time zero represent mean ± SD of normal skin. Activities: cathepsin D: μg-thyrosin/ml. Elastase: units/ml (1 unit produces an OD of 0.010 in 1 h under specific conditions). ß-glucuronidase: sigma U/ml/4h

Besides investigating enzyme activities in biopsy extracts, we also wanted to find out if there was any correlation between serum proteolytic activity (especially elastase) and inhibitors of PMN chemotaxis found in the serum of late Arthus reactions[10]. It could be assumed that enzyme activities which were locally released in the Arthus reactions may enhance the corresponding activities in the serum. However, elastase activity showed a remarkable continuous decrease most pronounced at 24 h. In contrast, serum β-glucuronidase and also lysozyme and myeloperoxidase (data are not shown) remained nearly unchanged during the reaction period under observation (Figure 91.5). We assume from these data that during the reaction time the inhibitory capacity of serum for elastase was increased.

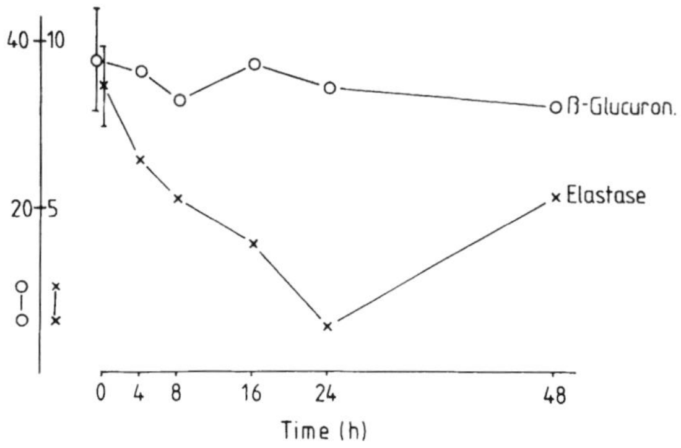


**Figure 91.5** Activities in serum during the reaction period. Data given at time zero represent mean ± SD of the serum activities in five untreated animals. Activities: β-glucuronidase: sigma U/ml/4h. Elastase: units/ml (1 unit produces an OD of 0.010 in 1 h under specific conditions)

## DISCUSSION

The phagocytosis of immune complexes has been demonstrated to cause a considerable release of lysosomal enzymes[17] from PMN *in vitro* including bactericidal activities as well as proteases (elastase). Because of the digestive properties of these enzymes such a release could account for a considerable quantity of the tissue injury observed in situations where immune complexes are deposited and accumulation of PMN occurs *in vivo*. However, a regulatory role for the proteases could also be proposed since many humoral or cellular aspects of acute inflammatory processes are influenced *in vitro* by these activities (see Introduction).

In a first attempt to elucidate the regulatory role of PMN lysosomal enzymes in acute immune complex mediated inflammation we demonstrated the occurrence of different hydrolytic activities in biopsies of Arthus reactions. The enzymes measured were probably released by immigrating inflammatory cells but, in part, were also present in unaffected skin. Although the biopsies were carefully sliced in order to avoid tissue damage, it can not be excluded that some cell destruction caused by the preparation procedure contributes to the activities detected in the extracts.

While lysozyme and MPO activities seem to reflect the well-known kinetics of cellular infiltration in the Arthus lesions, the activities of elastase and cathepsin D were remarkably different and point to two important aspects.[1] The delayed increase in cathepsin D activity and the appearance of the second peak of elastase may be caused by other cells than the early immigrating PMN, and (2) The decrease in biopsies of cathepsin D and elastase activities and of elastase activity in serum during the whole reaction time suggests an interaction of proteases with the inhibitors in tissue and serum. It is well-known that elastase is rapidly bound to the serum inhibitors alpha$_1$-antitrypsin and alpha$_2$-macroglobulin, thus being partly inactivated[18]. Since in our investigations the enzyme activities were measured by functional methods, we could not detect the inactive forms of the enzymes. With respect to the serum elastase activity, even an induction or enhancement of such inhibitory capacity seems to be possible.

Concerning the possible regulatory role of PMN lysosomal enzymes, the balance of the active enzymes and the corresponding inhibitors determines the resulting biological activity. Further investigations on the role of hydrolytic enzymes released by inflammatory cells *in vivo*, especially in relation to the inhibitors of chemotaxis which may limit the inflammatory response, should focus on this important aspect of biological homeostasis.

**Acknowledgement**
The technical assistance of Mrs H. Braun-Habscheid is gratefully acknowledged.

## References


1 Cochrane, C. G. (1968). Immunologic tissue injury mediated by neutrophilic leukocytes. *Adv. Immunol.*, **9,** 97

2 Weissmann, G., Smolen, J. E. and Hoffstein, S. (1978). Polymorphonuclear leukocytes as secretory organs of inflammation. *J. Invest. Dermatol.*, **71,** 95

3 Goldstein, I. M. (1976). Polymorphonuclear leukocyte lysosomes and immune tissue injury. *Prog. Allergy*, **20,** 301

4 Janoff, A. and Zeligs, J. D. (1968). Vascular injury and lysis of basement membrane in vitro by neutral protease of human leukocytes. *Science*, **161,** 702

5 Taylor, J. C., Crawford, I. P. and Hugli, T. E. (1977). Limited degradation of the third component (C3) of human complement by human leukocyte elastase (HLE): Partial characterization of C3 fragments. *Biochemistry*, **16,** 3390

6 Brozna, J. P., Senior R. M., Kreutzer, D. L. and Ward, P. A. (1977). Chemotactic factor inactivators in human granulocytes. *J. Clin. Invest*, **60,** 1280

7 Schmidt, M. E., Douglas, S. D., Quie, P. *et al.* (1978). Effect of neutral granulocyte proteases on human immunocompetent cells: Action of elastase-like protease and chymotrypsin-like protease on mononuclear phagocytes. In Havemann, K. and Janoff, A. (eds.) *Neutral proteases of human polymorphonuclear leukocytes*, p. 298. (Baltimore–Munich: Urban and Schwarzenberg)

8 Vischer, T. L., Bretz, U. and Baggiolini, M. (1976). In vitro stimulation of lymphocytes by neutral proteinases from human polymorphonuclear leukocyte granules. *J. Exp. Med.*, **144,** 863

9 Goetzl, E. J. and Austen, K. F. (1972). A neutrophil immobilizing factor derived from human leukocytes. I. Generation and partial characterization, *J. Exp. Med.*, **136,** 1564

10 Till, G., Debatin, K. M. and Gemsa, D. (1980): Regulatory mediators in Arthus reactions: demonstration of chemotactic factor inactivator and cell directed inhibitor activity. This volume, Chap. 90

11 Wroblewski, F. and La Due, J. S. (1955). Lactic dehydrogenase activity in blood. *Proc. Soc. Exp. Biol. Med.*, **90,** 210

12 Gordon, S., Todd, J. and Cohn, Z. A. (1974). In vitro synthesis and secretion of lysozyme by mononuclear phagocytes. *J. Exp. Med.*, **139,** 1228

13 Pütter, J. (1974). Peroxidasen. In Bergmeyer, H. U. (ed.) *Methoden der enzymatischen Analyse*, p. 725. (Weinheim: Verlag Chemie).

14 Fishman, W. H. (1974). β-glucuronidase. In Bergmeyer, H. U. (ed.) *Methoden der enzymatischen Analyse*, p. 964. (Weinheim: Verlag Chemie)

15 Bieth, J., Spiess, B. and Wermuth, C. G. (1974). The synthesis and analytical use of a highly sensitive and convenient substrate of elastase. *Biochem. Med.*, **11,** 350

16 Barrett, A. J. (1970). Cathepsin D. Purification of isoenzymes from human and chicken liver. *Biochem. J.*, **117,** 601

17 Ohlsson, K. and Olsson, J. (1977). The extracellular release of granulocyte collagenase and elastase during phagocytosis and inflammatory process. *Scand. J. Haematol,* **19,** 145

18 Ohlsson, K. (1978). Interaction of granulocyte neutral proteases with alpha$_1$-antitrypsin, alpha$_2$-macroglobulin and alpha$_1$-antichymotrypsin. In Havemann, K. and Janoff, A. eds. *Neutral proteases of human polymorphonuclear leukocytes,* p. 167. (Baltimore–Munich: Urban & Schwarzenberg)

# 92

# Effect of flurbiprofen on prostaglandin synthesis (Abstract)

V. KASSIS (DENMARK)

The inhibitory effect of topically applied flurbiprofen, a newer non-steroidal anti-inflammatory agent, on prostaglandin biosynthesis in human skin biopsies in primary irritant dermatitis was examined. The flurbiprofen treated areas synthesized significantly less $PGE_1$ (279 pg/mg dry weight) than placebo treated inflamed skin (626 pg/mg dry weight). The average inhibition in 11 treated patients was 55% ($p < 0.01$ using Wilcoxon's signed rank test). Furthermore, when the anti-inflammatory effect of flurbiprofen was clinically evaluated, a poor correlation was found between the reduction of prostaglandin synthesis and the clinical effects of flurbiprofen.

# 93

# Intrapleural injection of asbestos induces early sister chromatid exchanges increase in bone marrow cells (Abstract)

P. FRITSCH, J. P. PONCY, J. BIGNON AND
J. P. GIROUD (FRANCE)

---

Inflammatory processes have been suggested to induce genetic modifications. Measurement of sister chromatid exchanges (SCE) provides a very sensitive and quantitative assay, correlated with mutagenic action of most chemical or physical agents. A measure of SCE of bone marrow cells has been developed in rats. In controls from 3 months to 2 years old SCE is constant, 2.37/cell $\sigma = 0.22$. The kinetic response of SCE after intrapleural injection of 20 mg crocidolite has been studied. Increase of SCE is observed from 3–5 days after the injection with a maximum value of 3.68 $\sigma = 0.11$. Only carcinogenic and not mutagenic effects of asbestos have been established *in vivo*. Moreover this compound does not induce any increase of SCE *in vitro*. During the first few days, translocation of fibres to bone marrow is negligible. Thus bone marrow is not a target organ. From its transient aspect, SCE increase seems correlated with inflammatory reaction induced by intrapleural injection. This assumption is being substantiated. Preliminary results demonstrate a serum factor from treated animals that induces SCE increase in controls.

94

# The effect of an acute inflammatory process on the resistance to infections in mice

M. PELLETIER, M. PARANT, F. PARANT, J. M. JADIN, L. CHEDID AND J. P. GIROUD (FRANCE)

## INTRODUCTION

In 1975 we demonstrated that exudate from acute non-immunological inflammatory reaction could induce DNA synthesis in macrophages in culture[1-3]. Recently we have shown that during various acute inflammatory processes, macrophages are stimulated and become able to inhibit, *in vitro*, tumour cell proliferation[9]. On the other hand, we have shown that acute inflammatory sera are able to modify some cellular functions, in particular:

(1) The induction of both DNA synthesis and mitosis in peritoneal macrophages in culture[8].
(2) The inhibition of polymorphonuclear chemotaxis[11].
(3) The induction of spontaneous DNA synthesis in spleen cells and the modulating response of these cells to PHA[7].

In the present work we have investigated whether the development of a non-immunological acute inflammatory reaction is able to modify resistance of mice against bacteria, *Klebsiella pneumoniae,* and against parasites, *Trypanosoma cruzi.*

## MATERIALS AND METHODS

### Animals

C 57BL/6 × AKR mice were obtained from the Centre d'élevage du CNRS,

Orléans, France and Sprague–Dawley rats (180–200 g) pathogen-free were obtained from Elevage Depré, St Doulchard, France.

### Inflammatory reaction

An inflammatory reaction was obtained in mice and rats by injection of 1 ml 1% calcium pyrophosphate suspension in a pyrogen free NaCl 0.15 mol/l.

### Inflammatory sera

Blood was taken from the rats 2 h after the start of inflammation. After centrifugation at 4 °C sera were collected and sterilized by filtering through a millipore filter (pore size 0.45 μm). Control sera from normal rats were prepared using the same technique.

### Infections

*Klebsiella pneumoniae* were obtained from Institut Pasteur collection (number 7823). Infection was induced by intravenous injection of $2 \times 10^3$ *K. pneumoniae* in suspension in a pyrogen free NaCl 0.15 mol/l 1–8 days after the start of inflammation or 24 h after intravenous injection of serum harvested from rats presenting an acute inflammatory reaction.

*Trypanosoma cruzi* were isolated in Argentina by P. Kierszenbaum and have been maintained by serial syringe passages of infected blood in NMRI mice since 1975. Infection was induced by intraperitoneal injection of $1 \times 10^3$ *T. cruzi* 1–3 days after the beginning of inflammatory reaction.

## RESULTS

Results were expressed as percentage of mortality during 10 days for *K. pneumoniae* and 30 days for *T. cruzi.* After these times all mice survived.

### Influence of an acute inflammatory reaction on resistance of mice against *K. pneumoniae*

Inflammatory reaction was induced 1–8 days before infection. Results reported in Figure 94.1 show that in all cases the mortality of mice was decreased. When inflammatory reaction was induced 8 day or 1 day before infection, the mortality of mice was decreased by 18% and 28%, respectively. When inflammatory reaction was induced 3 or 2 days before infection, the mortality of mice was decreased by 50% and 77%, respectively. Similarly, when inflammatory reaction was induced 2 or 3 days before infection, there was a delay in the mortality of unprotected mice.

### Influence of serum harvested from rats presenting an acute inflammatory reaction on resistance of mice against *K. pneumoniae*

24 h before infection, mice received intravenously 0.5 ml of normal serum or

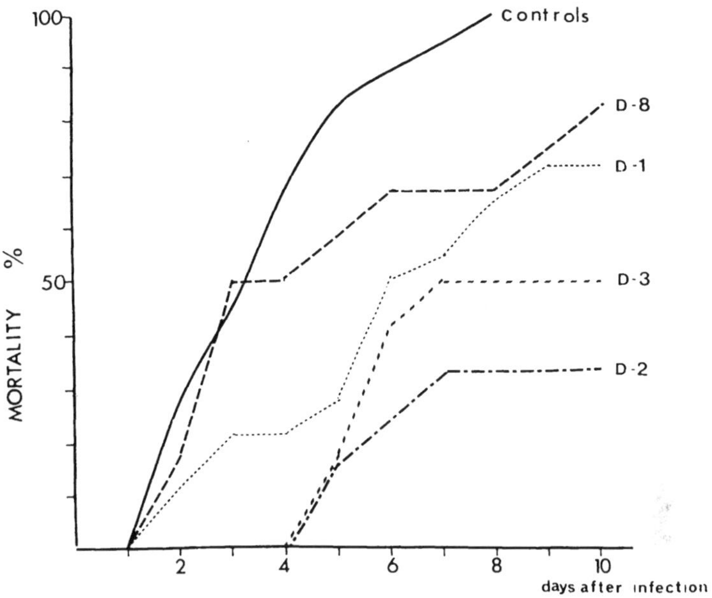


**Figure 94.1** Effect of an inflammatory process on mortality of mice infected with *Klebsiella pneumoniae*

serum obtained from rats 2 h after the beginning of inflammatory reaction. In Figure 94.2 it can be seen that, except for a slight delay in mortality of mice, the control serum of normal rats had practically no effect on mice mortality. After treatment of mice with the serum of inflamed rats, the mortality of mice decreased by 85%. Similarly it was established that there was an important delay in the mortality of unprotected mice.

**Influence of an acute inflammatory reaction on resistance of mice against *T. cruzi***

An inflammatory reaction was induced 1–3 days before infection. Results reported in Figure 94.3 show that when inflammation was induced 2 or 3 days before infection there was a marked decrease of the mortality of mice against *T. cruzi,* 52% and 60% respectively. In contrast, when inflammation was induced 1 day before infection the mortality of inflamed mice was identical to the mortality of normal mice, but it occurred more rapidly in inflamed mice.

## DISCUSSION

Many years ago Metchnikoff[10] reported that inflammatory reaction can

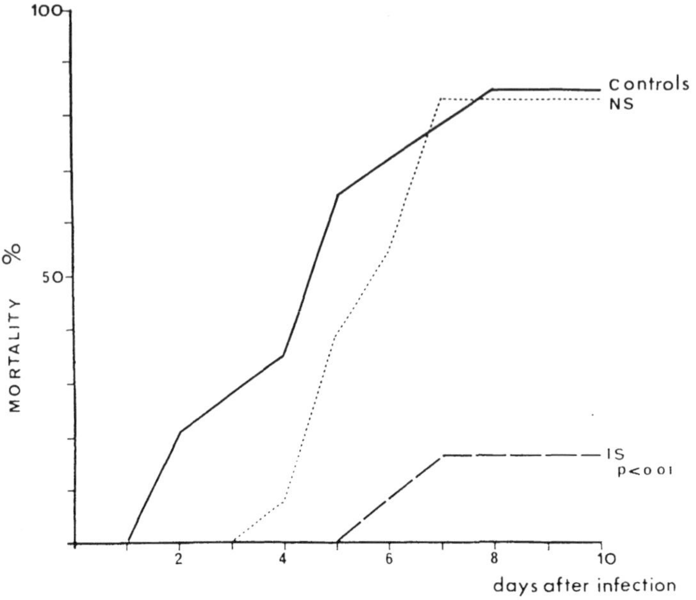


**Figure 94.2** Effect of an intravenous injection of inflammatory serum on mortality of mice infected with *Klebsiella pneumoniae*

stimulate resistance against infectious agents. In 1975 Fauve *et al.*[4] showed that chronic inflammation can increase the infection resistance of mice against *Salmonella typhimurium* or *Listeria monocytogenes*. More recently these authors have extracted from inflammatory granuloma a factor able to protect mice against *L. monocytogenes*[5,6].

In this work we have shown that an acute inflammatory reaction induced by intrapleural injection of calcium pyrophosphate 2 or 3 days before infection was able to enhance the resistance of mice against bacteria (*K. pneumoniae*) or parasites (*T. cruzi*). In the case of *K. pneumoniae* the protective effect can be transferred to normal mice by injection of serum obtained from animals presenting an acute non-immunological inflammation as early as 2 h after the beginning of inflammatory reaction.

These results suggest that a factor released in the serum during the inflammatory process was implicated in this protective effect. This factor was not specific of one type of irritant since the resistance of mice against *K. pneumoniae* was enhanced when inflammatory reaction was induced by intrapleural injection of Dextran (40 000 daltons) (unpublished data). It was also not specific of one type of bacteria since the resistance of mice against *L. monocytogenes* was enhanced by an acute inflammatory reaction (unpublished data). Furthermore, it was species non-specific, since injection of serum obtained

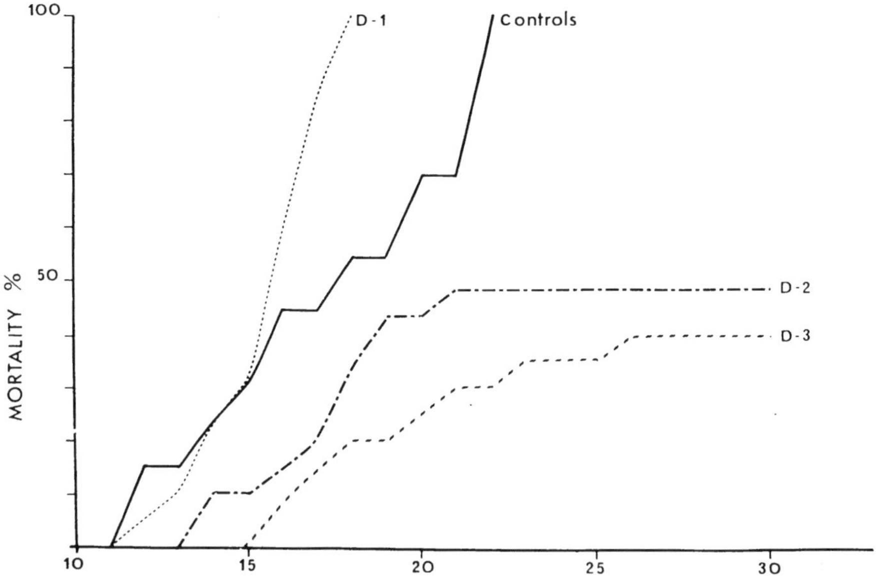


**Figure 94.3** Effect of an inflammatory process on mortality of mice infected with *Trypanosoma cruzi*

from rats undergoing an acute inflammatory reaction enhanced mouse resistance to infection.

This (or these) factor(s) released during acute non-immunological inflammatory reaction, which we have named Phlogokine(s), could be the counterpart of mediators released during delayed type hypersensitivity reaction, namely, lymphokines.

Purification of this (or these) factor(s) is in progress. In previous study we have shown that during various acute inflammatory processes, macrophages were stimulated and were able to inhibit, *in vitro*, tumour cell proliferation[9]. The marked degree of resistance against *K. pneumoniae* or *T. cruzi* acquired by mice during an inflammatory reaction could be also related to stimulation of macrophages.

**Acknowledgements**
This work was supported by a grant from INSERM number 78.1.182.2 and by a grant from DRET number 77/507. The technical assistance of Agnès Deslandres and Olivier Muntaner is gratefully acknowledged.

**References**

1 Adolphe, M., Fontagne, J., Pelletier, M. and Giroud, J. P. (1975) Induction of DNA synthesis in rat macrophages *in vitro* by inflammatory exudate. *Nature (London)*, **253,** 637
2 Adolphe, M., Fontagne, J., Pelletier, M. Giroud, J. P., Timsit, J. and Lechat, P. (1976).

Induction of DNA synthesis in rat peritoneal macrophages in culture by a pleural inflammatory exudate. *Agents Actions*, **6,** 114

3 Adolphe, M., Fontagne, J. Pelletier, M., Blondelon, D., Lechat, P and Giroud, J. P. (1977). Perspectives in Inflammation, Future Trends and Developments. In Willoughby, D. A., Giroud, J. P. and Velo, G. P. (eds.) *Proceedings of the Third International Meeting on Future Trends in Inflammation*, p. 469. (Lancaster: MTP Press)

4 Fauve, R. M. and Hevin, B. (1975). Influence d'une réaction inflammatoire sur la résistance de souris à l'infection par Listeria monocytogenes et Salmonella typhimurium. *C. R. Acad. Sci., Ser. D.*, **281,** 2037

5 Fauve, R. (1977). Inflammation and host resistance to pathogens. *Intensive Care Med.*, **3,** 237

6 Fauve, R. M. (1978). Inflammation and host resistance against pathogens in the Pharmacology of Immunoregulation. In Werner, Gitt and Floc'h, F. (eds.) *Proceedings of a Rhône-Poulenc Round Table Conference*, p. 319. (Academic Press)

7 Florentin, I., Pelletier, M. and Giroud, J. P. (1978). Lymphocyte proliferation induced *in vitro* by an acute non specific inflammatory exudate. Modulation of the response to phytohemagglutinin (PHA). *Eur. J. Rheumatol. Inflam.*, **1,** 316

8 Giroud, J. P., Pelletier, M. and Girre, C. (1977). Pouvoir mitogène de sérums de rats porteurs d'une inflammation aiguë vis-à-vis de macrophages en culture. *C. R. Acad. Sci.*, **285,** 1143

9 Kiger, N., Pelletier, M., Florentin, I., Mathe, G. and Giroud, J. P. (1978). Effect of a nonspecific acute inflammatory stimulus on macrophage activation and antibody - dependent - cellular - cytotoxicity. *Eur. J. Rheumatol. Inflam.*, **1,** 321

10 Metchnikoff, E. (1905). *L'immunité dans les maladies infectieuses.* Masson et Cie, p. 315–340

11 Giroud, J. P., Roch-Arveiller, M. and Bradshaw, D. (1978). Modification du chimiotactisme des polynucléaires de Rat au cours d'une réaction inflammatoire aiguë. *C. R. Acad. Sci.*, **286,** 721

# 95

# Interaction of inflammatory stimuli: diminished inflammatory response induced by cell accumulation at a distant site (Abstract)

W. LU AND D. M. WILLIAMS (UK)

A partial refractory period in polymorphonoculear leukocyte (PMN) emigration during inflammation was demonstrated through sequential stimulation of the rat peritoneal cavity (Lu, W., Scragg, M. A. and Williams, D. M. (1978). *Br J. Exp. Pathol.* **59,** 609): PMN accumulation in response to intraperitoneal injection (IP) of Brain–Heart infusion and proteose peptone (BHI/PP) was depressed by IP glycogen in saline (G) 4 h previously. This reduction may be due to (1) a change in the local endothelium rendering it refractory to a second stimulus; (2) reduced PMN availability in circulating blood; (3) mediators produced in the lesion leading to a local or central inhibition of PMN release or; (4) changes in PMN functional abilities such as adhesion to endothelial wall and chemotaxis.

To establish whether local inhibition of emigration or a centrally-acting mechanism is responsible for the diminished response, three groups each of 4 young adult male Sprague–Dawley rats received intrapleural injection (IPL) of 1 ml G followed 4 h later by IP BHI/PP. 2, 4 and 8 h after the IP injection, the total PMNs in both the pleural and peritoneal cavities were determined. Circulating PMNs were also monitored using tail vein blood.

The injection of G IPL significantly suppressed the accumulation of peritoneal PMNs in response to IP BHI/PP 4 and 8 h later ($p < 0.005$). Hence a systemic or central factor is important. This is further supported by the trend towards a reduction in the intrapleural PMN response 2 hours after IP BHI/PP (6 h after G IPL). Circulating blood PMN changes show the same trend as those in exudates; nevertheless, there are enough circulating PMNs at any time to mount a full response to G or BHI/PP, given alone or in combination. Hence the availability of PMNs in terms of number alone does not account fully for the reduction.

# 96

# Anti-inflammation in spontaneously arising animal cancers

S. NORMANN (USA) M. SCHARDT AND
E. SORKIN (SWITZERLAND)

## INTRODUCTION

Animals bearing transplanted cancers have defective monocyte accumulation both in the primary tumour and at distant sites [1-5]. Activated macrophages possess anti-tumour effector activity[6-9]. Consequently, an anti-inflammatory effect which alters the ratio of macrophages to tumour cells may interfere with host resistance and contribute to progressive cancer growth.

However, transplanted tumours may not be analogous to those arising spontaneously. For instance, transplanted tumours frequently produce a blood leukocytosis[2,10] that is not generally observed with spontaneously arising cancers of either animals or man. Transplanted tumours grow rapidly often with short or non-existent latency periods whereas spontaneous tumours arise from only a few cells and may exist for several months or years before clinical appearance. Furthermore, transplanted murine tumours are frequently infected with lactic dehydrogenase viruses that may lead to a wrong interpretation of valid results[11,12].

Accordingly, we have been investigating models of spontaneous animal neoplasms on the assumption that they more closely resemble human cancer than transplanted tumour models. In these studies, we have addressed two questions: (1) Does anti-inflammation directed against macrophages exist in spontaneously arising tumours and (2) if so, what is the relationship of the anti-inflammatory effect to tumour appearance.

Studies with spontaneous tumours have been facilitated by our ability to measure macrophage inflammatory responsiveness repetitively in the same animal[13]. Our test consists of the subcutaneous placement of a 13 mm diameter nitrocellulose filter of pore size less than 0.45 μm. After a suitable time interval (18 h for rats, 48–96 h for mice), the filters are removed, stained and the number of macrophages counted in 10 predetermined oil immersion fields. Although PMNs may appear on the filters, the predominating cell is the macrophage as judged by morphology and confirmed by non-specific esterase staining. Lymphocytes are rarely encountered. Since as many as 6 filters can be implanted into mice (12 for rats), the test permits sequential assessment of macrophage inflammatory responses before and during tumour appearance and growth.

## SPONTANEOUSLY INDUCED VIRAL TUMOURS

### Model 1: histiocytic lymphoma in SJL/J mice

Approximately 80% of SJL/J mice develop a spontaneous malignant lymphoma, histiocytic type (reticulum cell sarcoma) between 8 and 14 months of age. Mice were obtained at 2 months of age and maintained to up to 18 months of age. When sacrificed all mice were examined for lymph node enlargement, including inspection of inguinal, para-aortic, mesenteric, mediastinal, axillary and submaxillary nodes. Grossly enlarged nodes were dissected free and weighed collectively. Histologic sections were prepared from lymph nodes, liver, spleen, lung and kidney.

Apparently healthy SJL/J mice who were tumour free by histology had no evidence of deficient inflammatory responses either at 3 months or 1 year of age which might have predisposed them to develop malignancy. However, the macrophage inflammatory response of mice with tumours was depressed significantly over the control non-tumour bearing mice (Table 96.1). Tumour bearing animals were divided arbitrarily into two groups based on aggregated lymph node weights less than or greater than 1.5 g. All animals with large tumours had metastatic dissemination either to liver (90%), lung (73%) or kidney (75%). Animals with lymph nodes less than 1.5 g had infrequent metastatic dissemination. This partition enabled us to compare data obtained from animals of the same age but different sized tumours. An inflammatory effect was present in mice with very small tumours. The depression was similar whether these small tumours arose in young or aged mice.

We also examined the development of the anti-inflammatory effect in individual animals by sequential filter insertion. At the time of initial testing, some animals already had decreased inflammatory responses and of these several succumbed to their tumour within 2 months. Tumour palpation often failed to detect small tumours or even large ones if the tumour was disseminated in multiple lymph nodes. However, most mice progressively developed a more severe defect in macrophage inflammation over the 4 month period of

**Table 96.1** Depression of macrophage inflammatory response by spontaneously arising histiocytic lymphomas in SJL/J mice*

| *Condition* | *Age* (months) | *Mean weight lymph nodes* (g) | *Macrophages per oil immersion field* | *Degree of inhibition* |
|---|---|---|---|---|
| Non-tumour bearing † | 14–18 | 0.06±.01 | 168±10 | |
| Tumour bearing | 8–14 | 0.52±.13 | 106±11 | 37% |
| | 8–14 | 4.20±.42 | 97±7 | 42% |
| | 18 | 0.31±.10 | 86±9 | 49% |

* Data are reported as mean ± 1 standard error on 7 or more mice per group. Filters were removed after 96 h.

† These mice were from the same lot as those developing tumours and were tested concurrently. Tumour existence was determined by histology.

observation. In some animals the anti-inflammatory effect developed abruptly, whereas in others it occurred slowly and progressively.

From this study it was concluded that spontaneously arising malignant lymphomas in SJL/J mice do impair macrophage inflammatory reactions. However, the relationship between the inflammatory defect and the onset of spontaneously arising cancer remains unknown. The tumours arose internally and were often difficult to detect early. In addition, the tumour was usually multifocal, being present in spleen as well as in numerous lymph nodes.

**Model 2: acute lymphocytic leukaemia (ALL) in AKR mice**

The AKR mouse carries viral information necessary for leukaemia development at two different sites on its genome. Both sites appear to produce viruses (designated Akv viruses) which are indistinguishable[14] but the presence of the virus in blood or tissue is not sufficient to produce disease. Young mice produce large amounts of virus but do not develop leukaemia until after at least 5 months of age[15]. The leukaemia appears to be produced when a hybrid virus is formed by genetic recombination between the Akv virus and another endogenous virus[16]. Pathological changes first appear in the thymus[17], and neonatal thymectomy, but not splenectomy, markedly reduces tumour incidence[18]. Following lymphoma development in the thymus, the disease spreads to the spleen and mesenteric lymph nodes associated with appearance of abnormal lymphocytes in the peripheral blood (leukaemic phase). ALL develops in about 80% of AKR mice between the ages of 6 and 12 months. The leukaemic phase is conveniently monitored by the peripheral white blood cell (WBC) count.

Young 3-month-old mice without evidence of leukaemia were compared to age matched C57B1/6 mice as representative of animals who rarely develop tumours. As observed in Table 96.2, there was no significant difference between these two groups of mice. Thus, young AKR mice had normal macrophage responses despite the fact that they carried the endogenous Akv virus.

**Table 96.2** Depression of macrophage inflammatory responses by spontaneously arising lymphocytic leukaemia in AKR mice

| *Mouse strain* | Age (months) | *Condition* | *Macrophages per oil immersion field** | *Degree of inhibition†* |
|---|---|---|---|---|
| C57B1/6 | 3 | control | 116±7 | |
| AKR | 3 | non-leukaemic | 99±7 | NS |
| C57B1/6 | 6 | control | 128±8 | |
| AKR | 6–8 | non-leukaemic | 109±5 | NS |
| | 6–8 | leukaemic | 37±4 | 66% |

* Data are reported as mean ± 1 standard error on 7 or more mice per group. Data are for filters removed after 48 h.

† The % inhibition was calculated to compare age matched leukaemic and non-leukaemic AKR mice. NS means not significantly different from control C57B1/6 mice.

With appearance of leukaemia, however, abnormal responses were observed (Table 96.2). Macrophage responses in leukaemic mice were depressed by 66% when compared to AKR mice who had no elevation in peripheral WBC counts. Non-leukaemic mice had macrophage responses which were not significantly different from age matched control C57B1/6 mice. Thus leukaemia, rather than Akv leukaemia viruses, was associated with the depressed macrophage accumulation at inflammatory foci in the subcutaneous tissues.

By implanting filters sequentially, we measured the alteration in macrophage responses during development of leukaemia. The results of two such longitudinal studies are presented in Figure 96.1. They are representative of the observation that alterations in macrophage responses generally occurred either concurrently with, or immediately following, the onset of leukaemia. While abnormal macrophage patterns were observed in most mice with leukaemia, some mice had leukaemic episodes without concomitant depression in macrophage responses.

## EFFECT OF THE CHEMICAL CARCINOGEN 3-METHYLCHOLANTHRENE (3-MCA)

Among the well known potent chemical carcinogens is 3-MCA, a polycyclic aromatic hydrocarbon. This agent is considered a procarcinogen requiring metabolic conversion to form the actual carcinogen. While this agent is known to interfere with immunologic reactions[19], its effect on macrophages has not been thoroughly investigated. We have undertaken to study the effects of this chemical on macrophage mobilization in inbred DA strain rats.

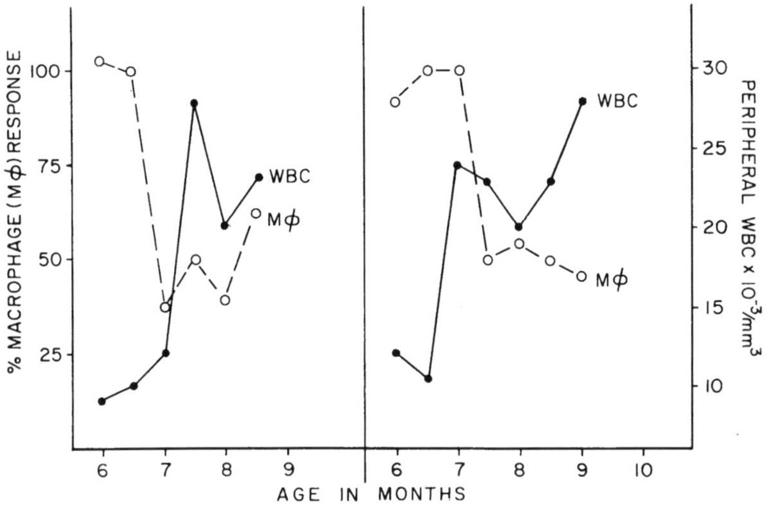


**Figure 96.1** Sequential evaluation of macrophage inflammatory responses in individual AKR mice during development of leukaemia

Paraffin pellets were impregnated with 3-MCA as described by Bartlett[20]. The carcinogen containing pellets were implanted subcutaneously into the thigh. Simultaneously, a second group of rats received control pellets consisting of paraffin but no carcinogen. Inflammation was evaluated at 5, 30 and 48 days after pellet implantation by filters inserted at remote sites on the upper back and chest. A macrophage response was considered abnormal if it was less than 2 standard deviations from the mean of age matched DA rats who had received neither carcinogen nor pellet implantation. The results are summarized in Table 96.3.

The presence of a paraffin pellet without carcinogen produced a low incidence of abnormal responses of less than 5% (1 out of 21 rats examined). In contrast, paraffin pellets containing carcinogen produced abnormal responses of 11% (5/45) on day 5 which increased to 23% on days 30 and 48. The latency period for tumour appearance is at least 6 months in DA rats with this dose of carcinogen. While it was concluded that 3-MCA does depress macrophage inflammatory responses, it is not clear for how long these abnormal responses will persist, although it is in excess of 90 days. Further, the correlation, if any, between abnormal macrophage responses and tumour incidence or latency interval is not yet resolved.

## CONCLUSIONS

Pike and Snyderman[21] and Hibbs *et al.*[22] have suggested that the macrophage is an anti-neoplastic surveillance cell whose function is subverted by factors

**Table 96.3** Depression or macrophage inflammatory responses by the chemical carcinogen 3-methylcholanthrene (3-MCA)*

| *Treatment* | *Ratio of abnormal responses to survivors* day 5 | day 30 | day 48 |
|---|---|---|---|
| Paraffin control | 1/23 4% | 1/21 5% | 0/20 0% |
| Paraffin containing 3-MCA (0.1%) | 5/45 11% | 10/43 23% | 9/40 23% |

* The carcinogen was administered by implanting paraffin pellets containg 3-MCA into the thigh musculature of inbred DA strain rats. Controls consisted of paraffin pellets without carcinogen. Inflammatory responses were determined at remote sites on the back and chest using subcutaneously placed nitrocellulose filters. Abnormal responses were defined as macrophage accumulation less than 2 standard deviations from the mean of age matched DA rats which received neither carcinogen nor paraffin.

elaborated by emerging tumours. In support of this hypothesis, macrophages are widely distributed in tissues and can be activated to kill tumour cells by a non-immunologic means under conditions wherein normal cells are spared[7,9]. Furthermore, abnormalities in macrophage inflammation leading to reduced accumulation of these cells within transplanted tumours have been reported[4]. Our most recent studies have extended these observations to spontaneous animal tumour models. In both spontaneously arising histiocytic lymphomas in SJL/J mice and acute lymphocytic leukaemia in AKR mice, the presence of the tumour depressed macrophage accumulation at inflammatory foci.

However, the critical question is whether these macrophage abnormalities are associated with tumour emergence or arise as a consequence of tumour bearing. The defect in SJL/J mice did appear early when the lymph nodes were only slightly enlarged, but such nodes may contain upwards of $10^8$ cells[23]. Unfortunately, it was not possible to quantitate the actual number of malignant cells in suspensions prepared from such nodes or on cytocentrifuge prepared slides. Leukaemic elevations in peripheral WBC counts did correlate with abnormal macrophage responses. However, this was not always seen, particularly during short cycles of leukaemia and remission. It may be significant that 3-MCA induces abnormalities prior to tumour development. Interpretation of this observation as support for the hypothesis that tumour related anti-inflammation ablates macrophage surveillance would be greatly enhanced if our additional studies demonstrate that the defects correlate with tumour emergence.

Recent studies have established that the anti-inflammatory effect is dependent upon tumour presence. The defect is rapidly corrected by surgical excision but reappears with metastasis[24]. This observation is consistent with the notion that Akv viral infection alone is not sufficient to depress macrophage responses but that the defects are associated with actual tumour presence. This conclusion is particularly interesting in light of studies showing that murine lactic dehydrogenase viral infection depresses peritoneal macrophage chemotaxis[25] and that a soluble, low molecular weight anti-inflammatory factor can be extracted from some but not all murine leukaemia viruses. However, actual infection of monocytes with viruses seems an unlikely cause of the abnormal inflammatory responses since monocytes from tumour bearing animals behave normally in non-tumour bearing recipients[27]. Nonetheless, a low molecular weight factor of viral or other origin remains a possible tumour related, anti-inflammatory mediator. Such a factor can be obtained from homogenates of whole tumours[28], peritoneal ascites fluids[29] and supernates of cultured tumour cells[30]. It is curious that such factors inhibit monocyte but not PMN chemotaxis *in vitro*[28] and show a similar cell selective inhibition of inflammatory responses *in vivo*[2,30].

## ACKNOWLEDGMENTS

This work was supported by grants from the National Cancer Institute, CA 22517 (USA) and from the Swiss National Science Foundation 3.213.77. We are grateful to Mr. Bosco Koncar for his excellent technical assistance.

### References

1 Bernstein, I. D., Zbar, B. and Rapp, H. J. (1972). Impaired inflammatory response in tumor-bearing Guinea Pigs. *J. Natl. Cancer Inst.* **49,** 1641

2 Normann, S. J. and Sorkin, E. (1976). Cell-specific defect in monocyte function during tumor growth. *J. Natl Cancer Inst.*, **57,** 135

3 Normann, S. J. and Schardt, M. (1978). A cancer related macrophage dysfunction in inflamed tissues. *J. Reticuloendothelial Soc.*, **24,** 147

4 Normann, S. J. and Cornelius, J. (1978). Concurrent depression of tumor macrophage infiltration and systemic inflammation by progressive cancer growth. *Cancer Res.*, **38,** 3453

5 Snyderman, R., Pike, M. C., Blaylock, B. L. *et al.* (1976). Effects of neoplasms on inflammation: depression of macrophage accumulation after tumor implantation. *J. Immunol.*, **116,**585

6 Stewart, C. C., Adles, C. and Hibbs, J. (1978). Cloned macrophages can be induced to kill tumor cells. *J. Reticuloendothelial Soc.*, **24,**107

7 Hibbs, J. B. Jr. (1976). Role of activated macrophages in nonspecific resistance to neoplasia. *J. Reticuloendothelial Soc.*, **20,** 223

8 Hibbs, J. B. Jr., Taintor, R. R., Chapman, H. A. *et al.* (1977). Macrophage tumor killing: influence of the local environment. *Science*, **197,**

9 Hibbs, J. B. Jr. (1976). The macrophage as a tumoricidal effector cell: A review of *in vivo* and *in vitro* studies on the mechanism of the activated macrophage non-specific cytotoxic reaction. In Fink, Mary A. (ed.) *The Macrophage in Neoplasia*, p. 83. (New York: Academic Press)

10 Eccles, S. A., Bandlow, G. and Alexander, P. (1976). Monocytosis associated with the growth of transplanted syngeneic rat sarcomata differing in immunogenicity. *Br. J. Cancer*, **34,** 20

11 Riley, V. (1968). Lactate dehydrogenase in the normal and malignant state in mice and the influence of a benign enzyme-elevating virus. In Bush, H. (ed.) *Methods in Cancer Research*, Vol. 4, pp.493–618. (New York: Academic Press)

12 Ryan, W. L. (1974). Erronous interpretation of valid experimental observations through interference by the LDH Virus. *J. Natl. Cancer Inst.*, **52,** 1673

13 Normann, S. J. and Schardt, M. (1978). A macrophage inflammation test using subcutaneous nitrocellulose filters. *J. Reticuloendothelial Soc.*, **23,** 153

14 Elder, J. H., Gautsch, J. W., Jensen, F. C. *et al.* (1977). Biochemical evidence that MCF murine leukemia viruses are envelope (env) gene recombinants. *Proc. Natl. Acad. Sci. (USA)*, **74,** 4676

15 Rowe, W. P. and Piecus, T. (1972). Quantitative studies of naturally occuring murine leukemia virus infection of AKR mice. *J. Exp. Med.*, **135,** 429

16 Hartley, J. W., Wolford, N. K., Old, L. J. and Rowe, W. P. (1977). A new class of murine leukemia virus associated with development of spontaneous lymphomas. *Proc. Natl. Acad. Sci. (USA)*, **74,** 789

17 Siegler, R. and Rich, M. A. (1963). Unilateral histogenesis of AKR thymic lymphoma. *Cancer Res.*, **23,** 1669

18 McEndy, D. P., Boon, M. C. and Furth, J. (1944). On the role of thymus, spleen, and gonads in the development of leukemia in a high leukemia stock of mice. *Cancer Res.*, **4,** 377

19 Prehn, R. T (1963). Function of depressed immunologic reactivity during carcinogenesis. *J. Natl. Cancer Inst.* **31,** 791

20 Bartlett, G. L. (1972). Effect of host immunity on the antigenic strength of primary tumours. *J. Natl. Cancer Inst.* **49,** 493

21 Pike, M. C. and Snyderman, R. (1976). Depression of macrophage function by a factor produced by neoplasms: A mechanism for abrogration of immune surveillance. *J. Immunol.*, **117,** 1243

22 Hibbs, J. B. Jr., Chapman, H. A. Jr., and Weinberg, J. B. (1978). The macrophage as an antineoplastic surveillance cell: Biological perspectives. *J. Reticuloendothelial Soc.*, **24,** 549

23 Normann, S. J., Schandt, M. and Sorkin, E. (1979). Anti-inflammatory effect of spontaneous lymphoma in SJL/J mice. *J. Natl. Cancer Inst.*, **63,** 825

24 Normann, S. J., Schardt, M. and Sorkin, E. (1979). Cancer progression and monocyte inflammatory dysfunction: Relationship to tumor excision and metastasis. *Int. J. Cancer* **23,** 110

25 Stevenson, M. M., Meltzer, M. S. and Steinberg, G. (1979). Alteration of macrophage function in mice with transplantable tumours: Evidence for virus-induced changes. *Fed. Proc.*, **38,** 1094

26 Gianciolo, G. J., Thiel, H. J., Bolognesi, D. P., and Snyderman, R. (1979). Macrophage accumulation inhibited by extracts of murine leukemia viruses (MLV). *Fed. Proc.*, **38,** 1364

27 Eccles, S. A. (1977). Studies on the effect of rat sarcomata on the migration of mononuclear phagocytes in vitro and in vivo. In James, K., McBride, B. and Stuart, A. (eds.) *The Macrophage and Cancer*, pp. 308–320. (Edinburgh: Econoprint)

28 Snyderman, R. and Pike, M. C. (1976). An inhibitor of macrophage chemotaxis produced by neoplasms. *Science*, **192,** 370

29 Normann, S. J. (1978). Tumor cell threshold required for suppression of macrophage inflammation. *J. Natl. Cancer Inst.*, **60,** 1091

30 Normann, S. J. and Sorkin, E. (1977). Inhibition of macrophage chemotaxis by neoplastic and other rapidly proliferating cells in vitro. *Cancer Res.*, **37,** 705

# 97

# Effect of tumour growth on inflammatory macrophages

D. NOLIBE, R. MASSE AND J. P. GIROUD (FRANCE)

## INTRODUCTION

Studies in many laboratories have led to the speculation that macrophages probably play a significant role in host defence against neoplasia. It has been shown both *in vitro* and *in vivo* that macrophages can destroy tumour cells via different pathways, specific[1] or otherwise[2]. On the other hand it has been demonstrated that patients with neoplasms have a depressed monocyte chemotactic responsiveness[3] and that macrophage accumulation in response to inflammatory stimuli is impaired during growth of experimental tumours[4,5].

Some authors suggest that this defect of macrophage response may contribute to the growth and diffusion of tumours. The present experiments investigated macrophage accumulation in response to inflammatory stimuli during the latent period of radio induced lung tumours. Radio induced tumours are of interest due to their long latent period similar to that of spontaneous tumours. Results were compared with macrophage response during growth of subcutaneously grafted radio induced or chemically induced tumours.

## MATERIAL AND METHODS

### Animals

Inbred Wistar AG rats, initially purchased from CNRS (Orleans la Source, France), were raised locally and maintained under conventional conditions.

## HARVEST OF MACROPHAGES

### Macrophage inflammation test (MIT)

The macrophage influx in tissue was quantified according to the method of Normann and Schardt[6] using nitrocellulose filter discs (Sartorius, 0.2 μm pore size) inserted subcutaneously. The inflammatory response was evaluated by counting cells on filters from ten predetermined oil immersion fields.

### Peritoneal exudate cells

Macrophages in peritoneal washings were counted 2 days after intraperitoneal injection of 2 mg of phytohaemagglutinin according to the technique of Normann and Schardt[7].

### Alveolar cells

Alveolar macrophages were obtained by broncho pulmonary lavages of isolated lungs. Ten lavages of 5 ml each were performed. After either peritoneal or pulmonary lavages, viable cell counts were rapidly performed and cytocentrifuge preparations made for morphological studies.

In some animals the three tests were carried out with the following timing: subcutaneous implantation of filters (day 0) removing of filters (day 2) PHA stimulation (day 9) peritoneal and pulmonary lavages (day 11).

## TUMOURS

Tumours were initially induced in the lungs of an inbred strain of Wistar AG. Two types of induction were utilized.

(1) Radio induction by chronic $\alpha$ irradiation of lungs by means of inhaled plutonium dioxide particles with a total dose delivered during latent period of 50–4600 rads.

(2) Chemical induction by combined effect of irradiation together with two intratracheal instillations of a mixture of benzopyrene (5 mg) and carrier dust ferric oxide $Fe_2O_3$ (5 mg) in 0.5 ml sterile 0.9% NaCl.

Four of the radio induced and one of the chemically induced tumours were serially transplanted subcutaneously in syngeneic, 6-month-old rats. Their histology and growth characteristics are summarized in Table 97.1. The number of animals per group is given in the legends of tables.

**Table 97.1** Characteristics of radio induced lung tumours

| | *Primary tumour* | | *Grafted tumour* | | |
|---|---|---|---|---|---|
| *Histologic type* | *α dose* (rads) | *Latent period* (days) | *Type of graft* | *Mean survival time of receivers* (days) | *Metastases* |
| Haemangiosarcoma (C 433) | 2000 | 425 | explants | 34 | +++ |
| Malignant fibro Histiocytoma (P 77) | 50 | 940 | established | 37 | +++ |
| Squamous Carcinoma (T 217) | 4600 | 470 | explants | 350 | ± |
| Bronchiolo-alveolar Carcinoma (T 243) | 1500 | 760 | explants | 110 | – |

## RESULTS

### Macrophage response in Wistar AG control rats

The kinetics of macrophage accumulation on filters was studied between 6 and 48 h after implantation of nitrocellulose discs. The results are reported in Table 97.2. After an early influx in the first 6 h, polymorphonuclear leukocytes disappeared and macrophages rapidly increased. After 48 h a uniform monolayer, consisting of more than 99% macrophage, was observed. Because of this, the 48 h time period was chosen for further experiments. For the controls (high power field) a mean number of 527±87 was counted per oil immersion fields.

**Table 97.2** Cell accumulation on filters

| *Time after filter implantation* (h) | *Macrophages* *Number* | *%* | *Polymorphonuclear leukocytes* |
|---|---|---|---|
| 6* | 9±2 | 20 | 36±8 |
| 12* | 120±69 | 44 | 150±82 |
| 18* | 481±101 | 83 | 98±19 |
| 24* | 339±72 | 87 | 52±18 |
| 48† | 527±87 | 96 | 24±21 |

Animals tested; *3; †5

When two filters were inserted in the same animal, differences in macrophage counts were less than 10% (Table 97.3). The main interest of the

**Table 97.3** Number of macrophages on two filters implanted in same animal

| *Animal* | *Filter 1* | *Filter 2* |
|---|---|---|
| Control 1 | 489 | 549 |
| Control 2 | 538 | 492 |
| Control 3 | 513 | 467 |

macrophage inflammation test using nitrocellulose filters was the possibility of repeating the measurement during growth of the tumours in grafted animals and in apparently healthy animals during the latent period of radio induced tumours.

The reproducibility of results was verified on a group of five animals (Figure 97.1) and suggested that the same animals could be implanted with one filter each per week, during 5 weeks, without modification of counts. The number of PHA-induced peritoneal macrophages in 6-month-old control rats was $26 \pm 3 \times 10^6$. The number of alveolar macrophages was $15 \pm 2.5 \times 10^6$ in the same animals.

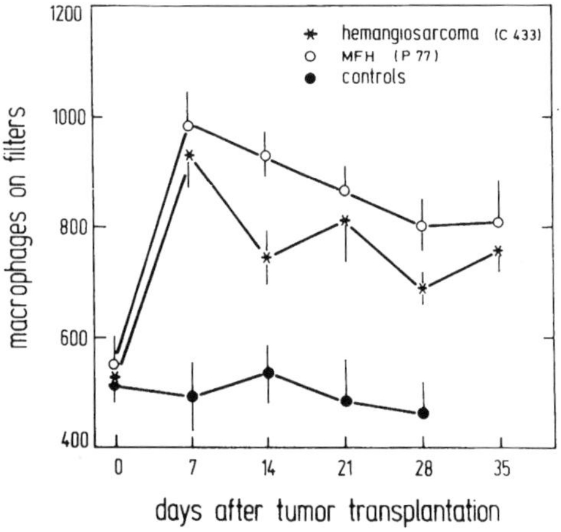


**Figure 97.1** Macrophage response to implanted filters in normal versus radio induced tumour bearing rats

**Macrophage response during latent period of radio induced tumours**

A group of 10 rats inhaled radioactive particles of plutonium dioxide (initial lung burden : 50 nCi). They were tested for their MIT response 18 and 24 months later during latent periods of lung tumours. With this initial lung burden a mean tumoural incidence of 25% and a latent period of between 400 and 800 days had been previously observed[8].

Among the 10 animals, only 3 died from lung tumours, 2 having bronchio-lo-alveolar carcinomas classified as $T_1$ and $T_2$ $N_0$ $P_1$ $M_0$ according to the TNPM classification in rats[8], i.e., tumours less than 5 mm in diameter without local invasion to lymph nodes and distant metastases. The other one was an epidermoid squamous carcinoma $T_3$ $N_1$ $P_1$ $M_0$, i.e. 1 cm in diameter with tracheo-bronchial lymph node invasion but no distant metastases. Results are reported in Table 97.4. No significant modification in the inflammatory macrophage response between the different groups was observed. Alveolar macrophage count was only affected in the 2 animals with bronchiolo-alveolar carcinomas and a non-significant increase (19.5 ± 3.5) was observed versus animals without tumours.

### Macrophage response during growth of grafted tumours

Four radio induced tumours were used for MIT evaluation. Characteristics of each of them are summarized in Table 97.1. They differed by histologic type and also by doubling time and metastatic potential. Two (C 433 and P 77) were fast growing highly metastatic tumours which killed the host between 28 and 45 days. Among the slow growing tumours which killed animals about 4 months after tumour implantation without any metastases, one (T 243) was a bronchiolo-alveolar carcinoma. Another, a squamous lung carcinoma (T 217) had a very slow growth and animals died after one year with very necrotic tumours and only 10% of the animals had any metastases.

**Table 97.4** Macrophage response during latent period of radio induced tumours

| | *Number of macrophages on filters in* | | |
|---|---|---|---|
| | | *Irradiated rats with* | |
| *Time after Inhalation* (months) | *Controls* (3 animals) | *Tumour* (3 animals) | *No tumour* (7 animals) |
| 18 | 589±44 | 540±47 | 549±96 |
| 24 | 494±52 | 615±78 | 663±119 |

In all cases (Table 97.5) a significant increase in inflammatory macrophage number was observed, respectively, 30% (C 433) 50% (P 77) 120% (T 217), 30% (T 243). In a second experiment, MIT response was performed each week in animals subcutaneously grafted with 5 $mm^3$ explants of haemangio-sarcoma, or with $10^6$ cells of the malignant fibrohistiocytoma. It was shown

**Table 97.5** Number of macrophages on filters inserted in four types of tumour bearing animals

| *Type of tumour* | *Time after tumour transplantation* (days) | *Number of macrophages* |
|---|---|---|
| Haemangiosarcoma* (C 433) | 28 | 688±29 |
| Malignant fibrohistiocytoma* (P 77) | 28 | 802±47 |
| Squamous lung carcinoma† (T 217) | 200 | 1162±75 |
| Bronchiolo-alveolar carcinoma† (T 243) | 90 | 688±31 |
| Controls‡ | — | 527±87 |

Animals tested: *5; †3; ‡10.

(Figure 97.1) that the number of macrophages increased rapidly in the first days after tumour graft, then decreased but remained significantly higher than in controls up to the death of the animals. P 77 tumour bearing animals also have a higher number of peritoneal (PHA induced) and alveolar macrophages (non-induced), Table 97.6.

**Table 97.6** Macrophage responses in P 77 tumour bearing animais (37 days after S.C. inoculation of $10^6$ tumour cells)

| *Type of macrophages* | *Number of macrophages* Controls | *Tumour bearers* |
|---|---|---|
| Filter induced tissue macrophages | 527±87 | 802±46 |
| PHA-induced peritoneal macrophages | $26 \pm 3 \times 10^6$ | $30 \pm 2 \times 10^6$ |
| Alveolar macrophages | $15 \pm 2.5 \times 10^6$ | $24 \pm 2.5 \times 10^6$ |

If only $10^3$ P 77 tumour cells were injected, the mean survival time of animals was 65±7 days, with a mean tumour weight of 105±10 g. In this case (Table 97.7) inflammatory tissue and peritoneal macrophages did not decrease significantly as compared to controls but did decrease significantly versus animals injected with $10^6$ cells. Alveolar macrophages were strongly reduced: $7 \times 10^6$ versus $15 \times 10^6$ in controls.

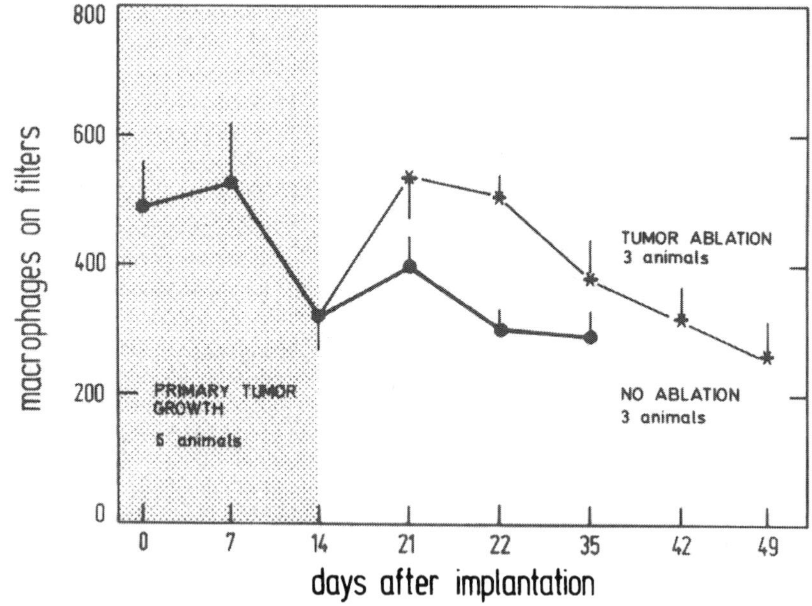


**Figure 97.2** Macrophage response to implanted filters in benzopyrene induced tumour bearing rats. Effects of tumour ablation

A more severe decrease of inflammatory macrophage response was observed during growth of a benzopyrene induced tumour (Figure 97.2). Further, a rapid enhancement after surgical removal of a primary tumour, with a new decrease during local tumour recurrence, were observed.

**Table 97.7** Macrophage responses in P 77 tumour bearing animals (62 days after S.C. inoculation of $10^3$ tumour cells)

| *Type of macrophages* | *Number of macrophages* |
|---|---|
| Filter induced tissue macrophages | 485±54 |
| PHA induced peritoneal macrophages | 21±5 × $10^6$ |
| Alveolar macrophages | 6.3±2.4 × $10^6$ |

## DISCUSSION

The results of this report demonstrate that no inhibition of inflammatory mononuclear cells is observed during the latent period of radio induced primary lung tumours. This is obtained with animals bearing relatively small but non-metastasizing tumours. However, the hypothesis that this inhibition requires a threshold number of tumour cells has not been confirmed by studies of animals bearing grafts of radio induced tumours. In fact, during subcutaneous growth of lung tumours an increase in inflammatory macrophages was observed. This increase occurs up to the death of animals, although the mean tumour weight is superior to 80 g. The effect is the same with metastasizing or non-metastasizing tumours.

On the other hand, as others have demonstrated with chemically induced tumours[4,5], a macrophage inhibition is observed in the case of a benzopyrene induced tumour. A good correlation between growth of neoplasm and macrophage inhibition effect is observed. Macrophage response is significantly restored by the surgical ablation of the primary tumour.

A lack of anti-inflammatory effect was previously described with some solid tumors (P 815 mastocytoma) in mice[9] and myeloid leukaemia in rats[10]. It seems that this is a general finding with radio induced lung tumours. Some data suggests that chemically induced tumours are distinct from radio induced tumours in the degree of tumour immunity.

Analysis of immunogenicity by surgical ablation of primary tumour followed by challenge tests shows that the four radio induced tumours tested are not detectably immunogenic. With the benzopyrene induced tumour, immunization made the animal resistant to lower challenge inoculum. Data from-Jamashi[11] in rats confirm that lung tumours induced by 7, 12-dimethylbenz (a) anthracene, 3-methylcholanthrene or benzopyrene have a high immunogenic potency. As macrophage infiltration in tumours increases with their immunogenicity it is possible that other macrophage functions differ according to the immunogenicity of tumours.

The same macrophage responses are observed in highly metastatic and in non-metastatic tumours; consequently it can be concluded that tumour growth as well as tumour dissemination are not the result of a defect in macrophage response. When this defect occurs, it is the last stage in the growth of tumours. It may well be important to determine in the experiment in progress whether it is a general result in all tumours, and why the inhibitory effect occurs later in radio induced than in chemically induced tumours. It might also be important to know why non-induced alveolar macrophages are more affected than inflammatory macrophages, although this last population provides the source of activated macrophages for expression of anti-tumoural immunity[12].

## References


1 Alexander, P. (1976). The functions of the macrophage in malignant disease. *Ann. Rev. Med.*, **27**, 207

2 Zbar, B., Bernstein, I. D., Bartlett, G. L., Hanna, N. G., and Rapp H. J. (1972). Immunotherapy of cancer: regression of intradermal tumors and prevention of growth of lymph node metastases after intralesional injection of living mycobacterium bovis. *J. Natl. Cancer Inst.*, **49**, 119

3 Snyderman, R., Seigler, H. F. and Meadows, L. (1977). Abnormalities of monocyte chemotaxis in patients with melanoma; effects of immunotherapy and tumor removal. *J. Natl. Cancer Inst.*, **58**, 37

4 Snyderman, R., Pike, M. C., Blaylock, B. L. and Weinstein, P. (1976). Effects of neoplasms on inflammation: depression of macrophage accumulation after tumor implantation. *J. Immunol.*, **116**, 585

5 Normann, S. J., Schardt, M. and Sorkin, E. (1979). Cancer progression and monocyte inflammatory dysfunction: relationship to tumour excision and metastasis. *Int. J. Cancer,* **23,** 110

6 Normann, S. J. and Schardt, M. (1978). A macrophage inflammation test using subcutaneous nitrocellulose filters. *J. Reticuloendothial Soc.*, **23,** 153

7 Normannn, S. J. and Schardt, M. (1978).A cancer related macrophage dysfunction in inflamed tissues *J. Reticuloendothelial Soc.*, **24,** 147–159

8 Nolibe, D., Masse, R., and Lafuma, J. (1980). The effect of neonatal thymectomy upon lung cancers induced in rats by 239 plutonium dioxide. *Radiat Res.* (In press)

9 Normann, S. J. and Cornelius, J. (1978). Concurrent depression of tumor macrophage infiltration and systemic inflammation by progressive cancer growth. *Cancer Res.*, **38,** 3453

10 Gauci, C. L., Wrathmell, A. and Alexander, P. (1975). The origin and role of blood born monocytes in rats with transplanted myelogenous leukemia. *Cancer Lett.* **1,** 33

11 Jamasbi, R. J., Nettesheim, P. and Kennel S. J. (1978). Demonstration of cellular and humoral immunity to transplantable carcinomas derived from the respiratory tract of rats. *Cancer Res.*, **38,** 261

12 Ruco, L. P. and Meltzer, M. S. (1978). Macrophage activation for tumor cytotoxicity: increased lymphokine responsiveness of peritoneal macrophages during acute inflammation. *J. Immunol.*, **120,** 1054

# 98

# Effect of an acute inflammatory process on tumour development

D. NOLIBE, I. FLORENTIN, M. PELLETIER,
R. MASSE AND J. P. GIROUD (FRANCE)

## INTRODUCTION

Since the pioneer work of Metchnikoff it has become well established that a non-immunological inflammation can increase host resistance against infection[1]. However, little is known about the efffect of such an inflammatory process on anti-tumour defences. Fauve *et al.*[2] demonstrated that an inflammatory reaction induced in mice by injecting talc particles embedded in a calcium phosphate gel, delayed Lewis carcinoma growth and inhibited metastatic spreading. In the present work, the influence of an acute non-immunological inflammatory reaction induced by an intrapleural injection of an irritant on tumour growth and metastasis of three tumour models in rats and mice has been investigated.

## MATERIALS AND METHOD

### Animals

Pathogen free rats on the inbred strain Wistar AG obtained from CNRS (Orléans la Source) were used. 3-month-old pathogen free C57BL/6 mice were purchased from OLAC (Bicester, England).

### Induction of the inflammatory reaction

Acute inflammation was induced under sterile conditions either in mice by intrapleural injection of 0.5 ml 12% dextran, or in rats by injection of 1 ml 1%

calcium pyrophosphate in saline, according to the technique previously described[3].

**Tumours**

Two models of tumour growth with spontaneous metastasis were used

(1) The 3 LL Lewis tumour is a lung carcinoma that arises spontaneously in a C57 BL/6 mouse and has been maintained by serial passages in the same strain. In the present experiment, tumour cells were obtained from lung metastatic foci and cultured into Falcon flasks in MEM medium supplemented with 0.1 mol/l glutamine and 10% foetal calf serum. After 48 h the medium was removed and replaced by fresh, protein free, medium. After 12 h incubation cells were harvested by scraping with a rubber policeman. Cell viability, assessed by the trypan blue dye exclusion test, was 90%. Viable tumour cells in 25 μl of MEM ($5 \times 10^4$) were injected subcutaneously into the left footpad. Tumour growth was followed daily by measuring footpad thickness increment. Animals were sacrificed on day 30 after tumour implantation, the lungs were removed, and the number of visible metastases were scored.

(2) A lung haemangiosarcoma (C 433) initially induced in Wistar AG rats by inhalation of plutonium dioxide insoluble particles ($\alpha$-emitter) was transplanted serially by subcutaneous implantation of calibrated small pieces of tumour tissue. In these experiments passages 39–40 have been used. At the death of the animals a complete autopsy was performed and the number of metastases in lungs and other organs was recorded.

One procedure of artificial metastasis (lung colony assay) was also used with P77 tumour cells derived from a malignant fibrohistiocytoma induced by irradiation in the same strain of Wistar AG rats. Viable tumour cells ($10^5$) were injected intravenously into the penis vein of syngeneic rats. After 28 days all animals were killed, and the number of metastases was recorded.

Throughout this paper the day of tumour inoculation is referred to as day 0. Details of protocols (number of animals per group, day of inflammatory treatment) are given with the results.

## RESULTS

### Influence of acute inflammation on growth and spontaneous metastasis of Lewis carcinoma in mice

Four groups of 10 mice were grafted s.c. with $5 \times 10^4$ 3 LL Lewis tumour cells on day 0. As shown in Figure 98.1, the tumour grew progressively in control animals. A significant acceleration of tumour development was observed when the inflammatory stimulus was applied 3 days before or at the same time as tumour cell inoculation. This phenomenon was detectable from day 10 to

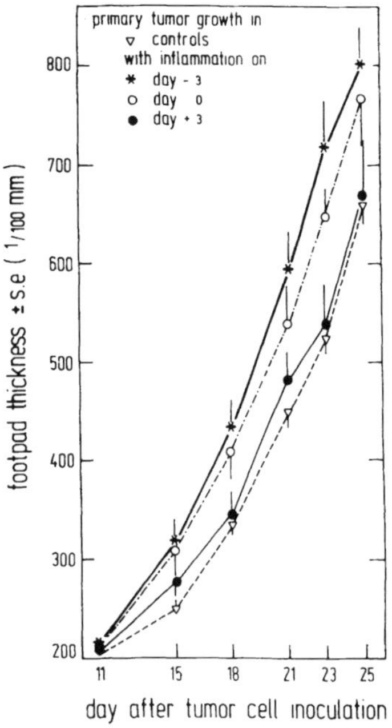


**Figure 98.1** Primary tumour growth of grafted 3 LL Lewis carcinoma in C 57 BL/6 mice

day 15 after tumour grafting. After this time the rate of tumour growth was similar in all groups of animals. Inflammation induced 3 days after tumour grafting did not significantly modify tumour growth. All animals were sacrificed on day 30, prior to natural death. As shown in Table 98.1, a significant increase in the number of lung metastases was observed in the groups of animals in which inflammation was induced 3 days before or on the same day as tumour grafting.

**Influence of acute inflammation on growth and metastasis of C 433 haemangiosarcoma in rats**

Four groups of 10 animals were grafted on day 0, with small calibrated pieces of lung haemangiosarcoma. In three groups acute inflammation was produced by intrapleural injection of calcium pyrophosphate at different times after graft. Mean survival time and mean tumour weight were recorded in each group and compared to controls without inflammation.

In controls, grafts resulted in progressive tumour growth leading to death of the host after 34 ± 7 days, by which time tumours had reached a diameter of approximately 35 mm and a weight of about 12 g (Figure 98.2). The tumour doubling time was approximately 4 days. No modification was observed for

**Table 98.1** Influence of an acute inflammation on s.c. injection of 5 × $10^4$ 3LL Lewis tumour cells

| *Day of application of the inflammatory stimulus* | *Mean number of lung metastasis ± SE* | *Mean spleen weight ± SE (mg)* |
|---|---|---|
| − 3 | 32.7 ± 7.2* | 200 ± 22 |
| 0 | 25.4 ± 6.9* | 252 ± 33 |
| +3 | 17.4 ± 3.4 | 149 ± 23 |
| controls | 11.4 ± 2.6 | 211 ± 26 |

*Significantly different from controls.

**Table 98.2** Influence of an acute inflammation on s.c. grafted haemangiosarcoma growth

| *Day of inflammatory stimulus* | *Mean survival time* (days) ± SE | *Mean tumour weight at death* (g) ± SE |
|---|---|---|
| 0 | 36 ± 2 | 13 ± 2 |
| 7 | 34 ± 2 | 15 ± 2 |
| 14 | 32 ± 2 | 12 ± 1 |
| controls (no inflammation) | 34 ± 2 | 12 ± 1 |

tumor development in treated groups. All controls and treated animals had the same growth curve (Figure 98.2) and their mean survival time and tumour weight at death were similar (Table 98.2).

All control animals had widespread spontaneous metastases, at time of death, principally in the lungs but also in other organs: kidneys, spleen and lymph nodes (Table 98.3). The influence of acute inflammation on the

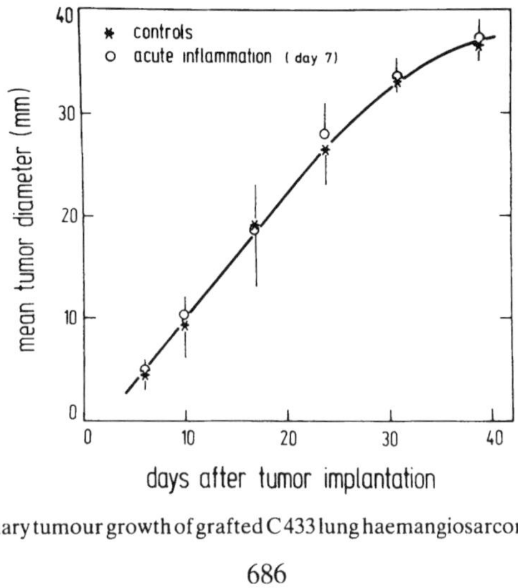


**Figure 98.2** Primary tumour growth of grafted C433 lung haemangiosarcoma in Wistar AG rats

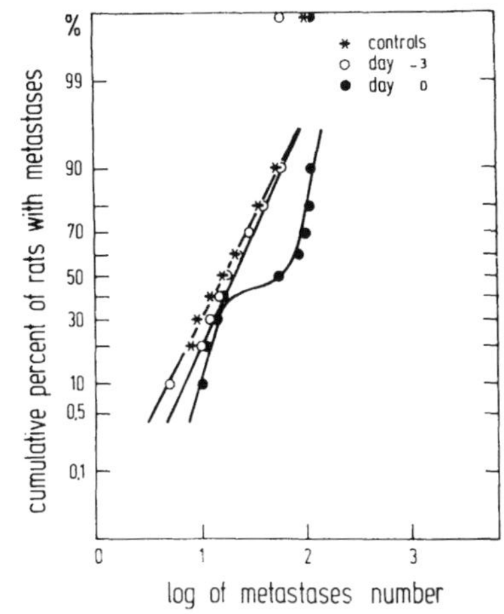


**Figure 98.3** Test for log normal distribution of lung metastases

metastasis process varied with time lapse between injection of the irritant and implantation of tumour.

If inflammation and tumour graft were performed on the same day, the total number of metastases decreased. In contrast, metastases increased when inflammation was induced 14 days after the tumour graft. No effect was observed at day 7 (Table 98.3). If the metastasis process in organs other than lungs is considered, a significant decrease was observed in all treated groups. However, it was more important when inflammation was delayed towards grafting (Table 98.3).

It was also possible with this same tumour model to increase the survival time of animals by surgical ablation of primary tumour and to study the development of metastases only. Time between implantation and surgical removal of the primary tumour illustrates kinetics by which the tumour controls the release of tumour cells and their development in distant organs. The primary

**Table 98.3** Influence of acute inflammation on spontaneous metastases of s.c. grafted haemangiosarcoma

| *Day of inflammatory stimulus* | *Mean number of metastases per animal ± SE* | | *Total number of others organs with macroscopic metastases/group* |
|---|---|---|---|
| 0 | 11± 1* | | 8 |
| 7 | 22 ± 3 | NS | 3 |
| 14 | 63 ± 11* | | 2 |
| controls (no inflammatory) | 19.5 ± 3 | | 14 |

*Significantly different from controls.

tumour was surgically excised in three groups of 10 animals 14 days after implantation. In spite of the ablation all animals died from lung metastasis, but had a prolonged median survival time (52 ± 9 days). 20 to 30% of recurrences occurred in each group and were eliminated as soon as they appeared.

No significant effect on the mean survival of animals was observed in inflamed animals as compared to controls. Nevertheless, the total number of metastases was enhanced in the group which received inflammatory stimulus and ablation on the same day. If inflammation occurred 3 days before ablation, the total number of lung metastases was less augmented (Table 98.4). However, in each group the dispersion of results was important: for example, 5 to 108 metastases in controls, 17 to 105 in group day 14. For this reason the differences in mean number of metastases per animal, respectively, 35 ± 32 (controls); 60 ± 33 (D 14); 46 ± 39 (D 11), were not statistically significant.

**Table 98.4** Effect of acute inflammation on sponteneous metastasis in animals surgically operated 14 days after implantation

| *Day of inflammatory stimulus* | *Mean number of metastases per animal ± SE* | *Total number of other organs with metastases/group* |
|---|---|---|
| 11 | 46 ± 12 (NS) | 3 |
| 14 | 60 ± 10 (NS) | 4 |
| controls (no inflammation) | 34 ± 10 | 9 |

**Influence of acute inflammation on experimental metastases (lung colony assay)**

Artificial metastases were induced by intravenous injection of $10^5$ P 77 tumour cells. Of three groups of 10 animals, two received an additional pleural inflammation the day of inoculation or 3 days before. Results are summarized in Table 98.5. They suggested a facilitation effect when inoculation and inflammation are concomitant. However, differences observed between groups were not significant because of the large dispersion of results. As is shown in Figure 98.3, where cumulative number of animals is plotted against

**Table 98.5** Effect of acute inflammation on artificial metastasis (lung colony assay) after intravenous injection of $10^5$ P 77 tumour cells

| *Day of inflammatory stimulus* | *Mean number of metastases per animal ± SE* |
|---|---|
| − 3 | 27 ± 6 (NS) |
| 0 | 75 ± 22 (NS) |
| controls (no inflammation) | 30 + 9 |

the logarithm of the number of metastases, populations obeyed a log normal distribution except for the day 0 group. For that group, two sub-populations were individualized: one with a high number of metastases (110 ± 58) and the other one with a low number (13 ± 2).

## DISCUSSION

It was observed in these different tumour models that an acute non-immunological inflammation is able to modify tumour behaviour. However, the effect varies according to the time of application of the inflammatory stimulus with respect to tumour inoculation. In the 3 LL Lewis tumour model, an acceleration of primary tumour growth was observed during the early phase of tumour development in mice developing the inflammation 3 days before or at the same time as tumour grafting. This increased tumour load may contribute to the higher number of lung metastases detected in these animals.

In the haemangiosarcoma model, enhancement or inhibition of the metastatic process could be observed according to the lapse time between tumour implantation and elicitation of inflammation. A decrease of lung metastases was observed when inflammation and tumour grafting were concomitant. In contrast, an enhancement was observed if inflammation was applied when the tumour was well developed (14 days after grafting). These data suggest that inflammation may be only active on a limited number of tumour cells. This hypothesis can be confirmed by the fact that in all treated animals metastases decreased in spleen, lymph nodes, kidney and liver. In contrast, with lungs, only few tumour cells are trapped in these organs.

With the model of artificial metastases, in the group in which injection of tumour cells and inflammation were concomitant, the existence of two populations, low and high responders to inflammatory stimulus or to development of metastases, could not be overlooked.

Conflicting results were observed with the 3 LL Lewis tumour model in mice and the haemangiosarcoma in rats when inflammation was induced at day 0. Two hypotheses are possible

(1) Differences in the response of the host, or differences in metastatic process of the two tumours. The latter is substantiated by the fact that haemangiosarcoma is a particular model in which tumour cells have direct access to the bloodstream. It is probable that the release of angiosarcoma cells in the circulation occurs more rapidly and in greater number than the release of Lewis tumour cells.

(2) The nature of inoculum: isolated cells (3 LL Lewis tumour) pieces of tissue (haemangiosarcoma) could induce some differences in the accessibility of tumour cells to effects of inflammation. Even in the same tumour

model, a large dispersion of the number of spontaneous metastases per lung is observed in animals without inflammation, However, the existence of several populations with different susceptibilities to metastatic process is not supported by mathematical analysis: all the animals of the different groups obey a log normal distribution. The conclusion, limited by a small number of animals, suggests a random phenomenon probably in relation to tumour development (vascularization, encapsulation).

Inhibition[3] or facilitation[4] of tumour growth by inflammation had been described previously. It seems that these conflicting results could be dependent on the kinetics of inflammation response and ratio between number of tumour cells and mediators of inflammation. Previous results suggest the following hypothesis: acute inflammation induces circulating factors[5] capable of activating macrophages[6] which become cytostatic to tumour cells[7]. This is also suported by preliminary experiments in which an increase of the latency period is observed in animals receiving a mixture of inflammatory macrophages and tumour cells (unpublished results). Poste *et al.*[8] have shown that the ability of inflammatory macrophages to destroy tumour cells is a short lived function. Thus the maintenance of effective macrophage cytotoxicity requires a constant new influx of activated macrophages by chronic inflammation.

## References


1 Fauve, R. M. (1977). Inflammation and host resistance pathogen. *Intensive Care Med.*, **3**, 237

2 Fauve, R. M. and Hevin, M. B. (1977). Inflammation et résistance antitumorale. I. Retard de croissance et inhibition du developpement des métastases de la tumeur de Lewis chez des souris porteuses d'une réaction inflammatoire distante d'un site d'inoculation des cellules malignes. *Ann. Immunol. (Paris)* **128 C,** 923

3 Willoughby, D. A., Dunn, C. J., Yamamoto, S., Capasso, F., Deporter, D. A. and Giroud, J. P. (1975). Calcium pyrophosphate induced pleurisy in rat: a new model of acute inflammation. *Agents Actions*, **5,** 35

4 Van Den Brenk, H. A., Stone, M. and Kelly, H. (1974). Promotion of growth of tumor cells in acutely inflamed tissues. *Br. J. Cancer*, **30,** 246

5 Giroud, J. P., Pelletier, M. and Girre, C. (1977). Pouvoir mitogène de sérums de rats porteurs d'une inflammation aiguë vis à vis de macrophages en culture. *C. R. Acad. Sci., Ser. D.* **285,** 1143

6 Pelletier, M. and Giroud, J. P. (1980). Effect of irradiation and cell reconstitution on the macrophage mitogenic activity of exudate and inflammatory serum. This volume, Chap. 121

7 Kiger, N., Pelletier, M., Florentin, I., Mathe, G. and Giroud, J. P. (1978). Effects of an non specific acute inflammatory stimulus on a macrophage and antibody dependent cellular cytotoxicity. *Eur. J. Rheumatol. Inflam.*, **1,** 321

8 Poste, G. (1979). The tumoricidal properties of inflammatory tissue macrophages and multinucleate giant cells. *An. J. Pathol.*, **96,** 595

99

# Role of endogenous pyrogen in the rabbit febrile responses to muramyl dipeptide (Abstract)

M. PARANT, G. RIVEAU AND L. CHEDID (FRANCE)

---

Muramyl dipeptide (MDP) is a low molecular weight synthetic adjuvant, analogue of a streptococcal peptidoglycan sub-unit. MDP was shown to represent the minimal active structure of peptidoglycan for both the adjuvant effect and the pyrogenicity. The immunoadjuvant activity of MDP is not strictly related to its pyrogenicity since synthetic analogues obtained with minor modifications are potent adjuvants without inducing any febrile response. Moreover, indomethacin completely inhibits the pyrogenic effect of MDP but does not modify the MDP-induced leucopenia. This treatment does not affect its immunostimulant properties. There is a general agreement that production of endogenous pyrogen by the host is the first step in the febrile response to bacterial pyrogens. Likewise the presence of transferable circulating endogenous pyrogen was demonstrated in the blood of rabbits made febrile with MDP. *In vitro* MDP is also able to release leukocytic pyrogen from rabbit phagocytic cells. As expected, production of endogenous pyrogen was not decreased in indomethacin treated animals. However, an injection of nitrogen mustard, which did not modify the febrile response to MDP, inhibited the production of endogenous pyrogen. This result has suggested that MDP fever can be caused by a direct action on thermosensitive brain structures.

# Discussion

**Dr H. Baart de la Faille (Netherlands)** reviewed his model of protoporphyria induced by DDC in hairless mice. He said that this appeared to be a good model for human erythropoietic protoporphyria (EPP), an inborn error of human porphyrin metabolism giving rise to an accumulation of protoporphyrin in the body. Both man and mouse showed severe hypersensitivity to violet light, the excess protoporphyrin acting as a photosensitizer. Photodermatitis developed after irradiation with distinct swelling and some erythema. Purpura was pronounced in man but not in the mouse. Light and electron microscopy had revealed endothelial damage ultimately leading to cell necrosis. There was exudation of a foamy appearing substance containing proteins, lipids and remnants of necrotic cells. In EPP they had found deposition of fibrin, immunoglobulins and complement factors. Mouse studies had shown lipid deposition in vessel walls shortly after irradiation, and after 24–48 h similar deposition was seen in epidermal cells. Alkaline phosphatase reactions in the capillary endothelium decreased or even disappeared 3–6 h following violet light exposure. The target molecules for light action lay in the cell membranes. The decrease in alkaline phosphatase suggested that the endothelial cell membrane became damaged. As yet one could only speculate as to which mediator systems were involved. Prostaglandins might be formed, following photo-oxidative damage of the membranes, and they might work together with kinins to produce the pain characteristic of the complaint. The deposition of complement factors might be indicative of activation of that system and blood clotting also evidently took place.

**Dr R. A. Wouterson (Netherlands),** continuing the description of these studies, said that the protoporphyric hairless mice were very sensitive to irradiation and their erythrocytes underwent haemolysis *in vitro* when exposed to violet light. Most investigators agreed that the important intermediate in reactions leading to photohaemolysis and photodermatitis included protoporphyrin in its excited triplet state and active oxygen species. There was evidence to suggest that besides singlet oxygen, superoxide and hydrogen peroxide might be formed during irradiation of protoporphyrin with light of 400 nm wavelength. In the presence of hydrogen peroxide and metal ions, superoxide could give rise to the even more toxic hydroxy radical. However, since scavengers for this radical did not cause any inhibition of photohaemolysis, it might not play an important role in the reaction. The primary effects in both photohaemolysis and photodermatitis appeared to be cell membrane damage. However, compounds such as beta-carotene, a scavenger for singlet oxygen which showed strong inhibition of photohaemolysis, hardly protected protoporphyric hairless mice against irradiation. Neither did cysteamine, an anti-oxidant with a still unknown mechanism, or diethyldithiocarbamate, an inhibitor of superoxide dismutase activity. Thus, it was clear that the reactions in irradiated protoporphyric skin were much more complicated than those in irradiated erythrocyte suspensions. They intended to use anti-inflammatory agents together with anti-oxidants in an attempt to protect against radiation damage but so far the results had not been impressive.

## DISCUSSION

**Professor J. L. Turk (Co-Chairman)** asked whether the effect of the anti-oxidant cysteamine was specific to the inflammatory reaction of protoporphyria or whether it would act in other sites of inflammatory lesions.

**Dr Wouterson** said that in the protoporphyria reaction the formation of superoxide or singlet oxygen took place within the cell. Thus one did not find an effect of superoxide dismutase as was found in other inflammatory reactions when the active oxygen species came from the surrounding fluid. He did not know in detail what happened when active oxygen species were formed within the cell. Some workers felt that damage was sustained by membrane proteins. Others believed that lipid peroxidation occurred. In his view, both the actions took place.

**Dr Baart de la Faille** said that attempts should be made to establish whether lipid peroxidation occurred in irradiated skin explants. Such systems might be preferable to examining skin *in vivo*, but certainly, if one had reasonable suspicion that active oxygen species were operative, then it was reasonable to use anti-oxidants.

**Dr W. Dawson (Chairman)** asked for comments on the purpural reaction in human beings. He wondered if its presence implied an effect on tissue cells as well as on red cells.

**Dr Baart de la Faille** said that the purpural reaction was a local event due to damaged blood vessels. He did not know why it was so pronounced, but histological examination showed very sparse leukocyte infiltration although extravasation of erythrocytes occurred very rapidly.

**Dr Dawson** commented that some of the substances which had been used, in addition to being scavengers, were also chelating agents and it was possible that some of the reactions observed might be due to chelation and removal of trace metals. If that were so, then penicillamine might be a more suitable treatment than a non-steroidal compound.

**Professor Turk** then turned attention to two presentations concerned with the Arthus reaction.

**Dr Lise L. Röckert (Sweden)** had tried to define *in vivo* the role of monuclear cells in a local inflammatory reaction. She had also wished to study the relationship between such local reactions and the serum antibody level. The rat had been chosen because of its steroid sensitivity and the ease of draining its thoracic duct. Ovalbumin was used as a sensitizing and challenging agent. In distinguishing between an Arthus response and a delayed-type reaction, they had found that the principle factor determining the reaction type was the time lapse between sensitization and challenge. For example, with 100 $\mu$g ovalbumin, a delay-type reaction was elicited after 7–9 days and an Arthus reaction from day 13 onwards. Between these periods, a mixed reaction was seen. The change to the Arthus reaction was correlated with increasing serum IgG levels starting on the ninth day. In the delay-type reaction and the mixed reaction, the majority of lymphocytes were positive to anti-T cell serum. The number of T cells increased from 12–24 h. In the Arthus reaction very few T cells could be identified from 4 h onwards. In all types of reaction, very few or no B cells could be identified. The T cell subsets involved remained to be investigated using monoclonal antibodies. Of particular interest in this connection was the lymphokine producing T cell, but so far no way of identifying this set had been described.

**Dr G. O. Till (Germany)** had been interested in regulatory mechanisms in leukocyte infiltration and as a model had used the reverse passive Arthus reaction. He had found that after an initial phase of complement activation, a second phase occurred with increasing amounts of chemotactic factor activity and cell directed inhibitor activity in the circulation as well as in biopsy material. Since lysosomal enzymes such as elastase and cathepsin could also inactivate chemotactic activity they had measured such enzyme activities in the biopsy extract and in the serum. They had so far shown activity for chemotactic factor inhibitor (CFI) and cell directed inhibitor (CBI). In the future they would purify these activities to show whether CFI, for example, was identical to the serum derived chemotactic inhibitor described by other workers. So far they could only speculate on whether the CBI was comparable to the neutrophil immobilizing factor or whether it was due to some other activity.

**Professor Turk** asked Dr Röckert how she had been able to ensure removal of antibodies from the anti-T sera. He wondered how she had been able to get sufficiently large supply of B cells to ensure absorption of all anti-B cell antibodies from the anti-T sera.

**Dr Röckert** said that for B cells they had used erythrocytes, macrophages and liver and thymus cells and had performed 13 absorptions. Subsequent reaction with spleen and lymph node preparations had not revealed the presence of any residual anti-B cell serum.

**Dr G. Faure (France)** noted that Dr Till had assayed both chemotactic activity and chemotactic inactivator activity in the same test sample. He asked whether methods were available to block the inactivator activity or whether the two were separated before the test.

**Dr Till** said that chemotactic activity in serum had a maximum value at 8 h at which time inactivator activity could not be found. Subsequently there was a sharp decrease of chemotactic activity and a steep increase in CFI. When CFI was present no chemotactic activity could be detected in serum. Even at 4 h, with low titres of CFI present, no chemotactic activity was found.

On being asked why he could not find chemotactic activity in biopsy material he said that he could only speculate. There might be an immune reaction in the vessel wall which activated complement. Complement activation products such as C5 derived chemotactic activity might reach the circulation. Locally deposited immune complexes might lead to high concentrations of these mediators which might in turn attract neutrophils.

**Professor Turk** said that very little work had been done on the Arthus reaction since it had been described 60 years previously; yet the Arthus reaction was a major cause of clinical disease which was the experimental model of immunologically induced vasculitis. There were many conditions, especially in infectious disease, producing reactions in the skin very much like the Arthus reaction. He was particularly interested in Dr Till's finding of active substances in sera of animals with the reaction. The condition of erythema nodosum leprosum was much like the Arthus reaction in patients with leprosy but there was no difference in the complement components compared to those in patients with the regular form of leprosy without vasculitis, except for the presence of C3 breakdown products. Levels of C1q reactive material in the sera and those of $CH_{50}$ were the same as in lepromatous leprosy.

**Professor D. A. Willoughby (UK)** said that they had used the reverse passive Arthus reaction but they had performed it in the pleural cavity since it was extremely difficult to quantitate the number of cells involved when it was performed in the skin. The reverse Arthus reaction could be used as a model to study the action of anti-inflammatory drugs. Using the Arthus reaction itself, the only drug showing effective suppression in the pleural cavity was dexamethasone. Nonetheless, the effects of carrageenin, which were very dependent on complement, were completely eliminated by compounds like indomethacin and the non-steroidal anti-inflammatory drugs such as propionic acid derivatives. This was obviously an effect worth further investigation. One had two systems, both of which were presumably producing an inflammatory response depending upon complement, yet they showed quite contrasting results when used to study the effects of anti-inflammatory agents.

**Dr Till** agreed that the dermal Arthus reaction had certain problems. They had recently started performing reverse passive Arthus reactions in the peritoneum with good results. They could separate cells easily and readily test for cell function.

**Professor Willoughby** said that very small numbers of lymphocytes entered the pleural cavity during the reverse passive Arthus reaction. They had performed time course studies from 15 min onwards because they had been interested in the leukocyte disappearance reaction. This reaction had been thought to be specific for cell mediated immunity but in fact it occurred with any irritant. At 4 h there was a large predominance of PMNs.

**Dr R. Vinegar (USA)** said that the lymphocytic reaction in the diaphragm might have been more intense. He wondered whether it had been examined.

**Professor Willoughby** said that he had not performed the reverse passive Arthus reaction in tissues subcutaneously. This was because, although one could obtain a subjective impression of the dominance of mononuclear cells, it was very difficult to quantitate.

**Professor Turk** said that unless one were performing a passive Arthus reaction one could not be sure that a mixed reaction was not occurring. In any active situation a cell mediated component was likely to exist. In addition, the presence of lymphocytes in the 24 h Arthus reaction was first emphasized in the 1930s. It was important to note that the lymphocyte was not pathognomonic of a delayed hypersensitivity reaction. Many such reactions showed the presence of more PMNs than lymphocytes.

**Dr P. Fritsch (France)** was invited to review his work on chromatid exchange. He said that inflammatory processes might be capable of producing genetic and phenotypic modifications. *In vitro* and *in vivo* studies suggested that inflammation could modulate and potentiate carcinogenesis induced by chemical or physical agents at the level of the target cell. Quantitiative study of genetic modification induced by inflammatory agents needed very sensitive genetic assays and recently sister chromatid exchange measures had been developed for this purpose. In normal cells, sister chromatid exchange occurred at a constant rate, as measured by uptake of an analogue of thymidine. Mutagenesis induced by physical or chemical agents increased this rate of exchange. To study the effect of local acute inflammation they had injected crocidolite into the pleural cavity of rats of various ages. Sister chromatid exchange was then studied in the bone marrow cells. There was no change in the exchange rate in 3 month old animals but for those 6 months or older there was a very significant increase following intrapleural injection. These preliminary results suggested that inflammatory-like reactions could produce genetic modification of cells that were not target cells for inflammation. The phenomenon seemed to correlate with substances present in the serum. The changes occurred only in older animals and further experiments were necessary to understand the mechanism by which inflammation could potentially modify induced carcinogenesis. He agreed that studies with standard mutagenic substances assaying for factors in the serum would be very valuable but so far the experiments were at a preliminary stage.

**Mme M. Pelletier (France)** reviewed the work of her group on the relation between inflammation and resistance to infection. Previous work had shown that during various acute inflammatory processes macrophages were stimulated which were able to inhibit tumour cell proliferation *in vitro*. They had therefore designed the present study to investigate whether the acute inflammatory reaction was able to protect mice against bacterial or parasitic infection. They found that an acute inflammatory reaction induced by intrapleural injection of calcium pyrophosphate 2–3 days before injection of *Klebsiella pneumoniae* or *Trypanosoma cruzi* increased the resistance of the mice. Similar results were obtained for inflammation induced by dextran, and infection by *Listeria monocytogenes*. In the case of *K. pneumoniae* infection, protection could be transferred to mice by injection 20 h before infection of sera obtained 2 h after the induction of inflammation. Thus it appeared that inflammation produced a factor in the serum which was able to protect mice against bacterial or parasitic infections.

**Dr W. Lu (UK)** was invited to review his work on the diminution of inflammatory responses. He said that earlier studies had investigated some of the factors which might account for the transient nature of the massive PMN emigration during inflammation. In particular, they had examined whether a change in the endothelial wall of the inflammation site might be rendered refractory to a second stimulus. By sequential stimulation of the rat peritoneal cavity they found that accumulation of PMNs in response to a strong stimulus was reduced by prior injection of a weak stimulus of a different nature into the same site. There were a number of possibilities for this effect, which could be divided into local and systemic factors. To establish whether the local or systemic influences were more important, they had injected the weak stimulus of 1% glycerol intrapleurally, and 4 h later, when the response in the pleural cavity was maximal, they injected the strong stimulant of a mixture of brain–heart infusion and peptone into the peritoneal cavity. Changes in PMN in the peripheral blood were monitored in blood samples collected from the tail vein. They had found that the accumulation of PMNs in the peritoneal cavity was reduced. Hence, a systemic factor appeared to be important. Changes in the peripheral blood followed the same pattern as changes in the exudate. At any time there were enough PMNs in the circulating blood to mount a full response to the weak or strong stimulants, given singly or together. Hence the reduction of emigration into the inflammatory site could not be explained by the number of PMNs in the blood alone.

**Dr Dawson** asked Mme Pelletier's research group whether they felt that they had been stimulating PMNs or monocytes or both to increase the phagocytosis of bacteria in the system.

**Mlle M. Parant (France)** said that they did not have a precise answer but it seemed that in *Listeria* infections the macrophages were implicated, whereas with *Klebsiella* both macrophages and PMNs seemed to be responsible for the effect.

**Dr Dawson** asked Dr Lu whether he had seen any increase in monocytes with stimulation. He also wondered whether the 'messenger' was derived from PMNs or whether it came from a tissue cell in the inflammatory site.

**Dr Lu** said that over the 8 h period in which he had studied sequential stimulation of the peritoneal cavity there appeared to be no appreciable change in monocyte patterns. The nature of the 'messenger' was a matter of speculation. Clearly a systemic mechanism was important, otherwise the introduction of two stimuli at the same site or at different sites would have different effects. It might be a parameter of the functional ability of the cell itself. It might be induced during acute inflammation or it might be both of these factors acting together.

**Dr R. Scheper (Netherlands)** drew attention to Mme Pelletier's finding of increased resistance to infections occurring some days after the onset of the inflammatory reaction.

**Professor J. P. Giroud (France)** said that changes in the peripheral blood after an acute inflammatory reaction occurred rapidly and disappeared by 48 h. Thus they might be inducing stimulation of macrophages or PMNs functions. Chronic inflammation was shown to modify infectious reaction and it seemed that in this case macrophages were involved. They had therefore attempted to show that these cells were also involved in the more acute inflammatory process, but the data were so far preliminary.

**Dr G. O. Till (Germany)** said that Dr Lu's observations were consistent with his own findings using the Arthus model. Using this model, at 4–12 h after the onset of the reaction they had been unable to elicit any further Arthus reactions in the same animal. Also, 12 h and later after the onset, they found the chemotactic factor inactivator and the cell directed inhibitor (CDI). Workers in Connecticut had shown that injection of complement derived chemotactic activity would increase CFI in the circulation and so he felt it likely that the inhibitory activity which Dr Lu had observed might be due to CFI or CDI.

**Dr Lu** said that several groups had described an 'anti-chemotactic factor' during acute inflammation. However, the relevance of the *in vitro* phenomenon of chemotaxis to an *in vivo* situation was not fully established.

**Mr M. A. Bray (UK)** said that *T. cruzi* was an obligative macrophage parasite, at least in the early stages of infection. It was well known that non-specific activation of the macrophage would enhance intracellular killing, which might be one explanation for the results. A second was an increase in hydrogen peroxide production which was one of the major features of the macrophage bearing *T. cruzi*.

**Dr Till** said that purified CFI injected together with antibody into the skin could totally suppress the accumulation. Thus CFI did seem to be a relevant mediator or regulator *in vivo*.

**Professor A. Sfikakis (Greece)** wondered whether the protective effect of the acute inflammatory reaction against infections could be due to stress related stimulation of ACTH and perhaps also to ACTH activation of the thymus.

**Professor Giroud** said that they had not performed experiments in adrenalectomized animals. Personally, he favoured a role for some low molecular weight substance having an effect on lymphocytes or macrophages or even being involved in the inhibition of chemotaxis.

**Professor S. J. Normann (USA)** was invited to review his work on inflammation and animal cancer. He said that activated macrophages would kill tumour cells in a non-specific way in conditions in which normal cells were usually spared. However, he and others had found that animals bearing transplanted tumours had a decreased stimulation of macrophages in inflammatory foci and within the tumour. Unfortunately, transplanted tumour models might not be analogous to spontaneous ones in latency-immunogenicity, peripheral leukocyte count and tumour cell numbers. Accordingly, they had examined spontaneous tumour models in the belief that these more closely resembled human cancer. They had examined two reticular neoplasms, a histiocytic lymphoma in SJL/J mice and a T cell lymphoma in AKR mice. In both of these models an anti-inflammatory effect against macrophages was observed at approximately the time at which the tumour could first be detected. In addition, the chemical carcinogen 3-methylcholanthrene increased the frequency of abnormal macrophage responses. The concept had been advanced that macrophages were surveillance cells whose function was subverted in the presence of tumours and the concept seemed to agree well with these experimental studies. However, their most recent investigations on mammary carcinoma in C3H mice did not support the concept, since no macrophage abnormalities were detected. He stressed that in examining any effects relevant to the surveillance hypothesis it was extremely important to examine events occurring very early, even prior to the appearance of the tumour. They had been doing so with a model of inflammatory response involving placement of a subcutaneous filter and enumerating the macrophages which appeared on the filter at appropriate times. This test could be used repetitively in the same animal and the results showed that in some but not all cancers which were arising spontaneously, abnormalities of inflammation did occur, although they were not yet certain how these findings related to the overall concept of surveillance.

**Dr D. Nolibe (France)** had also examined the effect of tumour growth on inflammatory macrophages. He had examined tumours induced by benzopyrene and those produced by a radioactive alpha-emitter. The macrophage inflammatory response had been measured using Professor Normann's implanted filter technique. With the benzopyrene tumour, macrophage depletion was concomitant with tumour growth and surgical ablation of the primary tumour suppressed the effect. However, with all types of radioactively induced tumour there was an increase in macrophage response despite the fact that the tumours were of different histological types, with different growth potential and metastatic potential. In a subsequent experiment they had studied the macrophage response during the 2-year latent period for the radioactively induced tumour and observed no change in this response. Thus, there was a clear difference between radioactively induced and chemically induced tumours in that precipitation of the former did not involve any defect in macrophage response. They also differed in other ways. The radioactively induced tumour with a latent period of 2 years was non-immunogenic. The benzopyrene induced tumour was immunogenic and had a latent period of only 130 days.

**Dr C. J. Dunn (France)** said that data presented earlier in the meeting also showed that immunological reactions reduced macrophage accumulation whereas non-immune reactions are without effect. Professor Normann's group had performed cross-transfusion of cell free sera and not found any factor released by the tumour or induced by the macrophage. However, an alternative explanation for results using the nitrocellulose disc method was simply that the macrophages were becoming less adhesive.

**Professor Normann** said that he would find it difficult to reconcile decreased adhesiveness with the yields of peritoneal macrophages coming from the pleural or peritoneal cavities. In addition, he often found that any abnormalities observed on the filter extended also to the cells in the cavities themselves. As to immunogenicity, he did not think that immunogenicity of the tumour exclusively determined whether it had an anti-inflammatory effect. He thought that further work would show that no single parameter was readily identifiable as the key to the host response.

**Dr Thompson (UK)** drew attention to recently reported results in which adjuvant arthritis and chemically induced tumours were mutually exacerbating. Thus, if the tumour were given after the adjuvant, then it increased, whereas if the adjuvant were given after the tumour, then the arthritis progressed. He felt that this might be connected with the inhibited monocyte response.

**Dr Nolibe** was then invited to describe his results on the effect of acute inflammatory processes on tumour development. He said that previous work had shown that during an acute non-immunological inflammation, factors were released which increased macrophage mitotic activity and rendered such cells cytotoxic to tumour cells *in vitro*. The present experiments had investigated the *in vivo* effect of an acute non-immunological inflammatory reaction on primary and metastatic tumour development. The inflammatory reaction was induced by intrapleural injection of dextran or calcium diphosphate. Results in three tumour models showed the effect varied according to the time of application of the inflammation with respect to tumour grafting. For example, with Lewis carcinoma, enhancement of primary and metastatic growth was observed when inflammation was produced 3 days before inoculation but not 3 days after. However, in a lung sarcoma model enhancement was observed if inflammation was induced on day 40. The interpretation of these differences was difficult but the general conclusion was that inflammation could exert an effect on tumour cell development.

**Professor Turk** commented that the effects of inflammation on resistance to infection were much more clear cut than the influence on tumour development. In the latter case one sometimes saw increased resistance but more often it was decreased. He wondered if Professor Giroud's group had examined a larger number of infectious organisms to which they might have found decreased resistance. Conversely, he wondered whether, if the numbers of tumours investigated had been increased, they might have found more direct evidence of increased resistance.

**Mlle M. Parant (France)** reported preliminary results on the pyrogenic effect of a synthetic adjuvant. The adjuvant, muramyl dipeptide (MDP) was a low molecular weight leukopeptide, an analogue of peptidoglycan. It represented the minimal active structure having both adjuvant and pyrogenic effect. It induced classical diphasic febrile responses in the rabbit and at the same time produced transferable circulating pyrogens. In rabbits made leukopenic with nitrogen mustard, MDP induced strong febrile response but failed to produce any circulating endogenous pyrogen. When given by the intraventricular route, no circulating antigen could be demonstrated although the pyrogenic effect was strongly increased. Both experiments indicated that MDP could have a direct pyrogenic effect, independent of production of endogenous pyrogens. Besides being a potent adjuvant, MDP represented a useful tool for studying fever. Indomethacin inhibited the febrile response to MDP but did not increase the other biological effects of the adjuvant.

**Professor Turk** asked whether MDP stimulated lymphokine release from lymphocytes *in vivo*. He wondered whether this might in part cause the pyrogen release.

**Mlle Parant** said that this was possible, because MDP could induce the production of pyrogens and at the same time the production of lymphocyte activating factor. However, the question had not so far been answered *in vivo*.

**Professor Turk** said that if lymphocytes were incubated with MDP and the supernatant produced a fever reaction then this suggested that at least part of the effect was due to lymphokine release.

**Dr W. Sluiter (Netherlands)** asked about the origin of the resident macrophages in the *in vitro* production of the pyrogenic factor. He also wished to know how many cells were being cultured.

**Mlle Parant** said that in experiments with rabbit peritoneal macrophages, the result with resident macrophages and induced macrophages were similar. As to cell numbers, they used $10^7$/ml.

**Dr Sluiter** said that for resident macrophages that was a large number. To his knowledge, one could harvest about $4 \times 10^6$ cells. This implied that the work was being carried out on rabbits which were not in a steady state. He also questioned Mlle Parant's conclusion from the nitrogen mustard experiment that MDP fever was caused by a direct action on the thermosensitive brain structures. To his knowledge, nitrogen mustard depleted the number of granulocytes and not the number of macrophages. They still remained and were the main source of the pyrogenic factor.

**Mlle Parant** said that one could not conclude that MDP did not affect macrophage numbers. There was a simultaneous decrease in PMNs and macrophages. In addition, after nitrogen mustard administration, when leukocyte counts were very low, fever occurred as in normal rabbits at a time when there was no circulating endogenous pyrogen.

# Section IX
# Lymphocytes

CHAIRMAN: C. M. Pearson
CO-CHAIRMAN: K. Trnavsky

# 100

# Comparative migration of guinea pig T and B lymphocytes from capillary tubes (Abstract)

R. J. SCHEPER, T. C. M. TH. VAN MAARSSEVEEN,
A. C. H. M. VAN DINTHER-JANSSEN AND
R. MULLINK (NETHERLANDS)

Using a capillary tube migration technique, a comparison was made between the random mobility of separated guinea pig T and B lymph node lymphocyte sub-populations and macrophage-rich peritoneal exudate cells. A decrease in random movement was found in that order, which would fit with the hypothesis that migration on a substrate is an adherence dependent phenomenon. In order to characterize a possible dichotomy between T and B cell locomotion, the effects of several factors which might interfere with their migration were studied. These factors included drugs which affect cell metabolism, cell surface ligands and some factors which may play a role in inflammatory foci (acidity, immune complexes and lymphokines). The results emphasize the similarity in the mode of locomotion of T and B lymphocytes. However, a remarkable difference was found in the stronger inhibition of B cell migration by pH values below pH 7.0.

# 101

# T lymphocyte sub-populations in rheumatoid arthritis

C. J. L. M. MEYER, G. J. M. LAFEBER, J. CNOSSEN, M. DAMSTEEG AND A. CATS (NETHERLANDS)

A variety of immunopathological findings indicate the involvement of the immune system in rheumatoid arthritis (RA), a disease of unknown origin. The finding of large numbers of T cells in the inflamed rheumatoid synovium[1,2] and the effect of T cell depletion by ductus thoracicus drainage during the course of the disease[3] suggests a role of the T lymphocyte in the pathogenesis of the disease. Recently human T lymphocytes have been classified[4] into two sub-populations with regard to the presence of receptors for immunoglobulin M or G. T lymphocytes with receptors for IgM ($T\mu$) contain a population of cells capable of enhancing immunoglubulin (Ig) synthesis by PWM stimulated B lymphocytes, whereas T cells with receptors for IgG ($T\gamma$) can suppress Ig synthesis in the same assay.

In the present study we investigated 24 RA patients with different degrees of activity for the presence of $T\mu$ and $T\gamma$ lymphocytes in the peripheral blood. Moreover, we tested these sera for lymphocytotoxic antibodies against T cell sub-sets. Lymphocytes were isolated from the peripheral blood by Ficoll–Isopaque density gradient centrifugation.

## T CELL SUB-POPULATIONS

B lymphocytes were characterized by the presence of surface Ig as earlier described[5]. T lymphocytes were assessed by their rosette formation with neuraminidase treated sheep erythrocytes (En). $T\mu$ and $T\gamma$ lymphocytes were detected by a recently developed mixed rosette assay using a combination of En and FITC labelled ox erythrocytes coated with either rabbit IgM or IgG antibodies[6]. Between the mean percentage of T lymphocytes in the peripheral blood of RA patients and of healthy donors no significant difference was found (75.5 ± 5.9 versus 71.7 ± 4.2). Also the mean percentage of B and Tγ lymphocytes of the RA patients did not differ from the healthy donors (for B lymphocytes 12.8 ± 1.3 versus 10.8 ± 2.0 and for Tγ 13.5 ± 4.1 versus 13.1 ± 1.3). The mean percentage of Tμ lymphocytes in the peripheral blood of the RA patients was significantly lower as compared with the healthy donors (30.6 ± 13.4 versus 57.4 ± 5.0).

Remarkable was the fact that very low percentages of Tμ lymphocytes were only found in patients with active disease as measured by BSE and Ritchie index. Table 101.1 presents the correlation between activity of the disease and mean percentages of Tμ and Tγ lymphocytes. These low values of Tμ lymphocytes were not caused by blocking of the Fcμ receptor by immune complexes since trypsin treatment of the lymphocytes followed by overnight incubation at 37 °C did not increase the percentage of Tμ lymphocytes.

**Table 101.1** Correlation between the mean percentage of Tμ and Tγ lymphocytes and degree of activity of rheumatoid arthritis

| | *Tμ* | *Tγ* |
|---|---|---|
| Active (BSE> 100, Ritchie index>20) $n = 7$ | 19 ± 8.3 | 12.4 ± 2.8 |
| Moderately active (BSE 50–100, Ritchie index 10–20) $n = 8$ | 26.8 ± 9.8 | 13.1 ± 5.5 |
| Not active (BSE<50, Ritchie index<10) $n = 9$ | 42.1 ± 8.4 | 14.6 ± 3.8 |
| Healthy donor $n = 10$ | 57.4 ± 5.0 | 13.1 ± 1.3 |

## CYTOTOXIC ANTIBODIES

Sera from patients with RA were tested for the presence of cytotoxic antibodies against lymphocyte populations from healthy donors and against lymphocyte populations enriched for T lymphocytes (% E rosette forming cells ≥ 95%), for Tμ lymphocytes (%Tμ lymphocytes ≥ 85%) and for Tγ lymphocytes (% Tγ lymphocytes ≥ 80%).

10 μl of cells (concentration $10 \times 10^6$c/ml) were incubated with 10μl test serum in microtitreplates for 1 h at 4°C. Next, 50 μl fresh rabbit complement was added and the mixture was incubated for 2 h at 15 °C. After staining with ethidium bromide the percentage of dead cells was scored.

The controls, including incubation with normal human serum and fresh rabbit complement or RA serum plus inactivated rabbit complement, never exceeded 10%. Anti-HLA activity could be excluded. Sera were considered to have cytotoxic activity when 30% or more dead cells were found. The results presented in Table 101.2 show that only patients with active disease had cytotoxic antibodies against Tμ lymphocytes. No cytotoxic activity against Tγ lymphocytes could be demonstrated.

**Table 101.2** Correlation between the mean percentage of Tμ lymphocytes and serum lymphocytotoxicity

| | | *Serum lymphocytotoxicity* | |
|---|---|---|---|
| *RA patients* | *Tμ* | *anti Tμ* | *anti Tγ* |
| Active | 19 ± 8.3 | 6/7 | 0/7* |
| Moderately active | 26.8 ± 9.8 | 2/8 | 0/8 |
| Not active | 42.1 ± 8.4 | 0/9 | 0/9 |

*One patient not tested.

## CONCLUSIONS

In patients with RA the percentage of Tμ lymphocytes in the peripheral blood is decreased as compared with the controls. Very low percentages of Tμ lymphocytes were associated with active disease and anti-Tμ antibodies. The finding of antibodies against T cell sub-sets in RA has also been demonstrated by Borel *et al.*[7] Low percentages of Tμ are not specific for RA because similar findings have been published for progressive systemic sclerosis and ageing humans[8,9].

Although the percentage of Tγ cells in the peripheral blood of the individual patients with RA varied more than in the control group, the mean percentage of Tγ cells in RA patients did not differ from the control group.

The finding that in patients with active RA the response of peripheral blood lymphocytes to PHA is decreased[10] correlates with the low percentage of Tμ lymphocytes in our patients, since this population contains the main proliferating cells after stimulation with mitogens[11].

### References

1 Bovel, J. A. van and Paget, S. A. (1875). Predominantly T cell infiltrate in rheumatoid synovial membranes. *N. Engl. J. Med.*, **293**, 517

2 Meyer, C. J. L. M., Putte, L. B. A. van de, Eulderink, F., Kleinjan, R., Lafeber, F. J. M. and Bots, G. TH. A. M. (1977). *J. Pathol.* **121**, 1

3 Wegelius, O., Laine, V., Lindstrom, B. and Klockars, M. (1970). *Acta Med. Scand.*, **187**, 539

4 Moretta, L., Webb, S. R., Grossi, C. E., Lydyard, P. M. and Cooper, M. D. (1977). Functional analysis of two human T cell subpopulations. *J. Exp. Med.*, **146**, 184

5 Putte, L. B. A. van de, Meyer, C. J. L. M., Lafeber, G. J. M., Kleinjan, R and Cats, A. (1976). Lymphocytes in rheumatoid and synovial fluids. *Ann. Rheum. Dis.*, **35**, 451

6 Cnossen, J., Lafeber, G. J. M., Damsteeg, W. G. M. and Meyer, C. J. L. M. (1980). Mixed rosette assay for the detection of Tμ and Tγ lymphocytes. *J. Immunol. Meth.*, **36**, 197

7 Borel, Y., Strelkaukas, A. J. Calley, R. T. and Schlossman, S. F. (1979). Anti T cell antibody

and loss of suppressor T cell in juvenile rheumatoid arthritis. *Arthritis Rheum.*, **23,** 595

8 Gupta, S. and Good R. A. (1979). Subpopulations of human T lymphocytes. X Alterations in T, B, Third population cells and T cells with receptors for IgM or IgG in ageing humans. *J. Immunol.*, **122,** 1214

9 Gupta, S. and Good, R. A. (1979). Subpopulation in human T lymphocytes. IX Imbalance of T cell subpopulations in patients with progressive systemic sclerosis. *Clin. Exp. Immunol.*, **38,** 342

10 Percy, J. S., Davis, P., Russell, A. and Brisson, E. (1978). A longitudinal study of *in vitro* tests for lymphocyte function in rheumatoid arthritis. *Ann. Rheum. Dis.*, **37,** 416

11 Hansen, G. S., Ruben, B. and Sprensen, S. F. (1977). Human leucocyte responses *in vitro*. I Transformation of purified T lymphocytes with and without addition of partially purified monocytes. *Clin. Exp. Immunol*, **29,** 295

# 102

# Enkephalins and the immune system (Abstract)

J. WYBRAN, T. APPELBOOM, A. GOVAERTS
AND J. P. FAMAEY (BELGIUM)

This study reports the *in vitro* influence of morphine, dextromoramide, levomoramide and methionine-enkephalin upon normal human T blood lymphocytes by using the active and total rosette tests, Morphine and dextromoramide inhibited the percentage of active T rosettes. This effect was completely reversed in the presence of naloxone, their specific antagonist. The specificity was further demonstrated by the absence of the effect of levomoramide, the inactive enantiomere, upon the rosette system. Methionine-enkephalin increased the percentage of active T rosettes. This effect was specifically inhibited by naloxone. These observations suggest that normal human blood T lymphocytes bear surface receptor-like structures for morphine, dextromoramide and methionine-enkephalin. Since non-opiate receptors have also been described on B lymphocytes, the 'two hits opioid lymphocyte receptor hypothesis' is presented. This theory postulates that opioid peptides can modulate the co-operation between T and B lymphocytes. Finally, such findings may provide a link betweeen the central nervous system and the immune system, and enkephalins may be the humoral mediators between the two systems.

# 103

# Experimental inhibition of E-rosette forming cells by *in vitro* incubation with adenosine, theophylline and verapamil

A. AUTERI, F. LAGHI PASINI AND T. DI PERRI (ITALY)

## INTRODUCTION

The E-rosette formation is a dynamic, energy-dependent property of human T lymphocytes. There is much evidence that critical metabolic processes such as oxidative phosphorylation[1], microfilament function[2], protein and nucleic acid synthesis[3], glycolysis[4], calcium intake[2] and intracellular nucleotide levels[5] are involved in this lymphocyte function. Therefore, the E-rosette formation may be inhibited *in vivo* as well as *in vitro* by any event that modifies one or more of these metabolic variables. It is well known that elevated intracellular levels of cAMP inhibit the E-rosette formation whereas elevated levels of cGMP augment the number of E-rosette forming cells[5,6].

Incubation of cholera toxin, dibutyril-cAMP, aminophylline or isoproterenol with human peripheral T lymphocytes markedly reduces the ability of these cells to form E rosettes[5,7], by an increase of intracellular cAMP. On the contrary, cholinergic agonists, by activating guanilate cyclase, are potent stimulators of E-rosette formation[8]. The activation of lymphocytes and the E-rosette formation seem to require the presence of divalent cations[2]; the transient opening of calcium channels is the crucial step for the induction of activation in T lymphocytes[9].

Moreover, it is well known that this lymphocyte sub-population is under thymic control, that is, mediated by humoral factor(s) produced by the epithelial cells of the thymus[10]. Recently, a pentapeptide (thymopoietin pentapeptide: TP5), synthesized by G. Goldstein, has been demonstrated to present the whole humoral property of thymic extract and to normalize T lymphocyte functions via a cGMP second signal (G. Goldstein, personal communication). As well as the thymic factor, levamisole, an anti-anergic chemotherapeutic agent, has been reported to normalize T lymphocyte functions and E-rosette formation by influencing cyclic nucleotide metabolism[11].

According to these premises, we have studied the *in vitro* effect of adenosine and theophylline (drugs known to interfere with nucleotide metabolism) and verapamil (a calcium channel blocker) on rosette forming cells (RFC). At the same time the possible role for levamisole and TP5 in reversing this inhibitory effect was investigated.

## MATERIALS AND METHODS

### E-rosette forming cells test

The E-rosette test was performed as described elsewhere[12]. *In vitro* effects of adenosine ($2.9 \times 10^{-5}$ mol/l final concentration), theophylline ($5.5 \times 10^{-5}$ mol/l final concentration) and verapamil ($2 \times 10^{-5}$mol/l final concentration) on RFC from healthy volunteers was evaluated. The drugs were incubated separately for 15 min at 37 °C with lymphocyte suspension, then the lymphocytes were washed three times in Hank's balanced salt solution (HBSS) before contact with sheep red blood cells (SRBC). *In vitro* effects of levamisole ($3.2 \times 10^{-5}$ mol/l final concentration) and TP5 ($1.33 \times 10^{-6}$ mol/l final concentration) on adenosine, theophylline and verapamil treated RFC was also evaluated. Lymphocyte suspension was incubated at the same time with adenosine, theophylline or verapamil and with levamisole or TP5. The incubation time was 15 min at 37°C; the lymphocytes were then washed three times with HBSS before the contact with SRBC. The effect of adenosine, theophylline and verapamil alone or with levamisole or TP5 on SRBC was also controlled. The drugs were added to the SRBC before contact with lymphocytes and were incubated for 15 min at 37 °C. Then SRBC were then washed three times in HBSS and added to lymphocyte suspension. The number of lymphocyte samples in the study were, respectively: adenosine and adenosine + levamisole = 29; adenosine and adenosine + TP5 = 5; theophylline and theophylline + levamisole or TP5 = 7; verapamil and verapamil + levamisole or TP5 = 6. The statistical analysis of the results was performed by the analysis of variance (one way).

## RESULTS

The results are shown in Figures 103.1–103.3. The incubation of lymphocytes

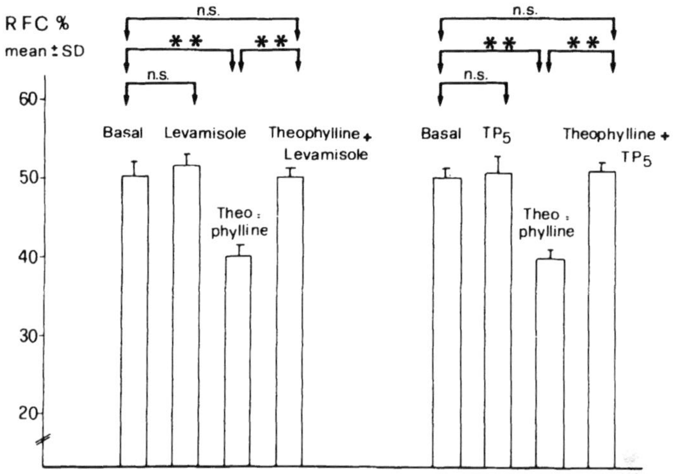


**Figure 103.1** Effect of TP5 and levamisole on theophylline-treated RFC

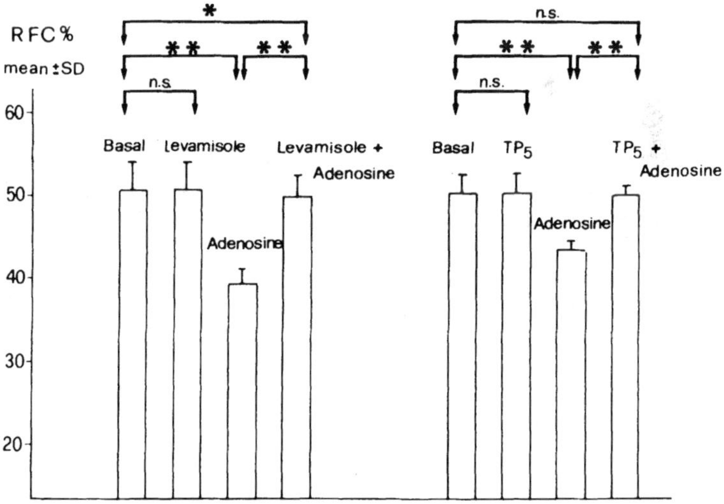


**Figure 103.2** *In vitro* effect of TP5 and levamisole on adenosine-treated RFC

from healthy subjects with adenosine or theophylline inhibits, in a statistically significant manner ($p = 0.000001$ and $p = 0.000001$), the number of E-rosettes. The quantitative inhibitory effect of the drugs seems to be very similar. In the same conditions levamisole or TP5 alone do not affect basal values. The inhibitory effect of theophylline is completely reversed by levamisole and TP5. The statistical analysis between basal values and theophylline plus levamisole or TP5 is not significant ($p = 0.26695$ and $p = 0.4890$). On the contrary, the difference of the means between theophylline-treated RFC and theophylline plus levamisole or TP5 is statistically highly significant ($p = 0.000001$ and $p = 0.000001$, respectively), thus showing a complete reversion of theophylline-induced inhibition of RFC. The same protective effect is shown by TP5 in adenosine-treated RFC: the difference of the means between basal values and adenosine plus TP5 is not significant ($p = 0.12230$), while the difference of the means between adenosine and adenosine plus TP5 is statistically highly significant ($p = 0.00009$). Levamisole also shows an effect on adenosine-treated RFC and there is a statistically significant difference between adenosine and adenosine plus levamisole ($p = 0.000001$), but there is also a residual statistically significant difference between basal values and adenosine plus levamisole, showing that levamisole is not able to reverse completely the inhibitory effect of adenosine ($p = 0.02693$). Verapamil inhibits in a highly significant manner the number of RFC ($p = 0.000001$). Neither levamisole nor TP5 restore the verapamil-inhibited RFC. The addition of the drugs to SRBC before the contact with lymphocytes does not modify the number of RFC.

## DISCUSSION

Our results show that *in vitro* addition of adenosine and theophylline markedly reduces the number of RFC. The effect of theophylline is probably mediated by the intracellular increase of cAMP due to the inhibition of phosphodiesterase, while adenosine acts by increasing the adenylate cyclase activity.

Levamisole and TP5 do not modify normal basal values but they are able to reverse the inhibitory effect of adenosine and theophylline in our experimental model. According to our premises, it seems to be likely that TP5 and levamisole act by restoring a normal intracellular cAMP/cGMP ratio or by preventing cAMP increase.

Verapamil, a calcium channel blocker, is able to inhibit *in vitro* the E-rosette formation. A transient opening of calcium channels seems to be a crucial step for the activation of T lymphocytes[9] and E-rosette formation could be correlated to intracellular concentration of calcium[2].

In lymphocyte mitogenic activation, calcium ions appear to act as a second

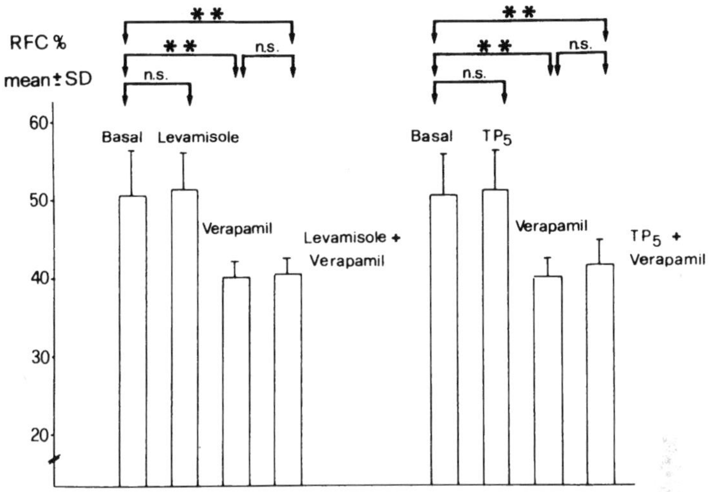


**Figure 103.3** *In vitro* effect of TP5 and levamisole on verapamil-treated RFC

messenger, associated with the effects mediated by cyclic nucleotides, Calcium ion is known to increase cGMP levels by activating guanilate cyclase[13]. On the other hand, calcium influx during lymphocyte activation is increased by dibutyril-cGMP and decreased by dibutyril-cAMP[9,14]. These findings show the complex inter-relationships that exist between cyclic nucleotide metabolism and intracellular calcium availability.

Levamisole and TP5 do not reverse the inhibitory activity of verapamil, thus confirming that they act at a different level of metabolic processes involved in E-rosette formation. The inhibition of RFC by the direct blocking of calcium transmembrane influx cannot be reversed by the modulating effect on cyclic nucleotide metabolism of TP5 and levamisole.

Our results confirm that E-rosette formation is a metabolic-dependent property of human T lymphocytes in which cyclic nucleotide metabolism and calcium intake are involved. Findings show that it is possible to anticipate an *in vitro* pharmacological manipulation that could clarify some physiological mechanism of lymphoid function.

**Acknowledgment**
The authors gratefully acknowledge Janssen Pharmaceutica-Beerse, Belgium, for the kind gift of TP5 synthesized by G. Goldstein.

## References


1 Bentwich, Z., Douglas, S. D., Siegal, F. P. and Kunkel, H. G. (1973). Human lymphocyte-sheep erythrocyte rosette formation: some characteristics of the interaction. *Clin. Immunol. Immunopathol.*, **1,** 511

2 Kersey, J. H., Hom, D. J. and Buttrick, P. (1974). Human T-lymphocyte receptors for sheep erythrocytes: conditions for binding including inhibition by cytochalasin B. *J. Immunol.*, **112,** 862

3 Bushkin, S. C., Pantic, V. S. and Incefy, G. S. (1974). Studies on the mechanism of human peripheral lymphocyte receptors formation in vitro. *Fed. Proc.*, **33,** 629

4 Jondal, M. G., Holm, G. and Wigzel, H. (1972). Surface markers on human T and B lymphocytes: I- A large population of lymphocytes forming non-immune rosettes with sheep red blood cells. *J. Exp. Med.*, **136,** 207

5 Chisari, F. V. and Edgington, T.S. (1974). Human T lymphocyte "R" rosette function. I- A process modulated by intracellular cyclic AMP. *J. Exp. Med.*, **140,** 1122

6 Gillette, R. W., Mckenzie, G. O. and Swanson, M. H. (1974). Modification of the lymphocyte response to mitogens by cyclic AMP and GMP. *J. Reticuloendothelial Soc.*, **16,** 289

7 Galant, S.P. and Remo, R. A. (1975). Beta-adrenergic inhibition of human T lymphocyte rosettes. *J. Immunol.*, **114,** 512

8 Strom, T. B., Lundin, A. P. and Carpenter, C. B. (1977). The role of cyclic nucleotides in lymphocyte activation and function. In Schwartz, R. S. (ed.) *Progress in Clinical Immunology*, Vol. 3 p. 115. (Grune and Stratton)

9 Freedman, M. H., Raff, M. C. and Gomperts, B. (1975). Induction of increased calcium uptake in mouse T lymphocytes by Concanavalin A and its modulation by cyclic nucleotides. *Nature (London)*, **255,**378

10 Dardenne, M. and Bach, J. F. (1973). Studies on thymus products. I- Modification of rosette forming cells by thymic extracts. Determination of the target RFC subpopulation. *Immunology*, **25,**343

11 Hadden, J. W., Coffey, R. G., Hadden, E. M., Lopez-Corrales, E. and Sunshine, G. H. (1975). Effects of levamisole and imidazole on lymphocyte proliferation and cyclic nucleotide levels. *Cell. Immunol.*, **20,** 98

12 Di Perri, T., Auteri, A., Laghi Pasini, F., Mattioli, F. and Volpi, L. (1978). A weekly oral dose of levamisole in the treatment of rheumatoid arthritis associated with E-rosette lymphocytes reduction. *Eur. J. Rheumatol. Inflam.*, **1,** 155

13 Hardman, J. D., Beavo, J. A., Gray, J. P., Chrisman, T. D., Patterson, W. D. and Sutherland, E. W. (1971). The formation and metabolism of cyclic GMP. *Ann. N.Y. Acad. Sci.*, **185,** 27

14 Whitney, R. B. and Sutherland, E. W. (1972). Enhanced uptake of calcium by transforming lymphocytes. *Cell. Immunol.*, **5,** 137

# 104

# Lymphocytes bearing Fcγ receptors in rheumatoid arthritis: binding properties of the Fc receptors detected by Facb rosettes and 'high avidity' EA rosettes

VIVIENNE R. WINROW AND N. D. HALL (UK)

## INTRODUCTION

The various immunological functions carried out by lymphocytes bearing receptors for the Fc portion of IgG (FcR) have become the subject of increasing research interest in recent years. These functions include regulation of the immune response[1] and antibody-dependent (K cell) cytotoxicity[2]. Such cells may therefore be important in the pathogenesis of diseases such as rheumatoid arthritis (RA), in which aberrant immune responses and tissue damage mediated by immunological mechanisms play a significant role.

A number of assays have been developed to identify FcR-positive cells, including binding of aggregated IgG[3] and EA rosette formation with IgG-coated ox erythrocytes[4] and human erythrocytes sensitized with anti-CD (Ripley) IgG[5]. More recently, several authors have demonstrated that different assay techniques measure different sub-populations of FcR-positive lymphocytes[6–9]. Such observations offer the opportunity to analyse the functions of particular FcRs on various cell types.

A number of reports have shown an increased proportion of FcR-bearing lymphocytes in the peripheral blood of patients with RA[10–12], although the cell population involved has not been identified. Recently, a novel assay has been described which uses rabbit Facb-sensitized calf erythrocytes to form rosettes with mononuclear cells[13]. This technique also detects an increased proportion of FcR-positive cells in rheumatoid patients. Further studies have demonstrated that the Facb rosette-forming cells form a sub-group of non-T, non-B, 'null' lymphocytes[14]. They appear to be similar to lymphocytes identified by other techniques as 'third population' cells[5], L cells[15] and UL cells[16]. Such lymphocytes are considered to express 'high avidity' FcRs, which bind monomeric IgG at 4 °C but not at 37 °C[15] and which form human EA (Ripley) rosettes[5,17].

Since the relationship of Facb-rosetting cells to those above is unclear, experiments were performed to compare the lymphocyte receptors detected by Facb rosettes and by 'high avidity' EA rosettes in terms of their sensitivity to incubation at 37 °C, and their binding specificity for various human and rabbit IgG preparations.

## METHODS

### Mononuclear cell preparation

Heparinized peripheral blood was obtained from patients with classical or definite rheumatoid arthritis receiving non-steroidal anti-inflammatory drug therapy only. Mononuclear cells were prepared from the blood by density flotation over Ficoll–Paque (Pharmacia)[18]. The interface cells were harvested, washed twice with phosphate buffered saline (PBS) and adjusted to $2 \times 10^6$ cells/ml in PBS. In some experiments, lymphocytes were incubated for 30 min at 37 °C as described by Pang and Wilson[8] to remove labile IgG from the cell membrane.

### Facb and 'high avidity' EA rosettes

Calf red blood cells (RBC) were obtained fromTissue Culture Services Ltd. (Slough) and were used to raise an anti-calf RBC serum in rabbits. The IgG fraction of the antiserum was purified on protein A–Sepharose CL-4B[19], and the Facb fragment prepared from this IgG by plasmin digestion[20]. This Facb was incubated with the calf erythrocytes and the sensitized cells used to form Facb rosettes with the rheumatoid lymphocytes as previously described[13]. Low levels of the IgG (anti-calf RBC) were treated similarly to form 'high avidity' EA rosettes.

When rosette inhibition studies were being carried out, the potential competitor was added in a small volume (20 μl) relative to the rosette assay mixture (400 μl) to give a final concentration of 40 μg/ml. Additions to the incubation tube were in the order: first competitor, then lymphocytes, and finally, coated calf erythrocytes. In each experiment, the percentage rosette formation in the absence of competitor was given the value 100, and the effect of the competitor related to this.

**Preparation of IgG and fragments**

Human IgG was purified from both healthy and rheumatoid serum by ion-exchange chromatography on DEAE-cellulose[21]. Samples of IgG were aggregated by incubation at 63 °C for 15 min. Myeloma sera of known IgG isotype were obtained either from the Royal United Hospital, Bath, or as generous gifts from other laboratories. We wish to thank Dr C J Elson (University of Bristol), Dr P M Johnson (University of Liverpool) and Dr P I Gaarder (Statensinstitutt fur Folkehelse, Oslo) for providing some of the IgG myeloma proteins used in this sudy.

IgG was also purified from normal rabbit serum by affinity chromatography on protein A–Sepharose CL-4B. Fragments of rabbit IgG were obtained following digestion with plasmin (Facb + pFc′), pepsin ($F(ab')_2$) and papain (Fab + Fc) as previously described[22]. All IgG samples and fragments were kept frozen in aliquots at −196 °C and were thawed once only before use in rosette inhibition studies.

## RESULTS

The effect of incubation at 37 °C on the proportion of cells binding Facb and 'high avidity' EA rosettes is shown in Table 104.1. It can be seen that Facb-rosette formation by rheumatoid lymphocytes was unaffected by this procedure. However, the formation of 'high avidity' EA rosettes was decreased in a number of samples following incubation.

**Table 104.1** Effect of incubation at 37 °C on the formation of Facb and 'high avidity' EA rosettes

| | *% Rosettes* | | | |
|---|---|---|---|---|
| | *Facb* | | *'High avidity' EA* | |
| *Patient* | *Pre-inc* | *Post-inc* | *Pre-inc* | *Post-inc* |
| Mi | 8 | 6 | 9 | 8 |
| Ha | 7 | 8 | 12 | 7 |
| Wh | 10 | 8 | 20 | 6 |
| Ri | 8 | 7 | 10 | 10 |
| Cu | 14 | 13 | 19 | 10 |

Lymphocytes from 5 rheumatoid patients were used to form Facb and 'high avidity' EA rosettes. Assays were set up before and after incubation of the lymphocytes for 30 min at 37 °C.

A comparison of the binding specificities exhibited by the receptors involved in both Facb and 'high avidity' EA rosette formation was undertaken using a number of IgG preparations to block the binding of the coated calf RBC. These was no difference in the actual rosette formation in the two assays in the absence of competitor. Mean values were 11% for Facb rosettes and 10% for 'high avidity' EA rosettes. The effect of various human IgG samples on the two assays is shown in Figure 104.1. Monomeric human IgG, either from healthy or from rheumatoid serum, did not block either rosette assay at the concentration used, but the same preparations were strongly inhibitory following heat aggregation. Using heat-aggregated myeloma proteins of known isotype, both receptors were shown to bind strongly to IgG3 and IgG1, weakly to IgG4 and not at all to IgG2. At least two different myeloma proteins of each isotype were used in these experiments.

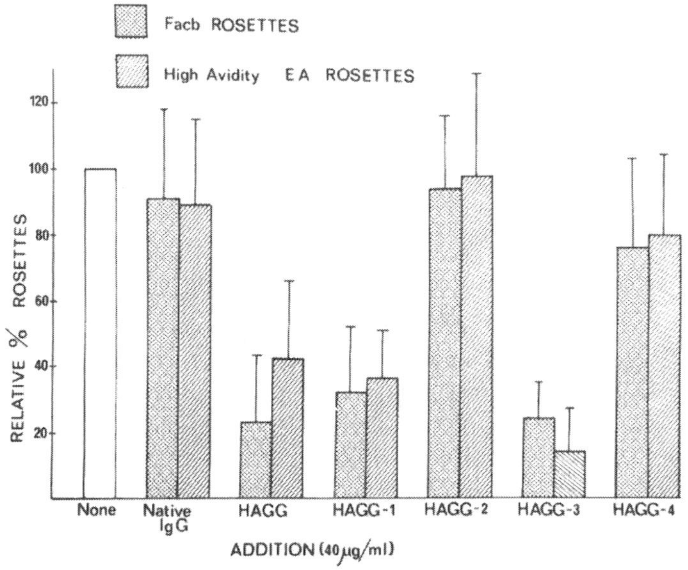


**Figure 104.1** Inhibition of Facb rosettes and 'high avidity' EA rosettes by various human IgG preparations. Lymphocytes from RA patients were used to form rosettes with Facb or IgG sensitized calf RBC. Competitor samples were included in the rosette assay at a final concentration of 40 μg/ml. Rosette formation in the presence of competitor was expressed relative to rosette formation in control assays in the absence of competitor (= 100). Each column and bar represents the mean ± 1 standard deviation of between 8 and 15 separate experiments. There was no difference in the actual proportion of Facb rosettes (mean 11%) and 'high avidity' EA rosettes (mean 10%) in the control assays. HAGG – heat aggregated serum IgG, HAGG – 1,2,3,4 – heat aggregated myeloma proteins of known isotype

Rosette inhibition assays similar to those with human IgGs shown in Figure 104.1 were also carried out with various rabbit IgG fragments. Results of these experiments are given in Figure 104.2. Native rabbit IgG monomer and Facb fragments inhibited both Facb and 'high avidity' EA rosette formation, but $F(ab')_2$ fragments were only inhibitory in the Facb rosette assay. The difference in the effect of $F(ab')_2$ on Facb rosette and 'high avidity' EA rosettes was significant ($p<0.01$). Fab fragments were inactive in both systems. As expected, Fc fragments inhibited both rosette assays, but the effect was much more marked on 'high avidity' EA rosettes ($p<0.01$). This selectivity of Fc fragments is thus opposite to that shown by $F(ab')_2$. The fragment of rabbit IgG consisting only of the Cγ3 domains – pFc' – did not affect Facb rosettes, but caused some enhancement of 'high avidity' EA rosette formation.

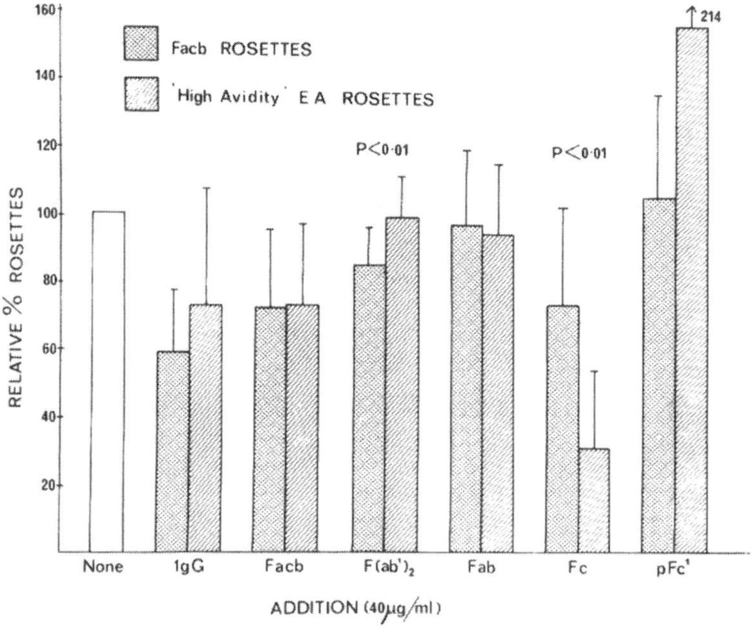


**Figure 104.2** Inhibition of Facb rosettes and 'high avidity' EA rosettes by various rabbit IgG fragments. Lymphocytes from RA patients were used to form rosettes with Facb or IgG sensitized calf RBC. Competitor samples were included in the rosette assay at a final concentration of 40 μg/ml. Rosette formation in the presence of competitor was expressed relative to rosette formation in control assays in the absence of competitor (= 100). Each column and bar represents the mean ± 1 standard deviation of between 8 and 15 separate experiments. There was no difference in the actual proportion of Facb rosettes (mean 11%) and 'high avidity' EA rosettes (mean 10%) in the control assays. Where indicated, groups of data were compared using the Student's t test

## DISCUSSION

This study was undertaken in order to investigate whether the Facb rosette technique identifies FcR distinct from those detected using more conventional assays such as calf RBC sensitized with low levels of IgG antibody or human erythrocytes + Ripley anti-CD antiserum ('high avidity' EA rosettes). The latter technique is considered to be a marker for non-T, non-B, 'null' lymphocytes[5,17,23]. The FcR on these cells (L cells) bind monomeric IgG at 4 °C but not at 37 °C[15]. The proportion of cells forming Facb rosettes was, however, unaffected by incubation at 37 °C and was not blocked by native human IgG at 4 °C. This suggests that the Facb receptor is not identical to that reported on L cells. The loss of some cells forming 'high avidity' EA rosettes on incubation at 37 °C may reflect the adherence of monocytes, since these cells have been reported to form human EA (Ripley) rosettes[24]. Removal of monocytes by phagocytosis of carbonyl iron has been shown not to affect Facb rosette formation[13].

The formation of both Facb and 'high avidity' EA rosettes was inhibited by aggregated human IgG far more effectively than by monomeric IgG. Both receptors showed specificity for $IgG_1$ and $IgG_3$, with little binding of $IgG_4$ and $IgG_2$. This pattern of isotype binding is similar to the FcR specificity of lymphocytes detected with human EA (Ripley) rosettes[25] and of monocytes[26] but differs from that of cytotoxic K cells[27–29]. However, when rabbit IgG fragments were used to block rosette formation, different patterns of inhibition were obtained, suggesting some differences in binding specificity of the receptors detected in the two rosette systems.

In molar terms, the 'high avidity' EA rosettes were inhibited equally by IgG and Fc, a result in close agreement with data obtained with human EA (Ripley) rosettes[25] and cytotoxic K cells[27]. The inhibitory effect of Facb fragment on the EA assay supports the conclusion of these authors that the FcR involved binds mainly to the $C\gamma 2$ region of the IgG. However, a rosette assay for FcR with $C\gamma 2$ specificity, Facb rosettes, shows a different spectrum of inhibition by rabbit IgG fragments. Fc was much less inhibitory in this assay than equimolar amounts of native IgG. Also $F(ab')_2$ fragments, but not Fab, were significantly active in blocking Facb rosette formation, indicating that the hinge region is part of the structure recognized by the Facb receptor. These results, together with data from the human IgG competition experiments, suggest that this receptor may show selective binding of immune complexes, or at least an altered structure in the hinge plus $C\gamma 2$ region of IgG.

This 'immune complex-like' structure is present in monomeric rabbit but not human IgG. A lymphocyte receptor with such specificity might have important functions both in cytotoxic mechanisms and in the regulation of immune responses by immune complexes. However, preliminary results suggest that Facb-rosetting cells do not have K cell activity[14]. Several other assays based on Facb rosette depletion are being undertaken to elucidate the function of this receptor and of the cells expressing it. Such studies should help to explain the increased proportion of these cells in the peripheral blood of rheumatoid patients and their role in the disease process.

**Acknowledgment**

This work was supported by a grant from the Arthritis and Rheumatism Council for Research.

## References

1 Moretta, L., Webb, S. R., Grossi, C. E., Lydyard, P. M. and Cooper, M. D. (1977). Functional analysis of two human T-cell subpopulations: help and suppression of B-cell responses byT-cells bearing receptors for IgM or IgG. *J. exp. Med.*, **146,** 184

2 Perlmann, P., Perlmann, H. and Wigzell, H. (1972). Lymphocyte-mediated cytotoxicity *in vitro*. Induction and inhibition by humoral antibody and nature of effector cells. *Transplant.Rev.*, **13,** 91

3 Dickler, H. B. and Kunkel, H. G. (1972). Interaction of aggregated γ -globulin with B lymphocytes. *J. Exp. Med.*, **136,** 191

4 Hallberg, T., Gurner, B. W. and Coombs, R. R. A. (1973). Opsonic adherence of sensitized ox red cells to human lymphocytes as measured by rosette formation. *Int. Arch. Allergy*, **44,** 500

5 Frøland, S. S. and Natvig, J. B. (1973). Identification of three different human lymphocyte populations by surface markers. *Transplant.Rev.*, **16,** 114

6 Clements, P. J. and Levy, J. (1978). Receptors for IgG (Fc receptors) on human lymphocytes: re-evaluation by mulitple techniques. *Clin. Exp. Immunol.*, **34,** 281

7 Gormus, B. J., Woodson, M. and Kaplan, M. E. (1978). Heterogeneity of human lymphocyte Fc receptors. I. Differential susceptibility to proteolysis. *Clin. Exp. Immunol.*, **34,** 268

8 Pang, G. and Wilson, J. D. (1978). Different rosette assays for detecting Fc receptor-bearing lymphocytes measure different subpopulations. *Immunology*, **35,** 407

9 Winchester, R. J., Hoffman, T., Ferrarini, M., Ross, G. D. and Kunkel, H. G. (1979). Comparison of various tests for Fc receptors on different human lymphocyte subpopulations. *Clin. Exp. Immunol.*, **37,** 126

10 Bach, J. -F., Delrieu, F. and Delbarre, F. (1970). The rheumatoid rosette. A diagnostic test unifying seropositive and seronegative rheumatoid arthritis. *Am. J. Med.*, **49,** 213

11 Sharpin, R. K. C. and Wilson, J. D. (1977). Increased EA-rosette formation by lymphocytes from patients with rheumatoid arthritis. *Clin. Exp. Immunol.*, **29,** 205

12 Wooley, P. H. and Panayi, G. S. (1978). Studies of lymphocytes in rheumatoid arthritis. I. Uptake of $^{125}$1-heat aggregated human IgG by Fc-receptor bearing lymphocytes. *Ann. Rheum. Dis.*, **37,** 343

13 Hall, N. D., Winrow, V. R. and Bacon, P. A. (1980). Lymphocytes bearing Fcγ receptors in rheumatoid arthritis. I. An increased subpopulation of cells in RA detected with Facb rosettes. *Ann. Rheum. Dis.* (In press)

14 Hall, N. D. and Winrow, V. R. (1980). Lymphocytes bearing Fcγ receptors in rheumatoid arthritis. III. Increased subpopulation of 'null' lymphocytes in RA detected by Facb rosettes. (Submitted for publication)

15 Horwitz, D. A. and Lobo, P. I. (1975). Characterisation of two populations of human lymphocytes bearing easily detectable surface immunoglobulin. *J. Clin. Invest.*, **56,** 1464

16 Dickler, H. B. (1976). Lymphocyte receptors for immunoglobulin. *Adv. Immunol.*, **24,** 167

17 Lobo, P. I. and Horwitz, D. A. (1976). An appraisal of Fc receptors on human peripheral blood B and L lymphocytes. *J. Immunol.*, **117,** 939

18 Böyum A. (1968). Isolation of mononuclear cells and granulocytes from human blood. *Scand. J. Clin. Lab. Invest.*, **21,** (Suppl. 97), 77

19 Hjelm, H., Hjelm, K. and Sjöquist, J. (1972). Protein A from Staphylococcus aureus. Its isolation by affinity chromatography and its use as an immunosorbent for isolation of immunoglobulins. *FEEBS Lett.*, **28,** 73

20 Stewart, G. A., Smith, A. K. and Stanworth, D. R. (1973). Biological activities associated with the Facb fragment of rabbit IgG. *Immunochemistry*, **10,** 755

21 Ishizaka, K., Ishizaka, T., Lee, H. L. and Fudenberg, H. H. (1965). Immunochemical properties of human γ A isohaemagglutinin. 1. Comparison with γ G and γM globulin antibodies. *J. Immunol.*, **95,** 197

22 Hall, N. D. (1978). Leucocyte migration inhibition with IgG-IgG complexes and rabbit IgG fragments in patients with rheumatoid arthritis. *Clin. Exp. Immunol.*, **34,** 219

23 van Oers, M. H. J., Zeijlemaker, W. P. and Schellekens, P. Th. A. (1977). Separation and properties of EA-rosette-forming lymphocytes in humans. *Eur. J. Immunol.*, **7,** 143

24 Shaw, G. M., Levy, P. C. and Lobuglio, A. F. (1979). Re-examination of the EA rosette assay (Ripley) for Fc receptor leucocytes. *Clin. Exp. Immunol.*, **36,** 496

25 Frøland, S. S., Michaelsen, T. E., Wisløff, F. and Natvig, J. B. (1974). Specificity of receptors for IgG on human lymphocyte-like cells. *Scand. J. Immunol.*, **3**, 509
26 Huber, H. and Fudenberg, H. H. (1968). Receptor sites of human monocytes for IgG. *Int. Arch. Allergy*, **34**, 18
27 Wisløff, F., Michaelsen, T. E. and Frøland, S. S. (1974). Inhibition of antibody-dependent human lymphocyte-mediated cytotoxicity by immunoglobulin classes, IgG subclasses and IgG fragments. *Scand. J. Immunol.*, **3**, 29
28 Simchowitz, L. and Schur, P. H. (1976). Antibody-dependent lymphocyte-mediated cytotoxicity. The nature of the effector cell and characterisation of its Fc receptor. *Scand. J. Immunol.*, **5**, 759
29 Spiegelberg, H. L., Perlmann, H. and Perlmann, P. (1976). Interaction of K lymphocytes with myeloma proteins of different IgG subclasses. *J. Immunol.*, **117**, 1464

# 105

# 'L' lymphocytes, immune complexes and the amplification of human T lymphocyte proliferation

D. A. HORWITZ AND E. M. CARVALHO (USA)

Immune complexes have an important role in the regulation of the immune response. IgG complexed to specific antigen can enhance or suppress lymphocyte proliferation *in vitro*. We have focussed our attention on augmentation of lymphocyte proliferation and have described the conditions required for enhancement by immune complexes, identified the lymphocyte population mediating this effect and have described a mechanism of action[1,2]. These studies will be summarized in this report. We will show that 'L' lymphocytes amplify T cell proliferation. 'L' lymphocytes are the C3 receptor negative sub-set of non-T non-B cells and comprise approximately 10% of blood lymphocytes in healthy individuals. The surface markers and functional properties of L cells have been well characterized[3,4].

Subjects were immunized with keyhole limpet haemocyanin (KLH) and lymphocytes from these sensitized donors were stimulated with either KLH alone or the antigen complexed to rabbit IgG anti KLH. In some experiments, cells from non-sensitized donors were used. A quantitative precipitin curve with $^{125}$I-labelled KLH was performed in order to calculate the amount of IgG required to prepare immune complexes at equivalence and to determine the antigen content of the precipitates. Lymphocytes were incubated in flat bottomed microwells in RPMI 1640 culture medium supplemented with antibiotics and 15% heat inactivated pooled human AB serum. The cells were incubated for 5 days, pulsed with tritiated thymidine and prepared for scintillation spectrometry.

Figure 105.1 shows the response of lymphocytes from sensitized and unsensitized donors to KLH (40 μg) and in a similar amount of antigen complexed to IgG after 3–6 days of culture. These studies revealed that lymphocytes from non-sensitized donors failed to respond to either antigen alone or IgG complexed to KLH. In some experiments, cells from non-sensitized donors were incubated with immune complexes in the presence of fresh serum. Although C3b activation by immune complexes can stimulate lymphocytes to produce lymphokines[5] we found no evidence that complement activation can stimulate lymphocytes to proliferate.

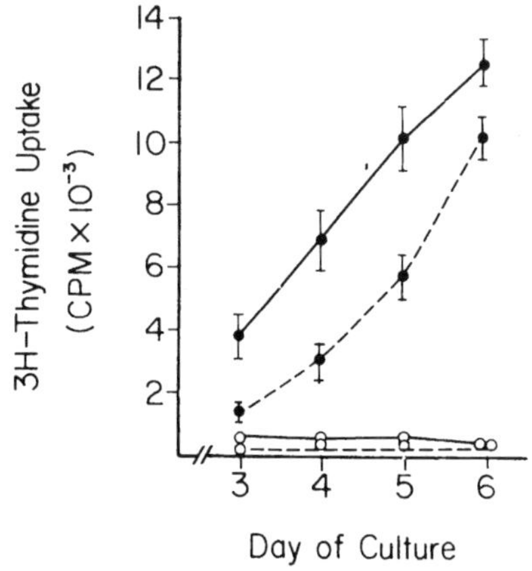


**Figure 105.1** Response of sensitized and non-sensitized lymphocytes to KLH and KLH-IgG–anti-KLH. 2 × $10^5$ mononuclear cells were stimulated with 40 μg KLH alone ( . . . ) or immune complexes of KLH-IgG–anti-KLH (———) containing the same amount of antigen. Cultures were harvested after a 4 h pulse with [$^3$H]thymidine on days 3 to 6. ● indicate studies with sensitized lymphocytes; ○ show studies with unsensitized lymphocytes. Counts/min of unstimulated cultures ranged from 240 ± 87 (day 3) to 596 ± 117 (day 6)

Figure 105.1 also shows that immune complexes stimulated lymphocytes from sensitized donors to proliferate 36 h earlier than cells stimulated by antigen alone. This augmentation of blastogenesis was much more pronounced during days 3 to 5 and began to disappear by day 6. Therefore, we harvested cells on day 5 in all of the succeeding experiments.

Figure 105.2 shows the effects of immune complexes prepared with various concentrations of KLH. Blastogenesis induced by these complexes was compared with that induced by an equivalent amount of antigen alone. These studies revealed three separate effects.

(1) The maximum stimulation of immune complexes was significantly greater than that induced by antigen alone.

(2) Marked enhancement of blastogenesis by immune complexes was evident at lower concentrations of KLH. When concentrations of KLH

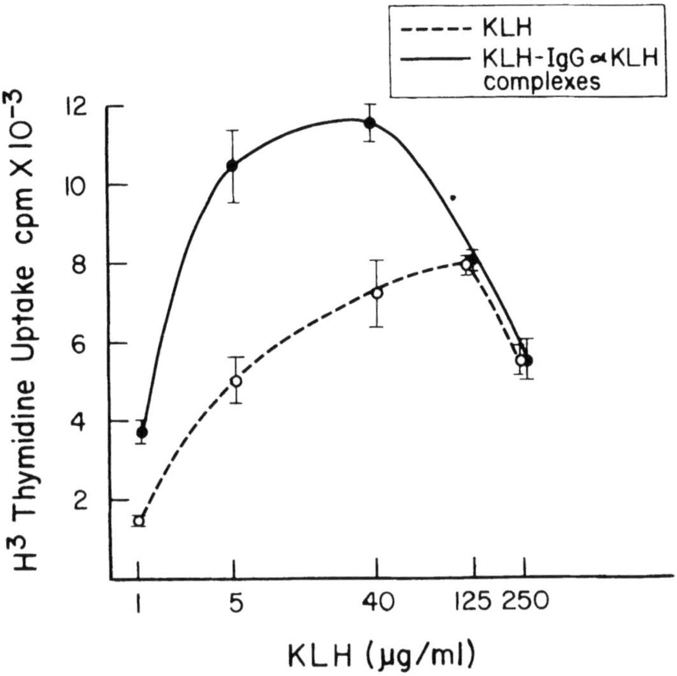


**Figure 105.2** Dose-response curve of the proliferative response of sensitized lymphocytes to KLH antigen alone, or to immune complexes of KLH-IgG–anti-KLH. $2 \times 10^5$ mononuclear cells in 0.2 ml were incubated with various concentrations of either stimulant for 6 days. [$^3$H] thymidine uptake in unstimulated cultures was less than 950 ct/min. Each point represents the mean of triplicate replicates ± standard error of the mean

one-tenth to one-half that required for the optimal response were complexed to IgG antibody, these complexes elicited a blastogenic response which was 2–4-fold greater than that induced by antigen alone

(3) When complexes were made with high concentrations of antigen, the enhancing effects of the complexes were abolished.

This last effect may be explained by reaching a threshold for activation of suppressor cells. Therefore, in the remainder of the experiments shown, complexes containing 40 μg of KLH were used. These complexes invariably produced enhancement of blastogenesis.

Figure 105.3 shows that lymphocytes with high avidity Fc receptors for IgG are required for the enhancement phenomenon. In these experiments, cells bearing Fc receptors for IgG were depleted by adherence to immobilized BSA–anti-BSA immune complexes, a procedure which depletes both monocytes and certain lymphocytes. Surface markers on the Fc receptor-depleted cells revealed an increase in E-rosette forming T cells and an increase in Ig positive B cells. Fc receptors on B cells detected by EA rosettes with IgG sensitized bovine RBC were demonstrated. However, high avidity Fc receptors detected by Ripley EA rosettes were absent. When monocytes were added back to Fc depleted cells, these preparations were able to respond well to antigen alone, but the enhancement phenomenon was abolished.

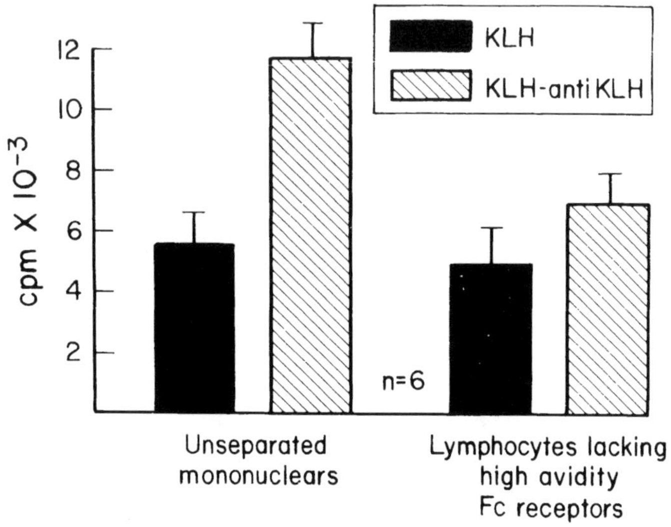


**Figure 105.3** Lymphocytes with high avidity Fe-IgG receptors were required for immune complex-induced enhancement. Mononuclear cells were depleted of monocytes and lymphocytes which attached to plastic-immobilized immune complexes, after which physiological concentrations of monocytes ($2 \times 10^4$ of 10%) were added back. Unseparated mononuclear cells were used as controls. Cells were stimulated with 40 μg of either uncomplexed or complexed KLH for 5 days. Counts per minute of unstimulated unseparated mononuclears was 528 ± 85, and Fc receptor depleted mononuclears was 543 ± 101

A role for 'L' cells in the enhancement phenomenon was revealed in the next series of experiments. Lymphocytes were fractioned into T cells by E rosetting and B and 'L' cells by negative selection. B cells were prepared by incubating non-T cells on petri dishes with immobilized BSA–anti–BSA immune complexes and harvesting the non-adherent cells. 'L' cells were prepared by incubating non-T cells on monolayers of EAC, and removing the C3 receptor negative non-adherent cells. In these studies only preparations containing T cells, 'L' cells and monocytes were able to show the enhancement phenomenon[2].

Previous studies from this laboratory have revealed that some Tγ cells possess high avidity Fc receptors for IgG[6]. Studies were undertaken to determine whether certain Tγ cells could also enhance lymphocyte proliferation. In these experiments KLH–anti–KLH immune complexes were immobilized to the flat bottomed wells of microtitre plates. Next, either the T cells or non-T cells were added to the wells in concentrations that would yield equivalent numbers of Tγ or 'L' cells sticking to the immobilized complexes. After the non-adherent cells were removed, a constant number of Fc receptor depleted lymphocyte preparations were added to the wells. Table 105.1 shows that wells containing Tγ cells failed to show enhancement but that 'L' cells were able to mediate this phenomenon.

**Table 105.1** Non-T lymphocytes are required for enhancement of blastogenesis mediated by immune complexes

| | | *Counts per minute ± SEM* | |
|---|---|---|---|
| *Step 1* | *Step 2* | *KLH* | *immobilized KLH* |
| None | unseparated mononuclear cells | 7,929 ± 137 | 15,933 ±2,402 |
| None | Fc-IgG receptor depleted lymphocytes | 6,557 ±402 | 8,538 ±554 |
| T γ cells adherent to immobilized immune complexes | Fc-IgG receptor depleted lymphocytes | | 8,821 ±200 |
| Non-T cells adherent to immobilized immune complexes | Fc-IgG receptor depleted lymphocytes | | 16,276 ±1,190 |

We considered the possibility that Tγ amplifier cells were present, but were masked by another sub-set of activated suppressor cells. In other studies lymphocytes were irradiated to inactive suppressor cells. The results, however, were identical to those with unirradiated cells.

Several possible hypotheses were entertained to explain the mechanism of 'L' cell-mediated enhancement of lymphoycte blastogenesis. The first was that immune complexes might stimulate 'L' cells to proliferate after binding to Fc receptors.The results shown in Table 105.2 do not support this suggestion and reveals that IgG antibody must be complexed to specific antigen for enhancement of blastogenesis. In these studies lymphocytes were cultured with bovine serum albumin (BSA)–anti BSA complexes. These immune complexes did not enhance lymphocyte proliferation. Moreover, an interaction of 'L' cells and BSA–anti–BSA complexes did result in the production of soluble factors potentiating the T lymphocyte response to KLH.

The second hypothesis considered was that stimulated T cells might induce 'L' cells to proliferate. The result shown in Table 105.3 exlude this possibility.

**Table 105.2** IgG antibody must be complexed to specific antigen for enhancement of blastogenesis

| *Additive* | *Counts/min* ± *SEM* |
|---|---|
| KLH | 6,297 ± 698 |
| KLH -anti-KLH | 15,909 ± 125 |
| BSA - anti-BSA | 54 ± 28 |
| BSA - anti-BSA + KLH | 5,229 ± 583 |

The values shown are after the counts per minute of unstimulated cells (954 counts/min) have been subtracted. 2 × $10^5$ mononuclear cells were added to each microwell.

**Table 105.3** L cells enhance T cell reactivity

| | *Counts per minute mean* ± *SEM* | | |
|---|---|---|---|
| | *Unstimulated* | *KLH* | *KLH – anti-KLH complex* |
| Unseparated mononuclear cells | 993 ± 23 | 7,123 ± 204 | 15,305 ± 107 |
| T cells | 1,083 ± 709 | 3,027 ± 602 | 5,050 ± 554 |
| T + L cells | 1,224 ± 290 | 5,622 ± 721 | 15,239 ± 818 |
| T + L cells (m) | 1,779 ± 113 | 5,002 ± 1,243 | 13,168 ± 885 |

L cells were treated with mitomycin 25 μg/ml.

In these experiments either T cells or 'L' cells were treated with mitomycin in order to block their capacity to divide. We observed that treatment of 'L' cells with mitomycin did not affect the magnitude of blastogenesis, whereas, as expected, mitomycin treatment of T cells completely abolished the proliferative response.These experiments demonstrated that 'L' cells do not participate in the blastogenic response, but instead they amplify T cell reactivity.

The third hypothesis considered was that 'L' cells might possess an accessory cell function similar to that of monocytes. Figure 105.4 shows the results of these studies.When T cells were mixed with monocytes the response to antigen was similar to that of unseparated mononuclear cells, but enhancement was not observed. T cell–'L' cell combinations responded poorly and the response observed could be explained by the small contamination of 'L' cell preparations with monocytes. A combination of 'L' cells, monocytes and T cells completely restored the enhancing effects of immune complexes. 'L' cell enhancement of T cell reactivity is, therefore, a monocyte-dependent event.

The ineffectiveness of monocyte–T cell combinations might be explained by insufficient numbers of functional monocytes. In additional studies not shown, cultures containing up to 20% monocytes did not respond to KLH–

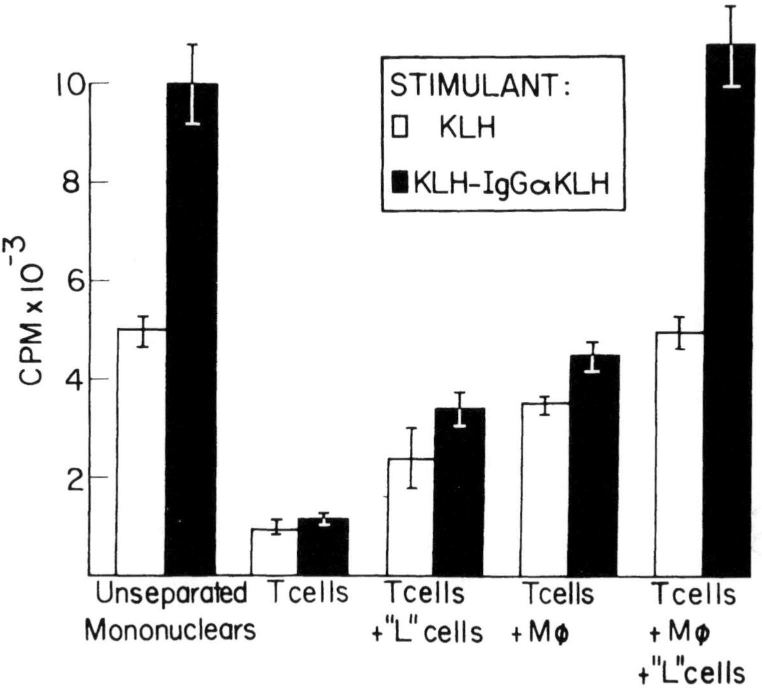


**Figure 105.4** Immune complex elicited enhancement of antigen-specific blastogenesis requires a combination of T cells, monocytes, and 'L' cells. T cells ($1.5 \times 10^5$) were incubated alone or with $2.5 \times 10^4$ 'L' cells and/or monocytes (Mø) and stimulated with uncomplexed KLH or IgG anti-KLH containing 40 µg/ml of antigen (see Materials and Methods). Values indicate the mean ± SEM of three separate experiments

anti–KLH immune complexes as well as unseparated mononuclear cells[2].

The fourth hypothesis considered was that 'L' cells might have a unique 'antigen-presentation' mechanism of action. In these studies either T cells, monocytes, or 'L' cells were incubated with either KLH or KLH–anti–KLH for 30 min at 37 °C and the antigen was removed from the cultures by repeated washing. These antigen-pulsed cells were transferred to microwells to which unseparated mononuclear cells were added. As reported by others, monocytes pulsed with antigen have the capacity to initiate a blastogenic response[7]. 'L' cells lack this capacity (Figure 105.5). Monocytes incubated with immune complexes can also trigger a proliferative response and the magnitude of this response was similar to that of uncomplexed antigen pulsed monocytes. 'L' cells pulsed with immune complexes trigger a proliferative response two-fold greater than that of monocytes.

These studies have revealed that 'L' cells can bind immune complexes to Fc receptors and present free antigenic determinants to other cells. It is possible

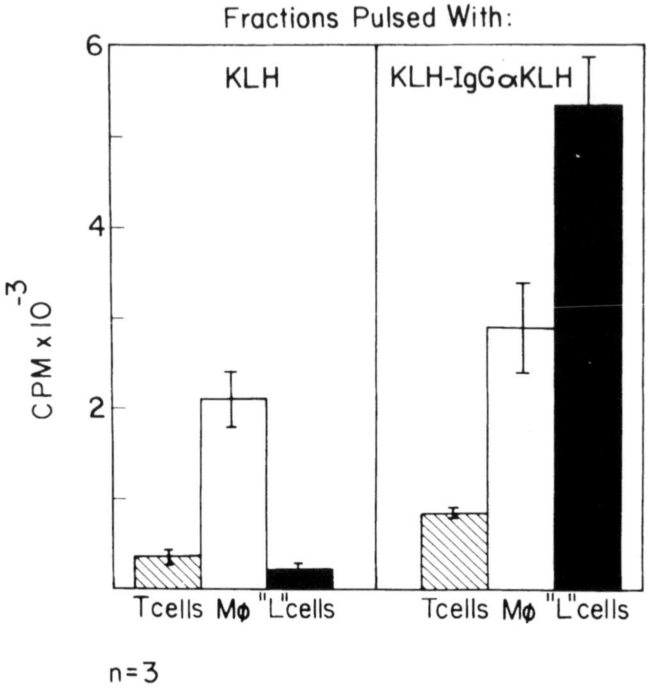


**Figure 105.5** A comparison of the antigen-presenting capacities of monocytes and 'L' cells. 5 × $10^4$ monocytes (Mø), 'L' cells or T cells were briefly exposed to either KLH alone or KLH-IgG-anti-KLH, washed, and added to microwells containing 2 × $10^5$ unstimulated, autologous mononuclear cells (see Materials and Methods). Values shown indicate the mean ± SEM of three separate experiments. Counts per minute of simultaneous cultures not stimulated with antigen have been subtracted from counts per minute of stimulated cultures

that passively bound antigen linked closely to *Ia* structures, present on approximately one-half of 'L' cells, may serve as recognition units for sensitized cells. It is important to emphasize that the effect of 'L' cells on T cell proliferation requires a macrophage intermediate. Further studies are required to define the specific sub-set of 'L' cells which mediate this effect and to define more precisely the 'antigen-presentation' mechanism. A perpetuation of T cell proliferation caused by 'L' cells that have interacted with certain immune complexes may be an important factor in the chronicity of some human inflammatory diseases.

The accessory function described in this report and the recently reported similarity between the cytotoxic properties of 'L' cells and monocytes[8] suggest a relationship between these two cell types. It is clear that blood 'L' cells can be distinguished from macrophages on the basis of electron microscopy[4], histochemical techniques (esterase and peroxidase staining)[3,4], and

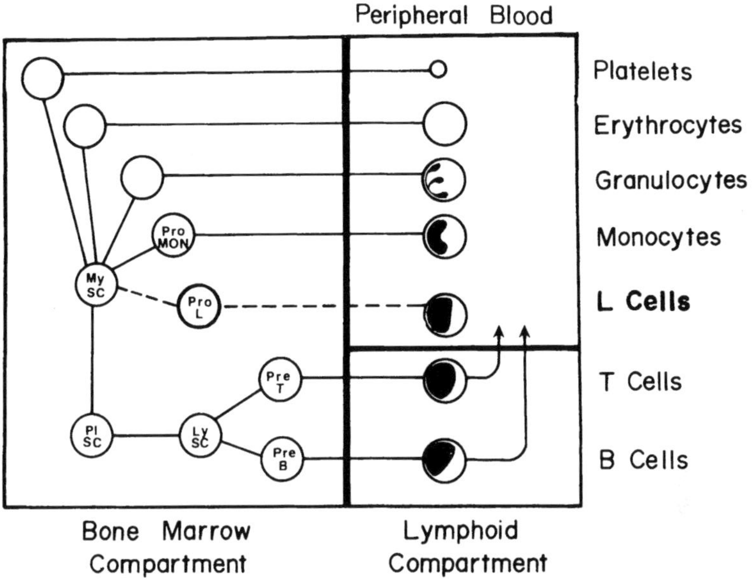


**Figure 105.6** Hypothesis for the origin of 'L' cells. Abbreviations: P1 SC, pluripotent stem cell; Ly SC, lymphoid stem cell; My SC, myeloid stem cell: Pro Mon. promonocyte; Pro L, precursor of 'L' cells

functional characteristics[3]. Moreover, there is no evidence that 'L' cells are monocyte precursors. 'L' cells lack the capacity to proliferate[3] and remain esterase negative and non-phagocytic after 4 days of incubation *in vitro* (unpublished observations). Figure 105.6 illustrates a probable origin of 'L' cells. These cells may be derived from a precursor in the bone marrow phylogenetically related to that of monocytes. The present 'L' cell precursor may reflect an incomplete differentiation from monocytes to lymphocytes and thus explain the fact that 'L' cells possess features common to both cell types.

## References


1 1 Carvalho, E. M., Davis, J. S. and Horwitz, D. A. (1979). Conditions required for Fc-dependent immune complex enhancement of antigen-specific lymphocyte blastogenesis. *J. Immunol*, **124,** 565

2 Carvalho, E. M. and Horwitz, D. A. (1980). Characterization of a non-T, non-B human blood lymphocyte that mediates the enhancing effects of immune complexes on lymphocyte blastogenesis. *J. Immunol*, **124,**

3 Horwitz, D. A. and Garrett, M. A. (1977). Distinctive functional properties of human blood L lymphocytes: a comparison with T lymphocytes, B lymphocytes, and monocytes. *J. Immunol.*, **116,** 437

4 Horwitz, D. A., Niaudet, M. F., Greaves, J. D. and Deteix, P. (1978). Surface markers and electron microscopy of human blood L cells: a comparison with T and B lymphocytes. *J. Immunol*, **121,** 678

5 Wahl, S. M., Iverson, G. M. and Oppenheim, J. J. (1974). Induction of guinea pig B-cell lymphokine synthesis by mitogenic and non-mitogenic signals to Fc, Ig and C3 receptors. *J. Exp. Med*, **140,** 1631

6 Horwitz, D. A., Cooper, M. and Carvalho, E. (1979). Binding characteristics of Fc receptors for IgG on human peripheral blood Tγ lymphocytes and 'L' lymphocytes: a technical report. *Clin. Immunol. Immunopathol*, **14,** 159

7 Rosenthal, A. S., Lipsky, P. E. and Shevach, E. M. (1975). Macrophage-lymphocyte interaction and antigen recognition. *Fed. Proc.*, **34,** 1743

8 Horwitz, D. A., Allison, A. C., Ward, P. and Kight, N. (1977). Identification of human mononuclear leucocyte populations by esterase staining. *Clin. Exp. Immunol.* **30,** 289

# 106

# Influence of anti-inflammatory drugs on PHA-stimulated lymphocyte proliferation with variable numbers of macrophages

H. MULLINK, MARY VON BLOMBERG-VAN DER FLIER, J. ZAAGSMA AND J. OORT (NETHERLANDS)

## INTRODUCTION

Together with macrophages, lymphocytes are known to be the predominant cell type in chronic inflammatory infiltrates. In order to establish the influence of anti-inflammatory drugs (AID) on the function of these cells, we studied the *in vitro* effect of AID in lymphocyte transformation tests (LTT) with phytohaemagglutinin (PHA). This mitogen is known to induce proliferation of T-lymphocytes nonspecifically.

The depressant effect of AID on lymphocyte proliferation has been shown in several reports[1-8]. Apart from an inhibitory effect at higher concentrations, one of the AID, indomethacin, has recently been shown to possess an enchancing effect at moderate concentrations[9-12]. We investigated a broad concentration range of eight AID on PHA-stimulated lymphocyte proliferation in order to establish both enhancing and inhibitory effects. The experiments revealed that four of the drugs did show both these effects.

It is well known that macrophages are necessary for lymphocyte activation[13-16], but recently suppressor effects of macrophages on lymphocyte functions have also been reported[17-20]. Often these suppressive effects are masked by the stimulatory effects, but in some clinical and experimental investigations they could be clearly demonstrated[21,22]. Since it has been reported that macrophages can secrete prostaglandins[19,23–25] and that prostaglandins depress the LTT[19,26,27], prostaglandins secreted by the macrophages are probably involved as suppressing agents.

To test if the enhancement of the lymphocyte proliferation obtained with moderate concentrations of the AID could be due to suppression of the secretion of these macrophage products, additional experiments were performed with variable proportions of macrophages present in the lymphocyte cultures.

## MATERIALS AND METHODS

### Preparation of cells

Lymphoid cell suspensions were obtained from outbred, female guinea pigs (TNO, Holland), weighing 250–350 g, 3–4 weeks after sensitization with Freund's complete adjuvant. Lymph nodes were removed aseptically and minced with scissors in culture medium. The dead cells in the lymphoid cell suspensions were removed by centrifugation through Ficoll–Isopaque cushions (density 1.077 g/ml; 20 min at 1000 *g*). After washing three times the cells were resuspended to a concentration of $4 \times 10^6$ cells per ml in culture medium[28]. Cell suspensions obtained in this way consisted of 4–7% macrophages and 20–25% B lymphocytes as was established by combined monocyte esterase staining and EAC rosetting[29]. 60–65% of the cells were T lymphocytes, which were identified by their ability to form rosettes with rabbit erythrocytes[30].

Macrophage-rich cell suspensions were obtained from the same animals 4 days after intraperitoneal injection of paraffin oil. The peritoneal cavity was washed out aseptically with 50–100 ml Hanks' balanced salt solution (BSS) and the obtained cell suspension was centrifuged for 10 min at 400 *g*. After washing three times with BSS these cells were also suspended in culture medium at a concentration of $4 \times 10^6$ cells/ml. The percentage of macrophages, which was 80–90%, was established by monocyte esterase staining in suspension, using a haemocytometer[29].

Lymphoid cell suspensions, containing 30% macrophages were obtained by mixing lymph node cell suspensions with peritoneal exudate cells in the required proportion. In all cell suspensions, cell viability was estimated in a haemocytometer by vital dye (eosin) exclusion. Medium RPMI 1640 containing 10% heat-inactivated fetal calf serum (Flow, Irvine, Scotland), 100 U penicillin and 75 μg gentamicin per ml was used as diluent and cell culture medium.

### Lymphocyte transformation test

$2 \times 10^5$ cells in 50 μl aliquots to which 100 μl of drug or control solutions were added, were cultured in round-bottomed microtitre plates (Linbro/Titertek,

Hamden, USA). Phytohaemagglutinin (PHA, Wellcome, Beckenham, England) was added to the cell suspensions immediately before filling the wells at a final dilution of 1:750. After 2 days of culture 0.4 $\mu$Ci [$^3$H]thymidine (Amersham/Searle, Chicago, USA) was added; the cultures were harvested 22 h later with a Titertek microharvester and [$^3$H] thymidine incorporation was measured by liquid scintillation counting and expressed as the mean counts per minute (ct/min) of sextuplicate cultures. In each experiment the ct/min of the cultures without drug were considered as control values and the mean mean ct/min of the cultures with drug expressed as a percentage of the control value.

**Drugs**

The following drugs were used: acetyl salicylic acid, indomethacin (gift from Merck, Sharp and Dohme), mefenamic acid (gift from Parke Davis), phenylbutazone and oxyphenbutazone (gifts from Geigy), benzydamine hydrochloride and hydrocortisone hemisuccinate (gifts from Organon) and dexamethasone. Immediately before use the drugs were dissolved in RPMI 1640, except mefenamic acid, which was first dissolved in 0.1 NaOH, diluted 1:5 with RPMI 1640, and neutralized with HCl. Then serial dilutions were made in culture medium.

## RESULTS

The effects of increasing concentrations of the anti-inflammatory drugs on PHA-stimulated guinea pig lymphoid cell cultures are evaluated as dose–response curves in which the 100% level represents the PHA-induced [3H]-thymidine uptake in the absence of drugs (Figures 106.1–106.3). As can be seen, some curves only show inhibition of lymphocyte proliferation, whereas in others this depressant effect is preceded by stimulation.

Looking at the inhibitory part of the curves, three different categories can be distinguished. First, the steroidal AID hydrocortisone and dexamethasone, which show a very gradually descending slope of the curve. Secondly, the non-steroidal drugs indomethacin, oxyphenbutazone and benzydamine, which all show a significantly steeper slope of the dose–response curve, and finally, acetyl salicylic acid, mefenamic acid, and phenylbutazone, showing a sudden onset of the inhibition and a very strong concentration-dependence.

The inhibitory part of the dose–response curve is preceded by a stimulatory part with four of the drugs (indomethacin, mefenamic acid, acetyl salicylic acid and phenylbutazone). This stimulation is rather strong in the case of mefenamic acid and less strong, although still significant, with the other three.

In order to test whether the stimulation observed in some of the dose-response curves might be due to a diminished secretion of inhibitory

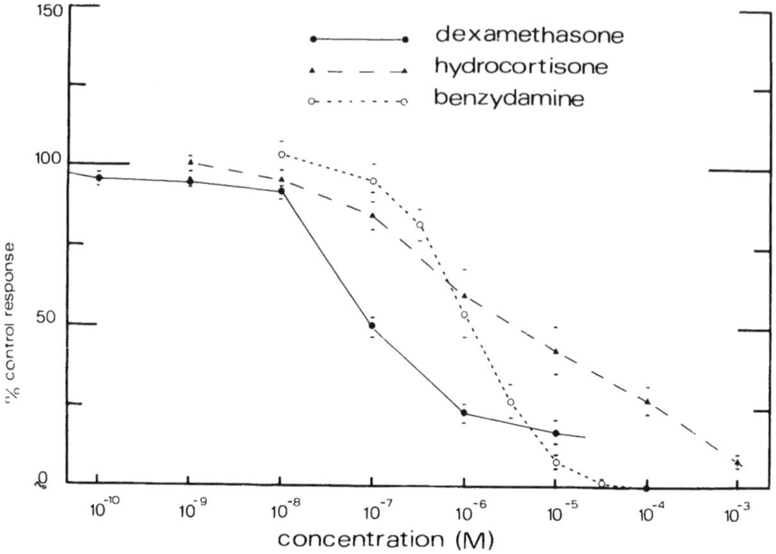


**Figure 106.1** Dose-dependent effects of benzydamine, hydrocortisone and dexamethasone on PHA-stimulated lymphocyte proliferation. The data are presented as the mean ± SEM of several experiments and are expressed as percentages of control cultures without drug

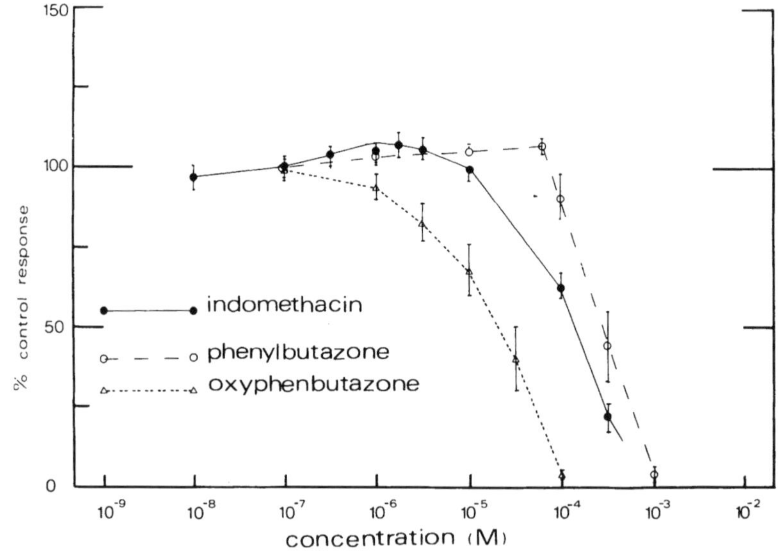


**Figure 106.2** Dose-dependent effects of phenylbutazone, oxyphenbutazone and indomethacin on PHA-stimulated LTT. The data are presented as in Figure 106.1

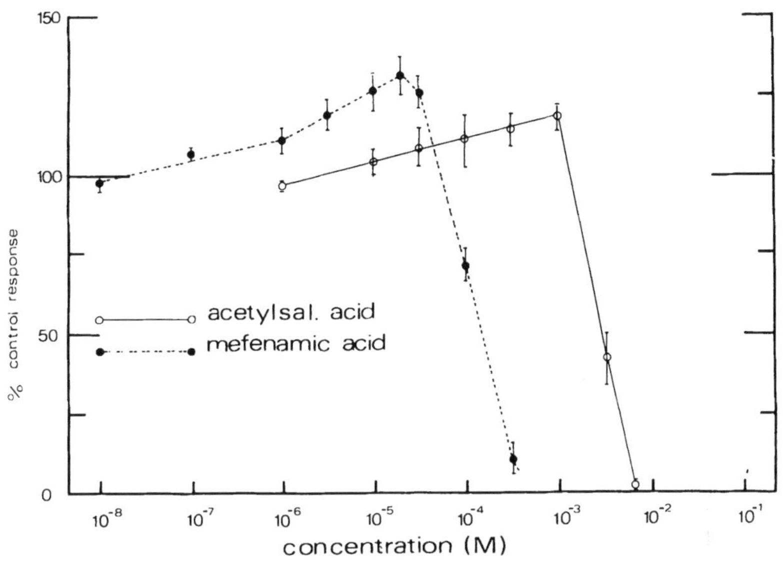


**Figure 106.3** Dose-dependent effects of mefenamic acid and acetyl salicylic acid on PHA-stimulated LTT. The data are presented as in Figure 106.1

mediators by the macrophages present, another series of lymphocyte cultures was studied. In these experiments autologous peritoneal macrophages were added to part of the lymph node cell suspensions, in such a way that two suspensions were obtained with 5 and 30% macrophages, respectively. The effects of AID on the PHA-induced lymphocyte proliferation of these cell suspensions were compared, and are shown in Figures 106.4–106.7. Here again, the data are expressed as percentages of ct/min of control cultures without drugs (n.b., Mean [$^3$H]thymidine uptake in lymph node cell cultures, 14 000 ct/min; mean [$^3$H]thymidine uptake in macrophage-supplemented cultures, 20 000 ct/min).

Figure 106.4 shows the results for indomethacin. The mean stimulation at the optimal concentration ($3 \times 10^{-6}$ mol/l) proved to be increased from 114 to 131% by the addition of macrophages. Figure 106.5 shows that the stimulation induced by mefenamic acid was increased from 116 to 134%. In contrast, with benzydamine, which did not show a stimulant effect in the original cell suspension (with 5% macrophages), a shift to the right of the dose-response curve was observed in the presence of 30% macrophages. Figure 106.6 shows a mean shift, at 50% inhibition from $1.6 \times 10^{-6}$ to $4.8 \times 10^{-6}$ mol/l. A different picture is seen in Figure 106.7, where the mean effect of acetyl salicylic acid on the PHA-induced proliferation of the two cell suspensions is shown. Here the most striking aspect is not the slight enhancement of the stimulation, but the shift of the inhibitory part of the

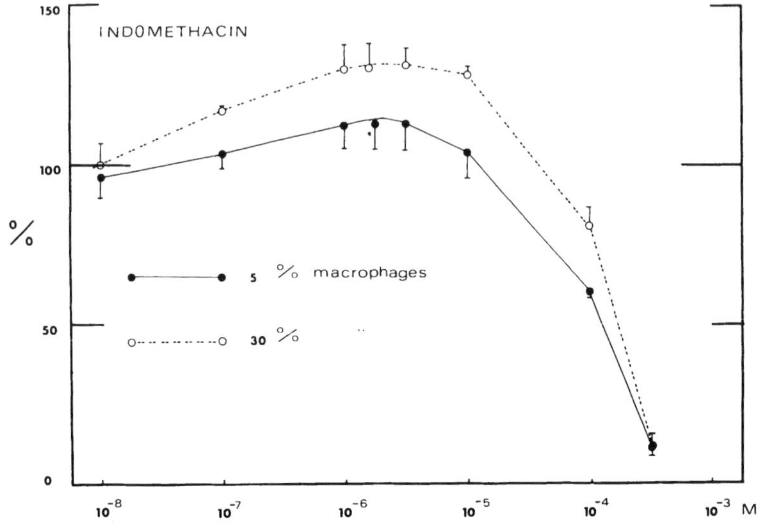


**Figure 106.4** Dose-dependent effects of indomethacin on PHA-stimulated LTT with 5 and 30% macrophages. Data are presented as the mean ± SEM of three experiments and are expressed as percentages of control cultures without drug

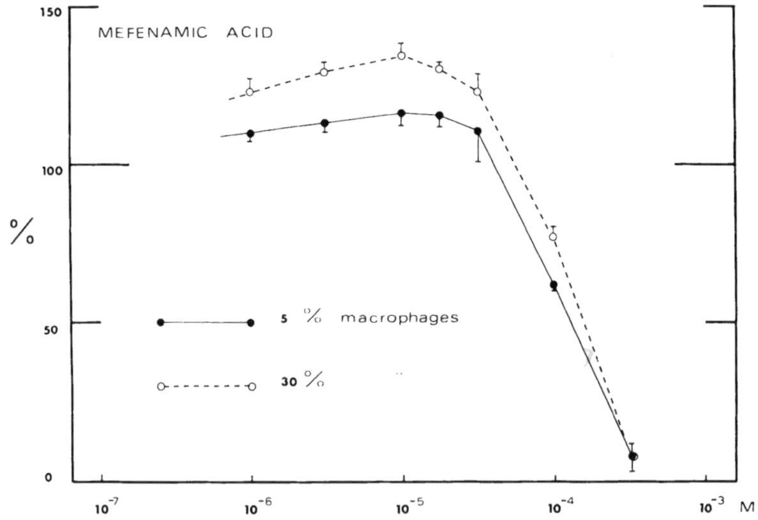


**Figure 106.5** Dose-dependent effects of mefenamic acid on PHA-stimulated LTT with 5 and 30% macrophages. Data are presented as in Figure 106.4

curve to the left. With dexamethasone, oxyphenbutazone and phenylbutazone no significant difference was found between the two cell suspensions. However, the effects of these drugs were only studied once (data not shown).

## DISCUSSION

Figures 106.1–106.3 show all drugs to be inhibitory to lymphocyte transformation at high concentrations. This immunosupressing effect of AID was considered at least partly responsible for the anti-inflammatory action of the drugs *in vivo*[1–6]. Recently, however, a number of other compounds have been shown to possess this property as well[7,52,53]. We are probably dealing with a non-specific, membrane-disordering effect. It is known that low concentrations of surface-active compounds (like AID) possess a membrane-stabilizing action but that higher concentrations are directly lytic to biological membranes[31]. In contrast, hydrocortisone, dexamethasone and benzydamine, with low $IC_{50}$ values of $3.6 \times 10^{-6}$, $10^{-7}$ and $10^{-6}$ mol/l (Table 106.1), respectively, probably have an immunosupressing effect at physiological concentrations. Preliminary experiments to detect the direct toxic action on PHA-stimulated lymphocyte cultures indeed showed a drug-induced cytotoxicity at concentrations which, for these three drugs, are considerably higher than the $IC_{50}$ values shown in Table 106.1. For the other drugs studied, these values seem to correspond with each other (unpublished data). It should be noted, however, that the well-known immunosupressive action of the corticosteroids found *in vivo* is partly due to a direct action on the lymphocytes[32–34].

As shown in Figures 106.4–106.7, stimulation of lymphocyte proliferation can be enhanced by adding macrophages to the cultures, which suggests that the stimulating action of moderate concentrations of the drugs is mediated by the macrophages present. It is well known that a minimum number of macrophages is required to induce lymphocyte proliferation, but higher numbers seem to be suppressive[15,20]. These two effects of macrophages on lymphocyte proliferation are reported to be dependent both on cell-to-cell contacts and on soluble factors[13,15,17,19,21].

The suppressing factors produced by the macrophages are probably prostaglandins of the E-type. These inflammatory modulators are known to be secreted by activated macrophages[19,23–25] and it has been found that they can inhibit lymphocyte functions[19,26,27,35–37]. Since mitogen-stimulated lymphocytes are able to produce lymphokines which in turn can activate the macrophages, a balance seems to exist between these two cell types and their products[38–41].

The drugs, which in our experiments appeared to enhance lymphocyte proliferation, are all well-known inhibitors of prostaglandin synthesis[25,42,43]

**Table 106.1** Inhibiting and enhancing effects of anti-inflammatory drugs on PHA-stimulated lymph node cell suspensions containing about 5% macrophages. The data are collected from Figures 106.1–106.4

| | *Inhibition* | *Enhancement* | |
|---|---|---|---|
| | $IC_{50}$ (mol/l) | *Concentration giving maximal enhancement* (mol/l) | *% enhancement* |
| Acetyl salicylic acid | $1.4 \times 10^{-3}$ | $1 \times 10^{-3}$ | 18 |
| Indomethacin | $1.26 \times 10^{-4}$ | $1 \times 10^{-6}$ | 8 |
| Phenylbutazone | $2.45 \times 10^{+4}$ | $6 \times 10^{-5}$ | 7 |
| Oxphenbutazone | $2 \times 10^{-5}$ | — | — |
| Mefenamic acid | $1.15 \times 10^{-4}$ | $2 \times 10^{-5}$ | 31 |
| Benzydamine HC1 | $1.15 \times 10^{-6}$ | — | — |
| Hydrocortisone h.s. | $3.65 \times 10^{-6}$ | — | — |
| Dexamethasone | $1 \times 10^{-7}$ | — | — |

Moreover, the sequence of drug concentrations producing maximal stimulation (indomethacin > mefenamic acid > phenylbutazone > acetyl salicylic acid corresponds with the reported potencies of these drugs for inhibition of prostaglandin synthesis[42]. These facts strongly suggest that the drug-induced enhancement is due to inhibition of prostaglandin secretion by the macrophages. Recent reports have described immunological enhancement by indomethacin under several experimental conditions as well as in clinical investigations[9–12,22,44–47]. When the enhancement by indomethacin found in our system is compared with some of these reports, it seems rather small, but, as indicated above, the interaction between lymphocytes and macrophages is dependent on many factors: the type of lymphocytes, the mitogen, the type and activation state of the macrophages etc.[9,13,15–17,20,48].

Considering that the dose–response curves, shown in Figures 106.4–106.7, are the resultant of two opposite effects, one of which reflects inhibition of lymphocyte proliferation and the other inhibition of prostaglandin production, then the influence of the increased number of macrophages can be explained readily. In Figures 106.4, 106.5 and 106.7, inhibition of prostaglandin secretion by indomethacin, mefenamic acid, and acetyl salicylic acid, respectively, starts at lower concentrations than those which cause inhibition of lymphocyte proliferation. With more macrophages present, the resultant curve shifts upwards, as shown in Figures 106.4 and 106.5. With benzydamine, however, which is a rather weak inhibitor of prostaglandin synthesis[43,49], the inhibition of lymphocyte proliferation already starts at concentrations not yet giving inhibition of prostaglandin synthesis. Here the addition of macrophages results in an overall shift to the right of the dose–response curve (Figure 106.6). Figure 106.7 shows the influence of macrophages on the effect of acetyl salicylic acid on lymphocyte proliferation. Again, a slight upward shift of the curve can be observed, but

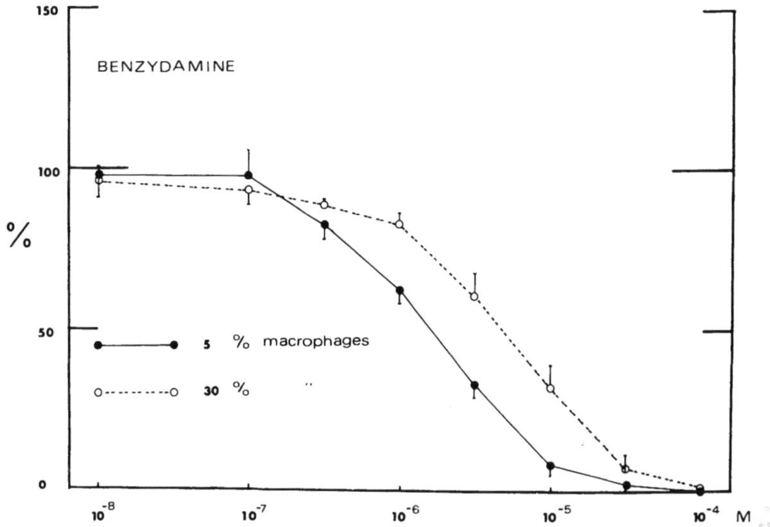


**Figure 106.6** Dose-dependent effects of benzydamine on LTT with 5 and 30% macrophages. Data presented as in Figure 106.4

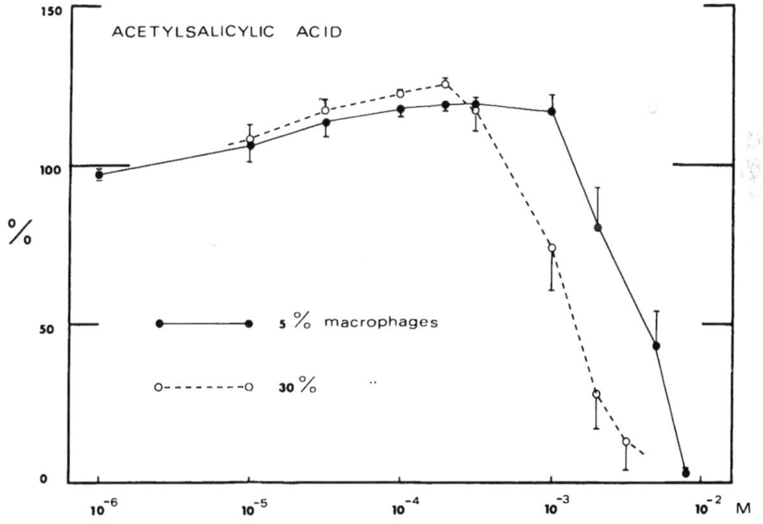


**Figure 106.7** Dose dependent effects of acetylsalicylic acid on PHA-stimulated LTT with 5 and 30% macrophages. Data presented as in Figure 106.4

more striking is the shift to the left of the inhibitory part of the curve. It looks as if this drug is more toxic to lymphocytes if more macrophages are present. This result seems rather puzzling, but there are reports showing the deviating behaviour of acetyl salicylic acid as compared to other anti-inflammatory drugs. For example, it is the only AID forming acetyl derivatives of serum proteins and other body constituents[50], an effect which is suggested to be responsible for the phenomenon described by Garcia a Leme *et al.*[51]. They found acetyl salicylic acid to be the only AID causing a permanent inactivation of a pro-inflammatory factor present in rat lymphocytes. As an explanation for the action of this drug in our experiments the possibility should be envisaged of lymphocytes being changed by acetyl salicylic acid in such a way that they become susceptible to destruction by macrophages.

**Acknowledgments**

We thank Mrs C. Montagne-Wajer, Mr D. van Romondt and Mr J. de Groot for excellent technical assistance, and Mr Y. C. Abraham–Dolman, and Mr W. R. Dolman for preparation of the manuscript.

**References**

1 Opelz; G., Terasaki, P. and Herata, A. A. (1973). *Lancet*, **2**, 478
2 Forbes, I. J. and Smith, J. L. (1967). *Lancet*, **2**, 334
3 Ambrose, C. T. (1966). *J. Exp. Med.*, **124**, 461
4 Winchurch, R. A., Foschi G. V. and Walz, D. T. (1974). *J. Reticuloendothel. Soc.*, **15**, 112
5 Park, S. K. and Brody, J. T. (1971). *Natl. New Biol.*, **233**, 181
6 Smith, J. L. and Forbes, I. J. (1967). *Nature (London)*, **215**, 538
7 Packman, M., Esterley, N. B. and Peterson, R. D. A. (1971). *J. Clin. Invest*, **50**, 226
8 Gabourel, J. D., Davies, G. H. and Rittenberg, M. B. (1977). *Clin. Immunol. Immunopathol.*, **7**, 53
9 Muscoplat, C. C., Rakich, P. M., Thoen, C. O. and Johnson, D. W. (1978). *Infect. Immun.*, 627
10 Goodwin, J. S., Bankhurst, A. D., Murphy, S. A., Selinger, D. S., Mussner R. P. and Williams, R. C. (1978). *J. Clin. Lab. Immunol.*, **1**, 197
11 Sohnle, P. G. and Collins-Lech, C. (1979). *Clin. Immunol. Immunopathol.*, **13**, 47
12 Barasoain, J. Rojo, J. M. and Portolés, A. (1979). *Immunopharmacology*, **2**, 83
13 Rosenstreich, D. L. and Mizel, S. B. (1978). *Immunol. Rev.*, **40**, 102
14 Mookerjee, B. K. (1977). *Transplantation*, **23**, 22
15 de Vries, J. E., Cavilles, A. P., Bont, W. S. and Mendelsohn, J. (1979). *J. Immunol.*, 1099
16 Hojo, K. and Hiramine, C. (1979). *Scand. J. Immunol.*, **9**, 381
17 Rinehart, J. J., Orser, M. and Kaplan, M. E. (1979). *Cell. Immunol.*, **44**, 131
18 Brondz, B. D., Khachikyan, E. Y. and Karaulov, A. V. (1979). *Bull. Exp. Biol. Med.*, **87**, 329
19 Goodwin, J. S., Bankhurst, A. D. and Messner, R. P. (1977). *J. Exp. Med.*, **146**, 1719
20 Lipsky, P. E. and Rosenthal, A. S. (1976). *J. Immunol.*, **187**, 1594
21 Lause, D. B. (1979). *J. Reticuloendothel. Soc.*, **26**, 775
22 Ansfield, M. J., Kaltreider, H. B., Caldwell, J. L. and Herskowitz, F. N. (1979). *J. Immunol.*, **122**, 542
23 Humes, J. L., Bonney, R. J., Pelus, L., Dahlgren, M. E., Sadowski, S. J., Kuehl, F. A. and Davies, P. (1977). *Nature (London)*, **269**, 149
24 Kurland, J. J. and Bockman, R. (1978). *J. Exp. Med.*, **147**, 952
25 Bray, M. A. and Gordon, D. (1978). *Br. J. Pharmacol.*, **63**, 635
26 Gordon, D., Bray, M. and Morley, J. (1976). *Nature (London)*, **262**, 401

27 Muscoplat, C. C., Klausner, D. J., Brunner, C. J., Sloane, E. D. and Johnson, D. W. (1979). *Infect. Immun.*, **26**, 311

28 von Blomber, M. and Scheper, R. J. (1980). *Immunology*, **39**, 291

29 Mullink, H., von Blomberg, M., Wilders, M. M., Drexhage, H. A. and Alons, C. L. (1979). *J. Immunol. Meth.*, **29**, 133

30 Stadecker, M. J., Bishop, G. and Wortis, H. H. (1973). *J. Immunol.*, **111**, 1834

31 Seeman, P. (1972). *Pharmacol. Rev.*, **24**, 583

32 Haynes, B. F. and Fauci, A. S. (1979). *Cell. Immunol.*, **44**, 157

33 Rosenberg, J. C. and Lysz, K. (1978). *Transplantation*, **25**, 115

34 Claman, H. N. (1972). *New Engl. J. Med.*, 388

35 Muraki Krishna Rao, K., Schwartz, S. A. and Good, R. A. (1979). *Cell. Immunol.*, **48**, 155

36 Goodwin, J. E. and Messner, R. P. (1979). *J. Clin. Invest.*, **64**, 434

37 Gordon, D., Henderson, D. C. and Westwick, J. (1979). *Br. J. Pharmacol.*, **67**, 17

38 Bonta, I. L. (1977). *Agents Actions Suppl.*, **121**,

39 Morley, J. (1974). *Prostaglandins*, **8**, 315

40 Goodwin, J. S. and Webb, D. R. (1980). *Clin. Immunol. Immunopathol.*, **15**, 106

41 Oort, J. and Mullink, H. (1974). *Proceedings of the 4th International Symposium of Medicinal Chemistry*, Maas, J. (ed.), pp. 1–15

42 Flower, R. J. (1974). *Pharmacol. Rev.*, **26**, 33

43 Moncada, S., Needleman, P., Bunting, S. and Vane, J. R. (1976). *Prostaglandins*, **12**, 323

44 Pelus, L. M. and Strausser, H. R. (1976). *Int. J. Cancer*, **18**, 653

45 Lynch, N. R. and Salomon, J. (1979). *J. Natl. Cancer. Inst.*, **62**, 117

46 Goodwin, J. S., Messner, R. P. and Bankhurst, R. P. (1977). *N. Engl. J. Med.*, **297**, 263

47 Goodwin, J. S., DeHoratius, R., Israel, H., Peake, G. T. and Messner, R. P. (1979). *Ann. Int. Med.*, **90**, 169

48 Ellner, J. J. and Spagnuolo, P. J. (1979). *J. Immunol.*, **123**, 2689

49 Flower, R. J., Cheung, H. S. and Cushman, D. W. (1973). *Prostaglandins*, **4**, 325

50 Hawkins, D., Pinckard, R. N., Crawford, I. P. and Farr, R. S. (1969). *J. Clin. Invest.*, **48**, 536

51 Garcia Leme, J., Ramos de Oliveira, J. C., Sudo, L. S. and Verissimo de Mello, S. B. (1978). *Br. J. Exp. Pathol.*, **59**, 345

52 Roux, F., Treich, I., Brun, C., Desrize, B. and Fournier, E. (1979). *Biochem. Pharmacol.*, **28**, 2419

53 Stites, D. P., Brecher, G., Schmidt, L. and Berger, F. (1979). *Immunopharmacology*, **2**, 39

# 107

# Influence of regional blood flow and inflammation on the localization of lymphoblasts in the small intestine of the mouse

C. A. OTTAWAY AND D. M. V. PARROTT (UK)

## INTRODUCTION

The ability of effector lymphocytes (lymphoblasts and their progeny) to act in a given tissue depends upon their localization within that tissue. Effector cells generated in lymphoid tissue in response to antigenic stimulation make their way to non-lymphoid tissue via the blood stream. Peripherally induced blasts, especially of the T cell line, have been found to have a propensity to localize in regions of inflammatory injury[1]. There is also a large body of evidence which indicates that, even in the absence of overt inflammation, there is a continuous repopulation of the gut tract with large numbers of both T and B lymphoblasts[2–6]. This is achieved by the deployment of effector lymphocytes which have arisen in Peyer's patches and mesenteric lymph nodes and have travelled by way of the thoracic duct and the blood stream to return to the gut.

Important changes can occur during an inflammatory process including hyperaemia, alterations in vascular permeability and the emigration of leukocytes and immune effector cells from the blood. Examination of how these processes interrelate could provide a basis for understanding the way in which expression of immunity can be influenced in sites of tissue injury. It has been pointed out that, in general, cellular emigration into an inflammatory site cannot be directly attributed to changes in vascular permeability[7], and in particular it has been shown that the accumulation of oxazalone-induced lymphoblasts in inflamed skin of the mouse is not related to vascular permeability changes alone[8].

In an effort to relate blood flow changes during inflammation to alterations in the level of representation of lymphoblasts within tissues, we have recently investigated the feasibility of using the distribution of $^{86}RbCl$ to measure the proportion of the cardiac output received by different organs of the mouse[9]. Application of this method to animals which have received labelied lymphoblasts can be used to assess the relationship of variations in regional blood flow to differences in the *in vivo* distribution of cells. We have reported that in mice at various stages of inflammation induced by a contact sensitizer, the localization of peripherally induced blast cells within the inflamed skin was positively correlated with the magnitude of the regional blood flow to the site[9]. This correlation of blast cell accumulation with regional blood flow was not antigen specific[9]. This suggests that the number of effector lymphoid cells found within a particular tissue can be influenced both by those properties which determine how the cells will interact with that tissue, as well as the probability that cells will be delivered to that site. Immune reactions may then be involved if antigens are present, either as primary or incidental participants at the inflammatory site, with which the accumulated effector cells can interact.

Here we wish to present the results of studies of cell localization and blood flow distribution within the small intestine. We have tested the hypothesis that variations in regional blood flow within the small intestine are related to the distribution of mesenteric lymphoblasts along the gut. Studies in normal animals demonstrate that there is such a relationship. During the development of a nematode induced enteritis in mice infected with *Trichinella spiralis*, this relationship undergoes alteration.

## METHODS

### Mice

7–14-week-old-mice of inbred NIH strain maintained in the department were used. Mice of the same age and sex were used within each experiment.

### Measurement of the cardiac output distribution (%CO)

Cardiac output distribution was measured by a method[9] developed from that originally described by Sapirstein[10]. Briefly, a known volume of $^{86}RbCl$ diluted with 0.9% saline was injected via an indwelling catheter in a lateral tail vein of the animal under study. This was flushed through with an equal volume of 0.9% saline and 45 s later the animal was sacrificed by injecting saturated KCl through the same cannula. The abdominal aorta and vena cava were then cut to allow exsanguination.

**Handling of tissues**

The tissues of interest were dissected out immediately following the cardiac output distribution determination for weighing and/or counting. The small intestine was removed in one piece and then cut into four equal lengths. Each length of small intestine was gently manipulated with forceps to remove faeces and chyme and washed in saline and then dried on filter paper. Peyer's patches were identified and excised from the small intestine prior to manipulation and counting.

**Preparation and labelling of cell suspensions**

Mesenteric lymph node cells (MLN) from untreated animals or from mice infected 4 days previously with *T. spiralis* were prepared at room temperature by gentle teasing of the nodes in RPMI-1640 medium containing 5% foetal calf serum (FCS). The cell suspensions were filtered through a 2 cm column of glass wool to remove fatty material and debris. The number of viable cells in suspension was determined by their ability to exclude 0.2% eosin. To label blast cells, MLN cells were incubated with the thymidine analogue [$^{125}$I]5-iodo-2-deoxyuridine [$^{125}$I]UdR) (Radiochemical Centre, Amersham, UK). Incubations were performed in RPMI-1640 with 5% FCS with 0.5 μCi/$10^7$ viable cells/ml for 60 min at 37 °C in a shaking water bath. After labelling, cells were washed three times in medium alone (RPMI-1640 without FCS). Injection doses of $1.5–2 \times 10^7$ viable cells were given through a lateral tail vein in a 0.4 ml volume. Multiple samples of each injection dose were kept for counting of the administered radioactivity. The distribution of blast cell label was determined when the animal was sacrificed at the time of assessing $^{86}$RbC1 distribution.

**Treatment of recipients**

Animals were either left untreated or infected with *T. spiralis* larvae at various times prior to cell transfer. Infective larvae recovered from a pepsin/HCl digest of the muscles of previously infected mice were administered by oral intubation (400–450 viable larvae to each mouse).

**Counting methods**

Radioactivity was measured by simultaneous counting on two channels as previously described[9]. We have shown that the two labels can be resolved and that cell localization estimates are not influenced by the presence of the $^{86}$Rb activity[9].

**Statistical methods**

The difference in means was assessed by Student's *t*-test. Regression analysis and correlation coefficients (*r*) were determined by standard methods[11]. The level of significance of correlation coefficients (i.e., the probability that the observed correlation could have arisen by chance) was assessed using

Student's *t*-test[12]. The assignment of confidence limits to the calculated regression equations followed the method of Moroney[12].

## RESULTS

### Mesenteric lymphoblast localization and regional blood flow along the small intestine

To assess the partition of blast cells and cardiac output within the small intestine, we studied both phenomena in the same animals. The pattern of localization of blast cells and the proportion of the cardiac output received by different segments of the small intestine is shown in Table 107.1. The fraction of the cardiac output received by the proximal small intestine was greater than that received by distal segments. The *in vivo* localization of [$^{125}$I]UdR MLN was also found to vary along the length of the small intestine (Table 107.1). The pattern of the proportion of injected MLN blasts found in a particular segment with the proportion of the cardiac output received by that segment (Figure 107.1) suggests that there is a relationship between these two distributions. Correlation analysis showed a significant positive relationship between MLN lymphoblast localization and regional blood flow within the small intestine which was unlikely to have arisen by a chance.

**Table 107.1** The 24 h localization of [$^{125}$I] UdR-MLN and the distribution of regional blood flow within the small intestine of normal mice (mean ± SD for six animals)

| | *% injected dose of cells* | *% CO* |
|---|---|---|
| Total small intestine | 4.2 ± 0.2 | 20.9 ± 2.4 |
| Proximal $SI_1$ | 1.4 ± 0.1 | 7.7 ± 1.5 |
| $SI_2$ | 1.5 ± 0.2 | 5.6 ± 1.1 |
| $SI_3$ | 0.9 ± 0.1 | 3.6 ± 0.6 |
| Distal $SI_4$ | 0.6 ± 0.1 | 3.1 ± 0.5 |

The distribution of cardiac output in that experiment was measured 24 h after the innoculation of labelled cells. The proportion of injected lymphoblasts which can be found in the small intestine is known to vary over the 24 h after injection of the cells[4,13]. Other experiments (data not shown) demonstrated that the correlation between blast cell localization and regional blood flow to intestinal segments is always significant regardless of the time after injection at which the measurements are taken.

### The effect of *Trichinella spiralis* infection

We have also examined the distribution of lymphoblasts and regional blood flow to the small intestine of mice undergoing a primary enteric infection with the nematode parasite *T. spiralis*. This produces a self-limiting enteritis in the

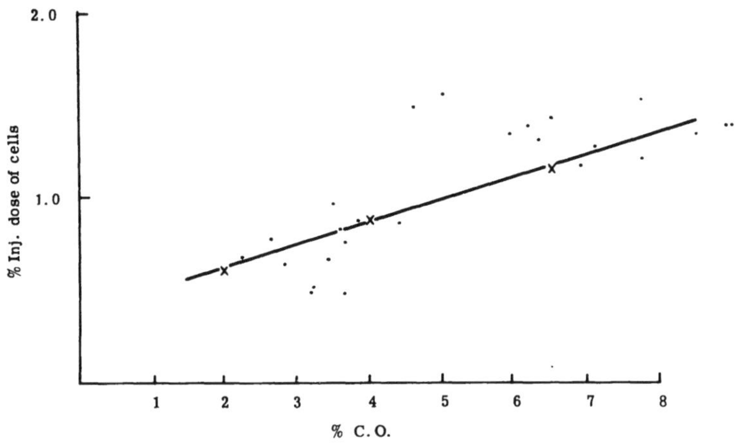


**Figure 107.1** The relationship of the localization of [$^{125}$I]UdR-MLN in a particular segment of small intestine and the percent of the cardiac output received by that segment in six normal animals. Regression analysis gave a correlation coefficient of $r = 0.77$ for the 24 segments with a probability that the correlation coefficient was due to chance of less than 0.01

mice during which enhanced lymphoblast localization occurs in the small intestine[13]. To investigate whether increased blast cell localization in the infected gut was a consequence of intestinal hyperaemia during the infection, the *in vivo* distribution of MLN lymphoblasts was studied in conjunction with the regional blood flow. The alterations found in blast localization 24 h after cell injection and regional blood flow to the small intestine compared to uninfected control animals are shown in Figure 107.2. The greatest change in cell localization occurred early in the infection (12–4 days), a time at which no significant alteration in the regional blood flow to the intestine was detected. The fraction of the cardiac output which goes to the small intestine was increased in the later stages of the infection (6–8 days), by which time morphological alterations in the small intestine have been found to be well established[14].

The relationship between blast cell localization along the intestine and regional blood flow was examined (Table 107.2). The blast cell and blood flow distributions within the intestine showed a significant correlation in uninfected animals as well as at 2 and 4 days after the initiation of the infection. At late stages of the infection (6–8 days), the nature of the relationship is altered and no significant correlation between blast localization and regional blood flow was found (Table 107.2).

To try to understand what alterations had occurred within particular regions of the small intestine, we compared the blast cell localization observed within segments of infected intestine to the level which would be expected if that segment were behaving in the same way as segments of uninfec-

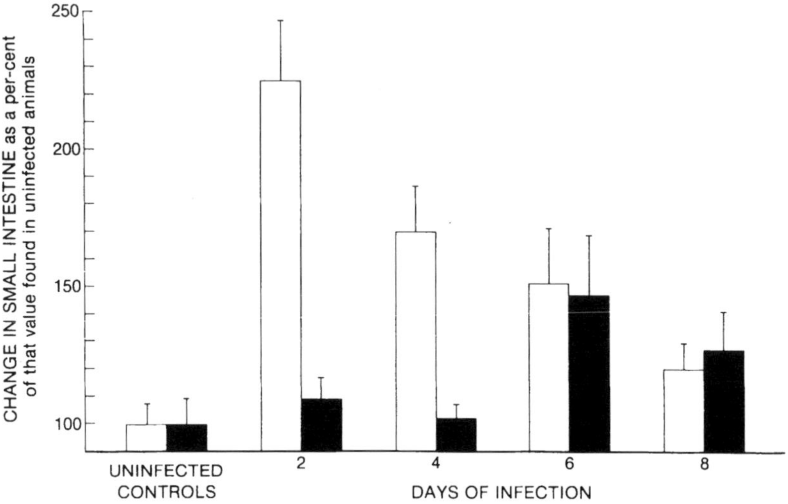


**Figure 107.2** The relative change in 24 h mesenteric lymphoblast localization (open areas) and the percent cardiac output (shaded areas) received by the small intestine during enteric infection with *T. spiralis*

**Table 107.2** Results of correlation analysis for 24 h [$^{125}$I] UdR-MLN localization and blood flow to small intestine at different stages of infection with *T. spiralis*

| *Experiment* | *Stage of infection* (days) | *r* | *n* | *p* |
|---|---|---|---|---|
| 1 | uninfected | 0.71 | 28 | <0.001 |
| | 2 | 0.63 | 24 | <0.001 |
| | 4 | 0.72 | 20 | <0.001 |
| 2 | uninfected | 0.60 | 20 | <0.01 |
| | 4 | 0.76 | 16 | <0.001 |
| | 6 | 0.43 | 16 | NS |
| | 8 | 0.08 | 24 | NS |

*r* = correlation coefficient; *n* = paired observations analysed (i.e., number of segments); *p* = probability that observed *r* is due to chance; slipe = slope of the regression line describing the relation between % inj. cells and % CO

ted intestine. A linear equation describing the pattern of blast localization observed in the control segments of intestine as a function of the per cent of the cardiac output received by those segments was constructed from the regression analysis. We then used the fraction of the cardiac output seen in infected segments to arrive at a prediction of what we would expect the level of blast localization to be, if they were behaving in the same way as the uninfected controls. One would expect that 95% of all observations which were behaving in the same way as the control group would fall within the range of the prediction ± 2 standard errors[12]. We did this for intestinal segments at various stages of the infection and scored the observations which were outside the predicted ranges. The results (Table 107.3) show that an excess of cells over what would be expected from the normal blast blood flow relationship appeared in different segments of the small intestine at different times of the infection. The regions of excess cell localization moved distally as the infection proceeded.

**Table 107.3** The distribution of increased blast cell localization within the small intestine during infection with *T. spiralis*

| *Stage of infection* | *Segments of small intestine* | | | | |
|---|---|---|---|---|---|
| | $SI_1$ (*proximal*) | $SI_2$ | $SI_3$ | $SI_4$ (*distal*) | *Experiment* |
| Uninfected | 0 | 0 | 0 | 0 | 1 |
| Controls | 0 | 0 | 0 | 0 | 2 |
| 2 days | ++ | ++ | ++ | 0 | 1 |
| 4 days | ++ | ++ | + | 0 | 1 |
| | + | ++ | 0 | 0 | 2 |
| 6 days | 0 | ++ | ++ | + | 2 |
| 8 days | 0 | 0 | + | + | 2 |

Scoring: + scored where observed localization was more than 2 SE greater than that predicted; ++ when more than 3 SE greater; and 0 when observed localization was within the level predicted ± 2 SE

## DISCUSSION

The purpose of this study was to investigate the role that regional blood flow variations may play as a modulator of lymphocyte effector cell localization within intestinal tissues. The distribution of $^{86}$RbC1 (per cent cardiac output) along the small intestine shows that the perfusion of the proximal small intestine is greater than that of the distal regions. To examine the possible contribution of these differences in regional blood flow to the pattern of lymphoblast migration observed in the small intestine, we measured *in vivo* lymphoblast migration and blood flow distribution concomitantly in the same animals. Examination of these phenomena in the normal small intestine shows that there is a significant positive correlation between them (Figure 107.1) and we have found that the degree of connection between lymphoblast distribution and blood flow distribution is not affected by the time at which the events are studied[15].

Immunoglobulin producing cells are known to have a non-uniform distribution along the length of the small intestine. In various mammals, including man[16], mouse[17], cow[18], pig[19], and the rat[20], it has been observed that immunoglobulin-containing cells are present in higher densities in the proximal small intestine with a gradient towards the distal end. Husband and Gowans[20] proposed that the increased numbers of immunocytes in the proximal small bowel resulted from stimulation by food antigens which encouraged their increased localization or retention there.

Our experiments suggest that, for the mouse, the efficiency of localization of blast cells along the normal intestine can be viewed as being the same on the average throughout the small intestine but that a gradient arises as a result of differences in the probability of blood flow being delivered along the intestine. Such a mechanism would provide for the deployment of effector cells to different regions in proportion to their physiological demands for perfusion without requiring any active solicitation by antigen.

We also wished to examine the interaction of blast cell distribution with the distribution of regional blood flow in the intestine under the influence of a natural inflammatory process. Infection with *T. spiralis* produces an enteritis which is associated with the development of villous atrophy and crypt hyperplasia. These morphological changes are maximal in the mid-jejunum at the time when worms are being cleared from the proximal small intestine[14].

The distribution of the intestinal infection with *T. spiralis* varies with time. For NIH strain mice, the infection lasts for about 12 days before the complete expulsion of the worm burden from the small intestine[14]. Between days 2 and 4 of the infection, approximately 80% of the worm burden resides in the proximal half of the small intestine. The worms move along the gut tract as the infection proceeds and by 8 to 10 days about 80% of the recoverable worms are found in the distal half of the intestine[14].

Examination of blast cell localization and regional blood flow in the small intestine during the infection showed changes in blast localization which occurred before any alteration in the delivery of blood flow (Figure 107.2) or vascular permeability of the small intestine[21]. The localization of blast cells in the intestine was markedly increased at day 2 and 4 of the infection, while alteration in the fraction of the cardiac output received by the small intestine did not occur until later stages of the infection (Figure 107.2).

The nature of the relationship between the distribution of lymphoblasts and blood flow was also altered during the infection. A significant correlation between blast cell localization and blood flow was found at 2 and 4 days after the infection as well as in uninfected animals (Table 107.2). The substantial increase in the level of cell localization found in the early stages suggests that the uptake of lymphoblasts or their retention was enhanced in infected intestine. In the later stages of the infection (6–8 days), no significant correlation between blast cell localization and blood flow was found along the intestine (Table 107.2).

Comparison of the individual segments of infected small intestine to those of uninfected animals (Table 107.3) showed that there was an excess localization of cells which could not be accounted for by the expected behaviour of the uninfected segments. This excess cell localization was found in different regions of the intestine as the infection proceeded, and is comparable to the manner in which the worm burden proceeds along the length of the small bowel[14]. This suggests that enhanced cell localization in a particular segment of the gut results from the presence of the parasite which somehow facilitates an alteration either in the uptake of blast cells from the blood or their retention in that region of the intestine.

How this enhancement of blast cell localization is produced is not known but it may have important consequences for the animals. Most of the lymphoblasts arriving in the blood stream from the thoracic duct at any given time have been stimulated in response to gut derived antigens. Factors which facilitate increased recruitment or retention of mesenteric lymphoblasts within an area of tissue containing the parasite could contribute to the immunological defence of the animal by concentrating effector cells capable of responding to various luminal antigens, including those of the parasite, in the disrupted area.

**Acknowledgment**
This work was supported by MRC grant 977/623/S(UK).

## References

1 Asherson, G. L. and Allwood, G. G. (1972). Inflammatory lymphoid cells: cells in immunized lymph nodes that move to sites of inflammation. *Immunology*, **22**, 493
2 Gowans, J. L. and Knight, E. J. (1964). The route of recirculation of lymphocytes in the rat. *Proc. R. Soc. London, Ser. B*, **159**, 257
3 Griscelli, C., Vassalli, P. and McCluskey, R. T. (1979). The distribution of large dividing lymph node cells in syngeneic recipient rats after intravenous injection. *J. Exp. Med.*, **130**, 1427
4 Hall, J. G., Parry, D. M. and Smith, M. E. (1972). The distribution and differentiation of lymph-borne immunoblasts after intravenous injection into syngeneic recipients. *Cell Tissue Kinet.*, **5**, 269
5 Guy–Grand, D., Griscelli, C. and Vassali, P. (1974). The gut associated lymphoid system: nature and properties of the large dividing cells. *Eur. J. Immunol.*, **4**, 435
6 McWilliams, M., Phillips–Quagliata, J. M. and Lamm, M. E. (1975). Characteristics of mesenteric lymph node cells homing to gut-associated lymphoid tissue in syngeneic mice. *J. Immunol.*, **115**, 54
7 Bohm, G. M. (1976). Vascular events in inflammations. *Agents Actions (Suppl. 3)*, 31
8 Rose, M. L. and Parrott, D. M. V. (1977). Vascular permeability and lymphoblast extravasation into inflamed skin are not related. *Cell. Immunol.*, **33**, 62
9 Ottaway, C. A. and Parrott, D. M. V. (1979). Regional blood flow and its relationship to lymphocyte and lymphoblast traffic during a primary immune reaction. *J. Exp. Med.*, **150**, 218
10 Sapirstein, L. A. (1958). Regional blood flow by fractional distribution of indicators. *Am. J. Physiol.*, **193**, 161
11 Dixon, W. J. and Massey, F. J. (1957). *Introduction to statistical analysis*, pp. 189–201. (New York: McGraw–Hill)
12 Moroney, M. J. (1951). *Facts from figures*, pp. 271–320. (Harmondsworth and New York: Penguin)
13 Rose, M. L., Parrott, D. M. V. and Bruce, R. G. (1976). Migration of lymphoblasts to the

small intestine. I. Effect of *Trichinella spiralis* infection on the migration of mesenteric lymphoblasts and mesenteric T lymphoblasts in syngeneic mice. *Immunology*, **31**, 723

14 Manson-Smith, D. F., Parrott, D. M. V. and Bruce, R. G. (1979). Villous atrophy and expulsion of intestinal *Trichinella spiralis* are mediated by T cells. *Cell. Immunol.*, **47**, 285

15 Ottaway, C. A. and Parrott, D. M. V. (1980). On the relationship between the localization of lymphoblasts and regional blood flow in the intestine. (Submitted for publication)

16 Crabbe, P. A. and Heremans, J. F. (1966). The distribution of immunoglobulin containing cells along the human gastrointestinal tract. *Gastroenterology*, **51**, 305

17 Crabbe, P. A., Bazin, H., Eyssen, H. and Heremans, J. F. (1968). The normal microbial flora as a major stimulus for proliferation of plasma cells synthesizing IgA in the gut. The germ-free intestinal tract. *Int. Arch. Allergy*, **34**, 362

18 Porter, P., Noakes, D. E. and Aller, W. D. (1972). Intestinal secretion of immunoglobulins in the preruminant calf. *Immunology*, **23**, 299

19 Allen, W. D. and Porter, P. (1977). The relative frequencies and distribution of immunoglobulin-bearing cells in the intestinal mucosa of neonatal and weaned pigs and their significance in the development of secreting immunity. *Immunology*, **32**, 819

20 Husband, A. J. and Gowans, J. L. (1978). The orign and antigen-dependent distribution of IgA-containing cells in the intestine. *J. Exp. Med.*, **148**, 1146

21 Rose, M. L., Parrott, D. M. V. and Bruce, R. G. (1976). Migration of lymphoblasts to the small intestine. II Divergent migration of mesenteric and peripheral immunoblasts to sites of inflammation in the mouse. *Cell. Immunol.*, **27**, 36

# 108

# Early lymphocyte activation and proliferative response induced by lectins: individual variations in man

A. KAHAN, A. POMPIDOU, P. MICHEL,
B. MACE AND D. ESNOUS (FRANCE)

## INTRODUCTION

An immunological inbalance was recently claimed in most of inflammatory rheumatic diseases, such as rheumatoid arthritis[1], SLE[2,3], ankylosing spondylitis and Reiter's syndrome[4–6]. Several methods were used but the criteria to assess immunological deficiency are not yet standardized. However, therapeutic use of immunomodulator drugs needs standardized criteria to show their action in patients. Therefore, we chose two tests to study the function of lymphocytes: early lymphocyte activation of the nucleus by the refringence test[7–9] and late lymphocyte activation by proliferative response ([$^{3}$H]thymidine incorporation).

Our preliminary studies and the data of literature showed a high variability of the proliferative response between individuals. Thus the first point was to determine the spontaneous variations in the same individual. This study was carried out on subjects with various immune diseases, particularly rheumatic diseases.

## MATERIAL AND METHODS

### Patients

22 healthy subjects (blood donors of St Vincent Hospital) were tested

monthly 2 to 4 times. Three subjects were taken off the study because of intercurrent disease.

**Lymphoblastic transformation test (LTT)**

The whole blood method was used[10]. Blood on calciparine (Choay) was diluted 1/40 in RPMI 1640 medium buffered with HEPES and antibiotics added. After 5 days culture (3 ml per culture) 1 $\mu$Ci/ml of [$^3$H]thymidine was incorporated for the last 18 h. Duplicates were done for control cultures as well as for each dose of lectin. Results are expressed either as index transformation (dpm mitogen/dpm control/dpm control) or as log (dpm mitogen /dpm control). The individual variation results are expressed as the difference of two successive values, $\Delta$ = log(dpm mitogen/dpm control).

**Nuclear refringence test (NRT)**

Lymphocytes were isolated from peripheral blood by Ficoll–Hypaque gradient. Platelets were removed by centrifugation in RPMI 1640 at 150 *g*. Suspensions containing 95% of lympho-monocytes were obtained and thermic equilibration was realized by incubation at 37 °C for 1 h. After 5 min cytocentrifugation (cytospin) at 1300 rev/min, smears were fixed wet in 5% acetic Zenker fluid at 22 °C. for 60 min and post-fixed in the same reagent for 10 min at 90 °C. After washing, drying and clearing in toluene, the smears were mounted in the mounting medium (Technicon) and observed with a phase contrast microscope. The refringence of 1000 cells is classified on a scale with three categories: The first one is represented by negligibly refringent cells (A), the second one by moderately refringent cells (B) and the third one by highly refringent cells (C). The refringence index is obtained according to Moebius formula using a coefficient determined by image intensity analysis (Cambridge Quantimet 720)

$$\mathrm{RI} = \frac{(\%\,\mathrm{A} \times 1) + (\%\,\mathrm{B} \times 2) + (\%\,\mathrm{C} \times 4)}{(1 + 2 + 4)}$$

This refringence index is very constant (27.5 ± 1.5) and has a normal distribution. Variations of the refringence index (RI) are expressed by the ratio to control, i.e.

$$100 - \frac{\mathrm{RI\ treated} - \mathrm{RI\ control} \times 100}{\mathrm{RI\ control}}$$

Incubations are performed in triplicate with $5 \times 10^5$ cells in 500 $\mu$l of medium in presence of lectin for 20 min at 37 °C. Viability is controlled by trypan blue dye exclusion (96 ± 3). Mean refringence index is calculated from triplicates and standard deviations tabulated. Statistical significance is evaluated by Wilcoxon test and Snedecor's *F* test. For individual variations, results are expressed as the difference of two successive values of ratio to control.

**Lectins**

The lectins used were phytohaemagglutinin M (PHA M Wellcome) at 2.5, 5, 10 and 100 $\mu$g per culture for LTT and for 5 × $10^5$ cells/ml for NRT, and concanavalin A (ConA Miles) at 6.25, 12.5, 25 and 50 $\mu$g per culture for LTT and 2.5 $\mu$g for 5 × $10^5$ cells for NRT. In both tests $Mn^{2+}$ and $Ca^{2+}$ at final concentration of $10^{-4}$ were added as activators of the reaction. Also used was Pokeweed mitogen (PWM Sigma) at dose 2.5, 5 and 10 $\mu$g/culture for LTT and 2.5 $\mu$g for 5 × $10^5$ cells for NRT.

## RESULTS

**Lymphoblastic transformation test**

The response to PHA is a dose–effect function for 2.5, 5 and 10 $\mu$g/culture ($y = 0.33 \times + 3.75$, $p <0.01$) (Table 108.1). There is a very slight dose effect for ConA at doses 6.25, 12.5 and 25 μg/culture ($p <0.05$). No dose effect was observed for PWM at the same doses as PHA.

**Table 108.1** Dose effect response to PHA

| | *Early activation (nuclear refringence test)* (NRT) | | *Proliferative response (lymphoblastic tranformation test)* (LTT) |
|---|---|---|---|
| *PHA* ($\mu$g/ml) | *Refringence index* | *Ratio to Control* | *Log (dpm PHA-dpm control)* |
| 0 | 26.9±1.4 | – | – |
| 2.5 | 25.6±1.6 | 94.5±3.1 | 3.88±0.60 |
| 5.0 | 24.6±1.8 | 91.4±4.9 | 4.33±0.43 |
| 10.0 | 24.0±2.1 | 88.9±5.7 | 4.53±0.43 |
| | $y = 280\,x + 95.85$ $p<0.01$ | | $y = 0.33\,x + 3.75$ $p<0.01$ |

The variations between different subjects are very important, whatever the dose, when results are expressed as transformation index (dpm PHA–dpm control/dpm control). Therefore we chose another mode of expression: log (dpm mitogen/dpm control) for both the variation between different subjects and in the same subject tested monthly. Under these conditions standard deviation does not exceed 0.60 for variations between different subjects and individual variations are lower than 0.7 of log (dpm mitogen/dpm control) in 82–93% of cases whatever the lectin or dose (Table 108.2).

**Nuclear refringence test (NRT)**

The response to PHA is a dose-effect function for 2.5, 5 and 10 $\mu$g/ml ($y = 280x + 95.85$, $p <0.01$) (Table 108.1). No dose-effect response is obtained with ConA and PWM. Individual variations are lower than 6% of the refringence index in 75% of cases (Table 108.2, Figures 108.1 and 108.2).

**Table 108.2** Human blood lymphocytes response to lectins: individual variations in man

| | *Early activation Nuclear refringence test (20 min incubation)* | | *Proliferative response thymidine incorporation (5 days culture)* | |
|---|---|---|---|---|
| *Lectins* (2.5 μg/ml) | *Ratio to control* | *Percentage of cases with individual variations <6%* | *log of ratio to control* | *Percentage of cases with individual variations <0.7 log ratio to control* |
| PHA | 89.89±5.29 | 80.77 | 3.88±0.60 | 82.76 |
| ConA | 87.37±6.28 | 84.85 | 3.68±0.63 | 75.86 |
| PWM | 93.11±6.38 | 74.19 | 3.74±0.62 | 72.30 |

No correlation between the two tests.

### Relation between LTT and NRT

Whatever the lectin used in LTT, at least 75% of healthy persons show a variation less than 0.7 of log (dpm lectin/dpm control) which is considered as the threshold. The same percentage (75–80%) was found for the NRT variation (less than 6%). However, no direct correlation was observed between LTT and NRT, whatever the lectin used, even considering both tests at optimal doses (Table 108.2).

## DISCUSSION

Lectins induce cellular activation mediated by glycoprotein surface receptors and cytosqueleton[11]. Early activation is shown by an intracellular GMPc increase[12,13] and by a nuclear refringence decrease, reflecting the chromatin dispersion[9]. Thus one nuclear refringence test in presence of lectins shows an early activation of the nucleus[7]. On the other hand, the proliferative response of lymphocytes to lectins shows a late activation of the nucleus and mainly a DNA synthesis. The absence of correlation between the two tests (LTT and NRT) also shows that they are implicated in different phases of nucleus acti-

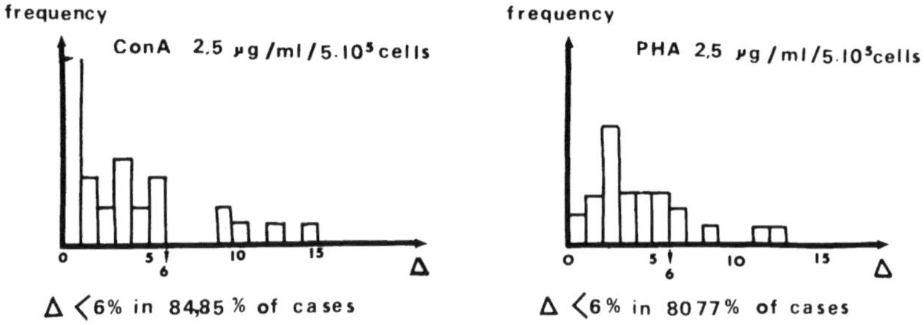


**Figure 108.1** NRT variations between individual values (Δ = percentage of nuclear refringence index)

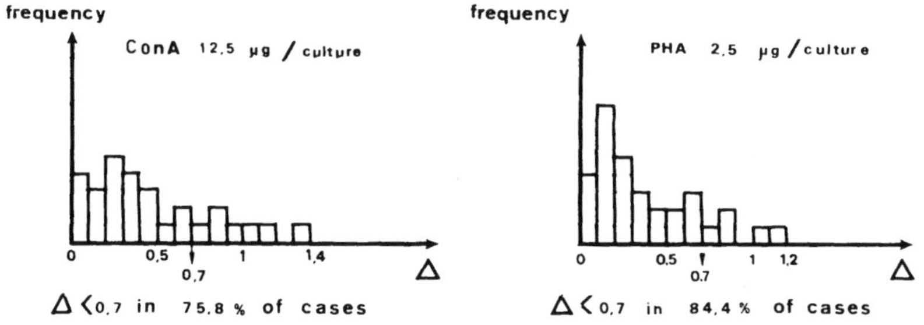


**Figure 108.2** LTT variations between individual values (Δ) of log (dpm mitogen/dpm control

vation, thus their simultaneous study will give more information about lymphocyte activation.

We used purified lectins at different doses in order to eliminate experimental variations and to obtain a better reproducibility of the results. Considering LTT in healthy subjects, an obvious dose-effect response was found for PHA, a slight dose effect for ConA, but none for PWM. These data suggest that sub-optimal doses of PHA should be used in order to discover an immunological deficiency in patients, but this is not so with ConA and PWM.

On the other hand, the lymphocyte response to different lectins, whatever the dose, shows, in a healthy population, large variation within monthly intervals. We could establish this variation up to a threshold of $\Delta = 0.7$ log(dpm lectin/dpm control), because 75% at least of the population had a variation below this point. Thus, to be able to establish an immunological deficiency or to assess the action of immunotherapy, the variations should exceed this threshold.

The data presented in literature generally do not take into account such variations in healthy subjects. Frobel *et al.*[5] suggest the existence of a cellular immune defect in AS and Reiter's syndrome, because they observed a lower response to sub-optimal doses of PHA (2.5 µg/ml) but in their study there is no dose-effect response in controls. Fan *et al.*[6] observed a diminution of the percentage of T lymphocytes in AS ($61.9 \pm 1.6$) compared to controls ($72.3 \pm 1.0$), but the response to optimal doses of PHA was normal.

On the other hand, the response of lymphocytes to lectins may be altered by seric factors such as lymphotoxic antibodies in SLE[14] or in scleroderma associated with myositis[15]. Furthermore, it should be realized that anti-inflammatory drugs may modify lymphocytes response *in vitro*[16]. Thus it is necessary to eliminate any susceptible factor to modify the response to lectins before assessing the immunological state by this test.

Considering the nuclear refringence test (NRT), the variations observed from one patient to another or in the same subject at monthly examination did not exceed 6%. This slight variation shows that the test is reliable and sensitive. We found for NRT a dose-effect response for PHA as well as for LTT.

This suggests that nuclear activation, either early or late, depends on lectin fixation of a greater or smaller number of membrane receptors which are activated.

## CONCLUSION

Repeated study of cellular immunity using LTT and NRT in the presence of lectins (PHA, ConA and PWM) permitted us to establish standardized criteria to assess the immunological state of patients. In our experimental conditions, normal limits are considered as 0.7 log(dpm lectin/dpm control) for LTT, but only 6% for NRT. These standardized criteria will permit us to make a criticai study of immune response and to assess the effect of immunotherapy in man.

**Acknowledgments**

We would like to thank Mrs C. Michalak and E. Gniazdowska for their valuable technical assistance. This work was partially supported by a grant INSERM ATP 69–78–101 and 79–1–518–2.

### References

1 Silverman, H. A., Johnson, J. S., Vaughan, J. H. and McGlamory, J. C. (1976). Altered lymphocyte reactivity in rheumathoid arthritis. *Arthritis Rheum.*, **19**, 509

2 Rosenthal, C. J. and Franklin, E. C. (1975). Depression of cellular mediated immunity in systemic lupus erythematosus. Relation to disease activity. *Arthritis Rheum.*, **18**, 207

3 Delbarre, F., Pompidou, A., Kahan, A. *et al.* (1971). Etude des lymphocytes du sang au cours de la maladie lupique. *Pathol. Biol.* **19**, 379

4 Christiansen, F. T., Hawkins, B. R. and Dawkins, R. L. (1978). J. Immune function in ankylosing spondylitics and their relatives: influence of disease and HLA B 27. *Clin. Exp. Immunol.*, **33**, 270

5 Frobel, K., Sturrock, R. D., Dick, W. C. and MacSween, N. M. (1975). Cell mediated immunity in the rheumatoid diseases. I. Skin testing and mitogenic response in seronegative arthritides. *Clin. Exp. Immunol.*, **22**, 446

6 Fan, P. T., Clements, P. J., Yu, D. T. Y., Opelz, G. and Bluestone, R. (1977). Lymphocyte abnormalities in ankylosing spondylitis. *Ann. Rheum. Dis.*, **36**, 471

7 Pompidou, A., Mace, B., Michel, P. and Esnous, D. (1979). Early modifications of lymphocyte nuclear refringence after stimulation by lectins and immunomodulators. In Preece, A. W. and Sabolovic, D. (eds.) *Cell Electrophoresis: Clinical Application and Methodology. INSERM symposium no. 11*, p. 149. (North Holland: Elsevier)

8 Pompidou, A., Touraine, J. L., Mace, B. and Hadden, J. W. (1979). Role of nucleic acid and cytosqueleton in nuclear refringence phenomenon of human blood lymphocytes. *Int. J. Immunopharmacol.*, **2**, 29

9 Pompidou, A., Mace, B., Esnous, D. and Michel, P. (1979). The nuclear refringence test, a new method for the evaluation of blood lymphocytes nuclei response 'in vitro' to lectins and immunomodulators in man. In Serrou, B. and Rosenfeld, D. C. (eds.) *New Trends in Human Immunology and Cancer Immunotherapy*.

10 Kahan, A., Perlik, F., Le Go, A., Delbarre, F. and Giroud, J. P. (1976). Adjuvant induced arthritis in four inbred strains of rats. An in vitro study of peripheral T and B lymphocytes. *Agents Actions*, **6**, 219

11 Cercek, L., Cercek, B. and Franklin, D. (1974). Biophysical differentiation between lym-

phocytes from healthy donors, patients with malignant diseases and other disorders. *Br. J. Cancer*, **29,** 345

12 Hadden, J. W., Hadden, E. M., Sadlik, J. R. and Coffey, R. G. (1976). Effects of Concanavalin A and succinylated derivative on lymphocytes proliferation and cyclic nucleotide levels. *Proc. Natl. Acad. Sci.*, **73,** 1717

13 Hadden, J. W., Coffey, R. G., Anathakrishan, R. and Hadden, E. M. (1979). Cyclic nucleotide and calcium in lymphocytes regulation and activation. *Int. J. Immunopharmacol.*

14 Glinski, W., Gershwin, M. E. and Steinberg, A. D. (1976). Fractionation of cells on discontinuous Ficoll gradient. Study of subpopulations of human T cells using anti-T-cell antibodies from patients with SLE. *J. Clin. Invest.*, **57,** 604

16 Lockshin, M. D. (1975). Aspirin and lymphocyte transformation. *N. Engl. J. Med.*, **292,** 809

# 109

# Lymphocyte responsiveness in acute and convalescent infectious mononucleosis (Abstract)

A. G. BIRD (UK) AND S. BRITTON (SWEDEN)

We have examined the ability of human peripheral blood lymphocytes from patients with acute infectious mononucleosis to mount an *in vitro* response to various mitogens. Antibody synthesis and secretion was analysed by use of a reversed plaque assay using staphylococcal protein-A coated sheep erythrocytes as target erythrocytes. The use of class specific anti-immunoglobulin developing sera allows detection of Ig class specific plaque forming cells. Unresponsiveness to pokeweed mitogen is a prolonged effect and recovery takes up to 12 weeks. The lack of T helper function detected, mirrors the already described unresponsiveness of mononucleosis T cells to T mitogens, as assessed by DNA synthesis.

We have analysed whether the T helper lymphocyte paralysis is the result of active suppression in acute disease. In experiments using cryopreserved lymphocytes mixed with convalescent cells of the same individual we can find no evidence of active suppressor cells in acute disease. We conclude that the absence of T helper function is the result of the turbulence in the immune system induced by EB virus and may be of potential pathological significance.

# 110

# Quantitative measurement of human leukocyte aggregation as a possible correlation with cell mediated immunity

B. ROUVEIX (FRANCE), P. BADENOCH-JONES AND J. L. TURK (UK)

## INTRODUCTION

The study of cell mediated immunity has been facilitated by the development of *in vitro* methods, especially in experimental animals. However, there are no wholly satisfactory *in vitro* methods for use with humans. Inhibition of migrating indicator cells resulting from the interaction of sensitized lymphocytes with specific antigen and the lymphocyte transformation test (LTT) are widely used. Both of these techniques have been extensively studied and compared with *in vivo* delayed hypersensitivity reactions, as assessed by skin testing[1-5]. They both have disadvantages. The migration inhibition is cumbersome, difficult to set up and is sometimes no better than semi-quantitative. In the lymphocyte transformation test, stimulation of antibody-producing cells by antigen may also be measured. It is not surprising, therefore, that the results obtained with these tests are not always correlated with each other and with skin test results[1,5-7]. The direct migration inhibition of leukocytes from sensitized subjects by specific antigen is thought to be due to release of lymphokines (leukocyte inhibitory factor, LIF) from lymphocytes which inhibits the spontaneous migration of mainly polymorphonuclear leukocytes. Indirect migration inhibition can be measured by assaying culture supernatants of sensitized lymphocytes and specific antigen on the migration of normal leukocytes.

An analogous situation exists in the guinea pig where the macrophage migration inhibition factor (MIF) can be measured in direct and indirect assays using peritoneal exudate cells (PEC) containing macrophages and lymphocytes. This has been well correlated with delayed hypersensitivity in the guinea pig[8]. It is well known that aggregation of normal macrophages by MIF containing culture media and of sensitized PEC by specific antigen is observed. This was first studied systematically by Lolekha *et al*[9]. and shown to correlate well with delayed hypersensitivity in the guinea pig. This was extended as an *in vitro* assay for transplantation immunity in the guinea pig[10] and it was also demonstrated that sensitized human lymphocytes cultured with specific antigen released macrophage aggregation factor (MAF) which could be assayed against guinea pig macrophages[11]. More recently, the direct aggregation of human leukocytes from sensitized subjects by specific antigen has been proposed as having a possible correlation with cell mediated immunity[12,13]. Aggregation in all these studies was measured subjectively by visual or microscopic examination.

We have recently developed a method for the quantitative measurement of direct and indirect macrophage aggregation in the guinea pig by measuring the light absorbance of stirred macrophage suspensions in a modified Born platelet aggregometer. This has been used to study the specificity, sensitivity and mechanism of aggregation[14,15]. We have now extended this method for the measurement of direct aggregation of human leukocytes by BCG sonicate and attempted to relate this to the LTT, direct LIF test and skin test reactions to tuberculin.

## QUANTITATIVE MEASUREMENT OF HUMAN LEUKOCYTE AGGREGATION

### Indirect measurement

Human lymphokine (LKY) was generated by culturing Ficoll purified lymphocytes from a PPD skin test positive subject with BCG sonicate (10 μg/ml) for 24 h in serum free medium. This aggregated human leukocytes, which could be measured quantitatively (Table 110.1). In addition, human lymphokine

**Table 110.1** Aggregation of human peripheral blood leukocytes by human BCG lymphokine. One batch of lymphokine was assayed against three separate cell preparations obtained from the same donor. Results are mean ± SE

| *Lymphokine concentration* | *Aggregation (cm) P–R* |
|---|---|
| 0.5 | 1.75±1.72 |
| 1 | 2.8 ±1.55 |
| 5 | 4.6 ±1.95 |
| 10 | 4.35±1.40 |

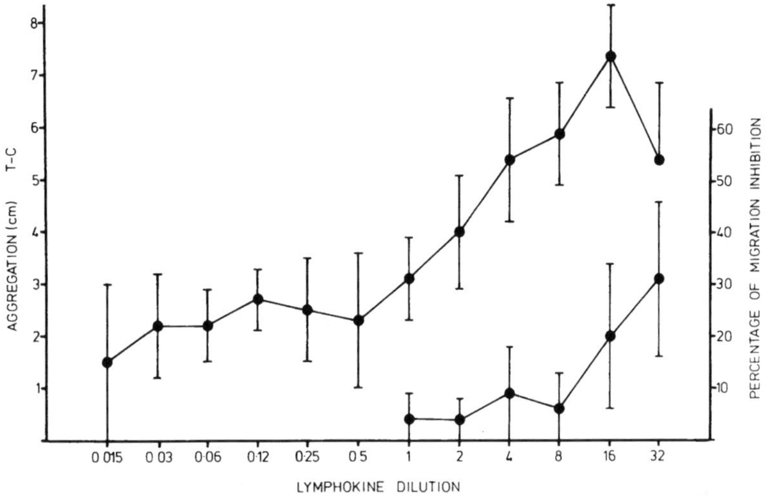


**Figure 110.1** Aggregation and migration inhibition of guinea pig peritoneal exudate cells by human concanavalin A induced lymphokine. One batch of lymphokine was assayed against five separate cell preparations. Results are mean ± SE

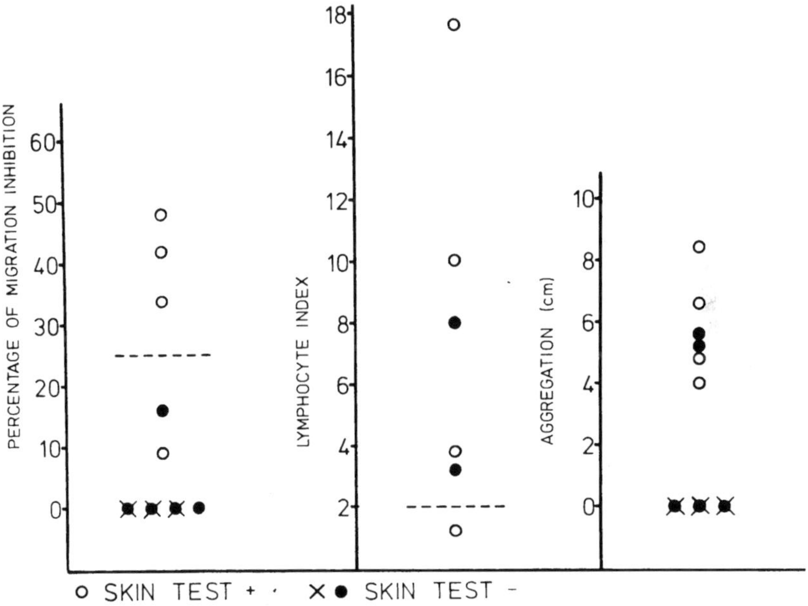


**Figure 110.2** Comparison of aggregation and migration inhibition of human leukocytes and lymphocyte transformation ([$^3$H]thymidine uptake) of human lymphocytes from skin test +ve(o) and −ve(●) subjects. 6 adults and 3 children under five (×) were tested. Antigen (BCG sonicate) concentration was 50 μg/ml in all cases. Migration inhibitions of >25%, aggregations of >2 cm and a transformation index >2−fold were considered significant

generated by stimulation of lymphocytes with concanavalin A aggregated guinea pig macrophages, and, in agreement with previous work on the guinea pig[14], this was more sensitive than the assay of MIF activity for the detection of lymphokine activity (Figure 110.1).

**Direct measurement**

Because human LKY generated by cultivating sensitized lymphocytes with BCG sonicate will aggregate normal leukocytes, the direct aggregation of leukocytes from PPD skin test positive and negative subjects by BCG sonicate was measured. LTT and migration inhibition were also measured in these subjects with this antigen. The results are summarized in Figure 110.2. This shows little correlation between the three parameters measured. As far as aggregation measurements are concerned the skin test negative children showed no leukocyte aggregation whereas aggregation was obtained in both skin test positive and negative adults. Thus these preliminary results indicate that quantitative measurements of direct leukocyte aggregation can be measured, although the relationship of this to other *in vitro* correlates of delayed hypersensitivity is not clear at the present time.

Potentially, measurement of direct leukocyte aggregation offers great practical advantages over the direct leukocyte migration inhibition assay and thus further work is being carried out using a number of different antigens, including viral bacterials and drug antigens.

## References


1 Fleer, A., Van der Hart, M., Blok-Shut, B. J. T. H. and Schellekens, P. T. H. A. (1976). Correlation of PPD and BCG-induced leukocyte migration inhibition, delayed cutaneous sensitivity, lymphocyte transformation in vitro and humoral antibodies to PPD in man. *Eur. J. Immunol.*, **6**, 163

2 Marsman, A. J. W., Van der Hart, M., Walig, C. and Eijsvoogel, V. P. (1972). Migration inhibition experiments with mixtures of human peripheral blood lymphocytes and guinea pig peritoneal exudate cells. *Eur. J. Immunol.*, **2**, 546.

3 Mitchell, C. G., Smith, M. G. H., Golding, P. L., Eddleston, A. L. W. F., and Williams, R. (1972). Evaluation of the leukocyte migration inhibition test as a measure of delayed hypersensitivity in man. Suppression of migration inhibition by puromycin. *Clin. Exp. Immunol.*, **11**, 535

4 Rosenberg, S. A. and David, J. R. (1970). Inhibition of leukocyte migration: an evaluation of this *in vitro* assay of delayed hypersensitivity in man to a soluble antigen. *J. Immunol.*, **105**, 1447

5 Thomas, J. H., Clements, D. and Grzybowski, S. (1971). *In vitro* lymphocyte responses and skin test reactivity following BCG vaccination. *Clin. Exp. Immunol.*, **9**, 611

6 Kaltreider, H. B., Soghar, D., Taylor, J. B. and Decker, J. L. (1969). Capillary tube migration for detection of human delayed hypersensitivity: difficulties encountered with "buffy coat" cells and tuberculin antigen. *J. Immunol.*, **103**, 179

7 Locksin, M. D., (1969). Failure to demonstrate leukocyte migration inhibition in human tuberculin sensitivity. *Proc. Soc. Exp. Biol. Med.*, **132**, 928

8 Bloom, B. R. (1971). In Bloom, B. R. and Glade, P. R. (eds.) *In vitro methods in cell-mediated immunity*, pp. 3–93. (New York: Academic Press)

9 Lolekha, S., Dray, S. and Gotoff, S. P. (1970). Macrophage aggregation in vitro: a correlate with delayed hypersensitivity. *J. Immunol.*, **104**, 296

10 Gotoff, S. P., Vizral, I. F. and Malecki, T. J. (1970). Macrophage aggregation *in vitro:* a model for transplantation immunity. *Transplantation*, **10,** 433

11 Gotoff, S. P., Lolekha, S., Lopata, M., Kopp, J., Kopp, R. L., and Malecki, T. J. (1973). The macrophage aggregation assay cell mediated immunity in man. Studies on patients with Hodgkin's disease and sarcoidosis. *J. Lab. Clin. Med.*, **82,** 682

12 Ford, P. M., Ford, S. E. and Gibson, G. (1977). Evaluation of antigen-induced buffy coat leukocyte aggregation as a simple test for allergic reactivity. *Int. Arch. Allergy Appl. Immunol.*, **53,** 56

13 Nicholls, E. M. (1974). Aggregation of buffy coat leukocytes. A simple sensitive assay for cell mediated immunity. *Clin. Exp. Immunol.*, **17,** 673

14 Rouveix, B., Badenoch-Jones, P. and Turk, J. L. (1979). A sensitive technique for measuring macrophage aggregation: a comparison with macrophage migration inhibition for the detection of lymphokine activity. *Immunology*, **36,** 589

15 Badenoch-Jones, P., Rouveix, B. and Turk, J. L. (1980). Studies on lymphokine-induced macrophage aggregation. Specificity and quantitative aspects. *Int. Arch. Allergy Appl. Immunol.*, **62,** 188

# Discussion

**Dr R. J. Scheper (Netherlands)** was invited to review his work on lymphocyte migration. He said that inflammatory reactions usually involved very few B lymphocytes, less than one would expect on the basis of their numbers in peripheral blood. They had therefore studied the *in vitro* capacity of lymphocyte classes to migrate. They had found that migration was dependent on the charge of the substrate and the charge of the cells. T cells migrated faster than B cells and he believed this was due to the more negative surface charge on the former than the latter. It was also important to note that in inflammatory reactions the pH was usually lower than 7 and they had found a small but significant difference between B and T cell migration as a function of acidity. They had also found that both T and B cells migrated further in activated serum than in fresh serum. Heat inactivation produced immune aggregates of IgG which behaved like immune complexes. They could mimic the aggregate induced chemokinesis or increased migration which occurred in heat inactivated serum by adding pre-formed heat inactivated immune complexes to fresh serum. In summary, their results showed that T cells had a higher locomotive capacity than B cells and that the latter were more inhibited by lower pH. Although the importance of these findings to the situation *in vivo* was not established, he felt that they did help to explain the low contribution of B cells to normal inflammatory reactions.

**Professor S. J. Normann** (USA) believed that only the blast-transformed cells participated in migration *in vivo*.

**Dr Scheper** said that his studies were performed on activated lymphocytes containing many blast cells and on those coming from chemically stimulated as well as unstimulated lymph nodes. At 18 h there was no difference in migration between activated and normal T cells or between normal and activated B cells. At 4 h, activated T cells had migrated somewhat further than normal T cells but the difference was not impressive.

**Dr C. J. Dunn (France)** said that he used lymphokine macrophage migration inhibition as a parameter of immunologically induced inflammatory processes. He wondered whether Dr Scheper had used lymphokines in the process and whether he regarded his findings as indicative of an inflammatory or anti-inflammatory effect.

**Dr Scheper** said that they had studied the effects of pH, of lymphokines and of immune complexes. Lymphokines did not have any effect on the migration of B or T lymphocytes although macrophages were inhibited in their migration. As to whether migration was a pro- or anti-inflammatory phenomenon, he did not know.

On being asked about the drugs utilized in his experiments he said that he had studied sodium azide, which in dogs inhibited B and T cells in exactly similar ways, colchicine, which inhibited the microtubule function as well as giving enhancement at low concentrations, and cytochalasin B, which again inhibited both T and B cell migration. So far their results with anti-inflammatory drugs were somewhat confused.

**Professor Normann** said that he had observed that heating the serum to 56°C enhanced the chemotactic activity, an effect which was not due to aggregation because the activity was in a fraction with a molecular weight of less than 150 000. Thus, when lymphocytes were reported to respond to heated serum he questioned whether this effect was necessarily due to aggregation.

**Dr Scheper** said that workers in Leiden, when studying immune complex mediated phenomena, always used immune aggregates prepared by heating serum for 20 min at 60°C. He had been able to mimic the enhanced migration in heat inactivated serum to exactly the same extent by adding immune aggregates to fresh serum. However, he had not fractionated the serum and he agreed that the evidence was indirect.

**Dr C. J. L. M. Meijer (Netherlands)** was invited to review his findings on T lymphocyte sub-populations in rheumatoid arthritis. He said that the inflammatory infiltrate in rheumatoid synovium was composed mainly of T cells and depletion of such cells by thoracic duct drainage had an effect on the course of the disease. For these reasons they investigated the T cell sub-populations in 24 rheumatoid patients. They found that there was a significant difference between the mean percentage of $T\mu$ lymphocytes compared to healthy controls. There was a negative correlation between clinical measurements of disease activity and the number of $T\mu$ lymphocytes. No such correlation was found between $T\gamma$ lymphocytes and disease activity, although the variation in $T\gamma$ lymphocytes was higher in patients than controls. They had found toxicity against $T\mu$ lymphocytes in 6 of 7 patients in the active disease group, but no such lymphocyte toxicity in the controls. In summary, there was a correlation between a lowered percentage of $T\mu$ lymphocytes and disease activity, and serum toxicity against $T\mu$ lymphocytes also appeared to be a feature of active disease.

On being questioned further about the cytotoxicity he said that in 2 patients toxicity was directed against both $T\mu$ and $T\gamma$. In toxic situations 50–80% of cells were killed, though never 100%. It was possible that this represented selective killing of the $T\mu$ fraction carrying the $Fc\mu$ marker.

**Dr M. D. Hall (UK)** said that the $T\mu$ plus $T\gamma$ populations did not appear to add up to the total T cell population.

**Dr Meijer** said that 25–30% of T lymphocytes did not have markers for either $Fc\gamma$ or $Fc\mu$ receptors. Of the 70% that did expose markers, 57% had $Fc\mu$ and 13% $Fc\gamma$.

**Professor D. A. Horwitz (USA)** said that the number of lymphocytes with Fc receptors for IgM could vary from 25%–80% with time and tissue culture. In the rheumatoid group there might have been delayed expression of the Fc receptor and longer culturing might have produced more positive cells.

**Dr Meijer** said that the cells were purified and tested on the second day. Certainly there were no differences in the $T\gamma$ lymphocytes between the first and second days. Nor had they found any increase in controls or patients in the percentage of $T\mu$ markers detected with a mixed rosette assay in lymphocytes examined immediately or 24 h after isolation. He did not feel that any inability to detect $Fc\mu$ markers was due to a blocking of antibodies on the $T\mu$ lymphocytes.

**Dr Horwitz** said that the precursor of the $T\mu$ cell was an esterase positive lymphocyte. He wondered whether esterases had been examined and if so what was the percentage of esterase positive cells in rheumatoids and normals.

**Dr Meijer** had not tested the esterase markers in these studies. However, in fractions used to study the purity of $T\mu$ lymphocytes, more than 95% had the characteristic dot-like staining. In the $T\gamma$ lymphocyte fraction this dot-like staining occurred in only 4–5%, the rest being negative or showing stippled staining.

**Mr M. E. J. Billingham (UK)** asked if there was any correlation between therapy and the $T\mu$ marker, and also enquired what was the function of the $T\mu$ cell.

**Dr A. Cats (Netherlands)** said that patients were treated with gold or penicillamine but they had found no correlation between the markers and drug therapy. Nor at present were they able to define the function of the $T\mu$ cell.

**Professor J. P. Famaey (Belgium)** was invited to review his work on enkephalins in the immune system. He said that because of the work of Professor Ferreira and others showing that enkephalins could have peripheral activity, they had decided to establish whether circulating enkephalins could react with lymphocytes using the Wybran rosetting model. They also decided to examine morphine and morphine-like compounds. To their surprise, they noted that morphine-like drugs reduced the number of rosettes while enkephalins increased the number. At present there was no explanation for this discrepancy except that increasingly the literature suggested that there were different enkephalin receptors. The $\mu$ receptors had greater affinity for morphine and less for methionine enkephalin while the $\delta$ receptors had greater affinity for this latter substance. The effect was totally reversed by the specific antagonist naloxone, which had no effect on the rosettes. They then examined the activity of dextromoromide and levomoromide and found that the former, active compound had an effect but not the latter, inactive one. These results suggested that there might be receptors for enkephalins and morphine-like compounds on T cells. Simultaneously, work in other laboratories had shown that specific receptors for beta-endorphins existed on B lymphocytes. However, these were non-opiate receptors not reversibly influenced by naloxone or other morphine antagonists. They would speculate that there was a co-operation between B and T lymphocytes as far as enkephalin effects were concerned. It was possible that enkephalins had a modulating effect on the immune system and since T lympohocytes shared a common antigen with the brain this also suggested that certain auto-immune neural diseases might be linked to the immune system.

**Professor C. M. Pearson (Chairman)** was not surprised that receptors for morphine or enkephalins existed on lymphocytes, if only because such cells had receptors for so many molecules. He wondered, in alluding to CNS disease, whether Dr Famaey was considering allergic enkephalic myelitis, schizophrenia or other conditions.

**Dr Famaey** said that they were interested in schizophrenia but binding studies would be required before one could be sure that the relevant receptors existed. There was, however, at least suggestive evidence that enkephalin could influence lymphocytes at concentrations totally compatible with those present in the serum.

**Dr Dunn** asked what action enkephalin might be expected to have in rheumatoid arthritis.

**Dr Famaey** said that Swedish studies showed changes in the basic level of enkephalin and endorphin during various diseases involving chronic pain. Rheumatoid arthritis was a good model for chronic pain and such molecules might be exerting some influence upon it. There was evidence that enkephalin-like activity was reduced in patients with trigeminal pain and rheumatoid arthritis might be similar.

**Dr Dunn** asked whether, apart from pain, enkephalins, by their attachment to lymphocytes, might directly affect the process of diseases in which lymphocytes were known to be pathogenic.

**Dr Famaey** did not know of any evidence for the effect on the disease process in RA but in other models it was suggested that competition existed between enkephalins and prostaglandins in producing changes in the level of cyclic AMP and GMP.

**Professor C. M. Pearson** said that following lymphocyte depletion by thoracic duct drainage two features which they had observed rapidly to disappear were morning stiffness and pain. He wondered whether these effects might be due to the removal of some receptors.

**Dr Hall** was invited to review his work on Fabc rosettes. He said that there had been much interest in recent years in the role of lymphocytes bearing receptors for the Fc portion of IgG. They had been implicated in the regulation of the immune response and in K cell cytotoxicity. Because Fc receptors were widely distributed on some T cells, B cells, other lymphocytes and monocytes it was not clear which assay detected Fc receptors on which cell sub-population. Accordingly they had limited the specificity of Fc receptors being detected.

The Fc portion of IgG contained Cγ2 and Cγ3 domains. They had developed an assay which detected only those cells with receptors for the Cγ2 region. This had been done by coating calf erythrocytes with rabbit Fabc fragments which were IgG molecules that had lost the terminal Cγ3 domains. Using the assay they had demonstrated an increased number of Fabc rosetting cells in the peripheral blood of rheumatoid patients compared to those with osteoarthritis, ankylosing spondylitis or healthy controls. Since the Fabc fragment did not bind to rheumatoid factor the assay was not complicated by possible interaction with antiglobulin factor on the lymphocyte surface. They had started to characterize the cell bearing the Fabc rosettes. It was neither a T nor a B lymphocyte. As to specificity of the receptor, it appeared to be blocked very effectively by immune complexes and not so effectively by native human IgG. It was inhibited by rabbit monomeric IgG but not very effectively by Fc fragments. This suggested a specific interaction between the receptor and immune complexes. The structure was not present in isolated Fc fragments. They were attempting to assess whether the cell had a particular biological function, but so far they had been unable to do so.

In response to questions about the cell type, he said that the receptors appeared to be borne by sub-population of null lymphocytes. On questioning about the interaction of antiglobulin complexes with Fabc formation he said that some of the receptors might be blocked, since trypsinizing the cells produced a higher proportion of them expressing the receptor. One could not automatically deduce that immune complexes were involved, however. Many other receptors were detected on treating the cell surface with an enzyme.

**Dr Horwitz** said that there was a relationship between these cells and what he called 'L' cells which did not make rosettes without T cells and which were Ig and C3 negative. He wondered whether the Fc receptor on the cells might have been modulated by some circulating immune complex so that it could not be detected but was still present. This would explain why there was no K cell activity.

**Dr Hall** said that the situation was complicated because different Fc receptors were expressed on the same cell, certainly with monocyte macrophages and possibly with these cells too. He had not tried deliberately to remove the receptors by incubating with immune complexes.

**Dr Leijh (Netherlands)** asked whether Fabc receptors could be detected on monocytes, because he understood from other work that monocytes needed the CH2 domain for Fc receptor binding.

**Dr Hall** said that they had depleted monocytes by incubation of blood with carbonyl ion and had found that the procedure did not alter the expression of Fabc rosettes. They had also purified monocytes by centrifugation and showed that such purified monocytes formed very few Fabc rosettes. The specificity of the Fabc receptor was somewhat controversial. Some workers suggested that the Cγ3 domain was the only one involved but others suggested some involvement of the Cγ2 as well.

**Dr Horwitz** was invited to review the work of his group on 'L' lymphocytes. He said that the work was designed to clarify the role of Fc receptors for IgG on antigen specific proliferation of human lymphocytes. Lymphocytes were taken from individuals immunized with keyhole limpet haemocyanin (KLH) and stimulated *in vitro* with either KLH or KLH complexed to IgG–anti-KLH. Immune complexes were found either to enhance or to suppress lymphocyte proliferation. They set out to establish the conditions under which such complexes would cause enhanced proliferation. Enhancement was found to be dependent on the Fc portion of the IgG immune complex and was mediated by a lymphocyte with a high avidity Fc receptor for IgG. There appeared to be two types of cell with this kind of receptor. One was a cell constituting about one-third of the Tγ cells forming E rosettes with sheep erythrocytes. The other type was the C3 receptor negative subset of the null cells which he had termed the 'L' cell. Selection experiments had shown that the L cell could mediate the effect whereas the Tγ cell could not. Further experiments suggested that the L cell was needed for the enhancement phenomenon. A programme designed to characterize the activity of the L cell showed that it could not be induced to proliferate by immune complexes. Stimulated T cells could not induce L cell proliferation; rather L cells seemed to enhance T cell reactivity, an effect which depended upon monocytes. It was known that monocytes exposed to KLH would trigger a proliferative response. No similar effect was found with L cells, but brief exposure to immune complexes produced a response 2–3 times that of similarly exposed monocytes. He therefore believed that the L cell had an accessory cell function in being able to present KLH determinants to monocytes and T cells in such a way that T cell proliferation was greatly enhanced. In this sense its response was more similar to that of monocytes than other lymphocytes, but so far they had been unable to induce monocytes to exert a similar enhancing effect. In summary, this small sub-set of cells, constituting 5% of human blood lymphocytes, had an accessory cell function in antigen specific proliferation.

**Professor Pearson** asked whether Dr Horwitz believed that L cells might be responsible for the propagation of the inflammatory response in rheumatoid arthritis.

**Dr Horwitz** said that that question was worth pursuing. There were now data from other laboratories suggesting that null cells were increased in synovial fluid. Another of their functions was non-specific cytotoxicity which was also increased in synovial fluid. It was possible that L cells increased in synovial fluid and in the presence of immune complexes they would perpetuate T cell proliferation.

**Dr Bray** asked whether there were any indications that the sub-population might produce soluble mediators in its helper function.

**Dr Horwitz** had looked for such mediators by investigating whether he could produce enhancement by different kinds of immune complex. Such experiments had given negative results.

**Dr J. Dingle (UK)** asked whether L lymphocytes, so far observed in man, existed in other species where they could be more closely defined.

**Dr Horwitz** said that Japanese workers had described a lymphocyte with similar characteristics in the mouse but he had not pursued the subject.

**Dr Scheper** asked Dr Horwitz to amplify his suggestion that B cells did not have Fc receptors. In addition, he wondered about the organ distribution of L cells.

**Dr Horwitz** said that B cells lacked the high affinity Fc receptor, which could be demonstrated using normal human serum at 4 °C. As to organ distribution, the L cells were found in the bone marrow and the spleen, not in peripheral lymph nodes.

**Dr R. Mullink (Netherlands)** was invited to review his work on the dose-dependent influence of anti-inflammatory drugs on PHA induced lymphocyte proliferation of guinea pig lymph node cells. These cultures consisted of 5% macrophages. Anti-inflammatory drugs appeared to cause inhibition at relatively high concentrations but most of the non-steroidal drugs caused enhancement at moderate concentrations. In order to investigate whether this enhancement involved the overriding of inhibitory mediators secreted by the macrophages, additional experiments were performed in which the proportion of macrophages was changed from 5% to 30%. Indomethacin and mefenamic acid again showed additional enhancement. For benzydamine a shift in the dose-response curve to the right was observed. Aspirin was exceptional in that the shift in the dose response curve was to the left. Such curves might be explained by regarding them as the resultant of two separate curves, one reflecting inhibition of prostaglandin production by macrophages resulting in enhancement of lymphocyte proliferation, the other reflecting a non-specific, perhaps partly toxic effect of the drug on the lymphocyte. Aspirin results, however, could only be explained by assuming that it induced effects on the lymphocytes, making them more toxic to macrophages.

**Dr Bray** said that this work confirmed much that had already been done on the influence of non-steroidal agents in lymphocyte transformation, in relation to prostaglandins. However, he doubted whether one could ascribe the inhibition with higher doses of non-steroidal agents to some toxic response. There might be other pathways of arachidonic acid metabolism which higher doses of drugs such as indomethacin would inhibit. Other workers had suggested that a balance existed between the various products of arachidonic acid metabolism in the lymphocytes.

**Dr Mullink** said that in preliminary experiments they had examined toxic influences on the lymphocyte and for most drugs there was good correlation between inhibitory effects and toxicity. For indomethacin for example an effect was seen at 0.1 mol/l.

**Dr Bray** said that at that dose one might expect inhibition of lipoxygenase products and so the influence of toxicity would be difficult to establish.

**Dr P. Bacon (UK)** questioned the relevance to the *in vivo* situation of culture systems in which PHA and drugs were added simultaneously to the cells. Paracetamoi, which was totally inactive clinically, would suppress PHA induced transformation *in vitro*. Experiments pre-dosing guinea pigs and then extracting the cells for further investigation seemed more appropriate.

**Dr Mullink** had not performed such experiments but he said that these effects had been demonstrated *in vivo* for indomethacin by others. There seemed to be an interaction between lymphocytes and macrophages and their products. The lymphocytes producing lymphokines stimulated macrophages which produced a range of products, some of them capable of enhancing lymphocyte proliferation, and others such as prostaglandin able to inhibit lymphocyte function.

**Dr F. Wong (USA)** said that if one were attempting to show enhancement of lymphocyte transformation one should start with a system which was already suppressed. Conversely, if one were looking for suppression then one should start with a normal lymphocyte system.

**Dr Mullink** said that they had not been specifically looking for enhancement. That was an additional effect revealed by their experiments. However, it was known that in some clinical systems in which immune suppression did occur some of the suppression was induced by factors produced by macrophages, for example prostaglandin.

**Dr C. A. Ottaway (Canada)** was invited to review his work on lymphoblast localization. He said that his group had been interested in the interrelationship between the accumulation of effector lymphoblasts in various tissues and regional blood flow variations, especially during inflammatory events. They had been investigating the feasibility of combining R686 studies of cardiac output with lymphoblast labelling to study the relationship between the two. In previous studies they had shown that accumulation of peripheral lymphoblasts in inflamed skin was directly proportional to the increase in the fraction of cardiac output going to the inflamed site. They had then proceeded to the gastrointestinal tract and had found that there was a normal gradient of blood flow along the small intestine but that the upper segment received more of the cardiac output than did the distal segments, even measured on a tissue weight basis. Thus, there were tissue specific differences in regional blood flow in the intestine. The distribution of lymphoblasts from the mesenteric lymph nodes to the small intestine correlated well with this distribution and so it seemed likely that immunocyte density along the small intestine might be attributable to differences in regional blood flow. In order to establish any influence of an inflammatory process in the small intestine they had produced enteritis in mice using the nematode parasite *Trichinella spiralis*. This parasite progressed down the bowel as it matured. Their findings had been contrary to expectations. There were no dramatic changes in blood flow in the early stages of infection but there were marked changes in lymphoblast localization. Lymphoblast accumulation doubled early in infection in a way unrelated to any demonstrable changes in regional blood flow. However, changes did occur in the efficiency with which these cells were interacting with the small intestine, even early in the infection. Such changes were at a maximum in the upper small intestine before any morphological alterations or change in vascular permeability were detectable. Lymphoblast accumulation was therefore a very early event in infection. Finally, in the intestine where mesenteric lymphoblasts were already primed to gut derived antigens, it would seem (at least in the natural infection) that the probability of subsequent immune interactions was very high, even if the inflammation was not primarily immune.

**Dr M. Ziff (USA)** asked whether the cells leaving the post-capillary venules were lymphocytes or blasts.

**Dr Ottaway** said that the cells escaped in the form of blasts, although there did not appear to be any specific morphological exit point.

**Dr Ziff** suggested that the cells might escape as small lymphocytes, meet the antigen in the extracellular space and undergo blastic transformation there.

**Dr Ottaway** said that he thought this was unlikely.

**Dr Ziff** said that in the perivascular regions of the rheumatoid synovial membrane one could detect small lymphocytes and collections of blasts could be seen in the neighbouring areas, which suggested that, in this disease at least, the cells regressed as small lymphocytes and then met the antigen and were converted to blasts. Dr Ottaway was providing blasts and so they egressed as blasts but in other diseases that was not the case.

**Dr Ottaway** said that the possibility existed that blasts might enter a tissue and then be converted into small cells. They were looking at a dynamic process and many changes might be occurring.

On being asked whether the blasts given were sensitized to the antigen involved in the gut infection he said that in this particular model the question was not critical. In these experiments he gave mesenteric lymph node blasts from animals undergoing infection only because it was possible to obtain a large number of blasts that way. However, similar results could be obtained with unstimulated blasts and even peripheral blasts gave some effect. All would enter the gut in a similar way.

**Dr A. Kahan (France)** was invited to review his work on lymphoblast activation in response to lectins. He said that immunological conditions in rheumatoid arthritis were not understood. Lymphocyte transformation (LTT) found in 60% of rheumatoid patients was considered low but the question of what was normal had not been resolved. Accordingly, they had studied such variation in normal individuals and had found the variation to be very large. Their group had also worked on a nuclear refringence test which seemed a good test for assessing immunomodulator action or for assessing the degree of immune deficiency in patients. Lectins put in the presence of lymphocytes for 20 min caused this index to fall, which meant that the chromatin which was previously very dense had become dispersed.

**Dr Horwitz** said that this work of Dr Kahan's was very important in that it attempted to assess lymphocyte stimulation by methods other than tritiated thymidine incorporation. Another way of studying such stimulation was to stain lymphocytes with acridine orange. This stained nuclear DNA green and RNA red and fluorographic recording revealed a variety of lymphocyte activation states before the cells actually divided.

**Dr B. Rouveix (UK)** was asked to describe his studies on aggregation of indicator cells. He said that they had developed a new method for assessing lymphokine activation by quantitative measurement of either direct or indirect macrophage aggregation in the guinea pig. They used a modified platelet aggregometer. They had attempted to establish the mechanism of such aggregation by measuring lymphokine activity in human BCG skin tests. This method had been compared with inhibition migration tests and with the lymphocyte transformation tests. Preliminary results suggested that the new method was more sensitive than the migration inhibition test in being more reproducible and easy to set up and he believed that it was suitable for the assay of a large number of samples.

# Section X
# Enzymes and Cell Secretion Products

CHAIRMAN: M. E. Billingham
CO-CHAIRMAN: M. U. Dianzani

# 111

# Macrophages as origin of factor increasing monocytopoiesis (FIM) (Abstract)

W. SLUITER, E. HULSING-HESSELINK, B. ELZINGA-CLAASEN and R. VAN FURTH (NETHERLANDS)

During the initial phase of an inflammatory reaction, a factor increasing monocytopoiesis (FIM)[1] in the bone marrow was found in the serum of mice. FIM is a protein without essential carbohydrates, has no colony stimulating activity, and is cell-line specific. The decrease in the number of monocytes during the second phase of an inflammatory response is probably governed by another humoral factor (monocyte production inhibitor, MPI)[2].

The aim of the present study was to establish the origin of FIM. Macrophages from different sources were studied, i.e. mouse peritoneal and alveolar macrophages, rabbit peritoneal macrophages, and two murine macrophage tumour cell lines. These cells were cultured for 48 h *in vitro*, and at various times the FIM activity was determined in culture fluid and extracts of lyophilized cells. The effect of phagocytosis on the FIM activity in culture fluid and cell extracts was also studied by allowing these cells to phagocytize opsonized polystyrene latex particles.

The FIM activity of a test sample was measured by determination of the increase in the number of monocytes in the circulation of mice after it had been injected intravenously and assessment of the effect on the proliferation rate of macrophage tumour cell lines. The results show that peritoneal macrophages have a high level of FIM activity. After these macrophages had phagocytized latex, their FIM activity decreased, whereas the activity in the culture fluid increased and remained demonstrable during at least 48 h of incubation of the cells, which indicates a continuous release and production of FIM by these macrophages. Similar results were obtained with alveolar macrophages and macrophage tumour cell lines, which supports the conclusion that FIM originates in macrophages.

**References**

1 van Waarde, D. *et al.* (1977). *Blood*, **50**, 141
2 van Waarde, D. *et al.* (1978). *Agents Actions*, **8**, 432

# 112

# Phagocytosis and enzymatic activity of $PGE_1$ treated rat peritoneal macrophages (Abstract)

D. VENZA-TETI AND A. MISEFARI (ITALY)

Various effects of prostaglandins (PGs) on macrophages and immunocompetent cells have been reported by different investigators. The present work has been undertaken to test functional activities of $PGE_1$ treated rat peritoneal macrophages. Peritoneal macrophages were collected from normal Sprague–Dawley albino rats. Adherent cells were cultured for 24 h at 37 °C in a humidified 5% $CO_2$ atmosphere. Cell viability was assayed by trypan blue dye exclusion test and by checking levels of lactic dehydrogenase.

Phagocytosis of zymosan, determined under phase contrast microscopy, was always lower when macrophages were pre-incubated with $PGE_1$ for 30 min at 37 °C. Also lysosomal activities, referred to β-glucuronidase and *p*-nitrophenyl-*N*-acetyl-β-glucosaminidase liberation, were lesser than in control, $PGE_1$-untreated macrophage cultures. These data indicate that $PGE_1$ induced marked functional changes of rat peritoneal macrophages and support the hypothesis for an *in vivo* modulatory effect of $PGE_1$ on macrophage function.

# 113

# Alterations in bone marrow leukocyte ultrastructure and alkaline phosphatase activity accompanying a peripheral inflammatory response in the rat (Abstract)

D. M. WILLIAMS, R. GILLETT AND J. E. LINDER (UK)

---

The alterations in leukocyte counts in peripheral blood which occur during a local inflammatory response are accompanied by changes in both mitotic activity and ultrastructural morphology of bone marrow precursors. In unstimulated marrow from young adult male Sprague–Dawley rats, alkaline phosphatase (AP) activity, as demonstrated by an osmiophilic method (Williams *et al*, 1979 *J. Histochem. Cytochem.* **27**, 665) is evident on the plasma membrane of eosinophils from the late promyelocyte stage onwards. Neutrophils are much less heavily labelled, the enzyme not being demonstrable until the metamyelocyte stage. Within 30 min of the subcutaneous injection of turpentine (4 ml/kg body weight) depletion of mature netrophils is apparent, becoming marked by 12 h. To compensate for this depletion, mitotic activity increases significantly after 12 h, involving all stages from the myeloblast, which is rarely seen dividing in resting marrow, to myelocyte. Additionally AP activity becomes evident in myeloblasts and promyelocytes. At 12 h dividing neutrophil precursors dominate the bone marrow, and although eosinophil numbers remain unchanged, they frequently fail to exhibit AP activity. By 20 h, as a consequence of earlier mitotic activity, numerous mature neutrophils are seen, many exhibiting AP activity, but mitotic activity appears less marked.

Ultrastructural changes are striking after 12 h in eosinophils and neutrophils. Both exhibit increased synthetic activity with more prominent dilated endoplasmic reticulum, persistence of the nucleolus, and, in eosinophils, a more florid Golgi. The significance of these changes remains to be assessed, although Pedersen and Hayhoe (1971, *Br. J. Haematol.*, **21,** 257) have suggested neutrophil AP levels are related to phagocytic ability. The appearance of AP positive neutrophil precursors in the marrow may thus reflect a heightened functional capacity of these cells, an aspect of the inflammatory response of obvious benefit to the host.

# 114

# *In vivo* inhibition of PMN migration by antimacrophage serum

S. H. FERREIRA, GLORIA E. P. DE SOUZA,
AND R. RIBEIRO DOS SANTOS (BRAZIL)

The aim of the present investigation was to evaluate the effect of rabbit anti-rat macrophage serum (AMS) on the oedema and cell migration induced by a preparation of *M. tuberculosis*. Inflammation induced by *M. tuberculosis* is known to recruit macrophages, and anti-macrophage serum was found to affect macrophages *in vitro* as well *in vivo*, and is becoming a valuable tool to study their various functions[1–4].

In the present study it was unexpectedly found that rats treated with AMS showed a reduced migration of polymorphonuclear cells to the *M. tuberculosis* inflamed paw. In contrast, AMS treated animals showed an enhanced oedematogenic response to the inflammatory stimuli. Since AMS had no effect on blood leukocyte count nor on mononuclear cell migration to the lesion and did not cross-react with PMN it was suggested that macrophages are involved in the control of PMN migration to the inflammatory site.

## EXPERIMENTAL PROCEDURES

### Preparation of AMS

Peritoneal exudate cells were obtained from Wistar rats 4 days after thioglycollate (10 ml, Becton-Dickinson & Co., USA) was injected intraperitoneally. The cells were collected in Eagle's medium pH 7.4 (MEM, Wellcome, England) containing 5 U/ml of heparin, placed in Erlenmeyer and incubated at 37 °C. Adherent cells were washed twice with the medium. The resuspended cells were washed three times and adjusted to $1–5 \times 10^6\,ml^{-1}$ viable (90–95%) macrophages/ml. New Zealand rabbits were treated weekly for 8 weeks with 2 ml of the cell suspension, injected subcutaneously into the back.

For the two initial injections the cell suspension was emulsified with an equal volume of Freund's complete adjuvant. The animals were bled 7–10 days after the last injection. The sera were complement-inactivated by heating to 56 °C for 30 min and subsequently absorbed with rat red blood cells and tissue acetone powder of several organs (brain, spleen, heart, lungs, liver and kidney). The sera were tested by indirect immunofluorescence reaction[5,6] with macrophages, spleen lymphocytes[7] and a predominant PMN peritioneal exudate obtained 4 h after an injection of 1 mg of carrageenin (Marine Coloides, USA). AMS reacted positively to the macrophages (1:320) while neither lymphocytes nor PMN reacted with a 1:20 dilution of AMS. AMS also inhibited phagocytosis of sensitized (IgG) sheep red blood cells[8].

Peritoneal macrophages were incubated at 37 °C with red cells in Eagle's medium, normal rabbit serum (NRS) and AMS. 100 cells were counted (phase microscopy) per coverslip. The percentage of cells showing phagocytosis was (1) 76 % in Eagle's medium, (2) 90% in NRS diluted 1:5, (3) 80% in NRS diluted 1:20, (4) 10% in AMS dilute 1:20 and (5) 5% in AMS diluted 1:5.

**Experimental animals**

Newborn Wistar rats were made tolerant to rabbit serum by receiving an intraperitoneal injection of 0.1 ml of NRS during the first 24 h of life. The efficacy of the induced tolerance was confirmed by the Gel immunodiffusion test[9], 5 days after the last treatment in rats which received 11 injections of NRS or AMS, given on alternate days.

**Experimental design**

Tolerant Wistar rats of both sexes (160–250 g) were divided into a control group (receiving NRS) and a test group (receiving AMS). The sera were administered on alternate days (0.1 ml, i.p.) throughout the duration of the experiments.

A culture of *M. tuberculosis* was heat-denatured for 30 min at 155 °C and delipidated with acetone[10]. This preparation (100 ng in 0.1 ml) was used as the phlogogenic stimulus, which was injected into the rat paw concomitantly with the third serum injection. The contralateral paw was injected with 0.1 ml saline. The volume of the paw was measured by a technique described elsewhere[11]. Cell migration to the paw was quantitated[12] by blind examination of tissue sections obtained from the central area of the lesion.

## RESULTS AND DISCUSSION

The rabbit antimacrophage sera used in our experiments had no effect on the peripheral blood total and differential white cell count during the period of observation. This is in accordance with several reports in the literature[2, 12]. Feldman *et al.*[13] explained the absence of effect of AMS on circulating monocytes (in contrast with the intense effect on peritoneal cells), suggesting that the antigen detected by AMS might be an antigen of differentiation associated with cellular maturity.

A general view of the several sections of the paws with low magnification showed an increase in cell infiltration after the administration of *M. tuberculosis* which tended to diminish after the third day. Cell infiltration was apparently less intense in animals treated with AMS. A careful blind analysis of the cell type present in the lesion in shown in Figure 114.1. In panel A, the increase in PMN in controls (NRS) is compared to that in AMS treated rats, when 500 cells were counted. The lower migration of PMN observed could result from an increased number of other cells. However, this does not seem to be the case, since a lower PMN count also occurred when the number of mononuclear cells counted were fixed in 100 (central panel). The number of mononuclear (panel C) cells was essentially the same in both groups, being higher only in the AMS-treated group on the third day. After the ninth day of inflammation there was a reduction in PMN and mononuclear cells contrasting with an increased number of fibroblasts which occurred in both groups of animals (NRS and AMS).

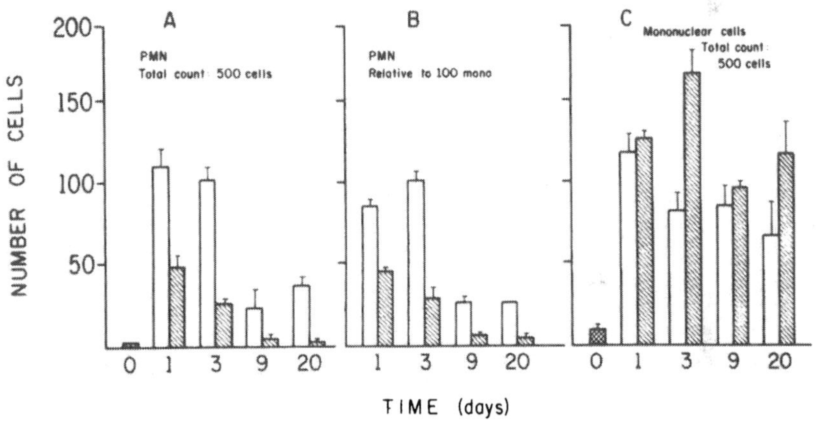


**Figure 114.1** Cell migration into the lesion induced by *M. tuberculosis*. Open and stippled bars indicate animals treated with normal and antimacrophage serum, respectively. The days after the inflammatory stimuli are indicated on the abscissa. Panel A; PMN population, when 500 cells were counted per paw ($n = 5$). Panel B; PMN population, when the number of mononuclear cells was fixed (100 cells, $n$=5). Panel C; Mononuclear population when 500 cells were counted per paw ($n = 5$). AMS treated rats showed a decrease in PMN population. The number of mononuclear cells was essentially the same in both groups.

Curiously, as shown in Figure 114.2, the oedematous response to *M. tuberculosis* was greater in animals treated with AMS. This might reflect the persistence of the trauma since there was a reduced migration of PMN and phagocytic activity of macrophages is probably reduced in these animals, AMS is known to strongly affect phagocytic activity *in vitro* and *in vivo*.

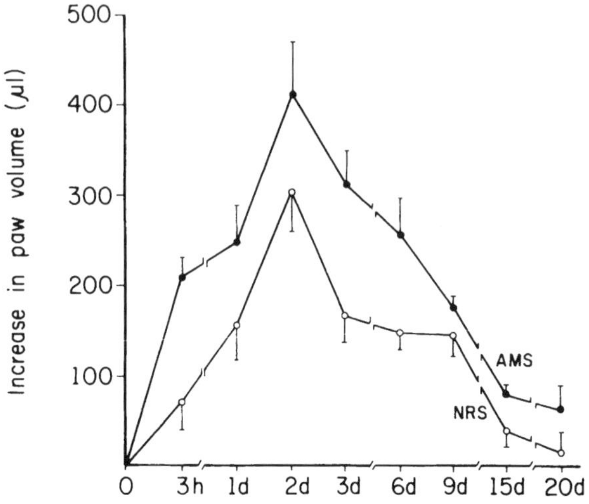


**Figure 114.2** Enhancement of the oedematogenic responses induced by *M. tuberculosis* by anti-macrophage serum. The open circles are for animals treated with normal rabbit serum ($n$ = 5). The break indicates a significant difference between groups ($p = 0.05$).

In conclusion, AMS- treated rats showed a significant reduction of PMN in the lesions. It seems that this is an indirect effect since AMS treatment did not change the number of peripheral PMN, and the serum, as shown by the immunofluorescence technique, did not cross-react against PMN. The existence of a factor controlling PMN released by macrophages was suggested by Kazmierowski[18] in the primate lung and by Russo (see Chapter 115) in the abdominal cavity of mice. These results are in line with Ferreira's[19] suggestion that resident macrophages might behave as 'tissue alarm cells', being an important element in the acute inflammatory reaction by triggering several lines of body defence.

## Acknowledgments

We thank Dr M. Mariano (Faculdade de Medicina Veterinária, USP) for comments and suggestions and FAPESP (Brazil) and Wellcome Foundation (England) for research grants.

## References

1 Unanue, E. R. (1968). Properties and some uses of antimacrophage antibodies. *Nature (London)*, **218,** 36
2 Hirsh, M. S., Gary, G. W. Jr. and Murphy, F. A. (1969). *In vitro* and *in vivo* properties of antimacrophage sera. *J. Immunol.*, **102,** 656
3 Argyris, B. F. and Plotikin, D. H. (1969). Effect of antimacrophage serum on antibody production and phagocytosis in mice. *J. Immunol.*, **103,** 372
4 Gallily, R. (1971). *In vitro* and *in vivo* studies of the properties and effects of anti-macrophage sera (AMS). *Clin. Exp. Immunol.*, **9,** 381

5 Coons, A. H. and Kaplan, M. H. (1950). Localization of antigen in tissues cells. II. Improvements in a method for the detection of antigen by means of a fluorescent antibody. *J. Exp. Med.*, **91,** 1

6 Ribeiro des Santos, R. S. and Hudson, L. (1980). *Trypanosoma cruzi*: Binding of parasite antigens to mammalian cell membranes. *Parasite Immunol.*, **2,** 1

7 Bøyum, A. (1976). Isolation of lymphocytes, granulocytes and macrophages. *Scand. J. Immunol.*, **5,** (Suppl. 5),

8 Stuart, A. E., Habeshaw, J. A. and Davidson, E. A. (1978). Phagocytes *in vitro*. In Weir, D. M. (ed.) *Handbook of Experimental Immunology, Vol. 2. Cellular Immunology*, pp. 1–30. (Oxford: Blackwell Scientific)

9 Ouchterlony, Ö (1958). Diffusion in gel methods for immunological analysis. *Prog. Allergy*, **5,** 1

10 Wadsworth, A., Maltaner, E. and Maltaner, F. (1931). The quantitative determination of the fixation of complement by the imune serum antigen. *J. Immol.*, **21,** 241

11 Ferreira, S. H. (1979). A new method for measuring variations of rat paw. *J. Pharm. Pharmacol.*, **31,** 649

12 Chalkley, H. W-. (1943). Method for the quantitative morphologic analysis of tissues. *J. Natl. Cancer Inst.*, **4,** 47

13 Feldman, J. D., Tubergen, D. G., Pollock, E. M. and Unanue, E. R. (1972). Distribution of a macrophage specific antigen. *Cell. Immunol.*, **5,** 325

14 Jennings, J. F. and Hughes, L. A. (1969). Inhibition of phagocytosis by anti-macrophage antibodies. *Nature (London)*, **221,** 79

15 Jasin, H. E., Lennard, D. and Ziff, M. (1971). Studies on antimacrophage globulin. *Clin. Exp. Immunol.*, **8,** 801

16 Despont, J. P. and Cruchaud, A. (1969). *In vivo* and *in vitro* effects of anti-macrophage serum. *Nature (London)*, **223,** 838

17 Kazmierowski, J. A., Gallin, J. I. and Reynolds, H. Y. (1977). Mechanism for the inflammatory responses in primate lungs. Demonstration and partial characterization of an alveolar macrophage-derived chemotactic factor with preferential activity for polymorphonuclear. *J. Clin. Invest.*, **59,** 273

18 Ferreira, S. H. (1980). Are macrophages the body's alarm cells? *Agents Actions*, **10,** 229

# 115

# Macrophage involvement in chemotactic response

M. RUSSO (BRAZIL)

## INTRODUCTION

Although polymorphonuclear leukocyte (PMN) migration is a cardinal event of acute inflammatory response the mechanisms by which these cells are recruited from the bloodstream and accumulate into sites of inflammation are not well understood.

Bacterial lipopolysaccharides (LPS) has among its large number of pathophysiological effects the capacity to induce diapedesis of neutrophils. It has been proposed that the C5a fragment, a highly active chemotactic factor generated via LPS activation of the complement (C) system, plays an important role in the early influx of PMN in inflammatory exudates[1]. However, in C5 deficient strains of mice, a delayed but still significant influx of PMN is observed after i.p. LPS administration[1,2].

A number of the host responses to LPS have been shown to be under genetic control. This aspect was clearly recognized in the C3H/HeJ strain of mouse, which is inherently refractive to many of the biological effects elicited by LPS. The C3H/HeJ mice are highly resistant to endotoxin shock[2,3], mount a poor immune response to LPS[4,5], are refractory to macrophage activation[6–8] and show decreased colony stimulating activity (CSA) response to endotoxin[9,10].

The present study was prompted by an observation noted while working with C3H/HeJ recipients that received i.p. C3He B/FeJ histocompatible peritoneal cells and challenged i.v. with LPS. It was found that the recipients' peritoneal cavity was densily populated by PMN cells. This finding was rather surprising since it is known that mice receiving a single i.v. LPS injection experience only small increases in the numbers of neutrophils in their peritoneal fluid[11]. This observation raised the question whether the chemotactic stimuli induced by LPS arises from its interaction with cells.

To evaluate this possibility C3H/HeJ recipients were injected i.p. with different C3He B/FeJ cell types and the peritoneal chemotactic response after i.v. LPS administration quantified. C3He B/FeJ donors were selected because, contrasting with the CeH/HeJ mice, they are susceptible to LPS and there are no measurable histocompatibility differences between donor and aceptor strains[12]. Evidence obtained with the experiments described herein suggests that macrophages play a role in the starting signal of extravascular neutrophilia induced after LPS injection.

## MATERIAL AND METHODS

### Animals

Genetically inbred female C3H/HeJ and C3HeB/FeJ mice, 20–25 g body weight were obtained from the Jackson Laboratory Bar Harbor, Maine.

### Endotoxin

LPS from *Salmonella abortus* equi Lot:613234, phenol-water extraction methods, from Difco Laboratories, Detroit, Michigan, was used throughout the experiments.

### Irradiation

Mice were irradiated with 720 rad in an acrylic plastic box by a Gammator M caesium -137 source (Radiation Machinery Corp., Parrisppany, New Jersey) delivering 630 rad/min.

### Preparation of cell suspension for the adoptive transfer

*Spleen cell suspension*

Spleens were aseptically removed and placed into serum-free MEM 199 (Grand Island Biological, Grand Island, NY). Spleen cell suspensions were prepared by squeezing the tissue through a hole of the splenic capsule. Cell clumps and debris were removed by filtering the supernatant through filters of silk stockings.

*Bone marrow cell suspension*

These were obtained as described previously[9], briefly, the marrows of femurs and tibias were flushed with 1 ml of MEM 199 and collected in plastic tubes kept on ice.

*Peritoneal cell suspensions*

Resident peritoneal cells were aseptically collected after i.p. injection of 3 ml $Ca^{2+}$, $Mg^{2+}$ free PBS. The cell suspensions were incubated in PBS supplemented with 20% heat inactivated foetal bovine serum for 30 min at room temperature in 60 mm Falcon tissue culture dishes. The non-adherent peritoneal cells were aspirated from the supernatant after repeated washing. The remaining adherent peritoneal cells were detached from culture dishes by treatment with 12 mmol/l lidocaine hydrochloride (Astra Pharmaceutical Co., Worcester, Mass.) for 10 min at room temperature followed by 10 squirts of PPS using a syringe (M. Rabinovitch, personal communication). The purity of non-adherent and adherent cell fractions consisted of 80% lymphocytes and 89% macrophages, respectively, as judged by morphological criteria.

All cell suspensions were washed once (900 rev/min for 10 min) and adjusted to the desired concentration. The cell viability assessed by trypan blue exclusion test was greater than 95%.

## RESULTS

### Production of chemotactic activity by adoptive transfer of different cell types after i.v. LPS administration

Previous work had suggested that C3HeB/FeJ peritoneal cells transferred to C3H/HeJ recipients induce an i.p. PMN influx after i.v. LPS administration. The initial experiments were carried out to confirm this observation and to determine whether other cell population from LPS-sensitive C3HeB/FeJ mice would also induce an extra-vascular neutrophilia in LPS-resistant C3H/HeJ recipients, after i.v. LPS injection.

Non-irradiated C3H/HeJ recipients were divided into four groups and injected i.p. with (1) saline, (2) $1.0 \times 10^6$ unseparated peritoneal cells, (3) $1.0 \times 10^6$ bone marrow cells, and (4) $1.0 \times 10^6$ spleen cells. 12 h after the cell transfer, the animals were challenged i.v. with 20 $\mu$g of LPS and 6 h later, the differential leukocytes count of the peritoneal exudate quantified. Figure 115.1 shows that the peritoneal cell population was the most effective in inducing PMN migration. The bone marrow cell population was less effective, as only one of the four tested animals showed a significant PMN influx, while the spleen cell population was almost ineffective, showing comparable values to the saline treated animals.

### Production of chemotactic activity by adoptive transfer of peritoneal cells after i.v. LPS administration

Once established that the peritoneal cell population was the more effective in inducing PMN migration, experiments were carried out with peritoneal cell population including additional control groups.

Non-irradiated C3H/HeJ recipients were inoculated i.p. with $2.0 \times 10^6$ unseparated peritoneal cells from C3HeB/FeJ or C3H/HeJ strains and 12 h later, the recipients were injected i.v. with 20 $\mu$g of LPS. 6 h after the LPS injection, the percent of PMN in the peritoneal exudate was quantified. Control

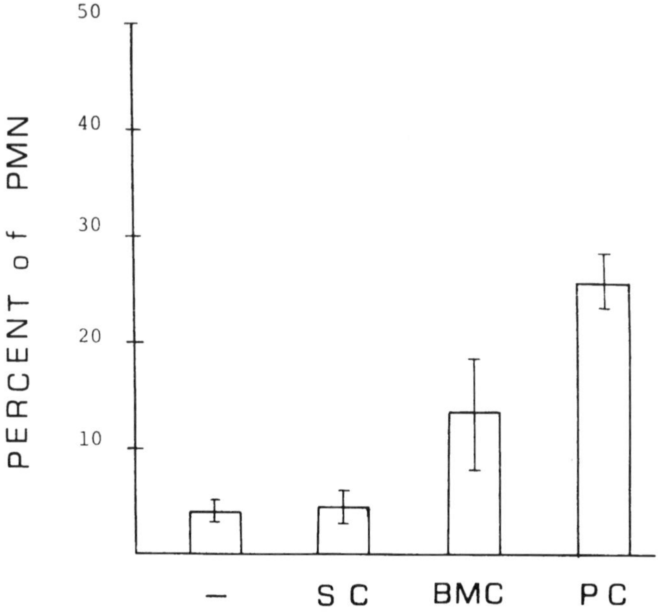


**Figure 115.1** Chemotactic response of C3H/HeJ recipients to i.v. LPS after i.p. injection of different C3HeB/FeJ cell population. C3H/HeJ mice were injected i.p. with (1) saline (–), (2) 1.0 × $10^6$ spleen cells (SC), (3) 1.0 × $10^6$ bone marrow cells (BMC) and (4) 1.0 × $10^6$ peritoneal cells (PC) obtained from C3HeB/FeJ donors. 12 h after the cell transfer, the animals were challenged i.v. with 20 µg of LPS and the peritoneal PMN migration quantified 6 h later. Values represent the mean ± SEM

groups did not receive LPS. As can be seen in Figure 115.2 the C3HeB/FeJ unseparated peritoneal cells again induced a significant influx of PMN into the peritoneal cavity of C3H/HeJ recipients after LPS challenge. Control groups, not injected with LPS, or C3H/HeJ recipients that received C3H/HeJ peritoneal cells showed only a minor increase in the PMN content of their peritoneal cavity (Figure 115.2).

**Production of chemotactic activity by adoptive transfer of different peritoneal cell types**

Results obtained above suggest that the C3HeB/FeJ peritoneal cell population mediate the i.p. influx of PMN observed in the C3H/HeJ recipients after systemic LPS administration.

In order to explore in more detail which type of peritoneal cells are responsible for the initiation of the chemotactic response and to minimize the recipients immunological response, experiments were performed in irradiated recipients which received i.p. different peritoneal cell types.

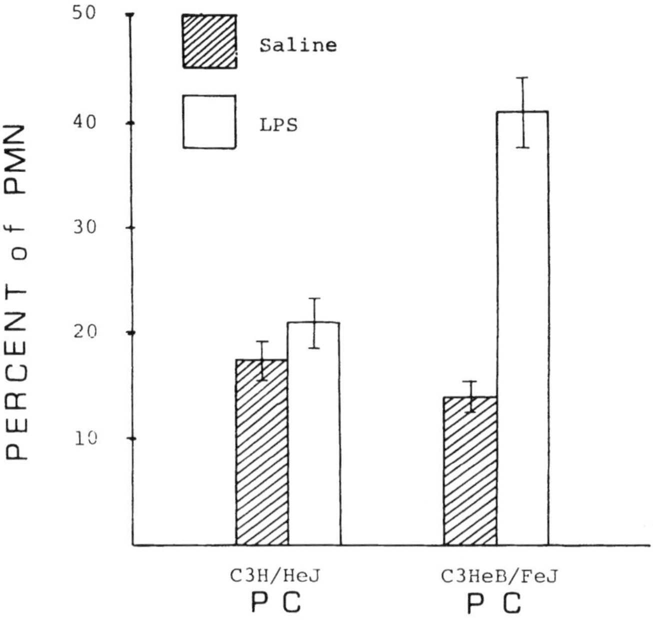


**Figure 115.2** Chemotactic response of C3H/HeJ recipients to i.v. with 20 μg of LPS. 6 h after the LPS injection, the peritoneal PMN migration was quantified. Values represent the mean ± SEM

C3H/HeJ recipients were lethally irradiated (720 rad) and 48 h later divided in three groups which received i.p. (1) $2.0 \times 10^6$ C3HeB/FeJ unseparated peritoneal cells, (2) $0.5 \times 10^6$ C3HeB/FeJ non-adherent peritoneal cells, and (3) $0.5 \times 10^6$ C3HeB/FeJ adherent peritoneal cells. 3 days after the cell transfer, irradiated recipients were challenged with 20 μg of LPS i.v. and their peritoneal cell exudate quantified 24 h later.

Figure 115.3 shows that $0.5 \times 10^6$ C3HeB/FeJ adherent peritoneal cells were as effective as $2.0 \times 10^6$ C3Heb/FeJ unseparated peritoneal cells in mediating the chemotactic response induced by LPS. In contrast, the C3HeB/FeJ non-adherent cells were not able to trigger the PMN influx.

These experiments corroborate the previous findings and suggest that the production of chemotactic activity starts after the interaction of LPS with adherent cell population.

## DISCUSSION

The experiments reported in this paper indicate that the C3HeB/FeJ adherent cell population are necessary for an effective chemotactic response

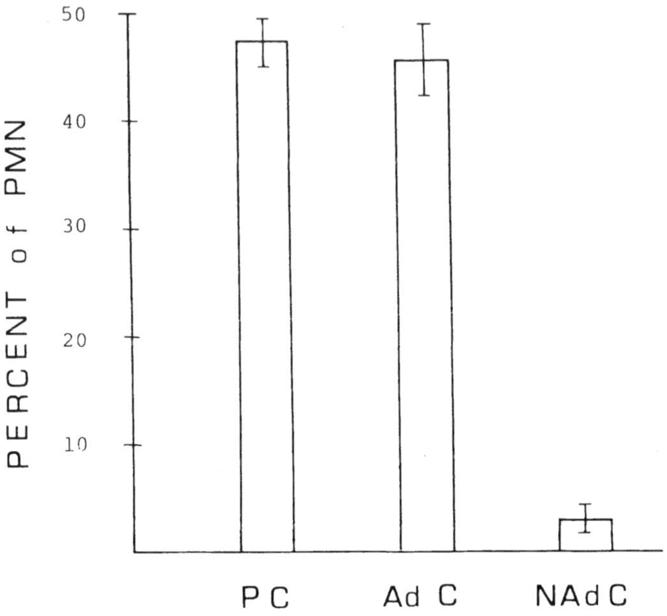


**Figure 115.3** Chemotactic response of irradiated C3H/HeJ recipients to i.v. LPS after i.p. injection of different C3HeB/FeJ peritoneal cell types. C3H/HeJ mice were irradiated (720 rad and injected i.p. 48 h later with (1) $2.0 \times 10^6$ unseparated peritoneal cells (PC), (2) $0.5 \times 10^6$ adherent peritoneal cells (Ad.C), and (3) $0.5 \times 10^6$ non-adherent peritoneal cells (N.Ad.C) obtained from C3HeB/FeJ donors. 3 days after the cell transfer the animals were challenged with 20 μg of LPS and the peritoneal PMN migration quantified 24 h later. Values represent the mean ± SEM

induced by LPS. It appears likely that the chemotactic activity arises from the interaction of LPS with macrophages, in the view of observations that (1) the adherent peritoneal cell population is mainly constituted by macrophages, and (2) the non-adherent peritoneal cell population, the spleen cell population that contains less than 10% of macrophages and bone marrow cells, rich in PMN and precursor cells, were almost ineffective in mediating the i.p. PMN influx.

At the present, little can be said about the chemical nature of the true chemotactic factor or the mechanism by which the chemotactic activity mediated by macrophages is generated. It will be interesting to learn whether the chemotactic factor is produced directly by a cell product or indirectly, by the interaction of the cell, or its products, with humoral factors.

The importance of C5 in the generation of complement dependent chemotactic activity *in vitro* as well as *in vivo* is recognized[1,13]. However, it is unlikely that the chemotactic activity mediated by macrophages observed in our experiments is due to the production of C5a, since LPS were administered i.v.

and thus generating a C5a chemotactic factor in the circulation and not in the peritoneal cavity. Furthermore, animals from C5 deficient strains or decomplemented by cobra venom factor were shown to exhibit a normal chemotactic response mediated by macrophages (M. Russo, unpublished observation).

A number of studies using different inflammatory agents have demonstrated a cell-derived chemotactic factor[14–17], but the relationship between the LPS induced macrophage mediated chemotactic activity and the cell derived chemotactic materials produced by other agents is unclear at the present.

The above data clearly established the requirement of adherent peritoneal cells for the production of chemotactic activity and suggest that a macrophage response to LPS is responsible for the initiation of the chemotactic response.

**Acknowledgments**
I would like to thank Ms. Maria de Lurdes Lorenzetti and Ms. Denise Correa Vilarinho for their excellent technical assistance. The numerous helpful discussions and the critically revised manuscript by Dr Mario Mariano is gratefully acknowledged. This work was supported by a grant from Fundaçao de Amparo à Pesquisa do Estado de São Paulo (78/1101).

**References**

1 Snyderman, R., Phillips, J. K. and Mergenhagem, S. E. (1971). *J. Exp. Med.*, **134**, 1131
2 Sultzer, B. M. (1972). *Infect. Immun.*, **5**, 107
3 Sultzer, B. M. (1968). *Nature (London)*, **219**, 1253
4 Watson, J., and Riblet, R. (1974) *J. Exp. Med.* **140**, 1147
5 Coutinho, A., Moller, G. and Gronowicz. E. (1975). *J. Exp. Med.*, **142**, 253
6 Chedid, L., Parrant, M., Damais, C., Parant, F., Juy, D. and Galelli. A. (1976). *Infect. Immun.*, **13**, 722
7 Bianco, C. and Edelson, P. J. (1977). *Fed Proc.* **36**, 1263
8 Ruco, L. P. and Meltzer, M. (1978). *J. Immunol.*, **120**, 329
9 Russo, M. and Lutton, J. D. (1977). *J. Cell. Physiol.* **92**, 303
10 Apte, R. N. and Pluznik, D. H. (1976). *J. Cell. Physiol.*, **89**, 313
11 Frumman, G. J. (1972). R.E.S., **12**, 62
12 Watson, J. and Riblet, R. (1975). *J. Immunol.*, **114**, 1462
13 Mergentagen, S. E., Snyderman, R., Gewurz, H. and Shin, H. S. (1969). *Curr. Top. Microbiol. Immunol.*, **50**, 37
14 Ryan, G. B. and Hurley, J. V. (1966). *Br. J. Exp. Pathol.*, **47**, 530
15 Borel, J.F. (1970). *Int. Arch. Allergy Appl. Immunol.*, **39**, 247
16 Zigmond, S. H. and Hirsh, J. G. (1973). *J. Exp. Med.*, **137**, 387
17 Kazmierowski, J. A., Gallin, J. I. and Reynolds, H. Y. (1977). *J. Clin. Invest.*, **59**, 273

# 116

# Determination of free lipid A and endotoxin (Abstract)

P. C. FINK AND J. KOZAK (W. GERMANY)

The wide spectrum of endotoxic activities among the different lipopolysaccharides has been shown recently to reside in the similar antigenic lipid A structure, which is an ubiquitous moiety in bacterial endotoxins (lipopolysaccharides). Based upon this concept, a heterogeneous enzyme-immunoassay to first determine free lipid A has been set up. Different antisera were obtained from rabbits and goats immunized with lipid A vaccine. The specificity of anti-lipid A IgG antibodies obtained after ammonium sulphate precipitation and DEAE-A-50 chromatography was assayed by passive haemolysis inhibition test.

Using a modified Limulus–Amoebocyte–Lysate (LAL) technique, standardized with endotoxin (ET) *Escherichia coli* 0113 PP–E-434 and detecting femtograms of endotoxin per ml, LAL positive reactions of 110 patients with different diseases were recorded spectrophotometrically. All normal controls, consisting of 51 healthy blood donors showed in comparison to the patient groups negative LAL reactions. For 33 post-operative patients with gram negative septicaemia, certified by positive blood cultures, ET equivalents ranging from 348 to 1020 pg/ml (mean concentration of 780 ± 112 pg/ml) were found. 20 patients with liver cirrhosis, spill-over phenomenon and negative blood cultures contained ET equivalents ranging from 320 to 810 pg/ml (mean concentration of 428 ± 84 pg/ml). 36 plasma samples from the umbilical vein of newborns induced LAL positive reactions in all cases in the range of 324 to 810 pg/ml (mean concentration of 396 ± 36). In 21 specimens taken simultaneously from the maternal peripheral venous blood ET equivalents demonstrated in the range of 312–840 pg/ml (mean concentration of 416 ± 32). The postnatal and maternal LAL positive reactions will be discussed in relation to the supernatants of sterile isolated lymphocytes and endotoxin plasma inhibitors.

# 117

# Mycoplasmas stimulate mouse peritoneal macrophages to secrete lysosomal enzymes and to be cytotoxic

H. U. SCHORLEMMER, M. KIST AND W. BREDIT
(WEST GERMANY)

## INTRODUCTION

The pathogenic mechanisms in mycoplasma infections are not fully understood. Several mechanisms may contribute to the recovery of animals from mycoplasma infections and resistance to reinfections. A feature of mycoplasma infections in the lungs and other sites is the associated mononuclear cell reaction. The infiltrating cells belong mainly to the lymphocyte and macrophage series. In bronchiolar exudates of mice infected with *M.pulmonis*[1,2] and hamsters infected with *M.pneumoniae*, macrophages are common. Serum antibodies transferred from mice recovering from pneumonia to recipient mice provides some protection against the development of pneumonia in these animals following inoculation of *M.pulmonis*[3]. According to the well-known view of Mackaness[4], immunity to infectious bacteria has two components.

The first is antigen specific and depends on T lymphocytes. When these react with the homologous bacterial antigen, they undergo blast transformation and liberate products that activate macrophages. The macrophages so activated are able to kill not only the bacteria that were used to stimulate the lymphocytes, but also antigenically unrelated organisms. There are several factors involved in the recruitment of mononuclear phagocytes. Those that facilitate entry of cells into sites of chronic inflammation and those that immobilize cells, allowing them to accumulate in lesions. Products of activate lymphocytes[5] presumably recruit macrophages into sites of delayed hypersensitivity reactions, including those elicited by microbial antigens. Also complement cleavage products active in macrophage chemotaxis have been described. There is some uncertainty whether C3a is chemotactic for macrophages but C5a is reported to be highly active[6]. The chemotactic activity of the C567 complex has long been known.

Moreover, many bacterial or fungal products are able to activate complement by the alternative pathway, generating C3b which activates macrophages to secrete hydrolytic enzymes[7]. In addition, the complement cleavage product C3a lyses various tumor cells and lymphoblasts[8,9] and appears to be important in having some microbicidal functions[10]. That activated macrophages more efficiently kill infectious organisms (viruses, bacteria, fungi and protozoa) than unactivated macrophages is well known, although the mechanisms involved have not yet certainly been identified. A possibility therefore arose that mycoplasmas might be able to stimulate the secretion of lysosomal enzymes and complement cleavage products by macrophages, and that these micro-organisms might be susceptible to the lytic effects of C/A. We want to analyse the role of macrophages in immunity to mycoplasma infections.

## RESULTS

### Mycoplasmas induce the selective release of acid hydrolases from cultured macrophages

*In vitro* studies with cultures of mouse peritoneal macrophages were designed to examine the capacity of stimuli with inflammatory properties, such as mycoplasmas, to induce selective release of acid hydrolases. Marked changes in the levels and distribution of the activities of lysosomal enzymes were induced by *Mycoplasma pulmonia* and *Mycoplasma homonis*. Two types of experiments were performed. In the first the effect of various concentrations on the level and distribution of enzyme activity in macrophage cultures after 24 h was measured. Secondly, the effect of a single concentration on the time course of changes in enzyme level and distribution in mouse macrophage cultures was determined. The organisms of *M.pulmonis* and *M.hominis* are rapidly taken up by phagocytosis and can be seen inside cultured macrophages after 3 h incubation at 37 °C. The ingestion is followed by marked selective release of lysosomal hydrolases into the culture medium.

Figure 117.1 compares the extent of the selective release of a representative lysosomal enzyme, *N*-acetyl-β-D-glucosaminidase, from macrophages exposed to two strains of mycoplasmas. They induce a dose-dependent increase in the amount of lysosomal enzyme in the culture medium. These levels increase from a base line amount of approximately 7% of total culture activity to nearly 70% in the presence of 200 μg/ml of *M.pulmonis*. The other organism, *M.hominis*, increased lysosomal enzyme release into the culture medium from the base line amount to about 45% of the total activity in the culture. Similar findings were made when two other representative lysosomal enzymes, namely β-glucuronidase and β-galactosidase were assayed. There was no evidence of any cytotoxic effect of either type of organism as indicated by measurement of lactate dehydrogenase levels in cells and culture media.

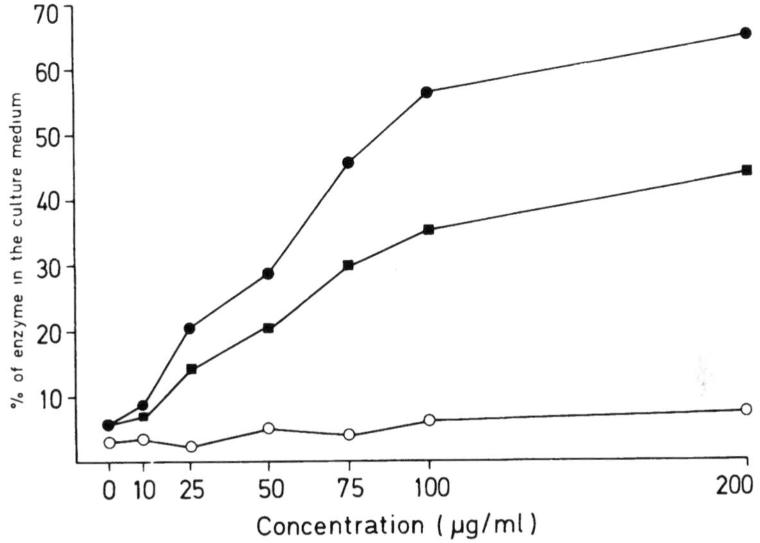


**Figure 117.1** Effect of 24 h incubation with various concentrations of *M. pulmonis* (●) and *M.hominis* (■) on the release of *N*-acetyl-ß-D-glucosaminidase and lactate dehydrogenase (○) from macrophages into the culture medium

The time course of enzyme production and release was studied in macrophage cultures maintained for various lengths of time up to 71 h, in the presence of a single dose of 50 μg/ml of *M.pulmonis* and *M.hominis*. The time dependence of the selective release of lysosomal enzymes caused by these stimuli is shown in Figure 117.2. Macrophage cultures exposed to the two micro-organisms showed by about 10 h a highly significant increase in the amount of β-glucuronidase in the medium. Subsequently, a rapid rise in the release of enzyme into the culture medium occurred so that by 71 h approximately 70% and 50% of the total enzyme activity was found in the culture medium with *M.pulmonis* and *M.hominis*, respectively. This time dependence of the selective release of lysosomal enzymes caused by these two mycoplasmas occurs with no detectable release of cellular lactate dehydrogenase into the culture medium.

**Induction of cytotoxic macrophages stimulated *in vitro* by mycoplasmas**

To mouse macrophages recovered from the peritoneal cavities without prior stimulation and cultured in a serum-free medium were added the two micro-

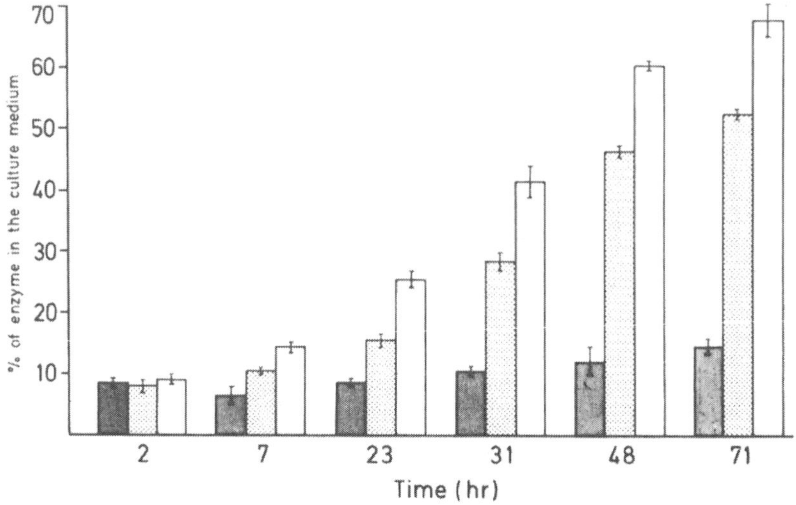


**Figure 117.2** The time dependent release of ß-glucuronidase from macrophages exposed to 50 μg/ml of the micro-organisms. ■ controls; ▦ *M. hominis*, and □ *M.pulmonis*

organisms *M.hominis* and *M.pulmonis*. The media of macrophages cultured with mycoplasmas (but not in the absence of these organisms) were found to contain material with cytotoxic activity. Stimulated macrophages might kill tumour cells by direct contact or by the release of a lytic factor. The presence of a lytic factor in the culture media of stimulated macrophages has been found in all our experiments. In several independent experiments, after 24 h incubation in the macrophage cultures stimulated by the mycoplasmas, the cytotoxic activity in the culture media for P 815 mastocytoma cells was significantly greater than in the controls. As is shown in Figure 117.3, the appearance of the lytic activity is dose dependent and *M.pulmonis* was the better stimulator tested.

The time course of lactate dehydrogenase release from mastocytoma cells incubated with normal and *M.pulminis* stimulated macrophages is illustrated in Figure 117.4. Macrophages were cultured in serum-free medium in the presence of *M.pulmonis* for 24 h. To each petri dish of cultured macrophages $1 \times 10^6$ target cells in 1 ml of fresh medium were added at the indicated times. The lytic activity progressively increased with time, and optimal cytotoxicity in the macrophage cultures was reached after 48 h. Normal macrophages were not cytotoxic.

**Treatment of mycoplasmas, P.mirabilis and L-phase variant with purified guinea pig C3a**

The results of incubating *M.pulmonis* with 25 μg of C3a for 30 min at 37 °C are shown in Figure 117.5. About 90% of the organisms were killed by C3a after

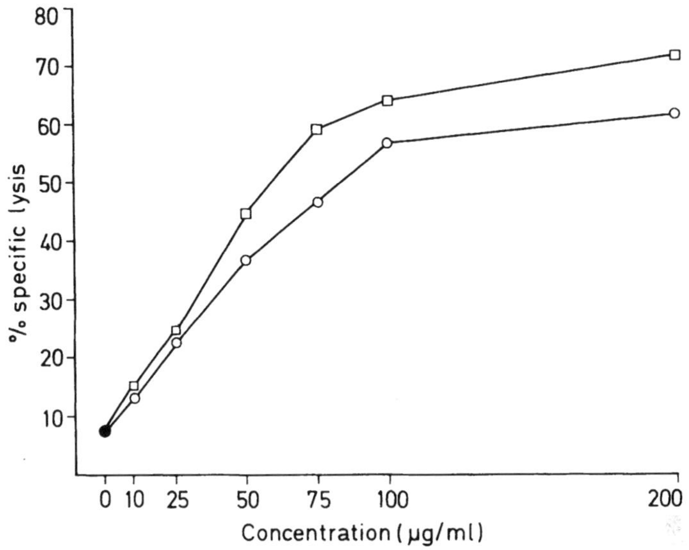


**Figure 117.3** Dose dependence of mycoplasma stimulation on macrophage cytotoxicity. Macrophage cultures grown in the presence of various concentrations of *M. pulmonis* (□) *or M. hominis* (○) for 24 h have shown a tumorolytic effect on labelled tumour cells used

this time. The effect of C3a on the viability of *M.hominis* organisms was even greater than on *M.pulmonis* organisms. As in the case of *M.hominis*, incubation of *P.mirabilis* L-phase variant with 25 μg/ml C3a for 30 min resulted in the killing of all the organisms. In contrast, the bacterial form was completely unaffected by the same treatment. Evidence that C3a lysed the L-phase variant organisms, rather than merely inhibiting their growth, was obtained in experiments showing release of DNA pre-labelled with $^{125}$IUdR from these cells by C3a. When the L-phase organisms were incubated with 10 μg/ml of C3a for 30 min, 92% of the label was released. On the other hand, when organisms were incubated with medium alone, only 6% of the label was released.

**Treatment of mycoplasmas with supernatants of macrophages activated *in vitro* by mycoplasmas**

In Figure 117.6 the results of incubating *M.pneumoniae* with two dilutions (1 : 2 and 1 : 10) of macrophage supernatants activated *in vitro* with *M. hominis* are shown for various periods of time. About 90% of the organisms were killed by this macrophage supernatant (1 : 10) after 15 min. There was a further loss of viability up to 30 min but not significantly after this time. More organisms were killed by using a dilution of 1 : 2 of the macrophage supernatant; 99% of them within 15 min and practically all after 2 h.

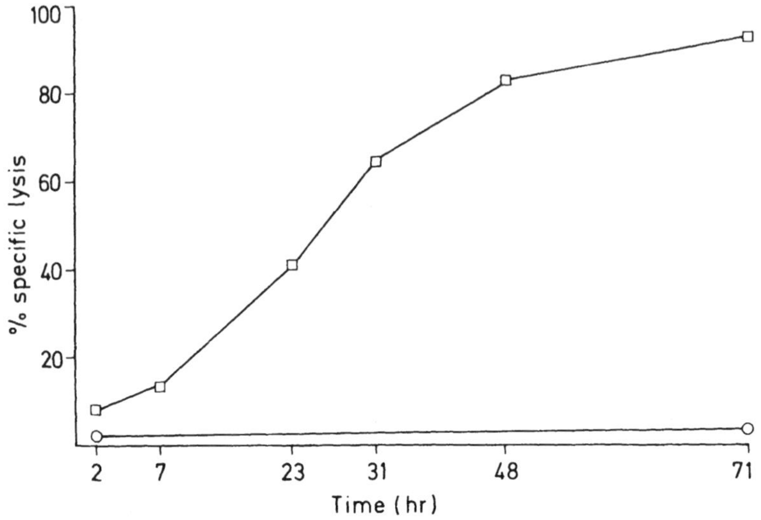


**Figure 117.4** The time course of lactate dehydrogenase release from mastocytoma cells incubated with normal (○) and *M.pulmonis* stimulated macrophages (□)

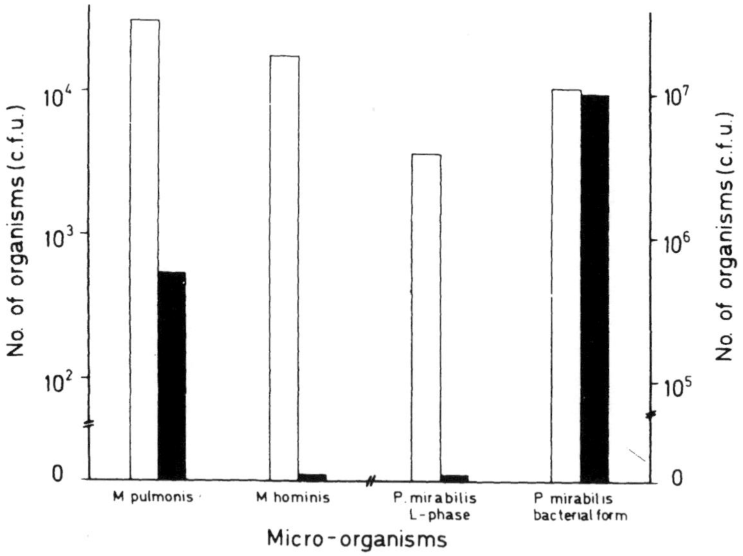


**Figure 117.5** The effect of C3a on mycoplasmas, L-phase organisms and bacteria. □ untreated micro-organisms; ■ micro-organisms treated with C3a

Evidence for the killing of mycoplasma organisms through lysis was sought by electron microscopic observations. *M.hominis* organisms before and after treatment with the lytic principle were centrifuged for 30 min at 20 000 *g* and the deposits observed. Intact organisms which had a characteristic unit membrane and cytoplasmic structure before treatment were never seen after treatment. Only membrane fragments remained, indicating that lysis had occurred.

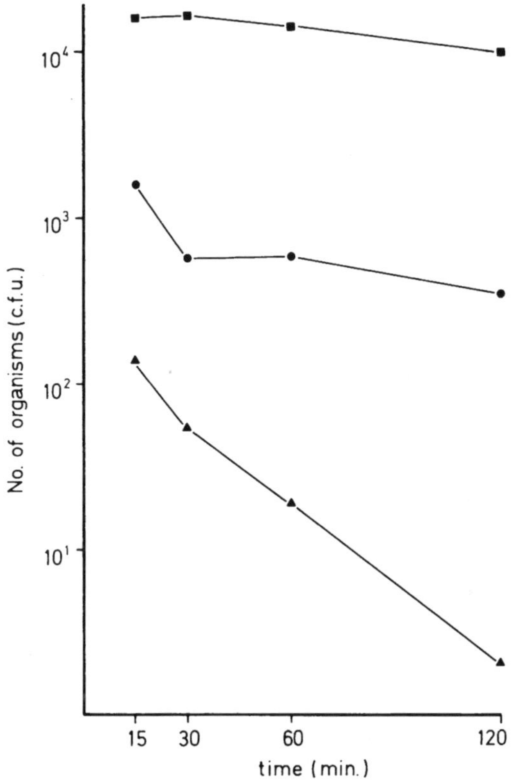


**Figure 117.6** The viability of *M.pneumoniae* after treatment with two dilutions (●) 1 : 10 and (▲) 1:2 of macrophage supernatants activated *in vitro* by mycoplasmas. The supernatant of untreated macrophages (■) is unable to kill *M.pneumoniae*

## DISCUSSION

A feature of mycoplasma infections in the lungs and other sites is the associated mononuclear cell reaction. A variety of microbial and other agents eliciting chronic inflammatory reactions induce the secretion of hydrolytic enzymes from macrophages[11]. We have found that mycoplasmas have similar effects on macrophages. The results of the experiments now reported show that mouse peritoneal macrophages, exposed *in vitro* to *M.hominis* or *M.pulmonis*, release large amounts of lysosomal hydrolases; the release is time and dose dependent and is not associated with loss of the cytoplasmic enzyme lactate dehydrogenase or any other sign of cell death. The release of enzymes may cause tissue damage and be a factor in the pathogenesis of some mycoplasmal diseases such as *M.pulmonis* induced chronic arthritis.

Normal macrophages have limited cytolytic and cytostatic activity, but activated macrophages acquire these capacities. Products of activated T lymphocytes stimulate macrophages to increased phagocytic activity and capacity to kill infectious bacteria[12]. Macrophages stimulated *in vitro* with *M.pulmonis* or *M.hominis* acquire the capacity to lyse added tumour cells. In addition, *M.pneumoniae* was sensitive to the supernatants of macrophages activated *in vitro* by mycoplasmas. In other experiments two species of mycoplasmas and a bacterial L-phase variant are sensitive to purified guinea pig C3a. The effect was a cytolytic rather than a cytostatic one, as shown by electron microscopy and release of labelled DNA. In contrast, intact bacteria were resistant to C3a.

Normal macrophages are known[13] to synthesize C3 and factor B of the alternative pathway[1] both of which are secreted intact. However, when the macrophages are activated they release cleavage products C3a and C3b or enzymes that cleave C3 in the medium[15] The mechanisms by which several agents exert their effects on macrophages and by which macrophages have cytotoxic effects on tumour cells and to become bactericidal are unknown. We have drawn attention to the fact that several stimulants of macrophages are able to activate complement by the alternative pathway[11]. The ways in which macrophages and components of complement may aid in recovery from infections by mycoplasmas are less well understood, but an important factor may be macrophage activation.

Several factors could trigger this process. Bredt[16] found that peritoneal macrophages were inefficient in phagocytozing *M.pneumoniae* organisms, but complement, activated by either the classical or alternative pathways, induced phagocytosis which might have been due to C3b on the surface of the organisms. *M.pneumoniae* cells are able to activate the alternative pathway of complement[17]. An early consequence of the activation is the cleavage of the native complement component C3 into a smaller fragment C3a and a large fragment C3b. The C3b formed is able to activate other macrophages whereas the C3a released appears to be important in the tumourolytic effects of macrophages as well as having some microbicidal functions. The activated macrophages could terminate mycoplasma infections by ingesting the organisms, a process favoured by having antibodies and/or C3b on their surface, and then killing and digesting them. Alternatively, the activated macrophages might release a lytic factor (C3a) to lyse the organisms. The relative importance of these mechanisms in recovery from different mycoplasma infections has yet to be established.

**Acknowledgment**

The authors wish to thank Mrs A Börner for her excellent technical assistance.

**References**

1 Lindsey, J. R. and Cassell, G. (1973). Experimental mycoplasma pulmonis infection in pathogen-free mice: models for studying mycoplasmosis of the respiratory tract. *Am. J. Pathol.*, **72,** 63

2 Taylor, G. and Taylor-Robinson, D. (1975). The part played by cell mediated immunity in mycoplasma respiratory infections. *Dev. Biol. Stand.*, **28,** 195

3 Taylor, G. and Taylor-Robinson, D. (1977). Factors involved in resistance to and recovery from mycoplasma pulmonis induced arthritis in mice. *Ann. Rheum. Dis.*, **36,** 232

4 Mackaness, G. B. (1962). Cellular resistance to infection. *J. Exp. Med.*, **116,** 381

5 Ward, P. A., Renold, H. G. and David, J. R. (1970). The production by antigen stimulated lymphocytes of a leukotactic factor distinct from migration inhibitory factor. *Cell. Immunol.*, **1,** 162

6 Showell, H. S., Tear, R. J., Zigmond, S. H., Schiffman, G., Aswanikumar, S. Corcoran, B. and Becker, G. L. (1976). The structure-activity relations of synthetic peptides as chemotactic factors and inducers of lysosomal enzyme secretion for neutrophils. *J. Exp. Med.*, **143,** 1154

7 Schorlemmer, H. U., Davies, P. and Allison, A. C. (1976). Ability of activated complement components to induce lysosomal enzyme release from macrophages. *Nature (London)*, **261,** 48

8 Ferluga, J., Schorlemmer, H. U., Baptisda, L. and Allison, A. C. (1976). Cytolytic effects of the complement cleavage product C3a. *Br. J. Cancer*, **34,** 626

9 Schorlemmer, H. U., Ferluga, J. and Allison, A. C. (1977). Interactions of macrophages and complement components in the pathogenesis of chronic inflammation. In Willoughby, D. A., Giroud, J. P. and Velo, G. P. (eds.) *Perspectives in Inflammation*, p. 191. (Lancaster: MTP Press)

10 Taylor-Robinson, D., Schorlemmer, H. U., Furr, P. M. and Allison, A. C. (1978). Macrophage secretion and the complement cleavage product C3a in the pathogenesis of infections by mycoplasmas and L-forms of bacteria and immunity to these organisms. *Clin. Exp. Immunol.*, **33,** 486

11 Schorlemmer, H. U., Bitter-Suermann, D. and Allison, A. C. (1977) Complement activation by the alternative pathway and macrophage enzyme secretion in the pathogenesis of chronic inflammation. *Immunology.*, **32,** 929

12 Mackaness, G. B. (1971). Resistance to intracellular infection. *J. Infect. Dis.*, **123,** 439

13 Lai A Fat, R. F. M. and van Furth, F. (1975). In vitro synthesis of some complement components (Clq, C3 and C4) by lymphoid tissues and circulating leucocytes in man. *Immunology.*, **28,** 359

14 Bentley, C., Bitter-Suermann, D., Hadding, U. and Brade, V. (1976). In vitro synthesis of factor B of the alternative pathway of complement activation by mouse peritoneal macrophages. *Eur. J. Immunol.*, **6,** 393

15 Schorlemmer, H. U., Hadding, U. and Bitter-Suemann, D. (1979). Effects of complement cleavage products released from stimulated macrophages in allergic diseases. *Eur. J. Rheum. Inflam.*, **2,** 130

16 Bredt, W. (1975). Phagocytosis by macrophages of mycoplasma pneumoniae after opsonization by complement. *Infect. Immun.*, **12,** 695

17 Bredt, W. and Bitter-Suermann, D. (1975). Interactions between mycoplasma pneumoniae and guinea pig complement. *Infect. Immun.*, **11,** 497

# 118

# Influence of colchicine derivatives on lysosomal enzyme release from polymorphonuclear leukocytes and intracellular levels of cAMP after phagocytosis of monosodium urate crystals

DANIELA MIKULÍKOVÁ AND KAREL TRNAVSKÝ
(CZECHOSLOVAKIA)

## INTRODUCTION

Colchicine and its analogues belong to the group of microtubular inhibitors[1]. Microtubules are involved in the transport of extracellular material wrapped in vesicles towards lysosomes. Drug-induced tubulostasis may lead to reduced digestion of phagocytozed material and could prevent metabolic transformation of this material. These events possibly play a role in the inhibition of the generation of inflammatory mediators[2]. Colchicine does not stabilize isolated lysosomes[3] and so its primary action on polymorphonuclear functions (release of lysosomal enzymes and chemotactic factors, motility etc.) is possibly mediated through its anti-microtubular activity[4].

Some of the colchicine derivatives exhibit similar effects to the parent compound, e.g. demecolcine and deacetylcholchiceine are equivalent to colchicine in antigout activity[5]. Deacetylcolchiceine is nearly as effective as colchicine in inhibition of urate-stimulated motility of PMN[6] and less active in urate-induced paw swelling in the rat[7].

Since enzyme release from PMN is probably crucial for the tissue injury in gouty arthritis[8] we studied the influence of colchicine derivatives – demecolcine and deacetylcolchiceine – on lysosomal enzyme release from PMN after phagocytosis of monosodium urate crystals (MSU). At the same time we assessed the intracellular level of 3,5-cyclic adenosine monophosphate (cAMP).

## MATERIALS

Demecolcine and deacetylcolchiceine were kindly supplied by Prof. F. Šantavý, Biochemical Institute of the Medical Faculty, Palacký University, Olomouc, Czechoslovakia. Both derivatives were checked for purity by thin-layer chromatography according to the method of Potěšilová *et al.* [30]. MSU microcrystals (0.5–30 μm) were a gift from Dr Továrek, University Hospital, Brno, Czechoslovakia.

## METHODS

### Separation of leukocytes

Leukocytes were obtained from the venous blood of healthy young men. 450 ml of blood was drawn into a plastic flask with 0.9 ml of heparin (5000 U/ml) and 90 ml of a 6% dextran solution. After gentle mixing, sedimentation was allowed to proceed in the same flask for 40 min at room temperature. The cell-rich supernatant was carefully transferred to centrifuge tubes and the cells were sedimented at 100 *g* for 8 min at room temperature. Supernatant fluid was removed, the erythrocytes were removed by hypotonic lysis (90 ml 0.85% NaCl for 30 s, add 270 ml distilled water for 20 s, add 90 ml 2.6% NaCl), and the leukocytes were washed twice more in 0.15 mol/l NaCl and resuspended in the buffered medium to a concentration of $5 \times 10^7$ leukocytes/ml of medium (1% glucose in phosphate buffer saline, pH 7.4, which contained 500 U of heparin per 100 ml). Neutrophils were 60–75% of the total leukocytes.

### Measurement of enzyme release

0.7 ml portions of cell suspension were dispensed into 10 × 75 mm plastic test tubes. The cells were incubated at 37 °C with gentle shaking with demecolcine or with deacetylcolchiceine in various concentrations (0.5 ml). Analogous serum was added to a concentration of 10%. After 1 h incubation the cells were exposed for 1 h to particles of microcrystalline monosodium urate (0.2 ml). The final concentration of urate was 0.5 mg/ml of medium. At the end of the experiment, the tubes were centrifuged at 755 *g* at 4 °C. The cell-free supernatants were used for enzyme determination. 0.5 ml of 0.05 mol/l Tris–HCl buffer pH 7.5 containing 4 mmol/l EDTA was added to the sediments (EDTA acts as phosphodiesterase inhibitor to prevent degradation of cyclic nucleotides by plasma enzymes). Samples were heated to 100 °C and centrifuged at low speed. Supernatants were stored at −20 °C for determination of cAMP.

**Estimation of enzymatic activities**

Lactate dehydrogenase (EC 1.1.1.27) was determined by the method of Bergmeyer *et al.*[10]. One unit of activity was defined as decrease of absorbance 0.001 value per min at 340 nm at 25 °C. Neutral proteases (EC 3.4.4.−) activity was estimated by the procedure reported by Ignarro[11]. Beta-glucuronidase (EC 3.2.1.31) activity was measured with phenolphthalein glucuronide as substrate[12] in 0.3 mol/l acetic acid–NaOH buffer, pH 4.5

Determination of total enzyme activities were made after cells were lysed by six freeze–thaw cycles. Broken cell preparation were centrifuged and enzyme activities were then determined. The cyclic nucleotide levels were estimated by cyclic AMP assay kit (The Radiochemical Centre, Amersham, England). Determination of cAMP is based on the competition between unlabelled cyclic AMP with a fixed quantity of tritium labelled compound for binding to a protein which has a high specificity for cyclic AMP[13]. Separation of the protein-bound cyclic AMP from the unbound nucleotide is achieved by adsorption of the free nucleotide on charcoal, followed by centrifugation[14].

## RESULTS

Polymorphonuclear leukocytes incubated with MSU crystals released lysosomal enzymes as well as the cytoplasmatic marker enzyme LDH (Tables 118.1 and 118.2). The pre-incubation with both colchicine derivatives in various concentrations resulted in a decrease of lysosomal enzyme release. The inhibition was dose dependent. The release of cytoplasmic enzyme LDH tended to decrease but not to such an extent as the release of lysosomal enzymes, especially in the experiment with demecolcine. Phagocytosis of MSU crystals induced the decrease of cAMP level (Tables 118.3 and 118.4). In the presence of tested colchicine derivatives, in concentrations $10^{-3}$ mol/l and $10^{-4}$ mol/l, there was an elevation in cAMP. This increase was dose dependent.

## DISCUSSION

Ultrastructural studies have shown that PMN actively take up crystals of MSU within phagosomes which merge with primary lysosomes[15]. Later, direct interaction of MSU crystals with lysosomes takes place, the organelle perforates, injuring the cell in general. Extracellular release of leukocyte

**Table 118.1** The effect of demecolcine (DEME) on release of lysosomal enzymes

| | *Lactate dehydrogenase* (units) | *Neutral protease* (μg tyrosine/18 h) | *β glucuronidase* (μg phenolphthalein/ 18 h) |
|---|---|---|---|
| Polymorphonuclear leukocytes (PMN) | 151.3 ± 8.4 (6.2%) | 453.02 ± 3.79 (7.5%) | 94.66 ± 1.76 (5.3%) |
| PMN + urate (U) | 426.5 ± 5.6 (17.5%) | 2146.66 ± 8.51 (35.4%) | 477.66 ± 8.02 (26.9%) |
| PMN + U + $10^{-3}$mol/l DEME | 335.4 ± 7.2 (13.8%) | 1067.00 ± 12.58* (17.6%) | 277.66 ± 3.84* (15.6%) |
| PMN + U + $10^{-4}$mol/l DEME | 375.5 ± 4.9 (15.4%) | 1574.33 ± 6.01* (25.9%) | 283.34 ± 2.03* (15.9%) |
| PMN + U + $10^{-5}$mol/l DEME | 406.7 ± 9.6 (16.7%) | 1848.50 ± 34.38* (30.5%) | 346.67 ± 2.40* (19.5%) |
| Total activity (100%) | 2433.9 ± 19.4 | 6065.10 ± 51.72 | 1778.33 ± 60.09 |

Each number represents the mean of five samples; *statistically significant difference $p < 0.01$. All activities were calculated for 5 × $10^7$cells.

**Table 118.2** The effect of deacetylcolchiceine (DAC) on release of lysosomal enzymes

| | *Lactate dehydrogenase* (units) | *Neutral protease* (μg tyrosine/18 h) | *β glucuronidase* (μg phenolphthalein/ 18 h) |
|---|---|---|---|
| Polymorphonuclear leukocytes (PMN) | 181.4 ± 6.6 (7.8%) | 214.68 ± 1.45 (3.4%) | 101.05 ± 2.08 (7.7%) |
| PMN + urate (U) | 343.7 ± 9.4 (14.8%) | 1705.33 ± 23.32 (27.0%) | 332.32 ± 3.28 (25.4%) |
| PMN + U + $10^{-3}$mol/l DAC | 228.6± 7.1* (9.9%) | 950.35 ± 8.11* (15.1%) | 121.70 ± 8.82* (9.3%) |
| PMN + U + $10^{-4}$mol/l DAC | 287.2± 7.7* (12.3%) | 1310.67 ± 17.73* (20.7%) | 197.05 ± 2.52* (15.1%) |
| PMN + U + $10^{-5}$mol/l DAC | 321.7± 8.3† (13.8%) | 1528.72 ± 9.12* (24.2%) | 262.65 ± 2.03* (20.1%) |
| Total activity (100%) | 2318.2 ± 33.4 | 6318.33 ± 4.41 | 1308.05 ± 41.60 |

Each number represents the mean of five samples; *statistically significant difference $p < 0.01$; †statistically significant difference $p < 0.02$. All activities were calculated for 5 × $10^7$ cells.

content induces tissue injury and inflammation[16]. Phagocytosis of MSU by human leukocytes leads to irreversible damage of the cell with simultaneous discharge of cytoplasmatic and lysosomal enzymes, events which differ from uptake of particles such as zymosan or immune complexes. These materials lead to selective extrusion of lysosomal but not cytoplasmic enzymes.

The release of lysosomal enzymes may be influenced by several pharmacologic agents[17]. Three major types of compounds have been studied.

(1) Those that interfere with the levels of cyclic nucleotides – elevation of cAMP cellular levels reduces the enzyme release. Accumulation of cGMP results in enhancement of enzyme release from PMN.

**Table 118.3** The influence of demecolcine (DEME) on cyclic nucleotide level

| | *Cyclic AMP* (pmol/5 × $10^7$ cells) |
|---|---|
| Polymorphonuclear leukocytes (PMN) | 16·13±0·26 |
| PMN + urate (U) | 15·47±1·18 |
| PMN + U + $10^{-3}$ mol/l DEME | 26·53±0·61* |
| PMN + U + $10^{-4}$ mol/l DEME | 26·30±1·14* |
| PMN + U + $10^{-5}$ mol/l DEME | 19·33±0·71 |

Each number represents the mean of five samples; *statistically significant difference $p < 0{\cdot}01$.

**Table 118.4** The influence of deacetylcolchiceine (DAC) on cyclic nucleotide level

| | *Cyclic AMP* pmol/5×$10^7$ cells) |
|---|---|
| Polymorphonuclear leukocytes (PMN) | 13·73±1·03 |
| PMN + urate (U) | 9·20±0·55 |
| PMN + U + $10^{-3}$ mol/l DAC | 16·27±0·52 |
| PMN + U + $10^{-4}$ mol/l DAC | 14·96±0·75 |
| PMN + U + $10^{-5}$ mol/l DAC | 9·87±0·64 |

Each number represents the mean of five samples; *statistically significant difference $p < 0{\cdot}01$.

(2) Agents which affect the state or function of cytoplasmic microtubules.

(3) Agents that are known to stabilize biomembranes.

Colchicine inhibits microtubule assembly both *in vitro* and *in vivo* by binding with high affinity to tubulin the major protein constitutent of microtubules. Malawista uses this mechanism for explanation of the fact that colchicine actively inhibits the extracellular relase of lysosomal enzymes[18–22]. Colchicine also potentiates the increase of cAMP in human leukocytes induced by beta-adrenergic agonists and phosphodiesterase inhibitors. Rudolph *et al.* and Malawista *et al.*[23,24] suppose that the generation of cAMP is normally restricted by an intact system of cytoplasmic microtubules. This constraint is relaxed by colchicine.

The structure–activity relationship of colchicine derivatives has been investigated in several models. The results do not support the unitary hypothesis for colchicine activity based on its interference with microtubular subunit protein aggregation. Deacetylcolchiceine, used in our study, is an active drug in acute gout, as is colchicine[25]. Deacetylcolchiceine has no effect on microtubular precursor protein and even in high concentrations has little or no antimitotic effect in a variety of cell systems *in vivo* and *in vitro*[26,27].

Deacetylcolchiceine is nearly as effective as colchicine in inhibiting the PMN motility *in vitro*, but[6] has no influence on the urate-induced paw swelling in mice[7]. Demecolcine, on the other hand, inhibits the urate-induced paw swelling in rat, as does colchicine[28,29]. Demecolcine is about equipotent to colchicine in inhibiting the uptake of nucleotide in various mammalian cell lines[26]. Deacetylcolchiceine did not inhibit the nucleotide transport. In our experiments the MSU crystal induced release of lysosomal marker enzymes from PMN was inhibited by both colchicine derivatives: deacetylcolchiceine and demecolcine. Pretreatment of the cells with both drugs resulted in an intracellular elevation of cAMP. In this respect tested derivatives were similar in their activity to colchicine. Considering differences in some of their biological effects we could not explain the inhibition of lysosomal enzymes release by one common mechanism. It seems that there is a certain correlation between the activity of these agents and the level of cAMP. This effect could be primary and may mediate later via the intracellular level of cyclic nucleotides the influence on the integrity of microtubular system.

## References


1 Brune, K. and Whitehouse, M. W. (1979). Cytostats with effects in chronic inflammation. In Vane, J. R. and Ferreira, S. H. (eds.) *Anti-inflammatory Drugs*, p. 531. (Berlin: Springer-Verlag).

2 Wright, D. G. and Malawista, S. E. (1972). The mobilization and extracellular release of granular enzymes from human leukocytes during phagocytosis. *J. Cell Biol.*, **53,** 788

3 Weissmann, G. (1966). Lysosomes and joint disease. *Arthritis Rheum.*, **9,** 834

4 Fitzgerald, T. J. (1974). Colchicine and allopurinol. In Scherrer, R. A. and Whithouse, M. W. (eds.) *Anti-inflammatory agents*, Vol. 1, p. 295. (New York: Academic Press)

5 Wallace, S. L. (1959). Colchicine analogues in the treatment of gout. *Arthritis Rheum.*, **2,** 389

6 Phelps, P. and McCarty, D. J. (1969). Crystal induced arthritis. *Postgrad. Med.*, **45,** 87

7 Fitzgerald, T. J., Williams, B. and Uyeki, E. M. (1971). Colchicine on sodium urate-induced paw swelling in mice: Structure-activity relationships of colchicine derivatives. *Proc. Soc. Exp. Biol. Med.*, **136,** 115

8 McCarty, D. J. (1979). Short-term drug control of crystal-induced inflammation. In Vane, J. R. and Ferreira, S. H. (eds.) *Anti-inflammatory Drugs*, p. 92. (Berlin: Springer-Verlag)

9 Zurier R. B., Hoffstein, S. and Weissmann, G. (1973). Mechanisms of lysosomal enzyme release from human leukocytes. *J. Cell Biol.*, **58,** 27

10 Bergmeyer, H. U., Bernt, E. and Hees, B. (1965). Lactic dehydrogenase. In Bergmeyer, H. U. (ed.) *Methods in Enzymatic Analysis*, p. 736. (New York: Academic Press)

11 Ignarro, L. J. (1974). Nonphagocytic release of neutral protease and β-glucuronidase from human neutrophils. *Arthritis Rheum.*, **17,** 25

12 Barrett, A. J. (1972). Lysosomal enzymes (Glycosidases). In Dingle, J. T. (ed.). *Lysosomes – a Laboratory Handbook*, p.116. (Amsterdam: North-Holland Publishing Company).

13 Gilman, A. G. (1970). A protein binding assay for adenosine 3, 5-cyclic monophosphate. *Proc. Natl. Acad. Sci. (USA)*, **67,** 305

14 Brown, B. L., Albano, J. D. M., Ekins, R. P. and Scherzi, A. M. (1971). A simple and sensitive saturation assay method for the measurement of adenosine 3′, 5′-cyclic monophosphate. *Biochem. J.*, **121,** 561

15 Schumacher, H. R. and Phelps, P. (1971). Sequential changes in human PMN's after urate crystal phagocytosis. *Arthritis Rheum.*, **14,** 513

16 Weissmann, G. and Rita, G. (1972). Molecular basis of gouty inflammation: interaction of monosodium urate crystals with lysosomes and liposomes. *Nature (London) New Biol.*, **240,** 167

17 Goldstein, I. M. (1976). Pharmacologic modulation of lysosomal enzyme release from polymorphonuclear leukocytes. *J. Invest. Derm.*, **67**, 622
18 Malawista, S. E. (1968). Colchicine: a common mechanism for its anti-inflammatory and antimitotic effects. *Arthritis Rheum.*, **11**, 191
19 Perper, R. J. and Oronsky, A. L. (1974). Enzyme release from human leukocytes and degradation of cartilage matrix: effects of antirheumatic drugs. *Arthritis Rheum.*, **17**, 47
20 Wright, D. G. and Malawista, S. E. (1973). Mobilization and extracellular release of granular enzymes from human leukocytes during phagocytosis: inhibition by cortisol and colchicine but not salicylates. *Arthritis Rheum.*, **16**, 749
21 Pesanti, E. L. and Axline, S. G. (1975). Colchicine effects on lysosomal enzyme induction and intracellular degradation in the cultivated macrophage. *J. Exp. Med.*, **141**, 1030
22 Andrews, R. and Phelps, P. (1971). Release of lysosomal enzymes from polymorphonuclear leukocytes after phagocytosis of monosodium urate and calcium pyrophosphate dihydrate crystals: Effect of colchicine and indomethacin. *Arthritis Rheum.*, **14**, 368
23 Rudolph, S. A., Greengard, P. and Malawista, S. E. (1977). Effects of colchicine on cyclic AMP levels in human leukocytes. *Proc. Natl. Acad.Sci. (USA)*, **74**, 3404
24 Malawista, S. E., Oliver, J. M. and Rudolph, S. A. (1978). Microtubules and cyclic AMP in human leukocytes: on the order of things. *J. Cell Biol.*, **77**, 881
25 Wallace, S. L. (1975). Colchicine and new anti-inflammatory drugs for the treatment of acute gout. *Arthritis Rheum.*, **18**, 847
26 Mizel, S. B. and Wilson, L. (1972). Nucleoside transport in mammalian cells. Inhibition by colchicine. *Biochemistry*, **11**, 2573
27 Lettre, H. and Fernholz, H. (1943). Beitrag zur Beziehung zwischen der Mitosegiftwirkung und der Konstitution von Colchicine Derivativen. *Z. Physiol. Chem.*, **278**, 175
28 Denko, C. W. and Whitehouse, M. W. (1970). Effects of colchicine in rats with urate crystal-induced inflammation. *Pharmacology*, **3**, 229
29 Trnavský, K. and Kopecký, Š. (1966). The influence of some anti-inflammatory drugs on the inflammatory reaction to sodium urate. *Med. Exp.*, **15**, 322
30 Potěšilová et al. (1967). *Collect. Czech. Chem. Commun.*, **32**, 141

# 119

# Biological and biochemical activities of *in vitro* differentiating murine bone marrow macrophages (Abstract)

V. KLIMETZEK (WEST GERMANY) AND H. G REMOLD (USA)

It is largely unknown which of the biological and biochemical activities of specifically activated macrophages are shared by young bone marrow derived macrophages and which ones are acquired after activation by lymphokines. We therefore studied the activities of *in vitro* differentiating bone marrow macrophages and their ability to respond to lymphokines at various time points.

Murine bone marrow cells grown for 16 days in the presence of CSF proliferated until day 10–12; afterwards the number of cells remained constant. Peroxidase positive cells decreased from 60% on day 3 to 3% on day 11. Non-specific esterase was detectable from day 8 onwards. Bone marrow macrophages secreted plasminogen activator, plasminogen independent proteinases, lysozyme, but no proteinase inhibitors. The amount of proteinases secreted during 24 h decreased with the age of the cells, whereas the amount of lysozyme remained constant. The rate of pinocytosis and phagocytosis varied with the age of macrophages. Peak activity was consistently found on day 12 to 13. 5 to 8-day-old macrophages showed low 5-nucleotidase activity, which increased substantially in older macrophages. 7 to 16-day-old macrophages responded to migration inhibitory factor. Their sensitivity to the lymphokine was independent of age. Incubation with lymphokines for 24 h also increased the protease secretion of macrophages. The experiments suggest that young bone marrow derived macrophages exhibit several biological and biochemical features typical of inflammatory macrophages, which are further accentuated after exposure to lymphokines.

# 120

# Effect of synovial tissue on the matrix of articular cartilage in organ culture (Abstract)

R. W. JUBB AND HONOR B. FELL (UK)

The experiments were made on the articular tissues of the metacarpophalangeal joints of young pigs. In organ culture the synovial tissue caused the breakdown of cartilage matrix[1] and inhibited the synthesis of its sulphated proteoglycan[2].

Breakdown was effected in two ways: (1) by a direct action on the matrix of living or dead (frozen:thawed) cartilage with which it was in contact, and (2) by an indirect action mediated through living chondrocytes from which contact was unecessary. Used synovial medium had a similar effect on isolated cartilage (3) as the indirect action.

Experiments on the uptake of radioactive sulphate ($^{35}SO_4$) showed that synovial tissue inhibited the incorporation of $^{35}S$ by living cartilage placed either in contact with or at a distance from the synovial explant; this had been demonstrated by biochemical analysis and autoradiography. If the synovium was removed, the cartilage regained its synthetic activity. Association of cartilage with synovial tissue did not prevent the formation of new cartilage beneath the cut surface of the original explant, but reduced its incidence.

**References**

1 Fell, H. B. and Jubb, R. W. (1980). *Arthritis Rheum.*, **20,** 1359
2 Jubb, R. W. and Fell, H. B. (1980). *Arthritis Rheum.* (In press)
3 Dingle, J. T., Saklatvala, J., Hembry, R., Tyler, J., Fell, H. B. and Jubb, R. W. (1979). *Biochem. J.*, **184,** 177

# 121

# Effect of irradiation and cell reconstitution on the macrophage mitogenic activity of exudate and inflammatory serum

M. PELLETIER AND J. P. GIROUD (FRANCE)

## INTRODUCTION

Our recent findings have demonstrated the existence of a mitogenic factor, for macrophages in culture, in acute inflammatory exudates (IMF) and sera of inflamed rats[1–3,8,14] which could be formed or released by cells[14]. The question arises whether the factors present in the exudate and in the serum have the same cellular origin and are identical chemical entities.

It has been shown that the molecular weight of seric factor is less than 2000 daltons, while the molecular weight of exudate factor is around 5000 daltons (unpublished data). On the other hand, the mitogenic activity of serum factor is still detectable after dilution of 1 : 4000, and the mitogenic activity of exudate factor only after dilution of 1 : 2000 (unpublished data).

In order to determine the origin, and explore the difference between these two factors, we have investigated the effect of irradiation and cell reconstitution on mitogenic activity, for macrophages *in vitro*, of exudates and sera obtained from inflamed rats.

## MATERIALS AND METHODS

### Animals

Male inbred Wistar rats, pathogen-free were used throughout.

**Irradiation**

Rats were exposed to 900 rad delivered at a rate of 1.42 rad/s by a Gravatom Industries RW 30/55 M caesium bomb irradiator. Both before and 5 days after irradiation peripheral blood leukocytes were counted using a Hycel automatic counter.

**Cell transfer studies (reconstitution)**

*Bone marrow cells*

Bone marrow cells were obtained from femurs of normal rats by dissection at the proximal and distal ends. An 18 G needle was inserted into one end of the open femur and the cells expelled by washing with medium 199. The cells were disaggregated by several gentle aspirations through the needle.

*Thymic cells*

The thymus of normal rats was removed and minced into small pieces in medium 199. After disaggregation of the thymic cells (as above), the cell suspension was filtered through a metallic grid to remove tissue fragments.

Both bone marrow cell and thymic cell suspensions were adjusted to a concentration of $4 \times 10^7$ cells/ml medium 199 and injected slowly into the tail vein of irradiated rats, in a volume of 0.5 ml/rat, between 2–3 hours after irradiation. Cells from rats presenting an acute inflammatory reaction were harvested by the same method, 4 h after the start of inflammatory reaction.

**Inflammatory reaction**

Inflammation was induced, under sterile conditions, by intrapleural injection of 1 ml 6% dextran (Pharmacia, France 40 000 daltons) 5 days after irradiation.

**Preparation of inflammatory exudates**

4 hours after the beginning of the inflammatory reaction exudate was collected in plastic tubes packed in ice. The exudate was centrifuged at 4 °C, and the supernatant passed through a millipore filter (pore size 0.22 $\mu$m). The filtered exudate was diluted to a final concentration of 50% with culture medium containing 20% newborn calf serum.

**Preparation of inflammatory sera**

Blood was collected 1 h after the start of the inflammatory reaction and centrifuged at 4 °C. The serum was sterilized by passing it through a millipore filter (pore size 0.22 $\mu$m) and supplemented with 20% newborn calf serum.

**Macrophage cultures**

Rat peritoneal macrophages were harvested, under sterile conditions, by washing the peritoneum twice with 10 ml medium 199 supplemented with 20% heat-inactivated newborn calf serum, penicillin 5 IU/ml, streptomycin

100 μg/ml and heparin 5 IU/ml. The cells were pooled in plastic tubes at 4 °C, counted using a haemocytometer, diluted to $1.5 \times 10^6$ cells/ml and cultured, in Leighton tubes containing glass coverslips, at 37 °C. After 3 h incubation the medium was discarded to remove non-adherent cells, and culture medium (as above without heparin) was added. 2 days after seeding the macrophages were treated with the exudate preparation or with the serum.

**Determination of DNA synthesis**

3 or 4 days after the addition of exudate or serum, the cells were incubated with 1 μCi/ml tritiated thymidine (sp. activity 25 Ci/mMol) for 3 h. Coverslips were washed with saline and fixed in methanol. The DNA synthesis was determined either by autoradiography or by counting in a liquid scintillation spectrometer.

**Autoradiography**

Fixed coverslips were mounted on slides and autoradiographs performed using the dipping technique. After exposure for 5 days they were developed and stained with haematoxylin and eosin. The labelling index (‰) was calculated on 2000 interphase cells from duplicate slides.

**Counting in a liquid scintillation spectrometer**

Coverslips were transferred to scintillation vials (4 vials for each assay) and 15 ml PCS (AMERSHAM France) were added. The samples were counted in a liquid scintillation spectrometer intertechniques SL3. The results were expressed as counts per minute. In order to compare the results obtained with both techniques they were expressed as percent of control response calculated according the following formula:

$$\frac{\text{labelling index macrophages} + \left.\begin{matrix}\text{exudate}\\ \text{or}\\ \text{serum}\end{matrix}\right\}\ \text{from irradiated rats}}{\text{labelling index macrophages} + \left.\begin{matrix}\text{exudate}\\ \text{or}\\ \text{serum}\end{matrix}\right\}\ \text{from unirradiated rats}} \times 100$$

$$\frac{\text{ct/min macrophages} + \left.\begin{matrix}\text{exudate}\\ \text{or}\\ \text{serum}\end{matrix}\right\}\ \text{from irradiated rats}}{\text{ct/min macrophages} + \left.\begin{matrix}\text{exudate}\\ \text{or}\\ \text{serum}\end{matrix}\right\}\ \text{from unirradiated rats}} \times 100$$

## RESULTS

The effect of irradiation on blood leukocyte counts and inflammatory leukocyte counts is shown in Figure 121.1. They indicate a suppression of 95% of

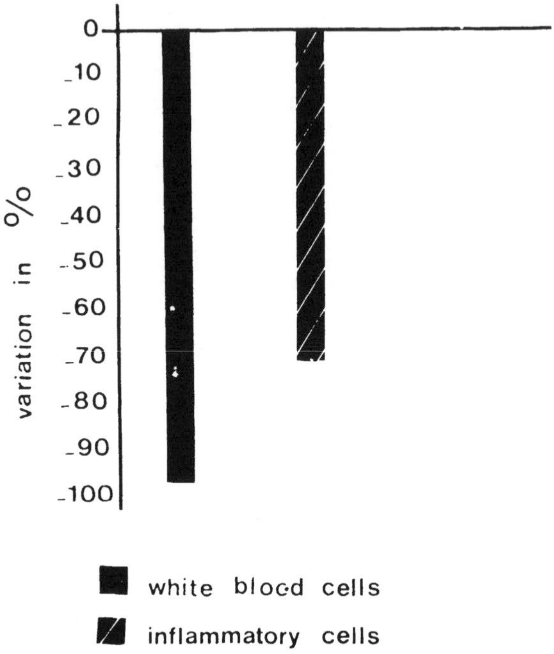


**Figure 121.1** Effect of irradiation (900 rad) on numbers of circulating leucocytes and inflammatory cells

peripheral blood leukocytes and 46% of exudate leukocytes following irradiation.

**Mitogenic activity of non-immunological inflammatory exudate and serum from irradiated rats**

Figure 121.2 shows that the mitogenic activity of inflammatory exudate from irradiated rats was 23% reduced when compared to the activity of an exudate from unirradiated rats. In contrast, a 68% increase of the mitogenic activity of the inflammatory serum was observed after irradiation.

**Mitogenic activity of non-immunological inflammatory exudate and serum after transfer of syngeneic bone marrow or thymic cells from normal rats to irradiated rats**

As shown in Figure 121.3, transfer of syngeneic bone marrow cells enhanced rather than abolished the effect of irradiation on mitogenic activity of exudate (38% decrease) and increased the mitogenic activity of serum (143%). Transfer of syngeneic thymic cells not only restored the mitogenic activity of inflammatory exudate from irradiated rats but also enhanced it (62%), and

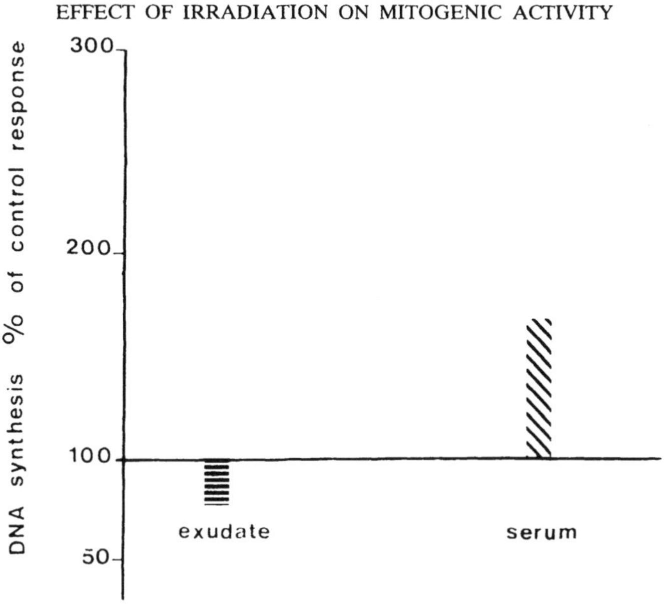


**Figure 121.2** Effect of irradiation on DNA synthesis of macrophages *in vitro* after treatment with inflammatory exudate or with inflammatory serum

enhanced the mitogenic activity of serum (198%) as well. Transfer of both cell types together fully restored the mitogenic activity of exudate and enhanced mitogenic activity of serum (259%).

**Mitogenic activity of non-immunological inflammatory exudate and sera after transfer of syngeneic bone marrow or thymic cells, harvested from rats presenting an acute inflammatory reaction, to irradiated rats.**

In figure 121.4 it can be seen that transfer of syngeneic bone marrow cells harvested from inflamed rats increased the mitogenic activity of exudate (32%) and of serum (218%). Transfer of thymic cells or both cell types from inflamed rats restored the mitogenic activity of exudate and also enhanced the mitogenic activity of serum (33% for thymic cells 427% for both cell types together).

## DISCUSSION

In the present study it has been shown to be unlikely that mitogenic activity of inflammatory exudate is influenced by irradiation and cell reconstitution in the same way as the mitogenic activity of inflammatory serum. So after irradiation and transfer of normal or inflammatory cells the mitogenic activity of

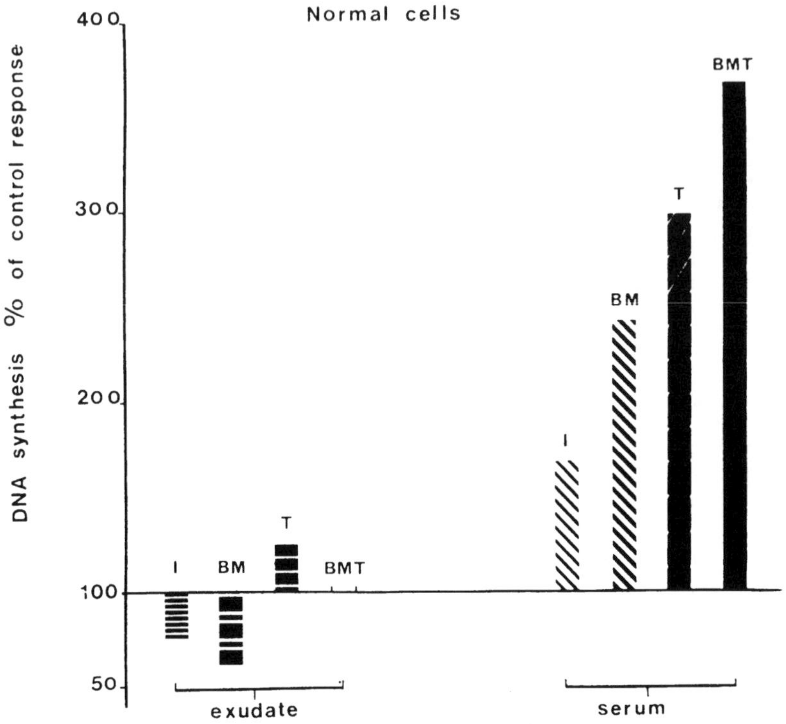


**Figure 121.3** Effect of irradiation (1) and bone marrow (BM) and thymus (T) normal cells reconstitution on DNA synthesis in macrophages *in vitro* after treatment with inflammatory exudate or with inflammatory serum

inflammatory serum is always enhanced while the mitogenic activity of exudate is either increased or decreased.

These results confirm that mitogenic factors from exudate and inflammatory serum may be of cellular origin[13,14]. Serum factor seems to be related to radio-resistant cells, since, after irradiation, the mitogenic activity of this factor increased. Transfer of normal or inflammatory cells facilitated release of seric mitogenic factor by radio-resistant cells.

Exudate factor could be related to radio-sensitive cells since after irradiation mitogenic activity of this factor decreased. Except for transfer of normal bone marrow cells, which emphasize the action of irradiation, transfer of normal or inflammatory cells could release a stimulating factor which helps to produce exudate mitogenic factor.

EFFECT OF IRRADIATION ON MITOGENIC ACTIVITY

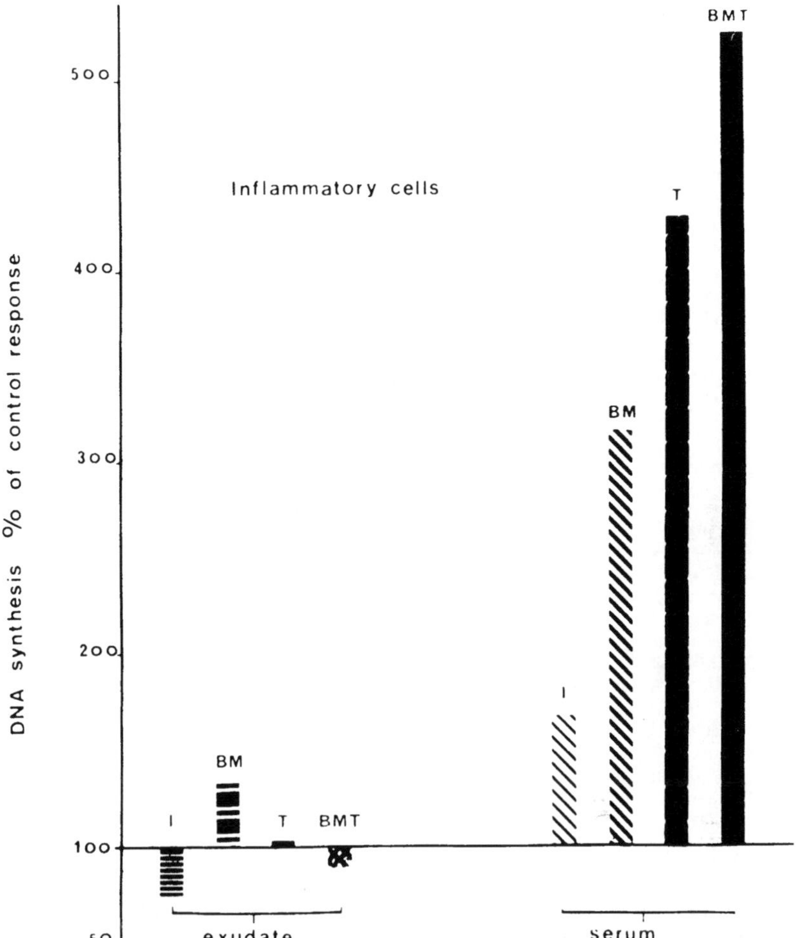


**Figure 121.4** Effect of irradiation (I) and bone marrow (BM) and thymus (T) inflammatory cells reconstitution on DNA synthesis in macrophages *in vitro* after treatment with inflammatory exudate or with inflammatory serum

A classical mechanism for macrophage division *in vivo* is thought to involve the release of soluble mediators (lymphokines) from sensitized lymphocytes upon challenge with antigen[4–6]. These factors are dependent on cell mediated immune reactions and may be derived from T lymphocytes[11,12]. In this way lymphocytes or their products may control the movement and multiplication of macrophages at the site of immunologically induced inflammation.

Hadden *et al.*[9–10] obtained evidence for macrophage mitogenic factor

(MMF) production by sensitized T lymphocytes upon challenge *in vitro* with an antigen.

The mitogenic factors from inflammatory exudate and serum could be a counterpart, in a non-specific inflammation reaction, of factors (lymphokines, MMF) released in a specific inflammatory reaction. For this reason we have named these inflammatory mitogenic factors phlogokines.

However, it is of great interest that these phlogokines are released or produced by the organism itself at an early stage during non-immunological inflammatory reactions.

## ACKNOWLEDGMENTS

This work was supported by a grant from INSERM No. 78–1–182–2 and by a grant from CNRS, ATP 651–39–51. We thank Doctor Irène FLORENTIN for performing the irradiations. The technical assistance of Brigitte Chanaud and Suzanne Strzalko is gratefully acknowledged.

### References

1 Adolphe, M., Fontagne, J., Pelletier, M. and Giroud, J. P. (1975). Induction of DNA synthesis in rat macrophages in vitro by inflammatory exudate. *Nature (London)*, **253,** 637

2 Adolphe, M., Fontagne, J., Pelletier, M., Giroud, J. P., Timsit, J. and Lechat, P. (1976). Induction of DNA synthesis in rat peritoneal macrophages in culture by a pleural inflammatory exudate. *Agents Actions*, **6,** 114

3 Adolphe, M., Fontagne, J., Pelletier, M., Blondelon, D., Lechat, P. and Giroud, J. P. (1977). In Willoughby, D. A., Giroud, J. P. and Velo, G. P. eds.) *Perspectives in Inflammation, Future Trends and Developments*. The Proceedings of the Third International Meeting on Future Trends in Inflammation, p. 469 (Lancaster: MTP Press)

4 Bloom, B. R., (1971). In vitro approaches to the mechanism of cell-mediated immune responses. *Adv. Immunol.*, **13,** 101

5 David, J. R. and David, R. R. (1972). Cellular hypersensitivity and immunity. *Prog. Allergy*, **16,** 300

6 Fidler, I. J., Darnell, J. H. and Budmen, M. B. (1976). In vitro activation of mouse macrophages by rat lymphocyte mediators. *J. Immunol.*, **117,** 666

7 Giroud, J. P., Fontagne, J., Blondelon, D., Adolphe, M., Dunn, C. J., Willoughby, D. A. and Lechat, P. (1977). Stimulation of macrophage DNA synthesis in culture by different types of acute non-immunological inflammatory exudates. *Biomedicine*, **27,** 19

8 Giroud, J. P., Pelletier, M., and Girre, C. (1977). Pouvoir mitogène de sérums de rats porteurs d'une inflammation aigue vis-à-vis de macrophages en culture. *C. R. Acad. Sci., Ser. D*, **285,** 1143

9 Hadden, J. W., Sadlik, J. R. and Hadden, E. M. (1975). Macrophage proliferation induced in vitro by a lymphocyte factor. *Nature (London)*, **257,** 483

10 Hadden, J. W. and Englard, A. (1977). Molecular aspects of macrophage activation and proliferation. In Hadden, J. W., Goffrey, R. G. and Spreafico, F. (eds). *Immunopharmacology*. (New York: Plenum)

11 McGregor, D. D. and Koster, F. T., 1971. The mediator of cellular immunity. IV. Cooperation between lymphocytes and mononuclear phagocytes. *Cell. Immunol.*, **2,** 317

12 North, R. J. and Mackaness, G. B. (1973). Immunological control of macrophage proliferation in vivo. *Infect. Immun.*, **8,** 68

13 Pelletier, M., Girre, C., Dunn, C. J., Willoughby, D. A. and Giroud, J. P: (1978). Induction of macrophage DNA synthesis in vitro by non-immunological inflammatory exudates: effect of irradiation and thymic or bone marrow cell reconstitution. *J. Pathol.*, **126,** 95

14 Pelletier, M., Girre, C., Lenfant, M., Fontagne, J., Adolphe, M. and Giroud, J. P. (1979). Inflammatory mitogenic factor (IMF): relation with T lymphocytes. *Eur. J. Rheumatol. Inflam.*, **2,** 124

# 122

# Effect of chronic inflammatory exudate on cell morphology and cell functions (Abstract)

M. KOH AND D. A. WILLOUGHBY (UK)

Granulomas induced by carrageenin have been shown to contain macrophages which persist at the sites of inflammation for prolonged periods. There has been extensive study on the pathology and biology of granuloma induction, progression and resolution, but no work has so far been reported on the functional characteristics of the exudate found in such lesions. We have shown in this study that exudate obtained from 10 days carrageenin granuloma exhibit certain effects on cells *in vitro*. Resting peritoneal cells when cultured in the presence of 50% exudate showed the following:

(1) The cells synthesised a fibrin-like mesh on which they spread extensively.
(2) Such cells divide at a higher rate than the controls.
(3) They also release more cytoplasmic enzyme than the controls.
(4) The above phenomena were not observed using heated chronic exudate (56 °C for 1 h).

These findings suggest that within chronic inflammatory lesions, mononuclear cells form fibrin on which they spread and become activated.

# 123

# Macrophages are activated by endocytosis of $\alpha_2$-macroglobulin–protease complexes to produce neutral proteases

T. L. VISCHER, D. BERGER AND E. D. FLORY (SWITZERLAND)

At sites of inflammation, proteases are released by inflammatory and tissue cells. The activation of the complement, the coagulation and the fibrinolytic systems produce additional proteases. Active proteases become inactivated by various inhibitors in the circulation and in tissues. Among the plasma protease inhibitors, alpha$_1$-antitrypsin and alpha$_2$-macroglobulin ($\alpha_2$M) are quantitatively the most important ones. In the circulation, proteases bound to alpha$_1$-antitrypsin are transferred to $\alpha_2$M[1]. The $\alpha_2$M–protease complexes are then taken up by the fixed tissue macrophages in liver and spleen[1,2]. In the experiments summarized in this paper, we have studied the effect of $\alpha_2$M–trypsin complexes on macrophages *in vitro*.

## UPTAKE OF $\alpha_2$M–TRYPSIN COMPLEXES BY MACROPHAGES

Both peptone-induced and non-elicited mouse peritoneal macrophages were exposed at room temperature in RPMI 1640 medium to human $\alpha_2$M, trypsin or $\alpha_2$M–trypsin complexes for 30 min. After washing, cytocentrifuge smears were prepared and stained with FITC-conjugated antibodies against $\alpha_2$M or trypsin. The macrophages exposed to $\alpha_2$M–trypsin complexes, but not those exposed to either native $\alpha_2$M or trypsin, contained small cytoplasmic inclusion positive for $\alpha_2$M or trypsin. From the results summarized in Table 123.1, we can conclude that macrophages take up only $\alpha_2$M–trypsin complexes but not free $\alpha_2$M. Similar results have been reported previously[3-5]. Neutrophil leukocytes containing $\alpha_2$M–trypsin complexes were not observed during these experiments. A detailed account of this work will be published elsewhere (E. Flory and T.L. Vischer, submitted for publication).

**Table 123.1** Endocytosis of $\alpha_2$M–trypsin complexes by mouse macrophages: summary of the results

| *Stimulants added to macrophages* | *Fluorescent markers* | |
|---|---|---|
| | *FITC-Rabbit anti-human $\alpha_2$M* | *FITC-Rabbit anti-human trypsin* |
| None | negative | negative |
| Trypsin | negative | negative |
| Native $\alpha_2$M | negative | negative |
| $\alpha_2$M–trypsin complexes | strongly positive | positive |
| Specificity controls by absorption of anti-$\alpha_2$M-serum with | | |
| Purified native $\alpha_2$M | negative | |
| Commercial IgG | positive | |

Since endocytosis of immune complexes activates non-elicited macrophages to produce neutral proteases such as plasminogen activator[6], we studied further macrophage activation.

## INDUCTION OF FIBRINOLYSIS IN CULTURES OF NON-ELICITED MACROPHAGES BY ENDOCYTOSIS OF $\alpha_2$M–TRYPSIN COMPLEXES

Non-elicited mouse peritoneal macrophages were cultured on Costar cluster dishes coated with [$^{125}$I]fibrin. When the cells were exposed to $\alpha_2$M–trypsin complexes or ovalbumin–anti-ovalbumin complexes, delayed fibrinolytic activity appeared, as measured as radioactivity released after 48 and 72 h of culture (Figures 123.1 and 123.2). The results were similar when the cultures were washed 2 h after exposure to the complexes indicating that neither release of lysosomal enzymes during endocytosis nor disintegration of non-endocytozed $\alpha_2$M–trypsin complexes were the cause of the increasing fibrinolytic activity. Protein synthesis was necessary for fibrinolytic activity as small doses of cycloheximide (0.25 μg/ml) inhibited it (Figure 123.2).

Therefore, progressive cell death can be excluded as a cause of fibrinolysis. Soybean trypsin inhibitor also blocked fibrinolysis. As collagenase or elastase from macrophages are not inhibited by it, release of plasminogen activator by the cells and digestion of fibrin by plasmin is the most likely expla-

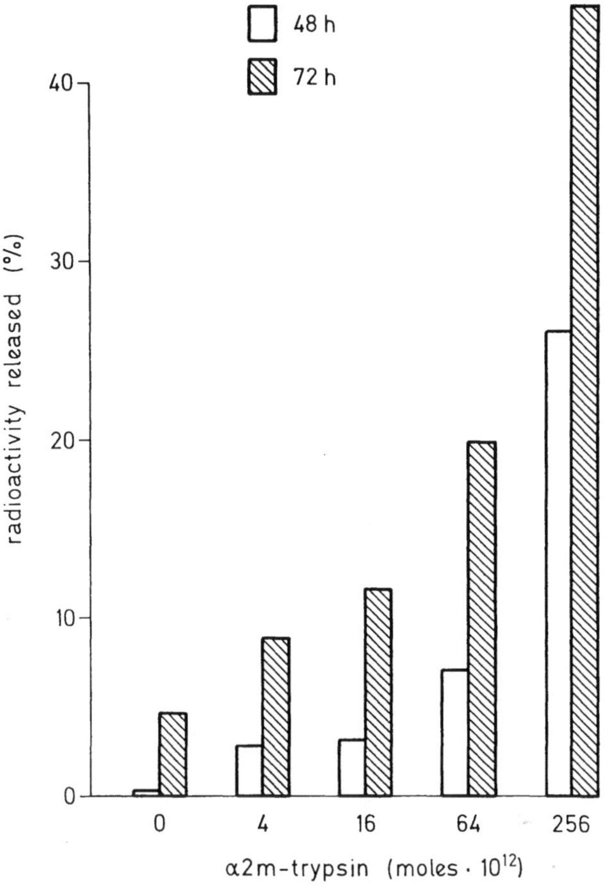


**Figure 123.1** Digestion of [$^{125}$I]fibrin by non-elicited peritoneal macrophages exposed to $\alpha_2$M–trypsin complexes

nation. The detailed account of these experiments has been published elsewhere[12]. We can conclude that non-elicited macrophages become activated by endocytosis of $\alpha_2$M–trypsin complexes to produce a protease corresponding probably to plasminogen activator. Like other proteases plasmin could activate the complement and kinin systems[7] or stimulate B lymphocytes[8] to potentiate inflammation. The removal of $\alpha_2$M–protease complexes formed during inflammation might be a participating factor in the mechanisms of self-perpetuation.

In order to establish whether such processes could occur *in vivo*, we looked for $\alpha_2$M–trypsin complexes in human synovitis.

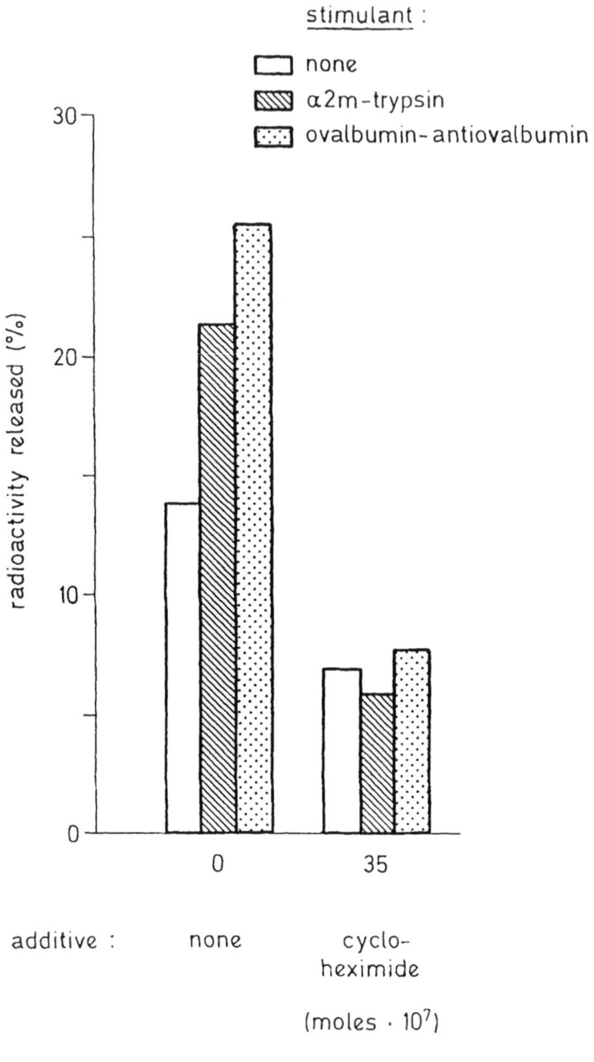


**Figure 123.2** Digestion of [$^{125}$I] fibrin by non-elicited macrophages exposed to $\alpha_2$M–trypsin or immune complexes: inhibition by cycloheximide. Fibrinolysis was measured after 72 h of culture

## $\alpha_2$-MACROGLOBULIN–TRYPSIN COMPLEXES IN SYNOVIAL FLUID CELLS

In synovial fluids, electrophoretic mobility of $\alpha_2$M is partially changed suggesting formation of $\alpha_2$M–protease complexes[9–11]. We therefore prepared cytocentrifuge smears of cells obtained from various synovial fluids aspirated from joints of patients with rheumatoid arthritis, ankylosing spondylitis, chondrocalcinosis or osteoarthrosis. Using an FITC-conjugated anti-human $\alpha_2$M antibody, cytoplasmic inclusions similar to those found in the previous *in vitro* experiments could be seen in monocytes. These results are summarized in Table 123.2. As native $\alpha_2$M was not taken up by the macrophages in the earlier experiments, we feel that the inclusions observed in the synovial fluid monocytes correspond to $\alpha_2$M–protease complexes. Thus, macrophage activation by endocytosis of these complexes might occur in human synovitis. Whether this process really contributes to the self-perpetuation phase of inflammation remains to be established.

**Table 123.2** Inclusions of $\alpha_2$-macroglobulin in monocytes from synovial fluids

| *Synovial fluids* | *WBC* ($mm^{-3}$) | *Monocytes* (%) | *Monocytes* (% with $\alpha_2$M) |
|---|---|---|---|
| Low inflammation $n = 15$ | 984 ± 891 | 57.7 ± 15.6 | 7.9 ± 5.6 |
| High inflammation $n = 11$ | 9118 ± 4075 | 20.3 ± 8.2 | 31.3 ± 22.1 |

## References


1 Ohlsson, K. and Laurell, C. B. (1976). The disappearance of enzyme-inhibitor complexes from the circulation of man. *Clin. Sci. Mol. Med.*, **51**, 87

2 Ohlsson, K. (1971). Elimination of $^{125}$I-Trypsin-$\alpha_2$-Macroglobulin complexes from blood by reticuloendothelial cells in dog. *Acta Physiol. Scand.*, **81**, 269

3 Dolovich, J., Debanne, M. T. and Bell, R. (1975). The role of $\alpha_1$-antitrypsin and $\alpha_2$-macroglobulin in the uptake of proteinase by rabbit alveolar macrophages. *Am. Rev. Resp. Dis.*, **112**, 521

4 Debanne, M. T., Bell, R. and Dolovich, J. (1975). Uptake of proteinase–$\alpha_2$-macroglobulin complexes by macrophages. *Biochim. Biophys. Acta*, **411**, 295

5 Debanne, M. T., Bell, R. and Dolovich, J. (1976). Characteristics of the macrophage uptake of proteinase-$\alpha_2$-macroglobulin complexes. *Biochim. Biophys. Acta*, **428**, 466

6 Gordon, S., Unkeless, J. C. and Cohn, Z. A. (1974). Induction of macrophage plasminogen activator by endotoxin stimulation and phagocytosis. *J. Exp. Med.*, **140**, 995

7 Gordon, S., Newman, W. and Bloom, B. (1978). Macrophage proteases and rheumatic diseases: Regulation of plasminogen activator by thymus-derived lymphocytes. *Agents Actions*, **8**, 19

8 Vischer, T. L. and Bertrand, L. (1976). Stimulating effect of neutral proteases on cells in vitro. *Agents Actions*, **6**, 180

9 Shtacher, G., Maayan, R. and Feinstein, G. (1973). Proteinase inhibitors in human synovial fluid. *Biochim. Biophys. Acta*, **303**, 138

10 Abe, S. and Nagai, Y. (1973). Evidence for the presence of a complex of collagenase with $\alpha_2$-macroglobulin in human rheumatoid synovial fluid: A possible regulatory mechanism of collagenase activity in vivo. *J. Biochem.*, **73**, 897

11 Ohlsson, K. and Skude, C. (1976). Demonstration and semiquantitative determination of complexes between various proteases and human $\alpha_2$-macroglobulin. *Clin. Chim. Acta*, **66**, 1

12 Vischer, T. L. and Berger, D. (1980). Activation of macrophages to produce neutral proteinases by endocytosis of $\alpha_2$M–trysin complexes. *J. Reticuloendothel.* Soc., **28**, 427

# 124

# A mitogenic factor for macrophages present in rat serum (Abstract)

N. S. CONNOR, A. W. FORD–HUTCHINSON AND M. J. H. SMITH (UK)

Rat macrophages, obtained from a mixed white cell population collected by peritoneal lavage, were plated out at $6 \times 10^5$ cells $cm^2$ in Medium 199 containing 20% fetal calf serum, 25 mol/l HEPES pH 7.4 and antibiotics and were aged for 3 days in culture. The cells were then cultured for a further 6 days in fresh medium containing 20% fetal calf serum, tritiated thymidine and 0–50% normal rat serum. Mitogenesis was assessed by counting the percentage labelled nuclei following autoradiography. Colony stimulating activity was assessed using thioglycolate elicited rat peritoneal macrophages harvested 3 days after injection. The cells were seeded at 600 cells/$cm^2$ in medium as above, in the presence or absence of rat serum or rat serum fractions and colonies were counted after 28 days incubation.

Concentrations of normal rat serum from 5–50% caused a significant increase in the percentage labelled nuclei following the 6 day pulse with tritiated thymidine. The optimal rat serum concentration was 25% which produced 40–60% labelled nuclei with a 75% increase in cell numbers over the 6 day culture period (control cultures contain <1% labelled nuclei).

Normal rat serum was also shown to contain colony stimulating activity but this could be distinguished from the mitogenic factor following chromatography on Sephadex G-75; the mitogenic factor having an apparent molecular weight of 50 000 daltons whilst the colony stimulating activity had an apparent molecular weight of 60 000–70 000 daltons.

This is the first report describing the presence of a macrophage mitogenic factor in normal serum and the factor appears to differ from that previously reported in inflammatory exudates which has an apparent molecular weight of <2000 daltons (Pelletier *et al.* (1979) *Eur. J. Rheum. Inflam.*, **2,** 124). This factor may be involved in the early events leading to granuloma formation in the absence of an immunological response.

# 125

# Secretion of plasminogen activator by mouse peritoneal macrophages elicited by injection of a suspension of killed streptococci

GENEVIÈVE LEMAIRE, J.–C. DRAPIER AND
J.–F. PETIT (FRANCE)

## INTRODUCTION

Certain populations of macrophages secrete neutral proteases such as plasminogen activator, elastase and collagenase. These enzymes, by contrast to lysozyme, are produced by macrophages only after induction (inflammation, endocytosis or immunological signal) and resident peritoneal macrophages show very little activity[1]. For plasminogen activator, the highest secretion rate has been observed in macrophages collected after injection of a non-specific irritant like thioglycollate broth[2]. However, all the substances used to obtain macrophage-rich exudates do not bring about a plasminogen activator production (after injection of fetal calf serum, mineral oil or endotoxin, the fibrinolytic activity of the macrophages is limited)[3].

We have found that in mice, an intraperitoneal injection of killed streptococci elicits macrophages which produce *in vitro* large quantities of plasminogen activator (Table 125.1).

4 days after injection of a suspension of killed *Streptococcus* $C_5$, inflammation of the peritoneal cavity is marked: the exudate contains $13 \pm 3 \times 10^6$ cells, 50% of which take up neutral red and the amount of soluble proteins recovered with the exudate is 2 to 3 times higher than for untreated animals.

After 4 h of *in vitro* cultivation (in medium 199 supplemented with 10% acid-treated fetal calf serum), the adherent peritoneal cells prepared from animals treated with streptococci contain less intracellular plasminogen acti-

**Table 125·1** Induction of plasminogen activator secretion

| In vivo *stimulation* | *Peritoneal cells/mouse* | *Plasminogen activator secreted* in vitro (*from 24 h to 72 h*) (Units/mg) |
|---|---|---|
| O | $3 \times 10^6$ | 0 |
| Thioglycollate | $18 \times 10^6$ | 5 |
| *Streptococcus* $C_5$ | $13 \times 10^6$ | 6·6 |
| *Streptococcus faecalis* | $9 \times 10^6$ | 2·3 |

Plasminogen activator was measured by a spectrophotometric assay[4] using a chromogenic substrate of plasmin. The activity is expressed as urokinase CTA units/mg of cellular protein.

vator than 'thioglycollate' macrophages but their production of activator, during *in vitro* cultivation, is higher and the percentage of enzyme secreted into the extracellular medium is greater (Table 125.2). Similar results have been obtained with streptococci of different groups: *Streptococcus pyogenes* $A_{22}$, *Streptococcus* $C_5$, *Streptococcus durans* $D_3$ and *Streptococcus faecalis*.

**125·2** Comparison of plasminogen activator production by thioglycollate or streptococci elicited macrophages

| In vivo | *Cultivation* in vitro 4 h | 48 h | | 96 h | | |
|---|---|---|---|---|---|---|
| *stimulation* | *Activator intracellular* | *Activator intracellular* | *secreted* | *Activator intracellular* | *secreted* | *Lysozyme secreted* |
| Thioglycollate | 32 | 30 | 2.4 | 60 | 13 | 140 |
| *Streptococcus* $C_5$ | 4 | 4.6 | 5.6 | 30 | 80 | 160 |

Activator: urokinase CTA units/mg intracellular protein. Lysozyme: μg of enzyme/mg intracellular protein. Cells were cultivated for 24 h in medium 199 with 10% acid-treated fetal calf serum and then transferred to serum-free medium (0·2% lactalbumin). At the end of the experiment conditioned medium was collected and cells recovered in 0·1% Triton.

As has been described for thioglycollate-elicited macrophages[4,5] the secretion of plasminogen activator by streptococci elicited macrophages is induced *in vitro* by the presence of serum and is inhibited by addition of WSA (water soluble adjuvant), an immunomodulator of mycobacterial origin. It is known that ingestion of poorly digestible material by macrophages increases the activity of lysosomal enzymes, and, in fact, in streptococci elicited macrophages we have found that, after adherence, the specific activities of β-glucuronidase, *N*-acetyl-β-glucosaminidase and acid phosphatase are multiplied by 2, 3 and 6, respectively, but streptococci elicited macrophages present other modifications which differentiate them from normal resident macrophages. They are cytostatic for syngeneic tumour cells (J.P. Tenu, personal communication), and, as we describe in this communication, they secrete large quantities of plasminogen activator. The action of streptococci in enhancing macrophage plasminogen activator production resembles that previously found for asbestos[6].

## References


1 Gordon, S. (1978). *Fed. Proc.*, **37,** 2754
2 Unkeless, J. C., Gordon, S. and Reich, E. (1974). *J. Exp. Med.*, **139,** 834
3 Gordon, S., Unkeless, J. C. and Cohn, Z. A. (1974). *J. Exp. Med.*, **140,** 995
4 Drapier, J. C., Tenu, J. P., Lemaire, G. and Petit, J. F. (1979). *Biochimie*, **61,** 463
5 Drapier, J. C., Lemaire, G., Tenu, J. P. and Petit, J. F. (1979). In Kaplan, J. G. (ed.) *The Molecular Basis of Immune Function*, (North Holland: Elsevier)
6 Hamilton, J., Vassali, J. D. and Reich, E. (1976). *J. Exp. Med.*, **144,** 1689

# Discussion

**Professor M.U. Dianzani (Co-chairman)** introducing the session, said that the measurement of secretion of enzymes and other products from cells during inflammation involved a number of problems. The first related to lysosomal enzymes which were re-absorbed, but re-absorbed at different rates. Thus in order to be sure that the lysosomal system was active, it was always necessary to refer to the activity of several enzymes simultaneously. In addition, membrane fluidity could influence lysosomal secretion. This was important to bear in mind because increasing the cholesterol content of membranes caused them to become more rigid. He then invited Dr Sluiter to describe his work on monocytopoiesis.

**Dr W. Sluiter (Netherlands)** said that during the initial phase of an inflammation induced in the mouse peritoneal cavity they had been able to demonstrate the presence of a factor increasing monocyte production in the bone marrow. The factor, referred to as FIM, had an action on the bone marrow monocyte precursors. After FIM administration *in vivo* the cycle time of promonocytes decreased and cell numbers increased indicating an effect upon the monoblasts. Normal peritoneal cells contained large amounts of FIM but during inflammation their activity decreased whereas FIM activity in serum increased. This suggested that cells released FIM during the inflammatory reaction. In order to establish in what type of cell the FIM originated, they cultured a variety of cells from different sources on a Teflon surface, the latter being used to prevent mononuclear phagocytes from adhering. Possible candidates for FIM production were lymphocytes, granulocytes and macrophages. The administration of latex to cell cultures produced monocytosis-inducing activity which depended on the number of macrophages present in the culture and was independent of the number of lymphocytes or granulocytes. The characteristics of the monocytosis-inducing activity were very similar to FIM. The molecular weight was between 10 000 and 25 000 daltons. There was no colony stimulating activity and the factor was highly thermolabile. These results suggested that macrophages were the origin of the factor increasing monocytopoiesis, a factor playing an important role in the regulation of monocyte production during inflammation.

**Professor Dianzani** said that Dr Sluiter had suggested that the factor stimulating monocytopoiesis was present even in tumour cells. He wondered whether any differences had been detected between tumour cells and normal macrophages.

**Dr Sluiter** had not observed differences for the tumour cell lines under study but he imagined that the amount of FIM activity in such macrophage cell lines would depend on activation, age and so on. After administration of latex to cultures of peritoneal macrophages a decrease in the amount of intercellular FIM was observed, and so it was possible that activated macrophages contained less FIM but were still producing it and releasing it to the medium.

**Dr D.M. Williams (UK)** described his findings on changes in leukocyte structure and activity in response to inflammation. He said that studies in rats and man had shown that alkaline phosphatase activity in neutrophils was inversely related to their age. The level of the enzyme in neutrophils was also sharply elevated in peripheral blood in the presence of an inflammatory response. The present study had been performed to determine precisely where the enzyme was localized in the neutrophils and to assess whether the increase in enzyme levels was attributable to large scale release of cells from the bone marrow. This was suggested because bone marrow neutrophils, at least in the rat, contained higher levels than blood neutrophils. Rat femoral bone marrow cells were collected 30 min to 20 h after the induction of an inflammatory response and an osmophilic staining method was used which allowed examination by light or electron microscopy. There was a depletion of mature cells in the bone marrow evident after 2 h, maximum after 6 h and persisting throughout the observation period. There was a doubling of the myeloblast promyelocyte population at 6 h when these cells accounted for 16% of the total nucleated cell population in the bone marrow. Only 1.1% of the total nucleated marrow cell population contained alkaline phosphatase. Within 2 h of the induction of the inflammatory response a 4-fold increase in alkaline phosphatase occurred in neutrophils and this change preceded any noticeable division of neutrophil precursors. This seemed to indicate increased enzyme production rather than an increase resulting from the fact that more enzyme positive cells were present. Striking ultrastructural changes also occurred, evident at 6 h and at a maximum at 20 h suggesting a synchrony between nuclear and cytoplasmic differentiation. This accelerated cytoplasmic development coincided in time with the period at which younger cells were beginning to appear in the circulation.

In answer to a question about the animals used he said that they were male Sprague–Dawley rats, 200–500 g in weight, thus 12 weeks or older.

**Dr C.J. Dunn (France)** said that turpentine which had been used as an irritant was an extremely toxic substance and he wondered how one could separate the effects of inflammation from those of toxicity.

**Dr Williams** had used turpentine because it produced a very marked neutrophilia very rapidly. However, similar, although less marked, results had also been obtained with other stimuli.

**Dr M.E.J. Billingham (Chairman)** said that eosinophils were usually markers of parasitic infection. He wondered why they should appear on injection of turpentine.

**Dr Williams** said that he had not quantitated the eosinophil response. Alkaline phosphatase positive eosinophils were seen in rat bone marrow and the increase in their numbers to this particular stimulus was very minimal. The change in their numbers was not comparable to that seen among the neutrophils and they might not be directly involved.

**Professor Dianzani** asked whether any biochemical measurements had been performed on alkaline phosphatase activity. If morphological determinations were carried out it was necessary to establish whether there was a real increase in enzyme activity or an increasing accessibility to the substrate.

**Dr Williams** said that he had conducted purely morphological observations but there were numerous studies equating such morphological findings with direct biochemical assays. In the conditions of his test an inflammatory stimulus had been given to one group and not to the other, and he felt it reasonable to interpret the increase in demonstrable levels of the enzymes to be a real phenomenon rather than a change in substrate accessibility.

**Dr M. Russo (Brazil)** reviewed his findings on macrophage involvement in the chemotactic response. He said that C3H/HeJ mice did not respond to the toxic immunological properties of bacterial lipopolysaccharide (LPS) whereas the histocompatible C3HeB/FeJ mice did respond. They had investigated the PMN migration into the peritoneal cavity induced after intravenous LPS administration in C3H/HeJ recipients that received different cell types from C3HeB donors. Spleen, marrow and peritoneal cells were injected intraperitoneally and 2 h after transfer the recipients were challenged with 20 μg i.v. LPS. 6 h later PMN migration into the peritoneal cavity was measured.

It was found that peritoneal cells were most effective in mediating chemotactic activity. LPS given i.v. did not in itself cause a significant PMN influx. To investigate in more detail which cell type was responsible for chemotactic activity, adherent and non-adherent peritoneal cells were injected separately and 3 days after cell transfer recipients were again challenged with 20 μg LPS. Adherent peritoneal cells were as effective as separated peritoneal cells. It was therefore proposed that the macrophages played a role in providing the starting signal for extravascular neutrophilia induced after LPS administration.

**Mr F. Visenten (Italy)** asked whether the chemotactic factor had been characterized. He wondered if it involved complement components or monokines secreted from macrophages or even lymphokines.

**Dr Russo** said that the complement levels in the various mouse strains were similar. As to the chemotactic factor itself, it might well involve monokines. He did not think it was complement because experiments in C5 deficient strains showed the same phenomenon. In addition, since LPS was given intravenously the C5a gradient would be in the circulation and not in the tissue.

**Dr P.C. Fink (Germany)** described his work on determination of free lipid A. He said that there had been considerable question about the specificity of the limulus-amoebocyte-lysate (LAL) test in the diagnosis of endotoxaemia. His study had attempted to evaluate the influence of pathological and stress leukocytosis using a very sensitive spectrophotometric LAL assay. The results showed a significant correlation between elevated white blood cell count and *Escherichia coli* endotoxin equivalents for patients with septicaemia or with liver cirrhosis. Supernatants isolated from lymphocytes prepared by sterile Ficoll gradient centrifugation gave positive reactions in a dose-response manner. Recognizing the restrictive clinical value of the test they set up an enzyme immunoassay technique to quantitate free lipid A, the supposed intrinsic moiety of the endotoxin molecule. It was found that lipid A shared common immune determinants between various endotoxin molecules. An enzyme immunoassay technique for quantitating free lipid A was thought to be a prerequisite for the quantitation of anti-lipid A antibodies in disease states.

**Dr T.L. Vischer (Switzerland)** asked how Dr Fink interpreted the finding of lipid A in the initial lymphocyte supernatant.

**Dr Fink** said that he had data showing that isolated neutrophils would give a positive LAL reaction and he thought that products secreted by lymphocytes as well as by neutrophils could non-specifically activate the LAL test.

**Dr Billingham** asked why patients with cirrhosis of the liver should show lipid A reactivity in their serum.

**Dr Fink** said that patients with cirrhosis had a diminished capacity to filter endotoxin derived from the gut. Lipid A was difficult to detect. Nonetheless, there was good evidence that during the detoxification process the immunogenic determinants of lipid A elicited anti-lipid A antibodies, so the quantitation of anti-lipid A antibodies would constitute the appropriate test for the future.

**Professor K. Trnavský (Czechoslovakia)** was invited to review his work on colchicine derivatives. He said that they had been studying the effects of two colchicine derivatives, demecolcine and deacetylcolchiceine on lysosomal enzyme release from human PNMs during the phagocytosis of urate crystals. Both substances were effective in gouty patients. Both drugs *in vitro* inhibited the release of lysosomal enzymes in a dose-dependent manner. At the same time there was an increase in cyclic AMP in the cells. These effects were not in themselves dramatic but it had to be remembered that deacetylcolchiceine was a drug that could be used in very high dosages. It differed from colchicine in several regards. It had no antimitotic effect. It did not influence microtubular proteins and it did not bind to serum protein, especially albumin, unlike colchicine.

**Professor Dianzani** asked whether lactate dehydrogenase had simultaneously been measured as a test of stabilization.

**Professor Trnavský** said that it had been measured and the results showed a total stabilization. Other evidence from the United States also suggested that such drugs stabilized against cell death. The case of deacetylcolchiceine was particularly interesting, since, in his experience and that of others, it did not bind to microtubular units and if from the point of view of microtubular function, colchicine might be expected to have the same activity as cyclic AMP.

**Dr Dunn** asked whether colchicine derivatives had been investigated in cases of calcium pryrophosphate accumulation, as in pseudo-gout.

**Professor Trnavský** had no experience of such studies but he did not think that colchicine was very effective in chondrocalcinosis; clinical experience had been negative.

**Dr S.H. Ferreira** was then invited to describe his findings on the use of anti-macrophage serum. He said the basic question was whether resident macrophages could control PMN migration to an inflammatory site. In rats they had stimulated cell migration with a *Mycobacterium* preparation and had found that they could effectively block PMN migration with anti-macrophage serum. Thus it seemed that resident macrophages were probably able to stimulate PMN migration to the site of the lesion.

In answer to a question he said that there was no modification in the levels of complement. He did not believe that complement was important in the reaction.

**Dr G. A. Higgs (UK)** said that on reducing PMN migration, oedema was observed. One interpretation of this finding was that acute cells were anti-inflammatory and thus it might be disadvantageous to inhibit their migration.

**Dr Ferreira** agreed that this might be so in the acute inflammatory state. In the chronic state however conditions might be different.

**Dr Higgs** enquired about the mechanism of enhanced oedema. He wondered if the cells were suppressing a mediator.

**Professor Ferreira** said that other experiments he had performed showed that *Mycobacterium* preparations were able to induce inflammation by releasing mediators, but the release appeared to stop after 7 days. Further injections of *Mycobacterium* would not then produce the same effects. In this it differed from carrageenin where a second full response could be induced. Thus it seemed that the *Mycobacterium* preparation, which was mainly protein, might be able to activate complement, and he did not believe that it was possible to exhaust complement with an anti-serum. But the *Mycobacterium* released mediators which caused vascular permeability and it continued to produce mediators, which was the reason for the enhanced phenomenon.

**Dr S.C.R. Meacock (UK)** said that macrophages originated in the bone marrow and some believed that a common stem cell existed between the PMN and the monocyte. He wondered whether the anti-serum had any effect on bone marrow cell precursors.

**Dr Ferreira** did not know. He thought it unlikely, however, since there was no change in the circulating cells.

**Mr P. Fox (Glasgow)** asked if any inflammatory changes were observed in the uninjected paw.

**Dr Ferreira** said that the control paw was injected with saline and the PMN response was almost non-existent.

**Dr N.S. Connor (UK)** asked how Dr Ferreira assessed that he had destroyed all the resting macrophages with the anti-macrophage serum.

**Dr Ferreira** said that they had paid particular attention to preparation of the anti-serum. Absorption, even in serum without dilution, had no effect on lymphocytes or neutrophils but the serum preferentially and very effectively blocked the reactions of macrophages.

**Dr Billingham** said that adjuvant arthritis induced in the rat by MTB could be blocked by giving small amounts of TB in saline some days previously, presumably because of the production of a blocking antibody. It might be that in Dr Ferreira's experiments similar blocking antibodies were being produced so that the second injection of tuberculosis would not be recognized by the same cells.

**Dr Ferreira** said that PMNs were far less important in the second reaction to MTB than were macrophages.

**Dr V. Klimetzek (Germany)** then described his work on macrophage differentiation. He said that during inflammation in the peritoneal cavity two effects proceeded simultaneously. One was an activation of the resident macrophages by lymphokine or other humoral factors. The other was an influx of bone marrow derived macrophages. A combination of these two processes was therefore always being observed in the peritoneal cavity. In order to establish which biochemical activities were specific for bone marrow derived macrophages, he had cultured bone marrow cells *in vitro* in the presence of colony stimulating factor and tested them from days 7 to 16. They had started so late in order to ensure that all granulocytes were out of the culture. The cells differentiated in three ways. Functions such as the secretion of lysosyme or reactivity to MIF remained stable over the whole period. Phagocytosis and monocytosis increased from days 7 to 12 and then decreased. 5′nucleotidase activity increased to day 12 then stayed constant, whereas chemotaxis increased until day 15 when 95% of the cells migrated through the membrane in response to C5a. Cultivated bone marrow macrophages thus appeared to behave like activated macrophages capable of further activation in response to lymphokines.

**Dr P.C.J. Leijh (Netherlands)** suggested that if bone marrow cells had been cultured in Teflon culture plates without adherence then cell activation might not have occurred.

**Dr Klimitzek** said that because Teflon plates were expensive he used a Teflon spray on normal plates. Cells adhered to these plates but in his experience and those of others to whom he had spoken, cells adhered to these membranes between days 8 and 10 and some substance such as EDTA had to be used to detach them.

**Dr Leijh** said that this depended upon the surface charge of the Teflon, which again depended upon the manufacturer. One preparation used in Belgium was negatively charged and macrophages would not adhere to it.

**Dr Klimitzek** said that Dr Leijh's technique had several disadvantages, including the need to assemble a large chamber. His own spraying procedure was very rapid and very cheap. For testing MIF for example, large numbers of cells were required which simply could not be produced in small Teflon chambers.

**Dr R.W. Jubb (UK)** described his work on the effects of synovium in organ culture on articular cartilage. He had found that the synovium could cause loss of proteoglycan and collagen by a direct effect on the cartilage matrix. It could also cause loss of proteoglycan and collagen by an indirect effect mediated through the living chondrocyte via the catabolin molecule. The synovium would cause reversible inhibition of proteoglycan synthesis by the chondrocyte, and in addition some of the chondrocytes could undergo a morphological change to take up an appearance resembling that of fibroblasts.

**Dr I.F. Skidmore (UK)** asked how much proteoglycan the culture would make in the absence of synovial tissue.

**Dr Jubb** said that in 14 days of culture the total amount of proteoglycan was increased by 70%. This level of increase was fairly consistent.

**Dr W.C. Dick (UK)** said that with a system as powerful as that being described, one might expect natural inhibitors to be present. He wondered if any had been detected.

**Dr Jubb** had found no such inhibitors. However, at present they did not know what controlled the system. He agreed that it seemed strange that starting with normal synovial tissue one should see such tremendously destructive effects on cartilage.

**Dr N.R. Ackermann (USA)** asked whether it had been possible to isolate the enzyme system responsible for inhibiting cartilage proteoglycan derived from the synovium. He also wondered how important was the catabolin induced breakdown as opposed to that induced directly by the synovium, independent of the chondrocyte.

## DISCUSSION

**Dr Jubb** had not examined specific enzymes within the cartilage released by the chondrocytes. Collagenase from the synovial tissue could be elevated with an increased breakdown of cartilage matrix by raising the oxygen tension in the cultures. As to the relative importance of the two breakdown mechanisms, he had not quantitated the two effects, but synovium cultured in contact with cartilage produced an almost total loss of cartilage matrix within 14 days. Synovium cultured in contact with dead cartilage produced complete loss of proteoglycan with only 20% loss of collagen. Thus, breakdown was maximal when the two systems acted together.

**Dr Barry (New Zealand)** said that there was a dynamic equilibrium of synthesis and breakdown occurring in cartilage and Dr Jubb was suggesting that the breakdown was enhanced while the synthesis was decreased. He wondered how one could be sure that both of these effects were happening simultaneously.

**Dr Jubb** said that inhibition of synthesis could be seen very early in culture. Within a few hours the uptake of sulphate had been severely inhibited. The loss of proteoglycan did not occur for some days and the loss of collagen was not seen until day 10. The breakdown of proteoglycan and the loss of collagen were associated with the fibroblastic transformation.

**Dr M. Koh (UK)** then reviewed his work on the effect of chronic exudates on cell morphology and cell functions. Resting rat peritoneal cells were cultured for 3 days in calf serum then for 3 days in a medium containing 50% chronic carrageenin exudate. After 4 days in the presence of exudate, a fibrin-like meshwork was observed at the bottom of the culture chamber. Histochemical tests suggested that the material was not actually fibrin but electron microscopic studies were being performed to establish the fact. In addition to the apparent fibrin formation, the exudate triggered cell spreading, mitosis and lysosomal enzyme release. On heating the exudate before adding it to the cell culture, spreading, mitosis and lysosomal release were inhibited.

**Dr Dunn** had performed similar experiments with similar results. He suggested that the role of the fibrin was to immobilize the cells and maintain them at the site of inflammation so that they could perform their functions.

**Dr Koh** said that although that might be true in acute inflammation, it did not seem to be the case in the chronic situation. Considerable deposits of fibrin-like material could be seen lining the cavity of a synovial joint.

**Dr Sluiter** enquired about the rate of cell division. His own work had shown that peritoneal cells would only divide to a very minor extent and he wondered what controls had been used.

**Dr Koh** said that control cells in newborn calf serum showed almost negligible division. In the presence of exudate, cell division was increased by 120%.

**Dr Russo** asked whether complement factors had been looked for.

**Dr Koh** said that zymosan had been used to remove C3 from the exudate, but although there had been a slight decrease in fibrin formation the effect had not been abolished completely.

**Dr F. Wong (USA)** had attempted to induce inflammation with carrageenin in the rat paw. Injection had been once a week for 3 months and he had seen no bone changes in the paws. Chronic inflammation induced by carrageenin was therefore quite different from that induced by *Mycobacterium*.

**Dr D. Berger (Switzerland)** described the work of his group on $\alpha_2$-macroglobulin. He said that macrophages could be activated by many compounds, one of which was a complex of $\alpha_2$-macroglobulin and proteinease. The complex induced macrophages to secrete more proteinase which could in turn be complexed with the most potent inhibitors present in plasma and at the site of inflammation. This explained, at least in part, the self-perpetuation of chronic inflammation.

**Dr Visentin** asked whether such macrophage complexes remained active. Secondly, he wondered whether macrophages themselves also synthesized, or at least released, $\alpha_2$-macroglobulins.

**Dr Berger** said that the proteinases within the inhibitors did stay active, at least for small molecular weight substrates. For large substrates there was steric hindrance and the activity was lost. Experiments with cyclohexamide had shown that inhibition of biosynthesis of protein within the macrophage culture led to loss of fibrinolytic activity. This fibrinolytic activity was not due to trypsin uptake by macrophages but to other neutral proteinases secreted by the macrophages themselves.

**Professor Dianzani** asked how long an incubation time was required to see a fall in proteolysis.

**Dr Berger** said that proteolytic activity appeared after 2 days and had a peak at 3 days.

**Dr N.S. Connor (UK)** then presented the work of his group on the detection of macrophage mitogenic activities in normal rat serum. Results showed that normal serum contained two mitogenic components, one stimulating resting peritoneal macrophages, as assessed by tritiated thymidine incorporation; the other stimulating elicited macrophage proliferation as assessed by colony and cluster formation. These activities were separable by Sephadex chromatography. The relevant molecular weights were 43 000 for the resting macrophage mitogenic factor and 56 000 for the colony forming factor. Since acute and chronic inflammatory exudates contained both of these mitogenic activities, it was postulated that they might be derived from circulating plasma entering the inflammatory site during periods of increased vascular permeability. In addition, they might be responsible for initiating non-immunological granuloma growth.

**Dr Sluiter** asked if the number of colony forming units had been measured in the peritoneal cavity of normal rats. Rats bred in open cages harboured many steady state infections, with consequent changes in inflammatory status.

**Dr Connor** said that animals housed in normal laboratory conditions and studies over a period of 2 years had shown very little difference in responses. If they were infected it was at a very basal level and he did not think that any such infection was related to the mitogenic responses being observed. However, colony forming cells were observed in the uninjected animals and so some basal infection might be occurring, although he had not been able to detect any incorporation of tritiated thymidine in the presence of normal serum in the cells of these animals.

**Dr Leijh** noted that in the labelling experiments Dr Connor reported 40–60% labelled nuclei with a 75% increase in cell numbers. He wondered whether this represented a heterogeneous population of macrophages with some cells dividing several times during incubation, or whether division of resident macrophages was being observed.

**Dr Connor** said that the population was fairly heterogeneous. Since the cycle time had been reported to be very long, within a 6 day period he would not expect to find successive replications of a single cell population. In addition, the number of labelled cells was distributed evenly over the surface, thus suggesting that a few individual cells were not repeatedly dividing.

**Dr Dunn** noted that the mitogenic factor reported by Dr Connor differed from that described in the exudate by Mme Pelletier's group. He wondered whether it also differed from their serum factor. He also enquired about the effects of inflammatory serum.

**Dr Connor** said that Mme Pelletier's group had not performed extensive molecular weight determinations on their inflammatory macrophage mitogenic factor, but since their preliminary reports gave it a molecular weight of some 5000 daltons it appeared to be a quite different material from his own. Inflammatory serum seemed to produce a yet different spectrum of activity. The factor was not usually found in normal serum using the inflammatory cell plus tritiated thymidine incorporation assay. Injection of endotoxin, however, rapidly stimulated elicited macrophage proliferation as detected with tritiated thymidine. Thus colony stimulating activity seemed to increase. He had no data on macrophage mitogenic activity in resting cells but he felt the situation might be similar.

**Dr G. Lemaire (France)** reviewed his work on plasminogen activator. Secretion of this activator was not a permanent property of peritoneal macrophages. It had to be induced by an appropriate stimulus, normally thioglycollate. To investigate the importance of ease of ingestion of stimulant materials they had injected suspensions of killed *streptococci*. Macrophages elicited in this way produced large quantities of plasminogen activator *in vitro*. After harvesting, *streptococci*-elicited macrophages contained 10 times less plasminogen activator than those elicited by thioglycoliate, but during *in vitro* culture produced more and secreted more into the extracellular medium. Certain features were common to both types of activation. For example, secretion was influenced by a water soluble adjuvant immunomodulator prepared from microbacterial cell walls.

**Dr Russo** asked why the water soluble adjuvant should block the release.

**Dr Lemaire** could not answer the question. Indeed, the action of immunomodulator was the reverse of what they had expected.

**Dr Billingham** then thanked all speakers for their participation.

# Index

GPSR Compliance

*The European Union's (EU) General Product Safety Regulation (GPSR) is a set of rules that requires consumer products to be safe and our obligations to ensure this.*

*If you have any concerns about our products, you can contact us on ProductSafety@springernature.com*

In case Publisher is established outside the EU, the EU authorized representative is:

Springer Nature Customer Service Center GmbH
Europaplatz 3
69115 Heidelberg, Germany

**Batch number: 10832080**

Printed by Printforce, the Netherlands